Handbook of
PHARMACEUTICAL
EXCIPIENTS

Handbook of
PHARMACEUTICAL
EXCIPIENTS

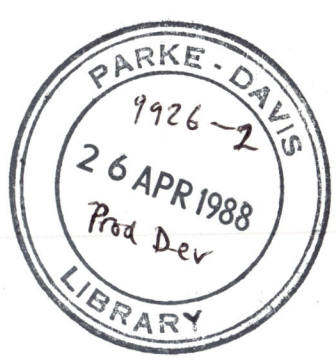
Published by

American Pharmaceutical Association
2215 Constitution Avenue, NW
Washington, DC 20037 USA

The Pharmaceutical Society of Great Britain
1 Lambeth High Street
London SE1 7JN, England

American Pharmaceutical Association Production Staff

James C. Boylan
Jack Cooper
Zak T. Chowhan

The Pharmaceutical Society of Great Britain Production Staff

Walter Lund
Ainley Wade
Robert F. Weir
Bernard J. Yates

Publication Production Staff

Marlene Povich, *Art and Production Manager*
Carol Niedzialek, *Production Coordinator*
John Covert, *Director of Publications*

Library of Congress Data

The use of portions of the text of *USP XXI/NF XVI* is by permission of the USP Convention, Inc. The Convention is not responsible for any inaccuracy of quotation or for any false or misleading implication that may arise from separation of an excerpt from the original context or by obsolescence resulting from publication of a supplement.

Selected structural formulas from *The Merck Index*, Tenth Edition, 1983, published by Merck & Co., Rahway, New Jersey, are reprinted with permission.

ISBN (U.S.): 0-917330-56-0
ISBN (U.K.): 0-85369-164-9

Printed in the USA

Table of Contents

Monographs

Committees

Members of Administrative Committee

James C. Boylan, Chairman
James B. Appino
Patrick P. DeLuca
George B. Griffenhagen
Arthur R. Mlodozeniec
Gerald J. Papariello
Ralph F. Shangraw

Members of the USA Steering Committee

Jack Cooper, Chairman
Zak T. Chowhan,
   Vice-Chairman
Gilbert S. Banker
Pramrod B. Chemburkar
John Haleblian
Saul S. Kornblum
Edward Lau
Jack Lazarus
Herbert Lieberman
Marvin H. Malone
Robert Mendes
Hyman Mitchner
Joseph A. Mollica
Boyd Poulsen
Christopher T. Rhodes
Bhogi B. Sheth
Bernard Sims

Members of the UK Steering Committee

R. F. Weir, Chairman
S. C. Jolly
T. M. Jones
W. Lund
J. E. Rees
W. G. Thomas

Corresponding Members of the Steering Committee

Pierre Buri
John A. Hersey
Hans Hess
Ryoichi Higuchi
Willi Lhoest
Brian Matthews
Tadashi Morioka
Shadir S. Nasir
Jerome Reinstein
Luigi Simioni
John Sjogren
Robert F. Weir

Members of the Monograph Committee

Ramesh N. Acharya
Michael J. Akers
Lloyd V. Allen
Shabir Anik
James B. Appino
Akira Asano
Albert Belmonte
Lyle D. Bighley
August Bruno
Albert E. Buckpitt
George Cohen
Robert E. Dempski
Robert Dusel
Robert Egidy
Henry Eisen
Milton Elefant
Stewart Ericksen
William Feinstein
Gordon C. Flynn
Charles Fox
Robert D. Gibson
Walter J. Gloor, Jr.
Frank W. Goodhart
Eugene E. Hamlow
Wesley Han
Dan Harpaz
Richard J. Harwood
Norman L. Henderson
Elvin A. Holstius
David Hsia
Richard Jones
Joseph L. Kanig
John S. Kent
Norman Kobayashi
John L. Lach
Jack Lazarus
James K. Lim
Robert Lipper
Irwin Lippman
Nicholas G. Lordi
Subhash K. Mallick
Shabir Z. Masih
James W. McGinity
F. Henry Merkle
Arthur R. Mlodozeniec
Don Monkhouse
Dan Mufson
Robert Nash
Noel O. Nuessle
James L. Olsen
Anthony Palmieri, III
Dan Pasquale
D. M. Patel
Garnet E. Peck
David G. Pope
Shankar D. Popli
James C. Price
Aquilar Rahman
Davis R. Reese
George Reier
Philip Reisberg
Arnold J. Repta
Martin Rieger
David Savello
Stanley Scheindlin
Lee C. Schramm
T. Werner Schwartz
John J. Sciarra
Eli Shefter
Efraim Shek
James T. Stewart
Julian J. Tagman
Murray M. Tuckerman
Paul Turi
Samuel Tuthill
Ravindra C. Vasavada
Deodatt A. Wadke
Seymour Weinstein
Harry T. Welles
Thomas A. Wheatley
Leon O. Wilken, Jr.
Karin Wolter
Andrew B. C. Yu
Cheng Der Yu

Corresponding Members of the Monograph Committee

James C. Cradock
Jerry Lanese
John F. Millar
Carl E. Rehm
Peter Tsai

UK General Collaborators

J. H. Bell
J. R. Bloor
I. Boyd
H. J. del. Cowe
J. T. Fell
A. G. Fishburn
A. T. Florence
J. Garnier
C. A. Johnson
H. Linton
N. Lynch
A. Parsons
H. Rees
J. Shatwell
R. L. Smith
J. Stevens
M. Sutherland
V. Watson
B. Welsh
S. B. Williamson

UK Scientist Collaborators

M. C. Allwood
N. A. Armstrong
M. E. Aulton
R. C. F. Baker
M. R. Billany
H. Burlinson
E. T. Cole
J. H. Collett
B. Croshaw
P. J. Davies
S. S. Davis
G. M. Eccleston
J. Emerson
B. Forrester
A. J. Grace
J. Hogan
R. L. Horder
J. E. J. Jeffries
T. M. Jones
A. J. B. Kayes
J. W. Kennerley
K. A. Khan

G. G. Liversidge
M. Lynch
S. Malcolm
M. C. Meyer
F. S. S. Morton
J. R. Nixon
J. F. Pickard
P. C. Record
R. M. E. Richards
K. Ridgway
R. C. Rowe
G. Rowley
A. B. Selkirk
F. E. J. Sendall
J. Staniforth
J. A. Stead
J. I. Wells
J. S. Wilde
S. B. Williamson
A. J. Winfield
H. E. C. Worthington
P. Wright

Members of the Academy HPE Laboratory Project

James B. Appino
John Callahan
Jens T. Carstensen
Zak T. Chowhan
Gary W. Cleary
Anthony G. Cusimano
Ray Daoust
Patrick P. DeLuca
Milton Elefant
Gordon L. Flynn
Charles Fox
Jeffrey L. Geisler
Alfonso R. Gennaro
Thomas P. Gillette
Herbert S. Grainger
Sophann Im
Gerald Kaplan
Lloyd Kennon

Terry T. Kensler
Robert G. Mendes
R. A. Miller
Robert A. Nash
Anthony Palmieri, III
Garnet E. Peck
James C. Price
George E. Rier
B. T. Roufail
Beverly J. Sandmann
S. Schiendlin
Joseph B. Schwartz
Joyoti A. Shah
Sy-Rong Sun
Arvind L. Thakkar
Paul Turi
Sriram Vemuri
Leon Wilkin

Preface

Experienced pharmaceutical formulators have for many years needed a systematic and comprehensive English language data resource on excipients: the additives used to convert pharmacologically active compounds into dosage forms suitable for administration to patients. The *Handbook of Pharmaceutical Excipients* was carefully planned and written to meet this need. It should serve as a reliable and useful source of technical information on the relationship between properties of excipients and the quality of dosage forms.

This volume includes 145 monographs in a uniform format on excipients most widely used in the preparation of pharmaceutical dosage forms. The technical information on these excipients was assembled from a wide, international range of scientific publications covering the physical, chemical and biological properties of these important materials. Examples of these properties include bulk and tap density, particle size distribution, crystal form, heat of adsorption, specific surface area, solubility, melting or boiling range, flowability, surface tension, sorption and desorption, photostability, etc. In addition, the *Handbook* includes information on documented interactions between excipients (sometimes still described as inert) and drug substances. These interactions may indeed create problems affecting the efficacy, safety and stability of pharmaceutical preparations.

Interest in excipients and their properties has expanded from a research perspective in line with the growing importance of bioavailability and bioequivalence. Among the factors known to affect drug absorption, the current revision of the *United States Pharmacopeia/National Formulary* mentions "the diluents and excipients used in formulating the dosage form, including fillers, binders, disintegrating agents, lubricants, coatings, solvents, suspending agents, and dyes." Although the monographs in this *Handbook* list many of the known interactions of excipients with drug substances, many other such interactions may not have been reported in the literature. Formulators are therefore advised to exercise caution and to undertake experimental studies before initiating clinical studies, particularly when dealing with new drug substances.

After the publication in 1974 of the *Katalog pharmazeutischer Hilfsstoffe* (*Catalog of Pharmaceutical Excipients*), which contains German-language monographs for nearly 100 Swiss pharmacopeial and non-pharmacopeial excipients, the idea of an edition in English was raised by United States and United Kingdom pharmaceutical scientists. This possibility was discussed at the 20th Annual Meeting of the American Pharmaceutical Association's Academy of Pharmaceutical Sciences in 1976. The goals established at that time included a recommendation to publish a Handbook of Pharmaceutical Excipients in the English language, structured in a format similar to the Swiss *Katalog*.

Noted British academic and industrial pharmaceutical scientists were contacted, and with their enthusiastic support, the cooperation of The Pharmaceutical Society of Great Britain was obtained. Their Industrial Pharmacists' Group Committee with the staff of the Department of Pharmaceutical Sciences of The Pharmaceutical Society of Great Britain then began collaborating with the APhA Academy of Pharmaceutical Sciences in the planning and preparation of the *Handbook of Pharmaceutical Excipients*. Aware of the Swiss connection, the publishers of the *Handbook* acknowledge the assistance and encouragement provided by the publishers of the *Katalog pharmazeutischer Hilfsstoffe*, namely, Ciba-Geigy, Hoffmann-La Roche, and Sandoz Ltd. in allowing an English translation of the *Katalog* to be made and used as a basis for the expanded *Handbook*.

To help expedite the publishing plan, steering committees in the U.S.A. and the U.K. were established to select excipients already officially recognized in *USP/NF* and *BP/EP* as well as to recommend non-official excipients which met the predetermined requirements for inclusion in the *Handbook*. The Steering Committees recognized the critical importance of distinguishing between information not requiring laboratory testing or evaluation and those parameters requiring laboratory testing. Examples of the latter include density, bulk and tap volume, particle size distribution, moisture sorption and desorption isotherms, mechanical properties, surface tension, viscosity and certain other properties of highly specific importance.

Scientific direction of the Handbook Project in the U.S.A. was the responsibility of an 18-member committee representing five schools of pharmacy and ten pharmaceutical companies under the chairmanship of Jack Cooper and Zak T. Chowhan. In the United Kingdom, the Pharmaceutical Excipients Project was directed by a committee of five academic and industry pharmacists under the chairmanship of Robert F. Weir.

Each monograph in the *Handbook* is divided into 20 sections as follows:

1. Nonproprietary Names
2. Functional Category or Categories
3. Synonyms
4. Chemical Names and CAS Registry Number
5. Empirical Formula and Molecular Weight
6. Structural Formula
7. Commercial Availability
8. Method of Manufacture
9. Description
10. Pharmacopeial Specifications
11. Typical Properties
12. Stability and Storage Conditions
13. Incompatibilities
14. Safety
15. Handling Precautions
16. Regulatory Acceptance
17. Applications in Pharmaceutical Formulation or Technology
18. Related Substances
19. Comments
20. Specific References
    USA: Authors and Reviewers
    UK: Authors and Reviewers

A number of monographs are "group monographs" containing description and technical information on two or more excipients belonging to a specific chemical series such as polyoxyethylene sorbitan fatty acid esters, polyoxyethylene stearates, and sorbitan esters. At the end of each monograph the author(s) and the reviewer(s) are acknowledged by * and **, respectively. Many of the monographs include scanning electron microphotographs taken at varying magnifications.

The compendial specifications for excipients with monographs in *USP XXI/NF XVI*, *BP* 1980, and *BP* Addenda 1982 and 1983 appear in Section 10. For details on pharmacopeial specifications which are currently applicable, the reader must refer to the latest revisions of the compendia as well as the latest addenda or supplements. Technical data from the APhA Academy of Pharmaceutical Sciences Handbook of Pharmaceutical Excipients Project which were generated between 1979 and 1980 by 34 laboratories representing pharmacy schools and pharmaceutical industry in the U.S.A. are summarized in Section 11 of the monograph. The Laboratory Methods used by these laboratories are summarized in Appendix II.

Completion of the Handbook Project will represent the results of years of work by numerous contributors who have provided invaluable experience in the compilation of the data in the monographs, 30 of which came from The Pharmaceutical Society of Great Britain. A total of 150 pharmaceutical scientists representing academic and industrial pharmacy in the U.S. and the U.K. volunteered their efforts for which we are most grateful. We also wish to extend our sincere thanks to James C. Boylan and Ralph T. Shangraw for their assistance in reviewing and correcting the galley proofs in cooperation with the staff of the American

Pharmaceutical Association, and to Ainley Wade of The Pharmaceutical Society of Great Britain for invaluable help in this connection.

The planning and implementation of the *Handbook of Pharmaceutical Excipients* was directed by the two Steering Committees in the USA and UK whose members are listed on page vii.

Notice to Readers

1. The *Handbook of Pharmaceutical Excipients* is a compilation of information obtained from the scientific literature, experiments as conducted by members of the APhA Academy of Pharmaceutical Sciences, and personal observations by authors of the individual monographs. The *Handbook* was written by volunteers from either the APhA Academy of Pharmaceutical Sciences or The Pharmaceutical Society of Great Britain. It is intended to be a convenient reference work generally descriptive of excipient products available at the time information for the *Handbook* was compiled. There is no intent, implied or otherwise, that any of the information contained within constitutes standards for the substances described. References are made in various monographs to the *USP/NF* and/or *BP/EP*. Diligent effort was made to use compendial information available as of January 1, 1985. However, since compendial monographs are frequently revised, the reader is urged to consult the most current compendium, or its supplement, for correct information.

2. During the preparation of the *Handbook of Pharmaceutical Excipients*, effort was made to determine all of the suppliers of the various excipients mentioned in the *Handbook*. This proved to be a very difficult task. The identification of known suppliers of an excipient product does not constitute an endorsement of the supplier or its product, and the lack of identification of any supplier of an excipient product is not intended to reflect adversely on that supplier or its product.

3. The data reported with regard to particular excipient products reflects only the results of testing of the particular batch or sample tested. The data reported may not necessarily be reflected in other batches or samples.

Acacia

1. Nonproprietary Name
NF: Acacia
BP/EP: Acacia

2. Functional Categories
USP: Tablet binder; suspending and/or viscosity-increasing agent; emulsifying and/or solubilizing agent
Other: protective colloid

3. Synonyms
Gum acacia; gum arabic

4. Chemical Name and CAS Registry Number
Acacia   [9000-01-5]

5. Empirical Formula
—

Molecular Weight
240,000 to 580,000

6. Structural Formula
—

7. Commercial Availability
USA

Brampton Co., J. W.
Colloides Naturels
Colony Imports & Export Corp.
Dormar Chemicals, Inc.
Indiana Botanic Gardens, Inc.
Ingredient Technology Corp. Flavor & Fragrance Div.
Ingredients International, Inc.
Dr. Madis Laboratories, Inc.
Meer Corp.
Neal & Co., M. F.
Paulaur Corp.
Ruger Chemical Co.
TIC Gums, Inc.

UK

Arthur Branwell & Co., Ltd.
Chemical Exchange (UK), Ltd.
Courtin & Warner, Ltd.
M. Hamburer & Sons, Ltd.
Impaq, Ltd.
John Kelly's, Ltd.
Kimpton Bros., Ltd.
L.J. Rickard, Ltd.
Steetley Chemicals, Ltd.
A.F. Suter & Co., Ltd.
Thew, Arnott & Co., Ltd.

8. Method of Manufacture
Acacia is obtained from trees of the genus *Acacia* which grow in the Sudan and the Senegal region of Africa. The Kordofan grade from *Acacia verek* is considered to be the most desirable. The bark of the tree is cut, and the exudate which appears is allowed to dry on the bark. The dried exudate is collected and graded. The material is then processed by removal of bark, sand and other particulate matter, followed by grading, sizing and blending to various specifications. The various types differ in mesh size, water-insoluble residue, solution color and clarity. A spray-dried form is also available.

9. Description
Thin flakes, spheroidal tears, or in powdered or granular form; white or yellowish-white color; odorless, and bland taste.

10. Pharmacopeial Specifications

	NF (Tears or Powder)	BP/EP (Powder)	BP/EP (Tears)
Botanic characteristics		+	+
Identification	+	+	+
Microbial limits	*Salmonella* NEG.	*E. coli* NEG	—
Water	≤15%	—	—
Total ash	≤4%	—	—
Acid-insoluble ash	≤0.5%	—	—
Sulfated ash	—	≤5%	≤5%
Insoluble residue	≤1.0%	≤0.5%	≤0.5%
Solubility	—	+	+
Loss on drying	—	≤15.0%	≤15.0%
Arsenic	≤3 ppm	—	—
Lead	≤0.001%	—	—
Heavy metals	≤0.004%	—	—
Starch & dextrin	+	+	+
Tannin-bearing gums	+	+	+
Agar & tragacanth	—	+	+
Agar & sterculia gum	—	+	+
Sucrose & fructose	—	+	+

11. Typical Properties

Academy HPE Laboratory Project Data		
Method	**Lab #**	**Results (%)**
MC-1	5	10.75[a]
MC-1	5	12.54[b]
MC-1	5	3.92[c]

Suppliers: Penick[a]; EM Labs[b]; Fisher[c]

Solubility: Water: 1 g in 2.7 g; alcohol: insoluble; glycerin: 1 g in 20 ml; propylene glycol: 1 g in 20 ml
pH (5% solution): 4.5-5.0.
Specific gravity: 1.35-1.49.
Viscosity of solutions: Variable; depending upon the source of the material, processing, storage conditions, pH and the presence of salts. Prolonged heating of acacia solutions results in a decrease of viscosity due to depolymerization or to particle agglomeration. The solutions exhibit Newtonian behavior.

12. Stability and Storage Conditions
Stored in a tight container in a cool, dry place. Solutions are subject to bacterial or enzymatic degradation. Powdered acacia should be preserved in an air-tight container.

13. Incompatibilities
Alcohol, adrenaline, amidopyrine, bismuth subnitrate, borax, cresol, eugenol, ferric salts, morphine, phenol, physostigmine, tannins, thymol, sodium silicate and vanillin. Many salts reduce the viscosity of acacia solutions, while trivalent salts may initiate coagulation. Acacia solutions carry a negative charge, and will form coacervates with gelatin and other substances. In the preparation of emulsions, solutions of acacia are incompatible with soaps.

14. Safety

Acacia is recognized as safe for general use as a food additive by the FDA and the Joint FAO/WHO Expert Committee on Food Additives. Although generally recognized as free from adverse reactions following ingestion, there have been a limited number of reports of allergenic reactions in man. It is not for parenteral use due to the danger of arabinosis.

15. Handling Precautions

None

16. Regulatory Acceptance

NF XVI; BP/EP 1980

17. Applications in Pharmaceutical Formulation or Technology

Use	Concentration (%)
Emulsifying agent	5.0-10.0
Suspending agent	5.0-10.0
Table binder	1.0-5.0 (Caution must be exercised to avoid prolonged disintegration time)

18. Related Substances

None

19. Comments

None

20. Specific References

1. G. O. Aspinal, Gums and Mucilages, *Advances in Carbohydrate Chemistry and Biochemistry*, 24, 333-379 (1969).
2. R. L. Whistler, "Industrial Gums," Academic Press, New York, N.Y., 1959.
3. F. Smith and R. Montgomery, "The Chemistry of Plant Gums and Mucilages," Rheinhold Publishing Co., New York, N.Y., 1959.
4. D. M. W. Anderson and I. C. M. Dea, Recent advances in the chemistry of acacia gums, *J. Soc. Cosm. Chemists*, 22, 61-76 (1971).
5. J. Swarbrick, Coarse dispersions. In "Remington's Pharmaceutical Sciences," Chapter 22, 15th Ed., Mack Publishing Co., 1975.
6. "Toxicological Evaluation of Some Food Additives." Food and Agriculture Organization (WHO), FAO Nutrition Meeting Report Series No. 53A, 316-318, Rome, 1974.
7. Food Additives, *Federal Register*, 41, No. 236, 53608-53609, December 7, 1976.
8. The chemistry and rheology of water-soluble gums and colloids, *SCI Monograph No. 24*, Society of the Chemical Industry, London, 1966.

USA: E. Shefter*; J. Cooper*; J. W. Boenigk**

Alcohol

1. Nonproprietary Name
USP: Alcohol
BP: Ethanol (96%)

2. Functional Category
USP: Solvent
Others: Preservative

3. Synonyms
Ethanol; ethyl alcohol; grain alcohol; methyl carbinol

4. Chemical Names and CAS Registry Number
Ethanol
Ethyl alcohol [64-17-5]

5. Empirical Formula
C_2H_5OH

Molecular Weight
46.07

6. Structural Formula
C_2H_5OH

7. Commercial Availability

USA
Ashland Chemical Co.
Bage, Inc.
Clinton Corn Processing Co., Div. Nabisco Brands, Inc.
Eastman Chemical Products, Inc.
Mallinckrodt, Inc.
McKesson Chemical Co.
Publicker Industries, Inc.
Shell Chemical Co.
Stoney-Mueller, Inc.
Thompson-Hayward Chemical Co.
Union Carbide Corp.
U.S.I. Chemicals Co.

UK
Alcohols, Ltd.
BP Chemicals, Ltd.
Distillers Co., Ltd.
James Burroughs, Ltd.
Methylating Co., Ltd.
Unalco, Ltd.

8. Method of Manufacture
Whey, cellulose pulp and substances rich in starch or sucrose are subjected to controlled enzymatic hydrolysis fermentation to produce a fermented liquid which contains about 15% alcohol. The fermented liquid is fractionally distilled to produce alcohol which is 94.9-96.0% v/v (USP). Ethyl alcohol is also manufactured by converting ethylene into diethyl sulfate and then hydrolyzing the ester.

9. Description
A clear, colorless, mobile and volatile liquid with a slight, characteristic odor. It has a burning taste.

10. Pharmacopoeial Specifications

Test	USP	BP
Identification	+	+
Acidity or alkalinity	+	—
Nonvolatile residue	≤1 mg/40 ml	≤5 mg/100 ml
Specific gravity	0.812-0.816 at 15.56°C	0.8062-0.8087 at (20°/20°)
Aldehydes and other foreign organic substances	+	—
Amyl alcohol and nonvolatile carbon-izable substances	+	—
Fusel oil constituents	+	—
Methanol	+	—
Water-insoluble substances	+	—
Aldehydes	—	≤10 ppm
Benzene	—	≤5 ppm
Clarity of solution	—	+
Reducing substances	—	+
Volatile impurities	—	+
Concentration range	94.9-96.0% v/v	96.0-96.6% v/v
Acetone and isopropyl alcohol	+	—

11. Typical Properties (All entries refer to dehydrated alcohol unless otherwise specified.)
Boiling point: 78.5°C (101.3 kN/m²); 78.15°C (101.3 kN/m²) minimum boiling point of azeotropic ethanol/water mixture.
Color: Hazen units—10 maximum (Pt-Co scale)
Flammability: Readily flammable, burning with a blue, smokeless flame.
Flash point (closed cup method): 12°C (100%); 14°C (96%)
Hygroscopicity: Absorbs water rapidly from the air.
Melting point: −117.3 to −114.1°C
Miscibility: (at 20°C): Water: Completely miscible, with rise of temperature and contraction in volume. Chloroform, acetone, ether and glycerin: Completely miscible.
Refractive index: 1.3611 (at 20°C)
Specific gravity: 0.7904-0.7935 (at 20°C); ≤0.7964 (at 15.56°C)
Surface tension: 22.75 mN/m (ethanol/vapor at 20°C)
Vapor density (relative): 1.59 (air = 1)
Vapor pressure: 5.3 kN/m² (at 19°C)
Viscosity: 1.20 mNs/m² (at 20°C)

12. Stability and Storage Conditions
Sterilized by autoclaving in sealed ampoules, or by filtration. Stable.
USP: Preserve in tight containers, remote from fire.
BP: Protect from moisture and store in a cool place.

13. Incompatibilities
In acidic solution, alcohol may react vigorously with oxidizing materials. Mixtures with alkali may darken in color due to the reaction with residual aldehydes in alcohol. Organic salts or acacia may be precipitated from aqueous solutions or dispersions.

14. Safety
Though alcohol has intoxicating properties, atmospheric concentrations sufficient to produce this effect are not generally reached in industry.

Threshold limit value (TLV) in workroom air in the United Kingdom is 1,000 ppm (of vapor by volume), or 1,900 mg/m^3. Exposure to concentrations of 5,000-10,000 ppm results in irritation of the eyes and mucous membranes of the upper respiratory tract. If continued for an hour, stupor and drowsiness may occur.

Preparations containing more than 50% ethanol may cause skin irritation when applied topically.

Systemically, alcohol is a CNS depressant. Sufficient doses can lead to nausea, vomiting, flushing, mental excitement or depression, drowsiness, impaired perception and incoordination. Severe overdosing can cause coma and death.

Oral LD$_{50}$ (rat): 13.7 g/kg of body weight.

15. Handling Precautions

Fire/explosion hazard, dangerous when exposed to heat or flame.

Auto-ignition temperature: 390-430°C.

Explosive limits: 3.3-19.0% v/v in air.

Fixed storage tanks should be electrically grounded when ethanol is transferred.

Recommended extinguishers: Foam, CO_2, dry powder.

16. Regulatory Acceptance

USP XXI; BP 1980

17. Applications in Pharmaceutical Formulation or Technology

Use	Concentration (% v/v)
Preservative, bacteria and mold inhibitor	≥ 10
Disinfectant bactericide	60-90
Extracting solvent in galenical manufacture	Up to 85
Solvent in oral liquids	Variable
Solvent in film coating	Variable

18. Related Substances

Dehydrated alcohol, USP. Similar to alcohol USP, but contains not less than 99.5% v/v of C_2H_5OH.

Ethanol, BP. Contains 99.4-100.0% v/v C_2H_6O.

Diluted alcohol, NF. Content of C_2H_5OH is between 48.4% and 49.5% by volume.

The BP lists eight strengths of dilute ethanols, i.e., 90, 80, 70, 60, 50, 45, 25 and 20% v/v.

In the United States, the title "denatured alcohol" is used for ethyl alcohol which has been rendered unfit for human consumption by the addition of denaturing agents such as methanol and methyl isobutyl ketone.

Denatured ethanols for external use in the United Kingdom are industrial methylated spirit, BP, and surgical spirit, BPC 1973.

19. Comments

In the *European Pharmacopeia*, the term "ethanol" used without other indication means ethanol 99.5% v/v. The term "alcohol" without other indication means ethanol 95% v/v. Where other strengths are intended, the term "alcohol" is used, followed by the statement of the strength. The second edition of the *European Pharmacopeia* lists ethanol, alcohol and aldehyde-free alcohol only as reagents.

20. Specific References

1. V.D. Gupta, Effect of some formulation adjuvants on the stability of benzyl peroxide, *J. Pharm. Sci.*, 71(5):585, 587 (1982).
2. A.J. Spiegel and M.M. Noseworthy, Use of nonaqueous solvents in parenteral products, *J. Pharm. Sci.*, 52:917 (1963).
3. C.L. Lautenschlager and H. Schmidt, in *Sterilizations—Methoden Für Die Pharmazeutische Und Ärztliche Praxis*, George Thieme, Verlag, 1954, p. 162.

USA: G.W. Radebaugh* Z. Chowhan**
 UK: R.B. Forrester*

Alginic Acid

1. Nonproprietary Name
NF: Alginic acid

2. Functional Category
USP: Tablet binder, tablet disintegrant.
Others: Viscosity-increasing agent.

3. Synonyms
Polymannuronic acid; norgine

4. Chemical Name and CAS Registry Number
Alginic acid may be described chemically as a linear glycuronoglycan, consisting mainly of β-(1-4) linked D-mannurronic and L-guluronic acid units in the pyranose ring form. Chemical Abstract Registry # [9005-32-7]

5. Empirical Formula
$(C_6H_8O_6)_n$

Molecular Weight
Approximately 240,000

6. Structural Formula

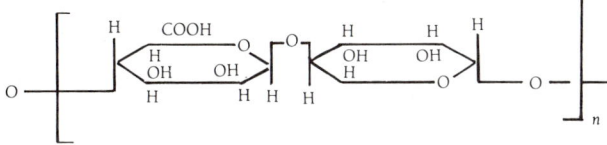

7. Commercial Availability

USA

Atomergic Chemetals Corp.
Colloides Naturels
Dormar Chemicals, Inc.
Edward Mendell Co., Inc.
Kelco Div. Merck & Co.
Pfaltz & Bauer, Inc.

UK

Alginate Industries, Ltd.
The British Ceca Co., Ltd.
Chemical Exchange (UK), Ltd.
Croxton & Garry, Ltd.

8. Method of Manufacture
Alginic acid is a hydrophilic colloid carbohydrate extracted with dilute alkali from various species of brown seaweed (Phaeophyceae).

9. Description
Alginic acid occurs as a white to yellowish-white, fibrous powder. It is practically odorless and tasteless.

10. Pharmacopeial Specifications

Test	NF	BP
Identification	+	+
Microbial limits	≤200/g tot. bact.	—
	NEG: *Salmonella*	
	species,	
	Escherrchia coli	—
pH (3% dispersion)	1.5-3.5	—
Loss on drying (4 hrs. at 105°C)	≤15% (w/w)	18%
Ash	≤4%	—

Test	NF	BP
Sulfated ash	—	≤7%
Lead	≤0.001%	≤10 ppm
Arsenic	≤3 ppm	≤3 ppm
Iron	—	≤300 ppm
Heavy metals	≤0.004%	—
Acid value	≥230	≥230

11. Typical Properties
Alginic acid is slightly soluble in water and insoluble in most organic solvents. It is soluble in alkaline solutions, resulting in viscous solutions. It is capable of absorbing 200-300 times its weight in water. Moisture content is approximately 7%.

Academy HPE Laboratory Project Data

Method	Lab #	Results
MC-8	18	7.01

Supplier: Mendell

12. Stability and Storage Conditions
Alginic acid, in warm storage areas, hydrolyzes very slowly, resulting in a decreasing molecular weight and lower solution viscosities. Store in a cool place in a well-closed container.

13. Incompatibilities
With the exception of magnesium, the alkaline earth metals and group III metals all form insoluble alginate salts.

14. Safety
Recorded toxicity:			
Intraperitoneal in rat	LD_{50}		1600 mg/kg
Intravenous in mouse	LD_{50}		1000 mg/kg

15. Handling Precautions
—

16. Regulatory Acceptance
NF XVI; BPC 1973

17. Applications in Pharmaceutical Formulation or Technology

Use	Concentration
Tablet disintegrant	1-5%
Tablet binder	1-5%
Viscosity-increasing agent	—

18. Related Substances
—

19. Comments
Some loss of viscosity usually occurs in a solution prepared from sterilized alginic acid. The extent of this loss may be influenced by the presence of other added substances.
Alginic acid is best incorporated or blended into a tablet granulation by dry-mixing processes.

20. Specific References:
1. Literature issued by Kelco Company, San Diego, CA.
2. Literature issued by Edward Mendell Co., Carmel, NY.

USA: J. W. McGinity*; M. R. Harris*; R. Dusch*; W. A. Vadino**; J. Cooper**

Ascorbic Acid

1. Nonproprietary Names
USP: Ascorbic acid
BP/EP: Ascorbic acid

2. Functional Category
USP: Antioxidant

3. Synonyms
Vitamin C; L-ascorbic acid

4. Chemical Names and CAS Registry Number
L-Ascorbic acid [50-81-7]
3-Oxo-L-gulofuranolactone (enol form)

5. Empirical Formula   Molecular Weight
$C_6H_8O_6$ 176.1

6. Structural Formula

CH₂OH
HCOH
HO   OH

7. Commercial Availability

USA

American International Chemical, Inc.
Byron Chemical Co.
Dormar Chemicals, Inc.
E.M. Chemicals, Inc.
Fallek Chemical Co.
Gallard-Schlesinger Chemical Mfg. Corp.
Hoffmann-LaRoche, Inc.
ICC Industries, Inc.
Ingredients International, Inc.
Knoll Fine Chemicals, Div. Knoll Pharmaceutical Co.
Pardee Co., The
Pfizer, Inc.-Chemical Div.
Reisman Corp., H.
Salsbury Laboratories, Inc., Chemical Dept.
S.S.T. Corp.
Takeda-Fallek Sales, Inc.
Uhe Co., George
United States Biochemicals Corp.
Vitamins, Inc.

UK

Grindsted Products A/S
E. Merck
Pfizer, Ltd.
Roche Products, Ltd.
Takeda Chemical Industries, Ltd.

8. Method of Manufacture

Ascorbic acid is prepared synthetically or extracted from various vegetable sources in which it occurs naturally, such as rose hips, black currants, the juice of citrus fruits and the ripe fruit of *Capsicum annuum L.* A common synthetic procedure involves the conversion of D-glucose to D-sorbitol by hydrogenation. The resulting D-sorbitol is oxidized by *Acetobacter suboxydans* to L-sorbose. A carboxyl group is added at C_1 by air oxidation of the diacetone derivative of L-sorbose, and the resulting diacetone-2-keto-L-gulonic acid is converted to L-ascorbic acid when heated with hydrochloric acid.

9. Description
White to light yellow, crystalline powder or colorless crystals with a sharp acidic taste and no odor. It is not hygroscopic. Upon exposure to light, it gradually darkens.

SEM: KY-8
Excipient: Ascorbic acid, USP fine powder
Manufacturer: Pfizer **Lot No.:** 9A-3/G92040-CO 146

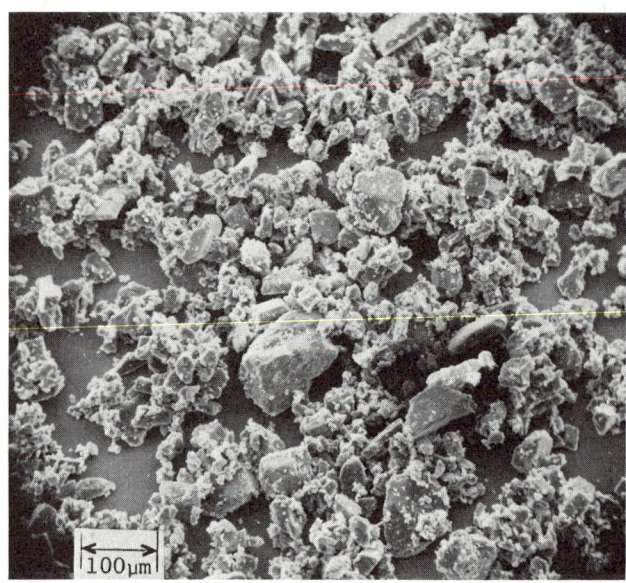

Magnification: 120× **Voltage:** 20 kV

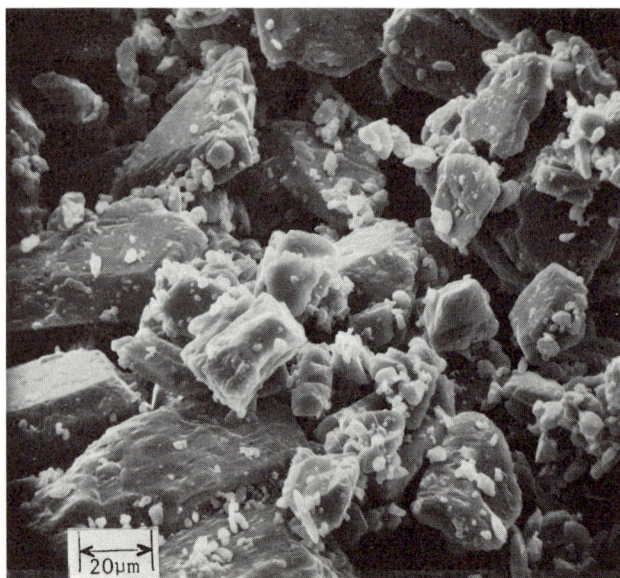

Magnification: 600× **Voltage:** 20 kV

SEM: KY-9
Excipient: Ascorbic acid USP granular
Manufacturer: Pfizer **Lot No.:** 9A-1/G01260-CO 140

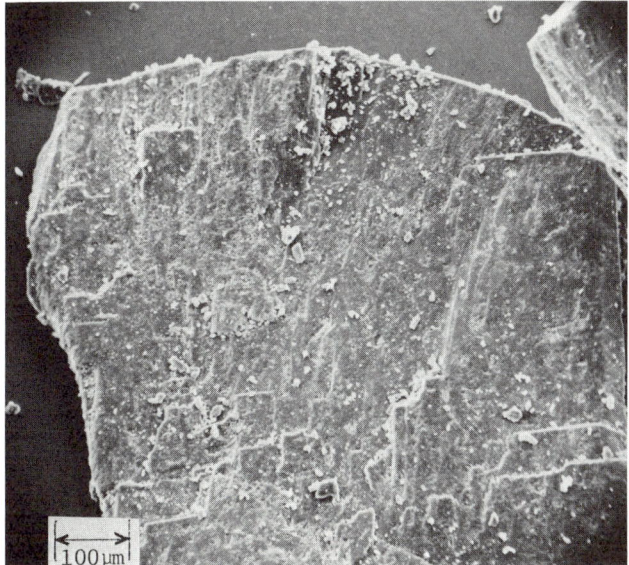

Magnification: 120× **Voltage:** 20 kV

SEM: KY-10
Excipient: Ascorbic acid, USP fine granular
Manufacturer: Pfizer **Lot No.:** 9A-2/G01280-CO 148

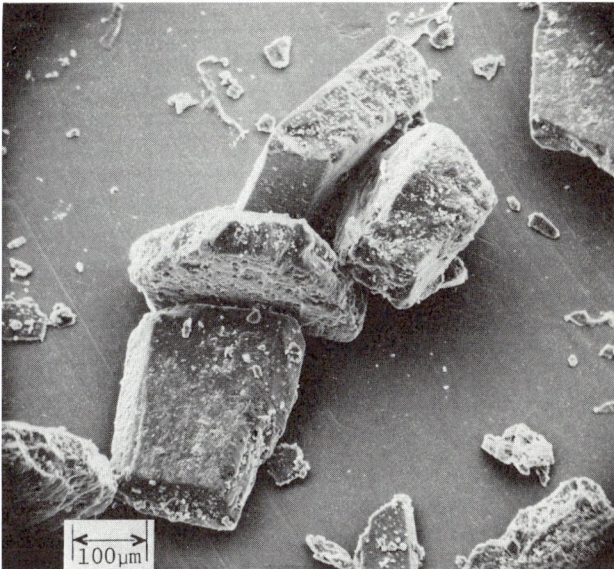

Magnification: 120× **Voltage:** 20 kV

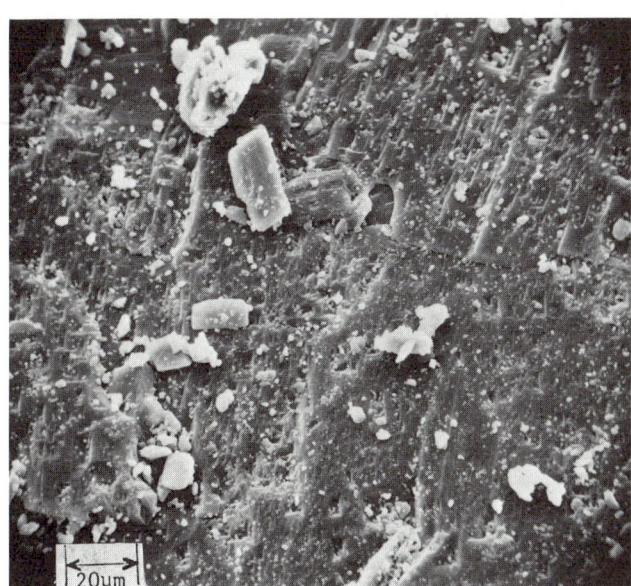

Magnification: 600× **Voltage:** 20 kV

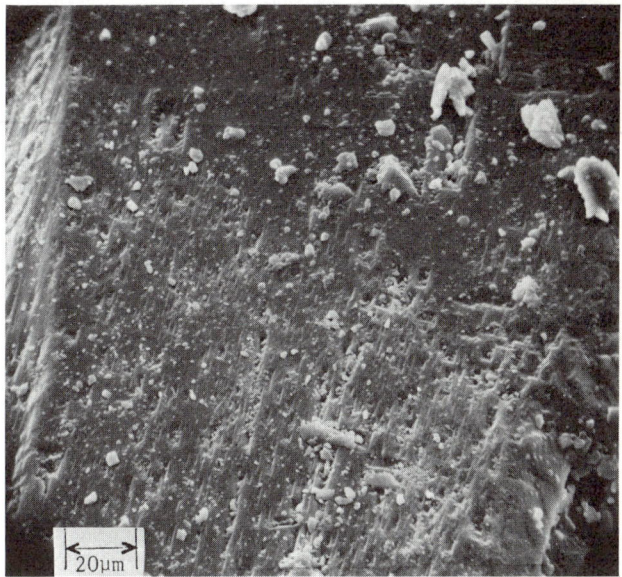

Magnification: 600× **Voltage:** 20 kV

SEM: UK-4
Excipient: Ascorbic acid, USP crystalline

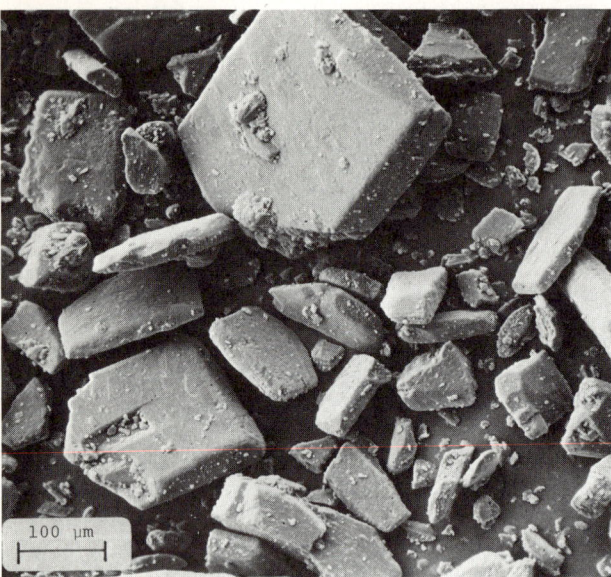

Magnification: 200×

SEM: UK-5
Excipient: Ascorbic acid, powder

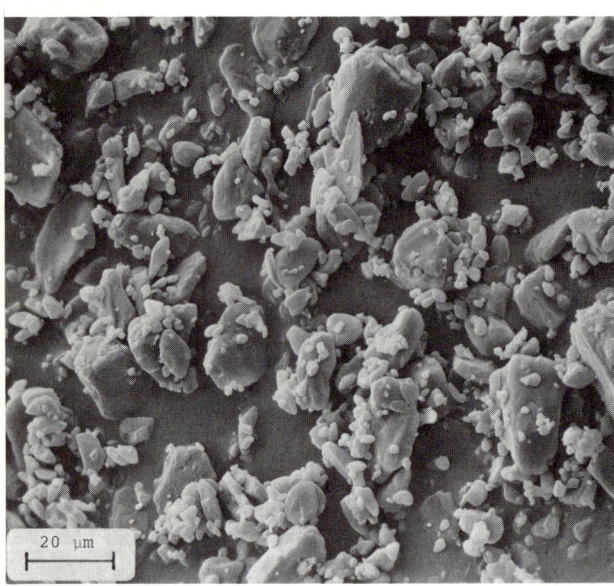

Magnification: 1000×

10. Pharmacopeial Specifications

Test	USP	BP/EP
Identification	+	+
Specific rotation	+20.5-+21.5	—
Residue on ignition	≤0.1%	
Sulfated ash	—	≤0.1%
Heavy metals	≤0.002%	≤10 ppm
Acidity (pH of 5% w/v sol)	—	2.2 - 2.5
Clarity & color of solution	—	+
Readily carbonizable substances	—	+
Assay	99.0-100.5%	≥99.0%

USP reference standard available

11. Typical Properties

Melting point: Melts with decomposition at about 190°C.
Solubility: Freely soluble in water (1 g in about 3 ml); soluble in alcohol (1 g in 30 ml), absolute alcohol (1 g in 50 ml), glycerin (1 g in 100 ml) and propylene glycol (1 g in 20 ml); insoluble in ether, chloroform, benzene, petroleum ether, oils, fats and fat solvents.
Poured bulk density: Crystalline: 0.7 - 0.9 g/cm³
Powder: 0.5 - 0.7 g/cm³
Tapped bulk density: Crystalline: 1.0 - 1.2 g/cm³
Powder: 0.9 - 1.1 g/cm³
Particle density: 1.65 g/cm³
Moisture content: 0.1% at ambient RH
Particle size distribution (typical values on sieve analysis):

Crystalline	Powder
10% < 106 μm	75% < 63 μm
30% < 150 μm	99% < 150 μm
50% < 212 μm	
65% < 250 μm	
80% < 300 μm	
95% < 500 μm	

12. Stability and Storage Conditions

Crystalline ascorbic acid is reasonably stable in air when dry. In the absence of oxygen and other oxidizing agents, it is heat-stable. It is unstable in solution, especially alkaline solution, readily undergoing oxidation even by atmospheric oxygen. The oxidation process is accelerated by light and heat and is catalyzed by traces of copper and iron. Solutions of ascorbic acid exhibit maximum stability at about pH 5.4. Store ascorbic acid in a tight container, free from contact with metals and protected from light.

13. Incompatibilities

Alkalis; heavy metal ions, especially copper and iron; oxidizing materials; methenamine; sodium nitrite; sodium salicylate; theobromine salicylate.

14. Safety

LD_{50} oral in mice: >6g/kg. LD_{50} intravenous in mice: 1.3 to 2.3 g/kg

15. Handling Precautions

Avoid excessive exposure to light, moisture and atmospheric oxygen, and keep free from contact with metals.

16. Regulatory Acceptance

USP XXI; BP/EP 1980

17. Applications in Pharmaceutical Formulations or Technology

Antioxidant in 0.01 - 0.10% concentration

18. Related Substances

Ascorbyl palmitate, NF; sodium ascorbate

19. Comments

—

20. Specific References

—

USA: A. Mlodozeniec*; J. L. Czeisler*; W. A. Vadino**; J. Cooper**.
UK: E. Cole*.

Bentonite

1. Nonproprietary Name

NF: Bentonite
BP: Bentonite

2. Functional Category

NF: Suspending agent and/or viscosity-increasing agent
Others: Adsorbent, gelling agent, emulsion stabilizer, clarifying agent

3. Synonyms

Wilkinite: wilhinite; soap clay; mineral soap; taylorite; bentonitum

4. Chemical Name and CAS Registry Number

Bentonite
Bentonite [1302-78-9]

5. Empirical Formula   Molecular Weight

$Al_2O_3 \cdot 4SiO_2 \cdot H_2O$ 359.16

Both bentonite and veegum are crystalline, clay-like minerals formed by devitrification and accompanying chemical alteration of glassy, igneous material. Both are essentially colloidal, hydrated aluminum silicates, with a higher rate of substitution of magnesium for aluminum in veegum. They are given the empirical formulae $Al_2O_3 \cdot 4SiO_2 \cdot H_2O$. Typical analyses show:

	Bentonite	Veegum
SiO_2	59.92%	61.1%
Al_2O_3	19.78%	9.3%
MgO	1.53%	13.7%
Fe_2O_3	2.96%	0.9%
CaO	0.64%	2.7%
Na_2O	2.06%	2.9%
K_2O	0.57%	0.3%

6. Structural Formula

—

7. Commercial Availability

USA

Beacon CMP Corp.
NL Chemicals/NL Industries, Inc.
Ruger Chemical Co.
Salomon & Bro., Inc., L.A.
Tamms Industries Co.
Thompson-Hayward Chemical Co.
Whittaker, Clark & Daniels, Inc.

UK

Bromhead & Denison, Ltd.
K&K Greeff Chemicals, Ltd.
Laporte Industries, Ltd.
Stecley Minerals, Ltd.

8. Method of Manufacture

A native, colloidal, hydrated aluminum silicate or clay, found in the Midwest, Wyoming and Canada.

9. Description

Very fine, odorless, pale buff or cream-colored to grayish powder, free from grit. May have a slight earthy taste. Consists of particles about 50-150 microns and numerous particles about 1-2 microns. Microscopic examination of samples stained with alcoholic methylene blue solution reveals strongly stained blue particles.

SEM: UK
Excipient: Bentonite

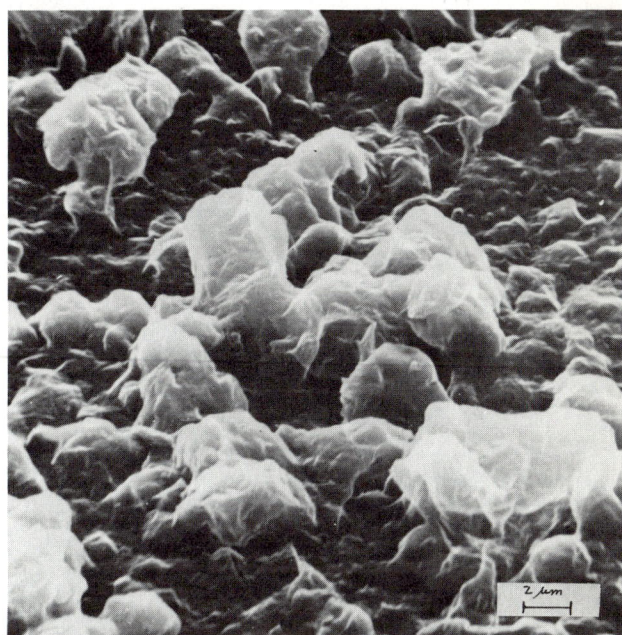

Magnification: 6500✕

SEM: KY-6
Excipient: Bentonite
Supplier: American Colloid Co.   **Lot No.** NMD 11780

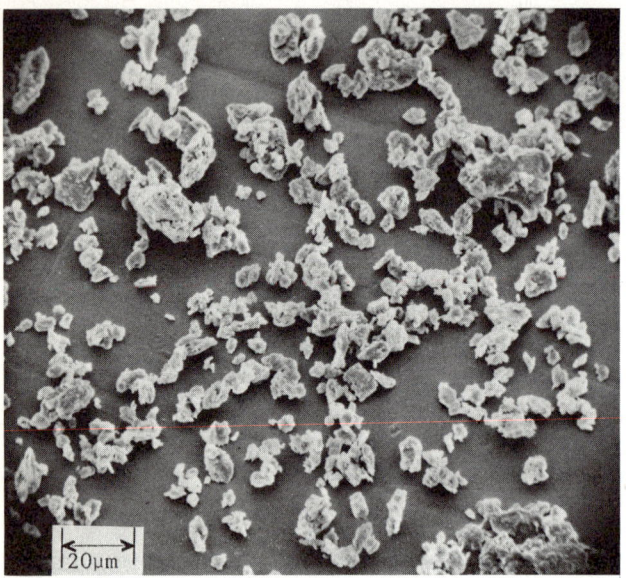

Magnification: 600×   **Voltage:** 10 kV

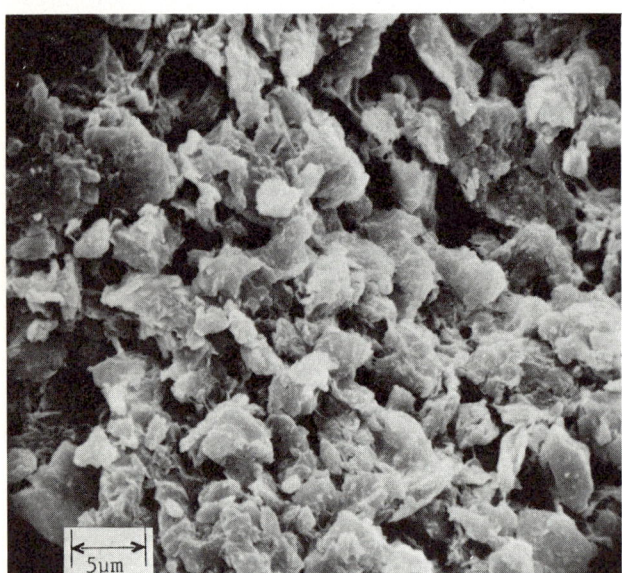

Magnification: 2400×   **Voltage:** 20 kV

10. Pharmacopeial Specifications

Test	NF	BP/EP
pH (4 g in 200 ml of H$_2$O)	9.5-10.5	—
Loss on drying	5-8%	5-12%
Gel formation	+	—
Swelling power	+	+
Fineness of powder	+	—
Microbial limit (*E. coli*)	absent	—
Identification	+	+
Alkalinity	—	+
Sedimentation volume	—	+
Coarse particles	—	+

11. Typical Properties

Bentonite consists mainly of montmorillonite, $Al_2O_3 \cdot 4SiO_2 \cdot H_2O$, but usually contains some magnesium and iron, together with small amounts of calcium carbonate and other minerals.

Analysis of Typical Moisture-Free Bentonite: Silica (SiO_2): 64.3%; alumina (Al_2O_3): 20.7%; ferric oxide (Fe_2O_3): 3.0%; ferrous oxide (FeO): 0.5%; titanium oxide (TiO_2): 0.1%; lime (CaO): 0.5%; magnesia (MgO): 2.3%; soda (Na_2O): 2.6%; potash (K_2O): 0.4%; sulfur (SO_3): 0.3%; water (bound H_2O): 5.1%; other constituents: 0.2%.

Solubility: Insoluble in water, but swells to approximately twelve times its volume when added to water. Insoluble in, and does not swell in, organic solvents—absolute alcohol, isopropanol, glycerin and fixed oils.

Sterilization: Sterilization is achieved by maintaining the solid at 150°C for 1 hour after drying at 100°C. Aqueous suspensions are sterilized by heating in an autoclave.

Academy HPE Laboratory Project Data

Method	Lab #	Results
MC-14	18	6.275%[a]
MC-14	18	5.70%[b]
FLO-1	14	No Flow[a]
EMC-1	18	Fig.18-EMC-1[b]

Supplier: [a]American colloid; [b]Whittaker Clark & Daniels

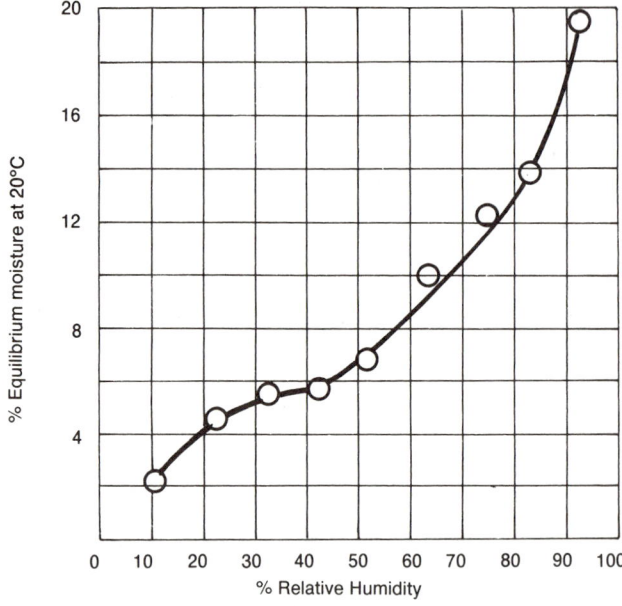

Figure: 18-EMC-1   **Method:** EMC-1
Bentonite NF Whittaker, Lot #NG3977

12. Stability and Storage Conditions

Bentonite is hygroscopic, and sorption of atmospheric moisture should be avoided following opening of the original package. Preserve in a tightly sealed container.

13. Incompatibilities

Aqueous preparations retain viscosity above pH 6, but are precipitated by acids. Acid-washed bentonite does not have suspending ability. Addition of significant amounts of alcohol to aqueous preparations will precipitate bentonite, primarily by dehydration of the lattice structure. It is incompatible with strong electrolytes, charged particles and solutions, sulfurated potash and acriflavine hydrochloride.

14. Safety

Bentonite is not absorbed from the gastrointestinal tract. No allergic responses following topical application have been reported.

15. Handling Precautions

—

16. Regulatory Acceptance

NF XVI; BP/EP 1980

17. Applications in Pharmaceutical Formulation or Technology

Use	Concentration (%)
Suspending agent	0.5-5.0
Emulsion stabilizer	1.0
Adsorbent (clarifying agent)	1.0-2.0

18. Related Substances

Bentonite magma: Preparation of bentonite and purified water used as a suspending agent. It contains 5% bentonite.

Hectorite: Magnesium bentonite, where magnesium replaces the aluminum in the molecule to produce a whiter product that has a greater swelling power in water. This is commercially available as *Veegum* (R. T. Vanderbilt Co.).

19. Comments

In high concentrations of calcium, sodium bentonite is converted to calcium bentonite, which tends to absorb less water. Bentonite may be used with concentrations up to 30% alcohol or isopropanol; 50% glycerin; 30% propylene glycol; or high molecular weight polyethylene glycols.

20. Specific References

1. J. C. Callahan, G. W. Cleary, M. Elefant, G. Kaplan, T. Kensler and R. A. Nash, Equilibrium moisture content of pharmaceutical excipients, *Drug Develop. and Ind. Pharm.*, 8:(3), 355-369 (1982).
2. F. Sadik, J. H. Fincher, and C. W. Hartman, X-Ray diffraction analysis for identification of kaolin NF and bentonite USP, *J. Pharm. Sci.*, 60:(6), 916-918 (1971).

USA: A. A. Belmonte*; K. R. Heimlich**; Z. Chowhan**
UK: A. J. Winfield*

Benzalkonium Chloride

1. Nonproprietary Name
NF: Benzalkonium chloride

2. Functional Categories
NF: Antimicrobial preservative; wetting and/or solubilizing agent
Others: Antiseptic detergent

3. Synonyms
—.

4. Chemical Names and CAS Registry Number
Ammonium-alkydimethyl (phenylmethyl)-chloride
Alkylbenzyldimethylammonium chloride [8001-54-5]

5. Empirical Formula   Molecular Weight
$[C_6H_5CH_2N(CH_3)_2R]Cl$ 360

6. Structural Formula (Graphical Formula)

R = Mixture of alkyls: n-C_8H_{17} to n-$C_{18}H_{37}$; mainly n-$C_{12}H_{25}$ (dodecyl), n-$C_{14}H_{29}$ (tetradecyl) and n-$C_{16}H_{33}$ (hexadecyl).

7. Commercial Availability

USA
Alcolac, Inc.
Armak Co., Industrial Chemicals Div.
Cyclo Chemicals Corp.
Danochemo A/S
Delamar, Inc.
Fellek Chemical Co.
HEXCEL Corp., Specialty Chemicals Div.
Hilton Davis Chemical Group
ICN K & K Labs, Inc.
Jordan Chemical Co.
Lonza, Inc.
Onyx Chemical Co.
Pfaltz & Bauer, Inc.
Rohm & Haas Co.
Ruger Chemical Co.
Sherex Chemical Co.
Sterling Organics, Div. Sterling Drug, Inc.
Tri-K Industries, Inc.

UK
ABM Chemicals, Ltd.
AKZO Chemie (U.K., Ltd.)
Albright & Wilson, Ltd.
Steetley Chemicals, Ltd.

8. Method of Manufacture
Benzalkonium chloride is formed by the reaction of a solution of N-alkyl-N-methyl-benzylamine with methyl chloride in an organic solvent suitable for precipitating the quaternary compound as it is formed.

9. Description
A white or yellowish-white, thick gel or gelatinous flakes with a mild aromatic odor. It is very bitter to taste; its aqueous solution foams when shaken. It is hygroscopic and affected by light and air.

10. Pharmacopeial Specifications

Test	NF
Identification	+
Water	≤15.0%
Residue on ignition	≤2.0%
Water-insoluble matter	+
Foreign amines	+
Ratio of alkyl components	+
Assay: (total alkylbenzyldimethyl-ammonium chlorides)	97.0-103.0%
(a)n-$C_{12}H_{25}$ homolog	≥40.0% of total
(b)n-$C_{14}H_{29}$ homolog	≥20.0% of total
(a) + (b)	≥70.0% of total

11. Typical Properties
Solubility: Very soluble in water, alcohol, and acetone. Insoluble in ether.
Chemical: Cation—active quaternary ammonium compound.
Antimicrobial: Active against Gram positive organisms. Not active against all the gram negative organisms. Ineffective against some *Pseudomonas aeruginosa* strains, *Mycobacterium tuberculosis, Trichophyton interdigitale* and *T. rubrum.* Combined with disodium edetate (0.01-0.1%), the activity against *Pseudomonas aeruginosa* is increased. In the presence of citrate and phosphate buffers (but not borate), activity against *Pseudomonas* can be reduced. It is relatively inactive against spores and molds, but active against some viruses, fungi and protozoa. Its activity increases with increasing pH, optimal activity occurring in the pH range of 4-10. The relatively inhibitory dilution as observed with a variety of micro-organisms is given in the following table:

Micro-organism	Dilution $\times 10^3$
Salmonella typhosa	1:256
Shigella dysenteriae	1:512
Escherichia coli	1:64
Aerobacter aerogenes	1:16
Salmonella paratyphi	1:64
Salmonella enteritidis	1:32
Proteus vulgaris	1:16
Pseudomonas aeruginosa	1:32
Vibrio cholerae	1:512
Staphylococcus aureus	1:800
Pneumococcus II	1:200
Streptococcus pyogenes	1:800
Clostridium welchii	1:200
Clostridium tetani	1:200
Clostridium histolyticum	1:200
Clostridium oedematiens	1:200

12. Stability and Storage Conditions
Solutions are stable at room temperature for prolonged periods, and may be autoclaved without loss of effectiveness.

Store in a cool place in an airtight container. Protect from light and prevent contact with metals. It may lose antimicrobial activity when the dilute solutions are stored in polyvinyl chloride and polyurethane foam containers.

13. Incompatibilities

Soaps, anionic surfactants, nonionic surfactants in high concentration, citrates, iodides, nitrates, permanganates, salicylates, silver salts, tartrates, zinc oxide, zinc sulfate, kaolin, aluminum, fluorescein, hydrogen peroxide, hydrous wool fat, sulfonamides, some rubber mixes, some plastics, cotton and protein.

14. Safety

Usually nonirritating and nonsensitizing and welltolerated in dilutions normally employed on the skin and mucous membranes. An occasional individual may be hypersensitive and may experience skin irritation on prolonged contact. Solutions stronger than 1:3,000 entering the eyes require prompt medical attention; concentrated solutions accidentally spilled on the skin may produce corrosive skin lesions with deep necrosis and scarring, and should be washed immediately with water, followed by soap solutions applied freely.

The fatal dose is estimated to be 1 to 3 g. An accidental intake can cause nausea and vomiting. Toxic symptoms include cyanosis due to paralysis of the respiratory muscles, dyspnea and asphyxia.

15. Handling Precautions

Repeated exposure of the skin to benzalkonium chloride may cause hypersensitivity.

16. Regulatory Acceptance

NF XVI

17. Applications in Pharmaceutical Formulation or Technology

1. Preservation of ophthalmic products: 0.01 - 0.02%; may be made more effective against resistant strains of *Pseudomonas* if used with polymixin B sulfate, 1000 USP units per ml, or combined with 0.1% disodium edetate.
2. Preservation of nasal and otic products: 0.002 to 0.02%, sometimes in combination with thimerosal, 0.002 - 0.005%.
3. Preservation of small-volume parenteral products: 0.01%, as usual concentration.

18. Related Substances

Benzalkonium chloride solution, NF XVI; BP 1980.

19. Comments

Addition of benzyl alcohol, phenyl propanol, or phenethyl alcohol enhances the microbial activity of benzalkonium chloride.

20. Specific References

1. R. A. Cowen and B. Steiger, *Cosmetic & Toiletries*, 92: 15 (1977).
2. R. M. Richards, *J. Pharm. Pharmacol*, 28: 264 (1976).
3. E. J. Lein, *J. Med. Chem.*, 19:849 (1976).
4. T. Tomlinson, C. M. Riley and T. M. Jefferies, *J. Chromatography*, 173: 89 (1979).

USA: S. Vemuri*; J. W. Boenigk**
UK: M. C. Allwood**

Benzoic Acid

1. Nonproprietary Name
USP: Benzoic acid
BP: Benzoic acid

2. Functional Category
USP: Antimicrobial preservative
BP: Antimicrobial preservative
Others: Bacteriostatic agent

3. Synonyms
Benzenecarboxylic acid; phenylcarboxylic acid; flowers of benzoin; phenylformic acid; dracylic acid; carboxybenzene

4. Chemical Name and CAS Registry Number
Benzoic acid [65-85-0]

5. Empirical Formula   Molecular Weight
$C_7H_6O_2$ 122.12

6. Structural Formula

7. Commercial Availability
USA
American International Chem., Inc.
Ashland Chemical Co.
Atomergic Chemetals Corp.
Baker Chemical Co., J. T.
Bentex Chemicals, Inc.
Browning Chemical Corp.
Delamar, Inc.
Floressence Perfumes Oils, Inc.
Gallard-Schlesinger Chemical Mfg.
Greeff & Co., R. W.
Kalama Chemical, Inc.
Mallinckrodt, Inc.
McKesson Chemical Co.
Pfaltz & Bauer, Inc.
Pfizer, Inc.—Chemical Div.
Ruger Chemical Co.
Sitco (Shah International Trading Corp.)
Tenneco Chemicals, Inc.
Thompson-Hayward Chemical Co.
Tri-K Industries, Inc.
Ungerer & Co.
United States Biochemicals Corp.
Velsicol Chemical Corp.

UK
Albright and Wilson Ltd.
Aldrich Chemical Co., Ltd.
Bayer UK Ltd.
BDH Chemicals, Ltd.
Hopkin & Williams
Koch-Light Laboratories, Ltd.
Kodak, Ltd.

8. Method of Manufacture
Benzoic acid is a naturally occurring substance. All commercial U.S. benzoic acid is prepared synthetically. One method of synthesis is by the continuous liquid-phase oxidation of toluene in the presence of a cobalt catalyst at 150-200°C and 5-50 atm. This process results in about a 90% yield. Benzoic acid can also be produced commercially from benzotrichloride or phthalic anhydride. Benzotrichloride, produced by chlorination of toluene, is reacted with one mole of benzoic acid to yield two moles of benzoyl chloride. The benzoyl chloride is converted to two moles of benzoic acid by hydrolysis. Yield is 75-80%. Phthalic anhydride is converted to benzoic acid in about an 85% yield by hydrolysis in the presence of heat and chromium and disodium phthalates. Crude benzoic acid is purified by sublimation or recrystallization.

9. Description
In bulk, benzoic acid appears as feathery, light, white crystals or powder. Individual crystals (monoclinic leaflets or needles) are colorless. Benzoic acid has a slight characteristic odor, suggestive of benzoin. It is essentially tasteless.

SEM: MF-13
Excipient: Benzoic Acid
Manufacturer: Merck Sharpe & Dohme International

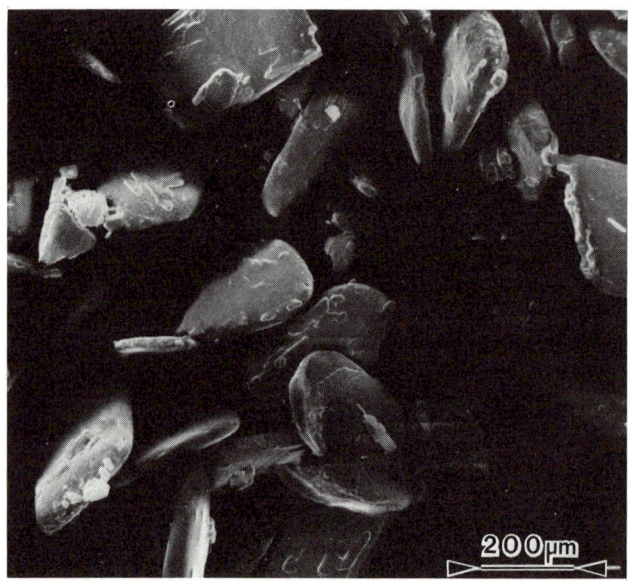

Magnification: 60✕

SEM: MF-13
Excipient: Benzoic Acid
Manufacturer: Merck Sharpe & Dohme International

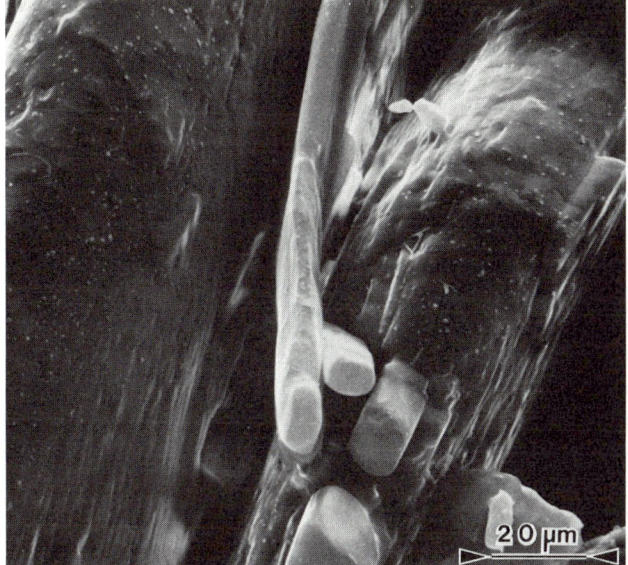

Magnification: 600×

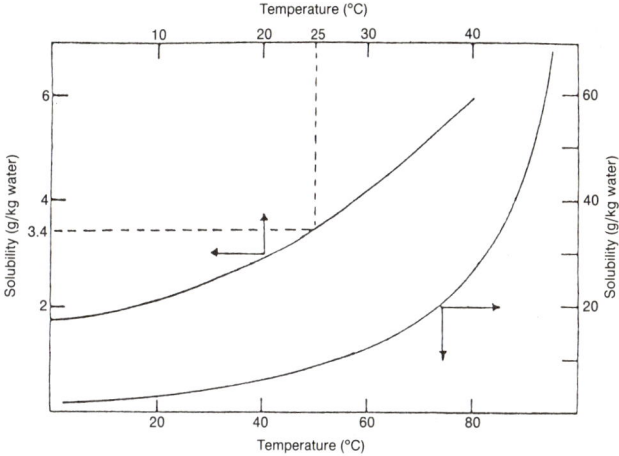

Aqueous solubility of benzoic acid as a function of temperature

Chemical: Benzoic acid exhibits reaction properties typical of organic acids. The carboxyl group is primarily *meta*-directing in further substitution of the aromatic ring. $K_a = 6.4 \times 10^{-5}$ (pKa = 4.19) at 25°C.

10. Pharmacopeial Specifications

Test	USP	BP/EP
Identification	+	+
Congealing range	121-123°C	–
Water	≤0.7%	–
Melting point	–	121-124°C
Residue on ignition	≤0.05%	–
Heavy metals	≤0.001%	≤10 ppm
Arsenic	≤3 ppm	–
Chlorinated compounds	–	≤0.07%
Sulfated ash	–	≤0.1%
Ash	-	+
Readily carbonizable substances	+	+
Readily oxidizable substances	+	+
Clarity and color of solution	-	+
Assay	99.5-100.5%	99.0-100.5%

11. Typical Properties

Physical:
Boiling point (at 760mm): 249.2°C
Flash point: 121-131°C
pH (sat'd sol. at 25°C): 2.8
Density: 1.316 g/cm³ at 24°C (solid)
Density: 1.075 g/cm³ at 130°C (liquid)
Refractive index: 1.53974 at 15°C (solid)
                  1.504 at 132°C (liquid)

Benzoic Acid Solubility[a] in Solvents Other Than Water

Solvent[b]	Volume (ml)[c]	Density (g/cm³)[d]
Acetone	2.3	0.79
Benzene	9.4	0.88
Carbon disulfide	30	1.26
Carbon tetrachloride	15.2	1.59
Chloroform	4.5	1.48
Ethanol, USP	3	0.80
Ethanol, absolute, 15°C	2.7	
Ethanol, absolute	2.2	0.79
Ethanol, absolute, boiling	1.5	
Ether	3	0.71
Methanol, 23°C	1.8	0.79
Toluene	11	0.87

[a] At 25°C unless otherwise specified.
[b] In addition to the list, benzoic acid is soluble in most fixed and volatile oils.
[c] Solubilities are expressed as milliliters of the solvent required to dissolve 1 g of benzoic acid.
[d] Densities are those of the solvents.

Antimicrobial activity: Bacteria: Moderate bacteriostatic activity against most species of gram positive bacteria. Typical MIC is 100 µg/ml. Less activity, in general, against gram negative than against gram positive bacteria. MIC for gram negative bacteria may be up to 1600 µg/ml. Inactive against spores. Molds: Moderate activity. Typical MICs are: 400-1000 µg/ml at pH 3; 1000-2000 µg/ml at pH 5. Yeasts: Moderate activity. Typical MIC is 1200 µg/ml. The addition of propylene glycol may enhance the fungistatic activity of benzoic acid.

Effect of pH: Only the undissociated acid shows antimicrobial properties, so the activity depends on the pH of the medium. Optimum activity occurs at pH values below 4.5; at values above pH 5, benzoic acid and sodium benzoate are almost inactive.

Academy HPE Laboratory Project Data

Method	Lab #	Results
DE-1	31	1.339 g/cm³ [a]
DE-1	31	1.315 g/cm³ [b]
MC-3	25	0.168 % [a]
MC-3	25	0.424 % [b]
SOL-5		*mg/ml*
Water (25°C)	11	3.04 ± 0.11
Water (37°C)	11	4.67 ± 0.07
Alcohol (25°C)	11	327.9 ± 24.3
Alcohol (37°C)	11	418.6 ± 26.3
Prop. glycol (25°C)	11	189.4 ± 15.1
Prop. glycol (37°C)	11	319.8 ± 5.4
Hexane (25°C)	11	9.6 ± 0.2
Hexane (37°C)	11	15.8 ± 0.12
SOL-6		*g/ml*
Water (25°C)	23	<0.001 b
Water (37°C)	23	<0.001 b
Alcohol (25°C)	23	0.334 b
Alcohol (37°C)	23	0.379 b
Prop. glycol (25°C)	23	0.225-0.325 [b]
Prop. glycol (37°C)	23	0.225-0.325 [b]
Hexane (25°C)	23	<0.001 b
Hexane (37°C)	23	<0.001 b
SOL-6		*g/ml*
Water (25°C)	23	<0.001 a
Water (37°C)	23	<0.001 a
Alcohol (25°C)	23	0.309 a
Alcohol (37°C)	23	0.380 a
Prop. glycol (25°C)	23	0.225-0.325 [a]
Prop. glycol (37°C)	23	0.225-0.325 [a]
Hexane (25°C)	23	<0.001 a
Hexane (25°C)	23	<0.001 a

Suppliers: [a] Humco; [b] Mallinckrodt, Inc.

12. Stability and Storage Conditions

Benzoic acid should be stored in a well-closed container. It has been reported (*Pharm. J.*, 1: 100, 1973) that no loss of benzoic acid or deterioration of its container occurred upon storage of a 0.1% aqueous solution for 8 weeks in polyvinyl chloride bottles.

13. Incompatibilities

Usual reactions with alkalis or heavy metals.

14. Safety

Ingested benzoic acid is conjugated with glycine in the liver to yield hippuric acid, which is then excreted in the urine. Benzoic acid is a gastric irritant and a mild irritant to the skin, eyes and mucous membranes. Human oral MLD: 500 mg/kg. Dog oral LD_{50}: 2000 mg/kg. Allergic reactions to benzoic acid have been reported. The WHO acceptable daily intake of total benzoates, calculated as benzoic acid, has been set at up to 5 mg/kg of body weight.

15. Handling Precautions

Benzoic acid should be handled with appropriate caution, since it is an irritant to eyes, skin and mucous membranes.

16. Regulatory Acceptance

USP XXI; BP 1980.

17. Applications in Pharmaceutical Formulation or Technology

Antifungal preservative and bacteriostat at values between 2.5 and 4.5. At a higher concentration in combination with salicylic acid, fungistatic activity is obtained.

18. Related Substances

Sodium benzoate (see separate monograph).

19. Comments

Benzoic acid is known to dimerize in many nonpolar solvents. This property, coupled with pH-dependent dissociation in aqueous media, comprises a classic textbook example of the effects of dissociation and molecular association on apparent partitioning behavior. The principles involved might be practically applied in determination of the total concentration of benzoate necessary to provide a bacteriostatic level of benzoic acid in the aqueous phase of an oil-in-water emulsion.

Solutions of benzoic acid or benzoate may be sterilized by autoclaving or by filtration.

The apparent aqueous solubility of benzoic acid is enhanced by the addition of citric acid or sodium acetate to the solution.

20. Specific References

1. E. R. Garrett and O. R. Woods. The optimum use of acid preservatives in oil-water systems: Benzoic acid in peanut oil-water, *J. Amer. Pharm. Assoc., Sci. Ed.*, 42: 736-739 (1953).
2. M. Grayson, Ed., "Encyclopedia of Chemical Technology," 3rd Ed., Vol. 3, John Wiley and Sons, New York, 1978, pp. 778-792.

USA: R. Lipper*; J. Cooper*; J. W. Boenigk**
UK: M. C. Allwood*; B. Crowshaw*; J. Emerson*

Benzyl Alcohol

1. Nonproprietary Names
NF: Benzyl alcohol
BP: Benzyl alcohol

2. Functional Category
USP: Antimicrobial preservative, solvent
BP: Local anesthetic; antiseptic

3. Synonyms
Phenylcarbinol; phenylmethanol; α-hydroxytoluene

4. Chemical Name and CAS Registry Number
Benzenemethanol [100-51-6]

5. Empirical Formula   Molecular Weight
C_7H_8O 108.14

6. Structural Formula

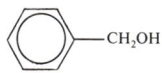

7. Commercial Availability
USA
Chemisphere Corporation
Florasynth, Inc.
Knoll Fine Chemicals, Inc.
McKesson Chemical Co.
Mitsubishi International Corporation
Monroe Chemical Co.
Norda Inc.
Orbis Products Corporation
Santell Chemical Co.
Stauffer Chemical Co.
Suburban Chemical Co.
Universal Oil Products Co.
Velsicol Chemical Corporation

UK
Albright Wilson, Ltd.
Aldrich Chemical Co., Ltd.
BDH Chemicals, Ltd.
Bush Boake Allen, Ltd.
Chemical Supply Co., Ltd.
Hopkin & Williams
Koch-Light Laboratories, Ltd.
Kodak, Ltd. (distributors for Eastman Organic Chemicals)
May & Baker, Ltd.
Tennants (Lancashire), Ltd.

8. Method of Manufacture
Benzyl alcohol is prepared by the distillation of benzyl chloride with potassium or sodium carbonate. It can also be made from benzaldehyde via the Cannizzaro reaction.

9. Description
Clear, colorless, oily liquid with a faint aromatic odor and a sharp, burning taste.

10. Pharmacopoeial Specifications

Test	NF	BP
Identification	+	+
Specific gravity	1.042-1.047	—
Distilling range	≥ 94% v/v distills at 202.5-206.5°	Distills below 200°C: ≥95% v/v distills at 203°-208°C
Refractive index (at 20°C)	1.539-1.541	1.538-1.541
Residue on ignition	≤0.005%	—
Chlorinated compounds	+	+
Benzaldehyde	≥0.2%	+
Assay limit	—	≥97.0% w/w
Acid value	—	≤0.5

11. Typical Properties
Acidity/alkalinity: Aqueous solutions are neutral to litmus.
Antimicrobial activity: Bacteria: Inhibiting agent with only modest bactericidal properties.
Gram-positive organisms: Moderately active; e.g., *Staphylococcus* spp. MIC = 3-5 mg/ml. Some organisms are very sensitive, having an MIC in the range 0.025-0.05 mg/ml. Gram-negative organisms: In general, poorer activity than against gram-positive species. MICs frequently greater than 3 mg/ml. e.g., *Pseudomonas aeruginosa*: MIC = 4.2-6.5 mg/ml; *Escherichia coli*: MIC = 4.5 mg/ml. Spores: Inactive, but may have enhanced activity in conjunction with heat. Benzyl alcohol 1% at pH 5-6 has been claimed to be as effective as phenylmercuric nitrate 0.002% against *Bacillus stearothermophilus* at 100°C for 30 minutes.
Molds and fungi: MIC = 3-5 mg/ml.
Yeasts: MIC = 2.5 mg/ml
Effect of pH: Optimum activity occurs when the pH is less than 5; little activity is shown at pH values above 8.
Boiling point: 204.7°C
Evaporation number: 1760 (ether-1)
Flash point: 103°C (open cup)
Partition coefficients (oil-water): Liquid paraffin-water = 0.2; peanut oil-water = 1.3
Solidification point: −15°C
Solubility/miscibility:

Solvent	Solubility
Water	(25°C) 4%
	(90°C) 7%
Ethanol (50%)	40%
Ethanol (absolute)	Miscible in all proportions
Chloroform	Miscible in all proportions
Ether	Miscible in all proportions
Fixed and volatile oils	Miscible in all proportions

Solubility at 20°C unless otherwise stated. g in 100 ml of solution.

Surface tension: 38.8 mN/m (38.8 dyne/cm)
Vapor density: 3.7 (air = 1)
Vapor pressure: 0.1 mm Hg at 30°C; 13.3 mm Hg at 100°C
Viscosity: 6 mNs/m^2 at 20°C (6cP)
Freezing point: 15°C
Volatility: Steam volatile

12. Stability and Storage Conditions

Oxidizes slowly in air to benzaldehyde and benzoic acid. Does not react with water. Can be stored in metal or glass containers. Plastic containers should not be used, except polypropylene or vessels coated with inert fluorinated polymers, e.g., Teflon. Store in an airtight container, remote from fire. Protect from light. Aqueous solutions can be sterilized by autoclaving. Some solutions may generate benzaldehyde during autoclaving.

13. Incompatibilities

Oxidizing agents and strong acids. Accelerates autooxidation of fats. Although antimicrobial activity is reduced in the presence of nonionic surfactants, e.g., polysorbate 80, the reduction is less than is the case with hydroxybenzoate esters or quaternaries. Benzyl alcohol is not bound by methylcellulose. It is only slowly sorbed by natural, Neoprene and butyl rubber closures the resistance of which can be enhanced by coatings of fluorinated polymers. A 2% aqueous solution in polyethylene containers may lose up to 15% of its benzyl alcohol content in 13 weeks at 20°C. Losses to polyvinyl chloride and polypropylene containers under similar conditions are usually negligible.

14. Safety

Acute toxicity: the oral LD_{50} has been estimated to be in the region of 1.2-3.1 g/kg for rats, 1.94 g/kg for rabbits and 1.58 g/kg for mice. The LD_{50} by the intraperitoneal route has been reported as approximately 0.4-0.8 g/kg in rats and guinea pigs. The liquid or vapor forms may give rise to local irritation and anesthesia of the skin, eyes and mucous membranes. Ingestion or inhalation may cause headache, vertigo, nausea, vomiting and diarrhea. Overexposure may result in CNS depression and respiratory failure.

When tested at a 10% concentration in soft paraffin, it provoked no sensitization reactions. However, there have been occasional reports of allergic response, particularly from injection of products containing 0.9% or more of benzyl alcohol. When injected or applied to mucous membranes, strong solutions may cause edema and pain. A hemolytic effect has been observed when red blood cells were rinsed with a large volume of sodium chloride (0.9%) solution containing 1.5% benzyl alcohol. The effect was attributed to the presence of benzyl alcohol.

15. Handling Precautions

Protect from ingestion, skin absorption and vapor inhalation.

16. Regulatory Acceptance

NF XVI; BP 1980

17. Applications in Pharmaceutical Formulation or Technology

Preservative: Up to 2% in aqueous or oily preparations; 0.9% in cortisone eye drops.
Solubilizer (5% or more): In aqueous or oily preparations. Local anesthetic and antiseptic in parenterals, cough products, ophthalmic solutions, ointments, and dermatological aerosol sprays.

18. Related Substances

None

19. Comments

Adverse reaction information regarding animals receiving LVPS containing benzyl alcohol is similar to information relating to human infants and is supported by preliminary but confirmatory tests in laboratory animals and by the consistency of the reported adverse effects with the established toxic syndrome of benzyl alcohol and related compounds. The use of benzyl alcohol in LVPS for human use ceased in the summer of 1982, and will also cease for veterinary products.

20. Specific References:

1. L.N. Elowe, *Ontario Coll. Pharm. Bull.*, 4: 45 (1955).
2. A.D. Russell, J. Jenkins and I.N. Harrison, *Adv. Appl. Microbiol.*, 9: 1 (1967).
3. D.V. Carter, P.T. Charlton, A.H. Fenton, J.R. Housley and B. Lessel, The preparation and the antibacterial and antifungal properties of some substituted benzyl alcohols, *J. Pharm. Pharmacol.*, 10: 149T (1958).
4. B. Croshaw, Preservatives for cosmetics and toiletries, *J. Soc. Cosmet. Chem.*, 3: 28S (1977).
5. A. Royce and G. Sykes, Losses of bacteriostats from injections in rubber-closed containers, *J. Pharm. Pharmacol.*, 9: 814 (1957).
6. M. Klein, E.G. Millwood and W.W. Walther, On the maintenance of sterility in eye-drops, *J. Pharm. Pharmacol.*, 6: 725 (1954).
7. K.H. Wallhauser, *Pharm. Ind.*, 36: 716 (1974).
8. R.P. Evans, Toxicity of intravenous benzyl alcohol, *Drug Intell. Clin. Pharm.*, 9: 154 (1975).
9. S.M. Harrison, B.W. Barry and P.H. Dugard, Benzyl alcohol vapor diffusion through human skin: dependence on thermodynamic activity in the vehicle, *J. Pharm. Pharmacol.*, 34: Suppl., 36P (1982).

USA: D.R. Reese*; A. Palmieri**; F.A. Restaino**
UK: M.C. Allwood*; B. Croshaw*; J. Emerson*

Butane

1. Nonproprietary Name

NF: Butane

2. Functional Category

USP: Aerosol propellant

3. Synonyms

n-Butane

4. Chemical Name and CAS Registry Number

n-Butane [106-97-8]

5. Empirical Formula   Molecular Weight

C_4H_{10} 58.12

6. Structural Formula

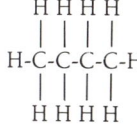

7. Commercial Availability

USA

Aeropres Corporation
Diversified Chemical and Propellant Company
Exxon Company
Industrial Hydrocarbons, Inc.
Phillips Chemical Company
Shell Chemical Company

UK

Air Products, Ltd.
Calor Group, Ltd.

8. Method of Manufacture

The hydrocarbons are natural products which are highly purified by passing through molecular sieves and removing most of the unsaturated compounds which may be present. They are separated from one another generally by fractional distillation.

9. Description

Butane is a liquefied gas and exists as a liquid at room temperature when contained under its own vapor pressure or as a gas when exposed to room temperature and atmospheric pressure. It is essentially a clear, colorless, odorless liquid, but may have a slight ethereal odor.

10. Pharmacopoeial Specifications

Test	USP
Identification	+
Water	≤0.001%
High-boiling residues	≤5 ppm
Acidity of residue	+
Sulfur compounds	+
Assay	≥97.0% C_4H_{10}

11. Typical Properties

Boiling point (°F): 31.1
Boiling point (°C): −0.5
Vapor pressure (psi at 21°C): 16.5; cm³
Liquid density (g at 70°F): 0.58
Kauri-Butanol value: About 25
Viscosity (cps): 0.173
Flammability in air: Lower limit (v/v %): 1.9; upper limit (v/v %): 8.5
Flash point (°C): −138
Solubility in water (v/v): 0.15 at 17°C and 770 mm
Solubility in alcohol (v/v): 18.0 at 17°C and 770 mm

12. Stability and Storage Conditions

All of the hydrocarbons used as propellants are extremely stable compounds. The hydrocarbon propellants are chemically nonreactive when used as propellants. They are flammable and explosive when mixed with certain concentrations of air. They should be stored in tight cylinders; exposure to excessive heat should be avoided.

13. Incompatibilities

Other than the lack of miscibility of the hydrocarbons with water, they do not have any practical incompatibilities with the usual ingredients used in aerosol pharmaceutical formulations. They are generally miscible with nonpolar materials and some semipolar compounds.

14. Safety

Acute toxicity data: Inhalation LD_{50} (rat) = 659 mg/kg. Butane is highly flamable and explosive.

15. Handling Precautions

These materials are liquefied gases and should be handled accordingly. They should be used in a well-ventilated room. It should be noted that the vapors do not support life; therefore, when cleaning large tanks, adequate provisions for oxygen must be provided for personnel cleaning the tanks. The hydrocarbons are highly flammable and explosive, and must be handled only in an explosion-proof room along with explosion-proof equipment. The room must be equipped with adequate safety warning devices. Personnel should wear rubber gloves, safety glasses and protective clothing.

16. Regulatory Acceptance

NF XVI

17. Applications in Pharmaceutical Formulation or Technology

Hydrocarbons such as butane, propane and isobutane are used for all topical pharmaceutical aerosols, with few exceptions. Depending upon the desired formulation, the concentration of propellant ranges from about 5% to 95% by weight. Foam aerosols generally use about 4-5% of a hydrocarbon propellant consisting of isobutane (84.1%) and propane (15.9%). Spray-type aerosols utilize a propellant concentration of 50% and higher. Only highly purified grades can be used for pharmaceuticals, since they may contain traces of unsaturated compounds which contribute a slight odor to the product.

18. Related Substances

Isobutane; propane

19. Comments

Due to recent changes in regulations, most pharmaceutical aerosols have been reformulated from a fluorochlorocarbon system to a hydrocarbon system.

20. Specific References

See trichloromonofluoromethane

USA: J. J. Sciarra*; J. W. Boenigk**
UK: P. J. Davies*

Butylated Hydroxyanisole

1. Nonproprietary Name
NF: Butylated hydroxyanisole
BP: Butylated hydroxyanisole

2. Functional Category
NF: Antioxidant
BP: Antioxidant

3. Synonyms
BHA; *Tenox*; *Embanox*

4. Chemical Names and CAS Registry Number
2-*tert*-Butyl-4-methoxyphenol
Phenol, (1,1-dimethylethyl)-4-methoxy-; *tert*-butyl-4-methoxyphenol [25013-16-5]

5. Empirical Formula   Molecular Weight
$C_{11}H_{16}O_2$ 180.25

6. Structural Formula

7. Commercial Availability
USA

Anachemia Chemicals, Inc.
Eastman Chemicals Products, Inc.
ICN Pharmaceuticals, Inc.
United States Biochemical Corp.
Universal Oil Products Co.

UK

Eastman Chemical International AG
May & Baker, Ltd.
Nipa Laboratories, Ltd.

8. Method of Manufacture
p-Methoxyphenol is reacted with isobutene.

9. Description
White or slightly yellow, waxy solid, having a faint, characteristic odor.

10. Pharmacopeial Specifications

Test	NF	BP
Identification	+	+
Residue on ignition	≤0.01%	—
Arsenic	3 ppm	—
Heavy metals	0.001%	—
Assay	≥98.5%	—
Hydroquinone	—	+
Sulfated ash	—	≤0.05%
Related substances	—	+

USP 3-*tert*- and 4-*tert*-butyl-4-hydroxyanisole reference standards are available.

11. Typical Properties
Antimicrobial activity: Activity is similar to that of the *p*-hydroxybenzoate esters (parabens). The greatest activity is against molds and gram-positive bacteria, with less activity against gram-negative bacteria.
Boiling range: 264-270°C at 733mm; 268.9°C at 745mm
Melting range: 48-57°C
Solubility: Insoluble in water. It is freely soluble in alcohol, propylene glycol, chloroform and ether.

Academy HPE Laboratory Project Data		
Method	Lab #	Results
SOL-7 at 25°C (Water)	32	0.32 mg/ml
SOL-7 at 37°C (Water)	32	0.78 mg/ml
SOL-7 at 25°C (Alcohol)	32	793.0 mg/ml
SOL-7 at 37°C (Alcohol)	32	834.0 mg/ml
SOL-7 at 25°C (Prop. Glycol)	32	467.0 mg/ml
SOL-7 at 37°C (Prop. Glycol)	32	456.0 mg/ml
SOL-7 at 25°C (Hexane)	32	48.0 mg/ml
SOL-7 at 37°C (Hexane)	32	10.0 mg/ml
DE-1	31	1.117 g/cm³

Viscosity, kinematic (at 99°C): 3.3 CST
Supplier: Eastman

12. Stability and Storage Conditions
Light causes discoloration and loss of activity. Preserve in a well-closed container protected from light.

13. Incompatibilities
Light and trace quantities of metal cause discoloration and loss of activity. Incompatible with oxidizing agents and ferric salts. It is a phenol and undergoes many of the reaction characteristics of phenolic compounds.

14. Safety
Toxicology LD_{50} in rats: 2.5-5.0 g/kg. Local and systemic tolerance: Estimated acceptable daily intake is up to 500 μg/kg of body weight as BHA, BHT or the sum of both.

15. Handling Precautions
To avoid any irritant effects during handling, the following precautionary measures are suggested: (1) Wear protective rubber gloves. In case of skin contact, wash immediately and thoroughly with soap and water. (2) Wear safety glasses to protect the eyes. If contact occurs, flush continuously with water for at least fifteen minutes and seek medical attention if irritation persists. (3) Use with ventilation adquate to maintain vapor concentrations below irritating levels when heating or spraying the antioxidant.

16. Regulatory Acceptance
NF XVI; BP 1980
BHA is being considered by the FDA for review as part of its program to reexamine the safety of food additives in the GRAS list.

17. Applications in Pharmaceutical Formulation or Technology
BHA is used to delay or prevent oxidative rancidity of fats and oils and to prevent loss of activity of oil-soluble vitamins.
For Vitamin A: 10 mg per 1,000,000 units
For β-carotene: 0.01%
For oils and fats: 0.02%
For essential oils and flavoring agents: 0.02-0.5%

18. Related Substances

Butylated hydroxytoluene; 2-5-butyl-hydroquinone; propyl gallate

19. Comments

None

20. Specific References

1. Tenox, Technical Data Publications, Eastman Chemicals Products, Inc.
Extending the shelf life of cosmetic and pharmaceutical products.

Improving the keeping qualities of flavoring materials.
For oils, fats and fat-containing foods.
Improving the stability of edible animal fats.
Increasing the shelf life of candy and chewing gums.
Preparation of emulsions.

2. Embanox, Food Grade Anti-oxidant, May & Baker, Ltd. (Official status, mechanism, detection, antimicrobial activity, solubilities, technical applications.)

USA: A. Asano*; J. W. Boenigk**
UK: J. R. Nixon*; W. Lund**

Butylated Hydroxytoluene

1. Nonproprietary Names
NF: Butylated hydroxytoluene
BP: Butylated hydroxytoluene

2. Functional Categories
NF: Antioxidant
BP: Antioxidant

3. Synonym
BHT

4. Chemical Names and CAS Registry Number
Phenol,2,6,-bis(1,1-dimethylethyl)-4-methyl-,
2,6-Di-tert-butyl-*p*-cresol [128-37-0]

5. Empirical Formula
Empirical Formula	Molecular Weight
$C_{15}H_{24}O$	220.35

6. Structural Formula

7. Commercial Availability
USA
Anachemia Chemicals, Inc.
ICN Pharmaceuticals, Inc.
Koppers Company, Inc.
United States Biochemical Corp.

UK
BTP Cocker Chemicals, Ltd.
Chance & Hunt
May & Baker, Ltd.
Eastman Chemical International AG

8. Method of Manufacture
p-Cresol is reacted with isobutylene.

9. Description
White crystalline solid, having a faint, characteristic odor.

10. Pharmacopeial Specifications

Test	NF	BP
Identification	+	+
Congealing temperature	$\geq 69.2°C$	—
Residue on ignition	$\leq 0.002\%$	—
Arsenic	3 ppm	—
Heavy metals	0.001%	—
Acid value	—	$\leq 0.05\%$
Sulfated ash	—	$\leq 0.1\%$
Freezing point	—	$\geq 69.2°C$
Assay	$\geq 99.0\%$	—

11. Typical Properties
Boiling point: 265°C (760 mm); 190°C (100 mm); 171°C (50 mm); 147°C (20 mm).
Refractive index: N_D^{75} 1.4859
Specific gravity: 20/4°C: 1.006; 80/4°C: 0.890; 90/4°C 0.883; 100/4°C: 0.875

Academy HPE Laboratory Project Data		
Method	Lab #	Results
SOL-7 at 25°C (water)	32	Insoluble
SOL-7 at 37°C (water)	32	Insoluble
SOL-7 at 25°C (alcohol)	32	108 mg/ml
SOL-7 at 37°C (alcohol)	32	147 mg/ml
SOL-7 at 25°C (hexane)	32	409 mg/ml
SOL-7 at 37°C (hexane)	32	514 mg/ml
SOL-7 at 25°C (propylene glycol)	32	Insoluble
SOL-7 at 37°C (propylene glycol)	32	Insoluble
DE-1	31	1.031

Supplier: Koppers Company, Inc.

12. Stability and Storage Conditions
Light causes discoloration and a loss of activity. Preserve in a well-closed container, protected from light.

13. Incompatibilities
Light and trace quantities of metal cause discoloration and a loss of activity. It is incompatible with oxidizing agents and ferric salts. It is a phenol and undergoes many of the reactions characteristic of phenolic compounds.

14. Safety
Toxicology: Oral LD_{50}: in rate: 1350-3900 mg/kg; in mice: 1040 mg/kg. LD_{100}: in cats: 940-2100 mg/kg; in rabbits: 2100-3200 mg/kg; in guinea pigs: 10,700 mg/kg.
Parenteral: A single intraperitoneal injection of 2.5 g/kg in mice produced respiratory distress and loss of responsiveness. An intracutaneous injection of 0.04-0.08 mg of BHT in ethanol induced local irritation and necrosis in guinea pigs.
Local and systemic tolerance: The solid material is slightly irritating to the skin or eyes if not promptly removed.
In animals, acute toxic doses of BHT induced salivation, mild miosis, restlessness, hyperexcitability, unsteadiness, increased urination, tremors, pronounced hindquarter paralysis and hemorrhage.
Allergenicity: Allergic contact sensitivity to BHT has been reported.
Maximum allowable concentrations: United States: BHT is permitted in limited concentrations (10-200 ppm) in specified foods. United Kingdom: 0.02% in fats and oils, vitamin oils, partial glyceryl esters and concentrates containing less than 100,000 IU vitamin A per gram. 0.01% in essential oils, isolates and concentrates. 0.001% in vitamin oils, preparations containing more than 100,000 IU vitamin A per gram. Estimated acceptable daily intake is up to 500 μg/kg of body weight as BHT, BHA or the sum of both.

15. Handling Precautions
To avoid irritating effects during handling, the following precautionary measures are suggested: (1) Wear protective rubber gloves. In case of skin contact, wash immediately and thoroughly with soap and water. (2) Wear safety glasses to protect the eyes. If contact occurs, flush continuously with water for at least fifteen minutes and seek medical attention if irritation persists. (3) Use with ventilation adequate to maintain vapor concentrations below irritating levels when heating the antioxidant.

16. Regulatory Acceptance

NF XVI; BP 1980

17. Applications in Pharmaceutical Formulation or Technology

BHT is used to delay or prevent oxidation, rancidity of fats and oils and loss of activity of oil-soluble vitamins. Suggested concentrations of BHT: For vitamin A: 10 mg per 1,000,000 units; for beta-carotene: 0.01%; for fats and oils: 0.02%; for essential oils and flavoring agents: 0.02-0.5%.

18. Related Substances

Butylated hydroxyanisole; 2-t-butyl hydroquinone; propyl gellate.

19. Comments

——

20. Specific References

1. S. M. Greenberg, L. M. Miller and J. E. Villaume, "A Review of the Food Additive, Butylated Hydroxytoluene" (Nov., 1978), Technical Panel, Manufacturing Chemists Association, Franklin Research Center.
2. TENOX, Technical Data Publications, Eastman Chemicals Products, Inc.
   "Extending the shelf life of cosmetic and pharmaceutical products."
   "Improving the keeping qualities of flavoring materials."
   "For oils, fats and fat-containing foods."
   "Increasing the stability of edible animal fats."
   "Increasing the shelf life of candy and chewing gums."
   "Preparation of emulsions."
3. EMBANOX, Food Grade antioxidant, May & Baker, Ltd. (Official status, mechanism, detection, antimicrobial activity, solubilities and technical applications).

USA: A. Asano,* J. W. Boenigk**
UK: J. R. Nixon,* W. Lund**

Butylparaben

1. **Nonproprietary Names**
   NF: Butylparaben
   BP: Butyl hydroxybenzoate

2. **Functional Category**
   USP: Antimicrobial preservative
   BP/EP: Antimicrobial preservative
   Others: Bacteriostatic agent

3. **Synonyms**
   Butyl chemosept, butyl parasept

4. **Chemical Names and CAS Registry Number**
   4-Hydroxybenzoic acid butyl ester
   n-Butyl-*p*-hydroxybenzoate [94-26-8]
   Butyl-4-hydroxybenzoate

5. **Empirical Formula**   **Molecular Weight**
   $C_{11}H_{14}O_3$ 194.23

6. **Structural Formula**

   HO —⟨ ⟩— COOCH$_2$(CH$_2$)$_2$CH$_3$

7. **Commercial Availability**

   USA

   Beta Chemical Corp.
   Inolex Chemical Co.
   Mallinckrodt, Inc.
   Napp Chemicals
   Nipa Laboratories, Inc.
   Protameen Chemicals, Inc.
   Tenneco Chemical, Inc.

   UK

   B.D.H. Chemicals, Ltd.
   Bofors (Great Britain) Co., Ltd.
   Bush Boake, Allen, Ltd.
   Nipa Laboratories, Ltd.

8. **Method of Manufacture**
   Butylparaben is prepared by esterification of *p*-hydroxy-benzoic acid with *n*-butanol.

9. **Description**
   White, crystalline, odorless powder.

SEM-MF-12
Excipient: Butylparaben

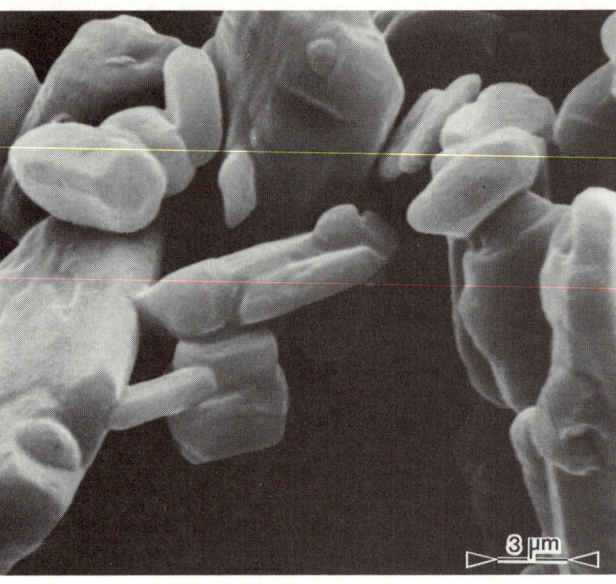

Magnification: 2400×

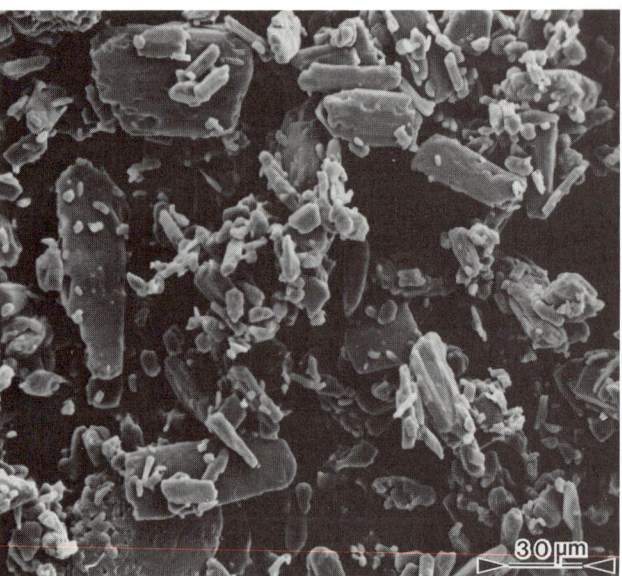

Magnification: 240×

10. Pharmacopeial Specifications

Test	NF	BP
Identification	+	+
Melting range	68–72°C	~69°C
Acidity	+	+
Loss on drying	≤0.5%	—
Residue on ignition	≤0.05%	—
Assay	99.0–100.5%	99.0–101.0%
Sulfated ash	—	≤0.1%

(USP reference standard available)

11. Typical Properties

Solubility: Almost insoluble in cold water (0.02% w/v at 25°C; 0.015% w/v at 80°C); readily soluble in ethanol (more than 50% w/v), propylene glycol (50% w/v), acetone, or diethyl ether; slightly soluble in natural fats, oils or glycerin.

Oil/Water Partition Coefficients: Mineral oil, 3.0; peanut oil, 280.0

Academy HPE Laboratory Project Data			
	Method	Lab #	Results
Solubility (water)	SOL-8	30	0.02%

12. Stability and Storage Conditions

Butylparaben should be stored in a well-closed container. Aqueous suspensions at pH 3-6 can be sterilized at 120°C for 20 minutes without decomposition. Aqueous suspensions at pH 3-6 are stable (less than 10% decomposition) for up to about four years at room temperature. Aqueous solutions at pH 8 or higher are subject to rapid hydrolysis (10% or more after approximately 60 days at room temperature).

13. Incompatibilities

The antimicrobial properties of Butylparaben are reduced in the presence of non-ionic surfactants. Adsorption to plastics is greater than that observed with methylparaben. Butylparaben is discolored in the presence of iron, and is subject to hydrolysis by weak alkalis and strong acids.

14. Safety

Butylparaben (5% in propylene glycol) when applied to the skin does not cause primary irritation. Butylparaben may elicit occasional skin sensitization, although repeated insult patch tests caused no allergic response in man. The acute and chronic oral toxicity of Butylparaben is low.

15. Handling Precautions

—

16. Regulatory Acceptance

NF XVI; BP/EP 1980

17. Applications in Pharmaceutical Formulations or Technology

Butylparaben (approximately 0.1%) alone, or in combination with other esters of *p*-hydroxybenzoic acid or with other antimicrobial agents, is used as a preservative in cosmetic and pharmaceutical preparations and in foods. As a rule, the preservative effect is increased in combination with other *p*-hydroxybenzoate esters.

18. Related Substances

Benzyl hydroxybenzoate BP (benzylparaben) is insoluble in water, but soluble in aqueous alkali hydroxides and ethanol. It is used as an antimicrobial preservative. Calcium salt of butylparaben is a crystalline powder which is 50 times more soluble than butylparaben. Ethylparaben. Methylparaben. Propylparaben

19. Comments

The following tabulation lists the minimal concentration (% in water) of butylparaben required to inhibit growth.

Aerobacter aerogenes ATCC 8308	0.04
Aspergillus niger ATCC 10254	0.02
Bacillus cereus var. mycoides ATCC 6462	0.0063
Bacillus subtilis ATCC 6633	0.0125
Candida albicans ATCC 10231	0.0125
Escherichia coli ATCC 9637	0.4
Penicillium digitatum ATCC 10030	0.0032
Rhizopus nigricans ATCC 6227A	0.0063
Saccharomyces cerevisiae ATCC 9763	0.0063
Staphylococcus aureus ATCC 6358P	0.0125

The effectiveness decreases with increasing pH due to the formation of phenolate anion.

20. Specific References

1. S. M. Blaug and D. E. Grant, Kinetics of degradation of parabens, *J. Soc. Cosmet. Chem.*, 25, 495 (1974).
2. J. Schimmel and M. N. Slotsky, Preservation of cosmetics. In: "Cosmetics, Science and Technology," Vol. III, 2nd Ed., M. S. Balsam and E. Sagarin, Eds., Wiley-Interscience, New York, 391-470 (1974).
3. H. Sokol, Recent developments in the preservation of pharmaceuticals, *Drug Standards*, 20:89 (1952).
4. C. Matthews *et al.*, *p*-Hydroxybenzoic acid esters as preservatives, *J. Am. Pharm. Assoc.*, 45:260 (1956).
5. *Ibid.*, p-Hydroxybenzoic acid esters as preservatives III, 45:268 (1956).
6. T. R. Aalto *et al.*, p-Hydroxybenzoic acid esters as Preservatives, *J. Am. Pharm. Assoc. Sci.*, 42:449 (1953).
7. K. Kakemi, H. Sezaki, E. Arakawa, K. Kimura and K. Ikeda, Interactions of parabens and other pharmaceutical adjuvants with plastic containers, *Chem. Pharm. Bull.*, 19:2523-2529 (1971).
8. E. L. Richardson, Preservatives: Frequency of use in cosmetic formulas as disclosed to FDA, *Cosmetic and Toiletries*, 92:85-88 (1977).

USA: M. Rieger*; P. Kotwal*; Z. Chowhan**
UK: M. C. Allwood*

Precipitated Calcium Carbonate

1. Nonproprietary Names

USP: Precipitated calcium carbonate
BP/EP: Calcium carbonate

2. Functional Category

USP: Tablet and/or capsule diluent

3. Synonyms

Precipitated chalk; precipitated carbonate of lime

4. Chemical Name and CAS Registry Number

Carbonic acid, calcium salt (1:1)
Calcium carbonate (1:1) [471-34-1]

5. Empirical Formula   Molecular Weight

$CaCO_3$ 100.09

6. Structural Formula

—

7. Commercial Availability

USA

Baker Chemical Co., J.T.
Beacon CMP Corp.
Chrystal Co., Charles B.
Gallard-Schlesinger Chemical Mfg. Corp.
Henley & Co.
KV Pharmaceutical-Desmo Chemical
Mallinckrodt, Inc.
McKesson Chemical Co.
Paulaur Corp.
Pfaltz & Bauer, Inc.
Ruger Chemical Co.
Thompson-Hayward Chemical Co.
Tri-K Industries, Inc.
Whittaker, Clark & Daniels, Inc.

UK

Allen and Sons (Chemicals), Ltd., Frederick
Chalk Products, Ltd.
Croxton and Garry, Ltd.
Hughes and Hughes, Ltd.
Johnson Matthey Chemicals, Ltd.
Luscombe, W. R.
Sturge, Ltd., John & E.
Tonra, Ltd.

8. Method of Manufacture

Prepared by double decomposition of calcium chloride and sodium carbonate in aqueous solution. Density and fineness are governed by the concentration of solutions, and heavy and light forms are available on the market.

9. Description

Fine, white, odorless, tasteless powder or crystals.

SEM:KY-3
Excipient: Precipitated calcium carbonate
Manufacturer: Whittaker, Clark & Daniels   **Lot No.:** 15A-3

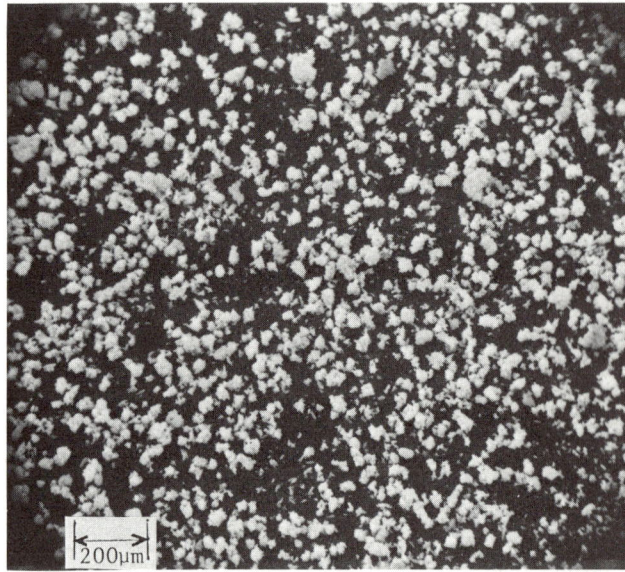

Magnification: 600× **Voltage:** 20 kV

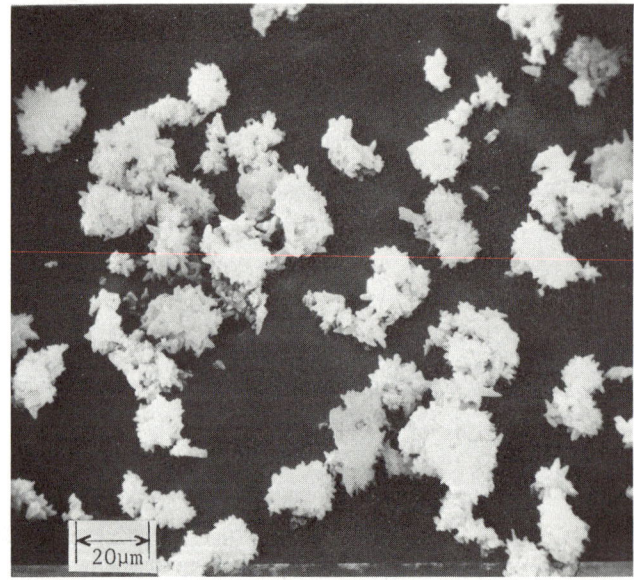

Magnification: 2,400× **Voltage:** 20 kV

SEM:KY-4
Excipient: Precipitated calcium carbonate
Manufacturer: Whittaker, Clark & Daniels   **Lot No.:** 15A-4

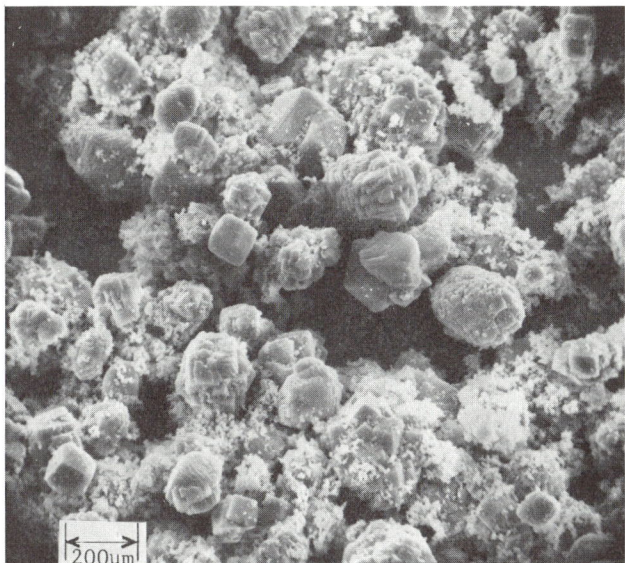

Magnification: 600×   **Voltage:** 20 kV

SEM:KY-5
Excipient: Precipitated calcium carbonate
Manufacturer: Whittaker, Clark & Daniels   **Lot No.:** 15A-2

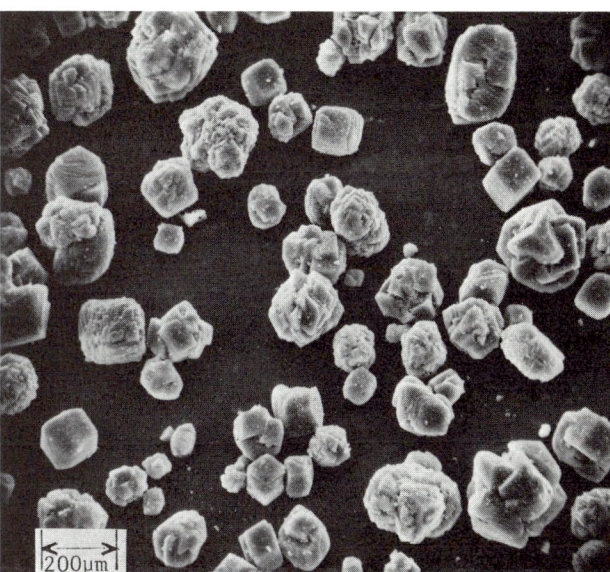

Magnification: 600×   **Voltage:** 20 kV

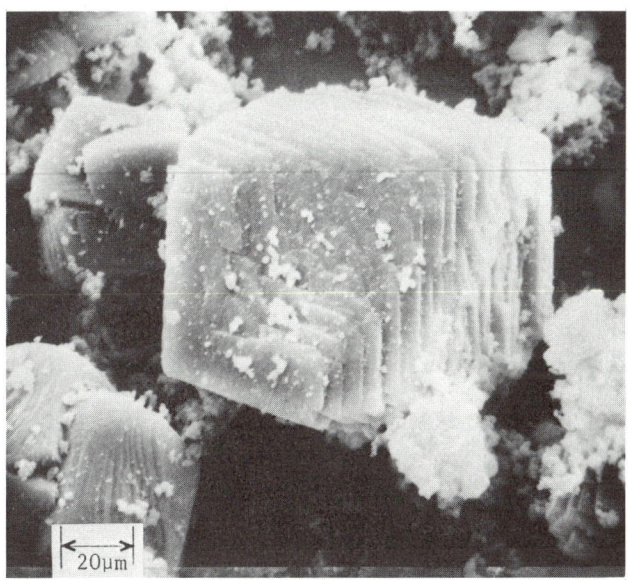

Magnification: 2,400× **Voltage:** 20 kV

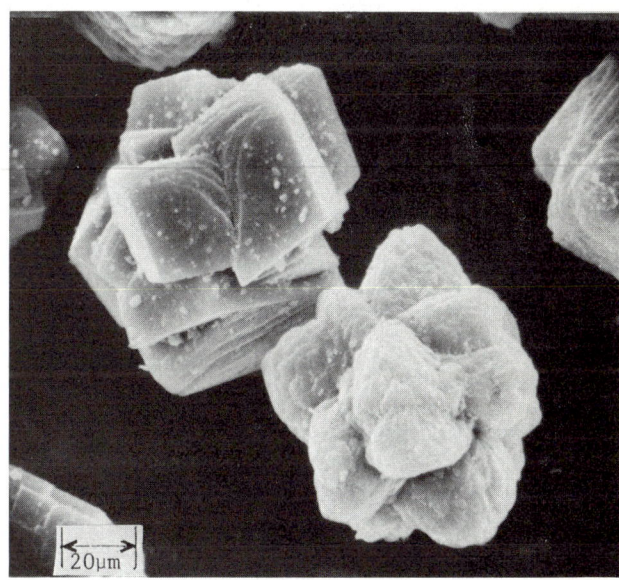

Magnification: 2,400× **Voltage:** 20 kV

10. Pharmacopeial Specifications

Test	USP	BP
Identification	+	+
Loss on drying	≤2.0%	≤2.0%
Acid-insoluble substances	≤0.2%	—
Substances insoluble in acetic acid	—	≤6 mg/3G
Fluoride	≤0.005%	—
Arsenic	≤3 ppm	≤4 ppm

Test	USP	BP
Barium	+	+
Lead	≤0.001%	—
Heavy metals	≤0.003%	≤20 ppm
Chloride	—	≤250 ppm
Sulfate	—	≤0.25%
Iron	—	≤200 ppm
Magnesium & alkali metals	≤1.0%	≤10 mg/G
Assay	98.0-100.5%	≥98.5%

11. Typical Properties

Academy HPE Laboratory Project Data

	Method	Lab #	Results
Bulk/tap density	BTD-8	36	B: 0.391 g/ml[a] T: 0.485 g/ml
Particle size dist.	PSD-5B	21	Less than 44µm-99.8%[a]
COM plot	COM-5,6	29	Fig. 29-COM-12[b]
COM plot	COM-4,5,6	20	Fig. 20-COM-11[b]
Compression	COM-7	12	Capping at 2,500 lbs.[b]
Compression	COM-7	12	Capping at 2,500 lbs.[b]
Compression	COM-7	12	No compacts formed[b]
Compression	COM-2	21	Compacts only at 52.7 MN/m²[c]

Suppliers: Chrystal[a]; Whittaker[b]; Clark & Daniels[c]

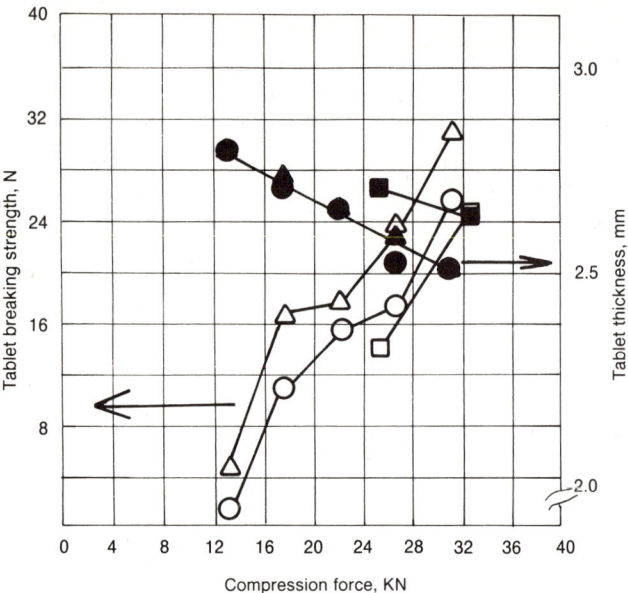

Calcium carbonate, precipated (Lot #64)

    ○ ● : Unlubricated, Carver Laboratory Press (COM-5)
    △ ▲ : Lubricated, Carver Laboratory Press (COM-6)
    □ ■ : Lubricated, Instrumented Stokes, Model F—
           Single punch press (COM-4)

Figure: 20-COM-11   **Method**: COM-4,5,6

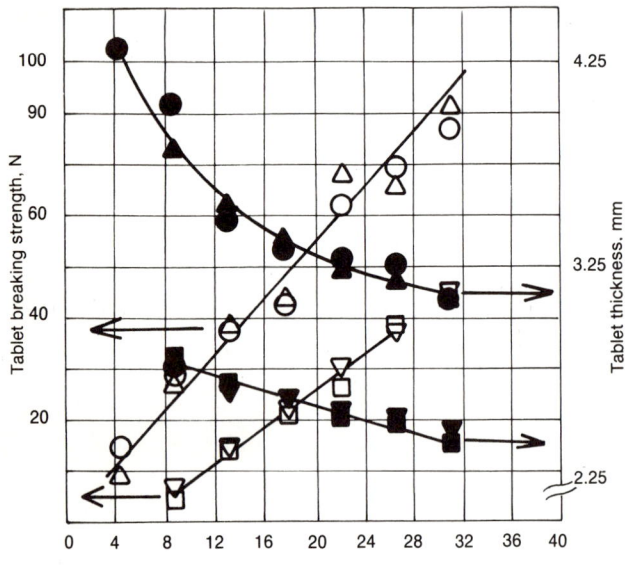

Calcium carbonate, precipated (Lot #300)

    ○ ● : Unlubricated, Carver Laboratory Press (COM-5)
    △ ▲ : Lubricated, Carver Laboratory Press (COM-6)

Calcium carbonate, precipated (Lot #2064)

    ○ ● : Unlubricated, Carver Laboratory Press (COM-5)
    △ ▲ : Lubricated, Carver Laboratory Press (COM-6)

Figure: 29-COM-12   **Method**: COM-5,6

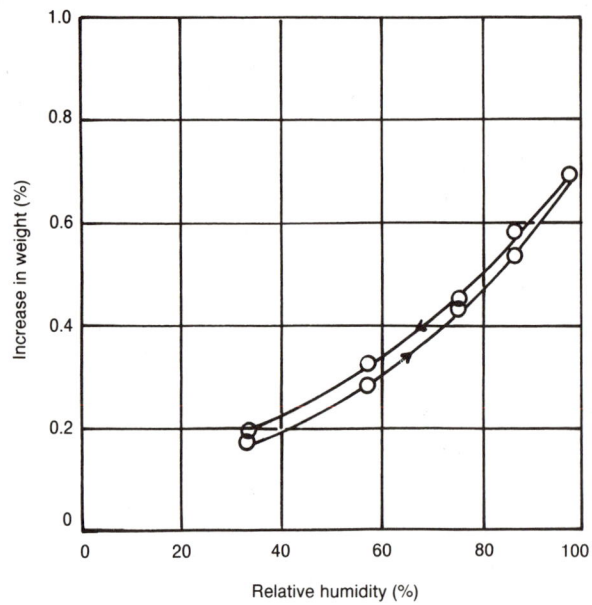

Figure: UK-SI-2 Precipitated calcium carbonate

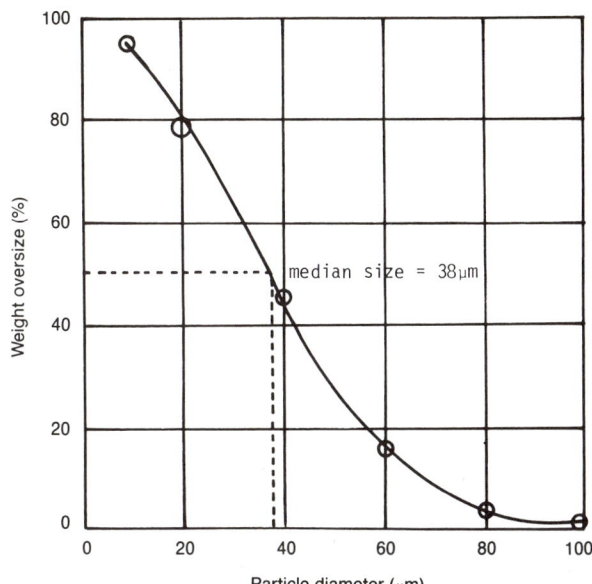

Figure: UK-PSD-2 Precipitated calcium carbonate

UK HPE Laboratory Project Data

Compression characteristics: Machine: Manesty E2; *Speed of compression:* 50 strokes per minute (since punches and die were lubricated after each compression cycle, tablet production was not continuous; however, the speed of entry of the punch into the die was similar to that of a continuously running machine).

Diameter: 12.5 mm
Weight range of tablets: 900 ± 10 mg
Tablet strength instrument: Schleuniger
Results:

Compressing Pressure MN−m²	Mean Crushing Strength (N)	Range (N)
60	< 9.8	—
104	< 9.8	—
152	< 9.8	—
182	17.7	9.8–27.5

Density: Particle: 2.32 g/cm³ (helium pycnometry); bulk: 0.76 g/cm³; tapped: 1.14 g/cm³ (1,250 taps)

Flowability: Cohesive
Melting Point: Non-fusible
Moisture Content: (a) 0.3% (Karl Fischer); (b) sorption isotherm (Fig. UK-SI-2)
Particle size distribution: Figure UK-PSD-2
Solubility: (a) Water: Less than 1 in 50,000; (b) Aqueous buffers (*Teorell* and *Stenhagen* citrate-phosphate-borate, pH 2-9 at 25°C and 60°C): pH 2 and pH 4: incompatible; pH 7 and pH 9: less than 1 in 50,000; (c) ethanol (100%): insoluble; (d) propan-2-ol: insoluble
Specific surface area: 1.81 m²/g (Micromeritics, Model 2205)

12. Stability and Storage Conditions

Stable in air. Preserve in a well-closed container. Precipitated calcium carbonate absorbs less than 1% moisture at 25°C at relative humidities up to 90%.

13. Incompatibilities

Acids; alum; ammonium salts

14. Safety

Excess use can result in hypercalcemia, renal impairment, constipation and stimulation of gastric secretion.

15. Handling Precautions

None

16. Compendial/Regulatory Status

USP XXI; BP/EP 1980

17. Applications in Pharmaceutical Formulation or Technology

Diluent in solid dosage forms
Basis for medicated dental preparations

18. Related Substances

None

19. Comments

None

20. Specific References

None

USA: R. Egidy*; J. L. Czeisler*; J. W. Boenigk**
UK: N. A. Armstrong*

Dibasic Calcium Phosphate

1. Nonproprietary Names

USP: Dibasic calcium phosphate, anhydrous
          Dibasic calcium phosphate, dihydrate
BP/EP: Calcium hydrogen phosphate, dihydrate
          Dibasic calcium phosphate, dihydrate

2. Functional Category

USP: Tablet and/or capsule diluent
Others: Direct compression excipient

3. Synonyms

Calcium hydrogen orthophosphate; dicalcium orthophosphate; secondary calcium phosphate; *Ditab*; *EmcomPress*

4. Chemical Names and CAS Registry Number

Phosphoric acid, calcium salt (1:1)
Dibasic calcium phosphate, anhydrous [7757-93-9]
Dibasic calcium phosphate, dihydrate [7789-77-7]

5. Empirical Formula

	Molecular Weight
Anhydrous: $CaHPO_4$	136.06
Dihydrate: $CaHPO_4 \cdot 2H_2O$	172.09

6. Structural Formula

—

7. Commercial Availability

USA

Baker Chemical Co., J.T.
Browning Chemical Corp.
Gallard-Schlesinger Chemical Mfg. Corp.
Mallinckrodt, Inc.
McKesson Chemical Co.
Mendell Co., Edward
Monsanto Co.
Pfaltz & Bauer, Inc.
Ruger Chemical Co.
Stauffer Chemical Co.
Thompson-Hayward Chemical Co.

UK

Albright and Wilson, Ltd.
Charles Page and Co.
K&K Greeff Chemicals, Ltd.
Steetley Chemicals, Ltd.

8. Method of Manufacture

A phosphate mineral such as apatite is dissolved in sulfuric acid and filtered. The addition of calcium hydroxide precipitates dibasic calcium phosphate. The substance has also been prepared from calcined animal bones.

9. Description

A white, odorless, tasteless powder or crystalline solid.

SEM: KY-1
Excipient: Calcium phosphate dibasic dihydrate (*EmcomPress*)
Manufacturer: Mendell   **Lot no.** 16A-3 (B-392X)

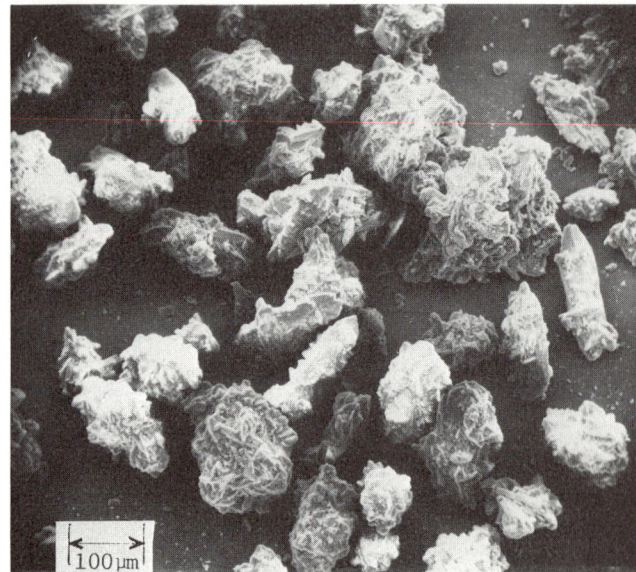

Magnification: 120×   **Voltage:** 20 kV

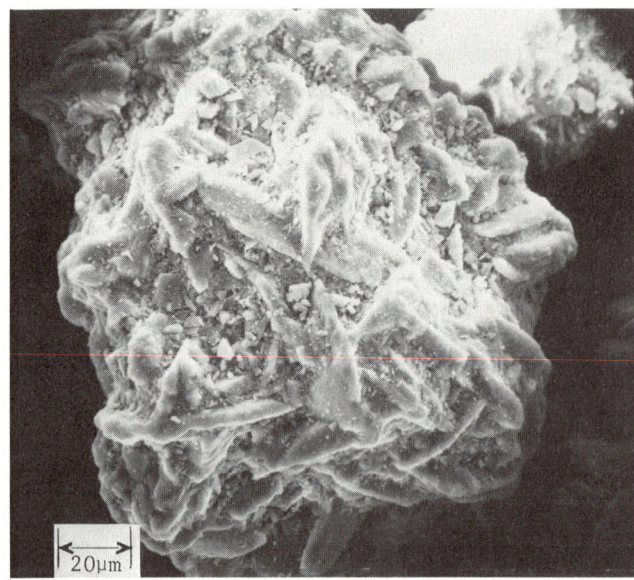

Magnification: 600×   **Voltage:** 20 kV

SEM: KY-2
Excipient: Calcium phosphate dibasic dihydrate
Manufacturer: Stauffer   **Lot no.** 16A-1 (89)

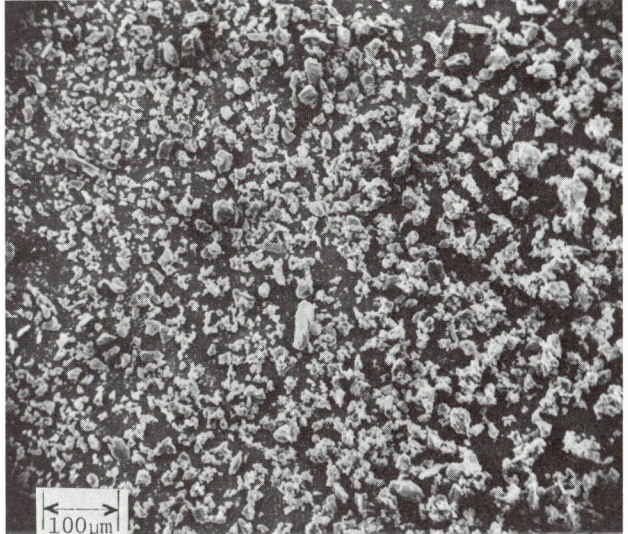

Magnification: 120× **Voltage:** 20 kV

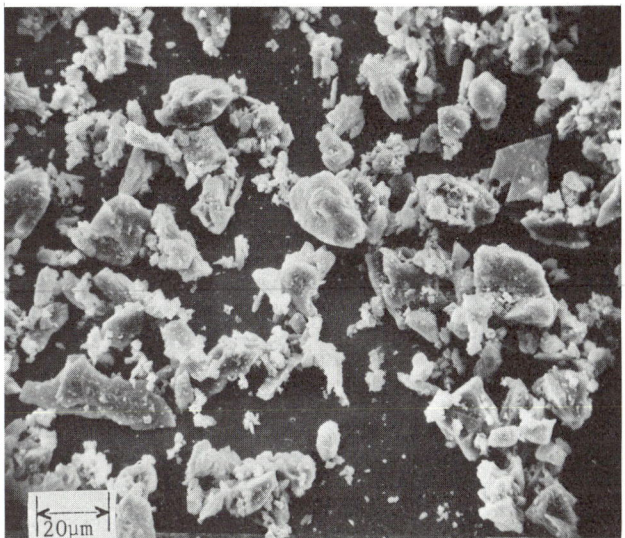

Magnification: 600× **Voltage:** 20 kV

10. Pharmacopeial Specifications

	Dihydrate USP	Dihydrate BP/EP
Identification	+	+
Loss on ignition	24.5-26.5%	—
Acid-insoluble substances	≤0.2%	—
Carbonate	+	+
Chloride	≤0.25%	≤330 ppm
Fluoride	≤0.005%	≤100 ppm
Sulfate	≤0.5%	≤0.5%
Arsenic	≤3 ppm	≤10 ppm
Barium	+	+
Heavy metals	0.003%	≤40 ppm
Iron	—	≤400 ppm
Monocalcium & tricalcium phos.	—	+
Assay	30.0-31.7% of Ca++	98.0-105.0% of CaHPO$_4$.2H$_2$0

11. Typical Properties

Solubility: Very slightly soluble in water. Soluble in dilute hydrochloric and nitric acids. Slightly soluble in dilute acetic acid.

Melting point: Anhydrous: Decomposes at red heat. Dihydrate: Decomposes at <100°C (loss of water).

Absolute density: Dihydrate: 2.35 g/cm^3

Tapped density: Anhydrous: 0.85 g/cm^3; Dihydrate (milled): 0.95 g/cm^3; Dihydrate (unmilled): 1.14 g/cm^3; *Emcompress:* 0.783-0.838 g/cm^3.

pH (20% slurry): 7.4

Particle size distribution: Anhydrous: Residue on 200 USS - 0.03%; Residue on 325 USS - 0.3%. Dihydrate (milled): Residue on 200 USS - 0.01%; Residue on 325 USS - 0.3%. Dihydrate (unmilled): Residue on 60 USS - 20.0%; Residue on 200 USS - 50.0%. *EmcomPress:* Residue on 250 USS - 95.0%.

Academy HPE Laboratory Project Data (Anhydrous)

	Method	Lab #	Results
Density	DE-1	31	2.873 g/cm^3[a]
Moisture content	MC-28	18	0.142%[b]
Moisture content	MC-12	18	0.149%[b]
Moisture content	MC-23	21	0.187%[a]
Moisture content	MC-20	14	0.100%[b]
Bulk/tap density	BTD-8	36	B:0.971 g/cm^3[a] T:0.71 g/cm^3[a]
Particle size dist.	PSD-7	24	9.4μm[a]
EMC plot	EMC-1	2	Fig:2-EMC-1[b]
SI plot	SI-1	13	Fig:13-SI-1[a]
COM plot	COM-2	21	Fig:21-COM-26[a]

Suppliers: Van Waters[a]; Monsanto Co.[b]

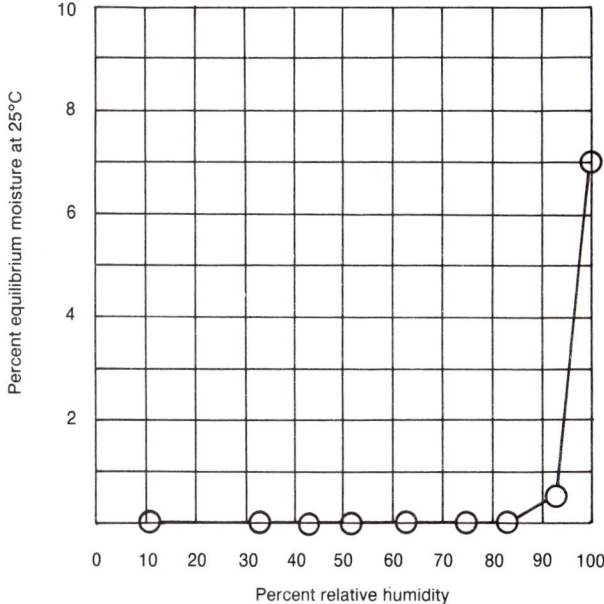

Dicalcium phosphate anhydrous, USP.

Figure: 2-EMC-1   **Method:** EMC-1 (Monsanto, Lot #RNB 476S)

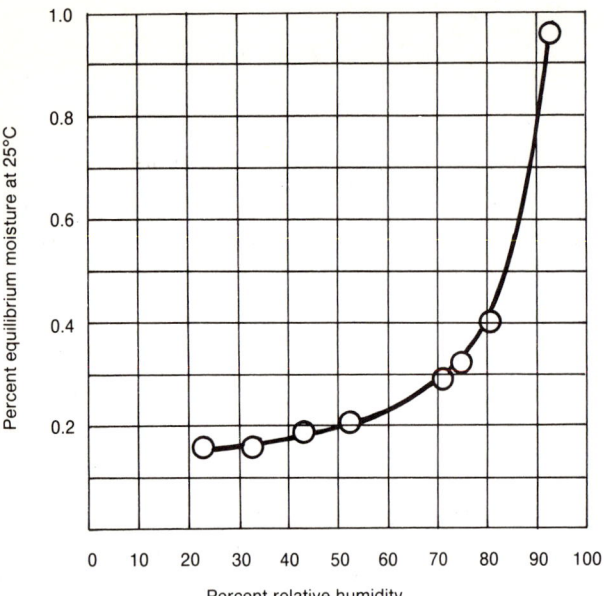

Dicalcium phosphate anhydrous.
Figure: 13-SI-1   **Method:** SI-1 (Van Waters, Lot #DK9)

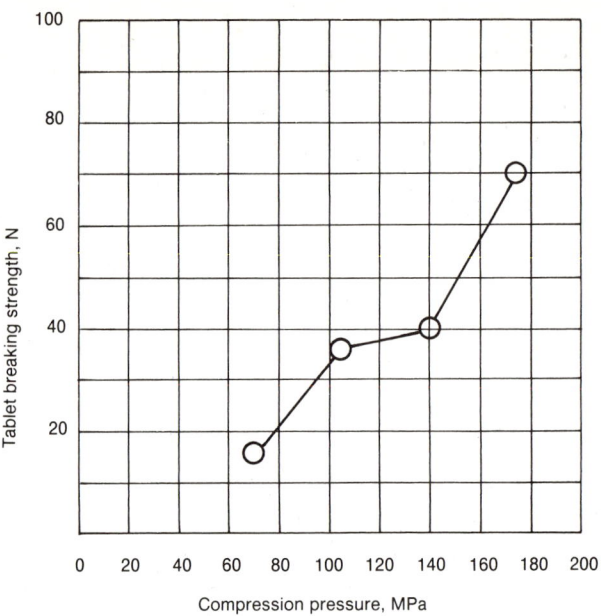

Calcium phosphate, dibasic, anhydrous
Tablet weight: 750 mg
Figure: 21-COM-26   **Method:** COM-2 (Van Waters & Rogers, Canada, Lot #DK9)

Academy HPE Laboratory Project Data (Dihydrate)

	Method	Lab #	Results
Density	DE-1	31	2.597 g/cm[3c]
Density	DE-1	31	2.305 g/cm[3a]
Moisture content	MC-20	10	1.1%[b]
Moisture content	MC-20	10	8.0%[c]
Moisture content	MC-25	15	20.36%[b]
Bulk/tap density	BTD-8	36	B:0.815 g/cm[3a]
			T:0.904 g/cm[3a]
Bulk/tap density	BTD-8	36	B:0.565 g/cm[3b]
			T:0.772 g/cm[3b]
Bulk/tap density	BTD-6	8	% consolidation[c]
			9.5% volume
			10.0% weight
Particle size dist.	PSD-7	24	4.2 μm[c]
Particle size dist.	PSD-5B	21	100% $\leq$44 μm[c]
Particle size dist.	PSD-5A	21	3% <44 μm[a]
Particle size dist.	PSD-5A	21	4% from 44-74 μm[a]
Particle size dist.	PSD-5A	21	47% from 74-149 μm[a]
Particle size dist.	PSD-5A	21	26% from 149-177 μm[a]
Particle size dist.	PSD-5A	21	18% from 177-250 μm[a]
Particle size dist.	PSD-5A	21	2% from 250-420 μm[a]
PSD plot	PSD-5A	21	Fig:21-PSD-1[a]
Average flow rate	FLO-3	24	No flow[c]
Average flow rate	FLO-3	24	6.0392 g/sec[a]
Friability index	PE-1	36	0.019[a]
EMC (unmilled)	EMC-1	2	Fig:10-EMC-1[c]
EMC (milled)	EMC-1	10	Fig:10-EMC-1[b]
Sorption isotherm	SI-1	13	Fig:13-SI-2[c]
Sorption isotherm	SI-1	13	Fig:13-SI-2[a]
Compression plot	COM-4,5,6	29	Fig:29-COM-13[a]
Compression plot	COM-All	20	No compression[c]

Suppliers: Edward Mendell Co.[a]; Monsanto Co.[b]; Stauffer Chemical Co.[c]

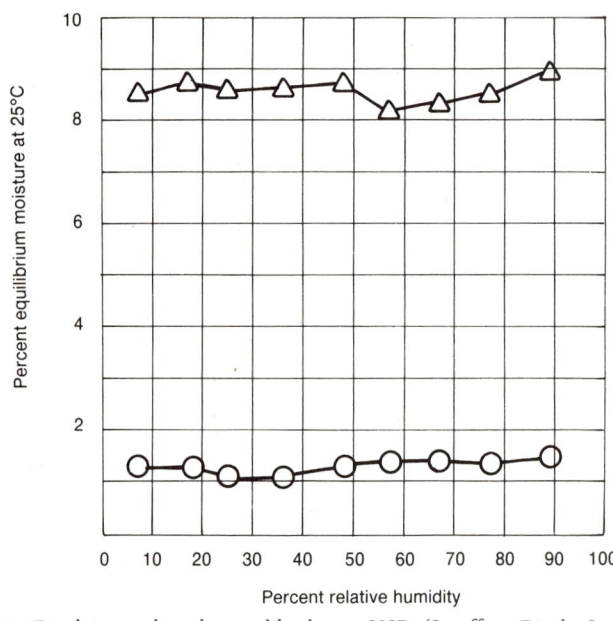

O: Dicalcium phosphate, dihydrate, USP (Stauffer, *Ditab*, Lot #16)
△: Dicalcium phosphate, dihydrate, USP (Monsanto, 250 grade, Lot #05587)
Figure: 10-EMC-1   **Method:** EMC-1

12. Stability and Storage Conditions

Relatively stable. Store in a well-closed container in a cool, dry place.

13. Incompatibilities

Acids; may interfere with the absorption of tetracyclines.

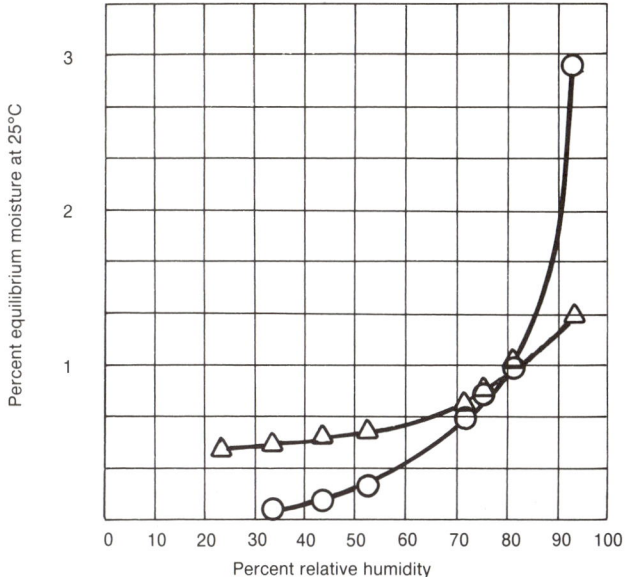

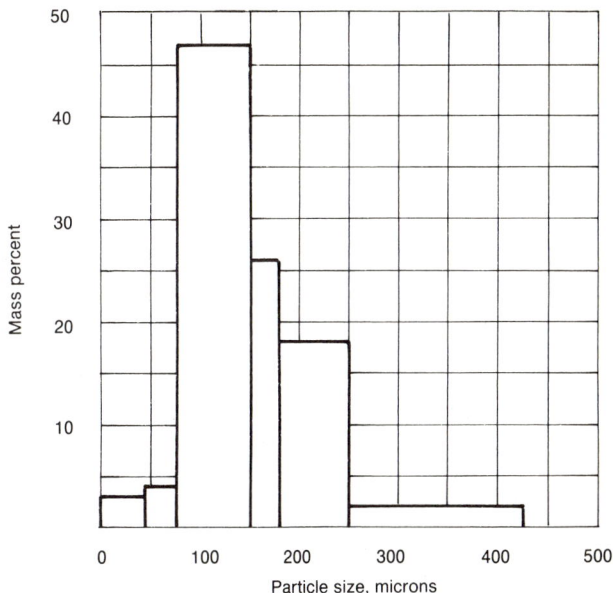

O :Calcium phosphate, dihydrate (Stauffer, Lot #89)
△ :Calcium phosphate, dihydrate, *EmcomPress* (Mendell, Lot #B-392X)
Figure: 13-SI-2   **Method:** SI-1

Calcium phosphate, dibasic, (Mendell, Lot # B-392X)
Figure: 21-PSD-1   **Method:** PSD-5A

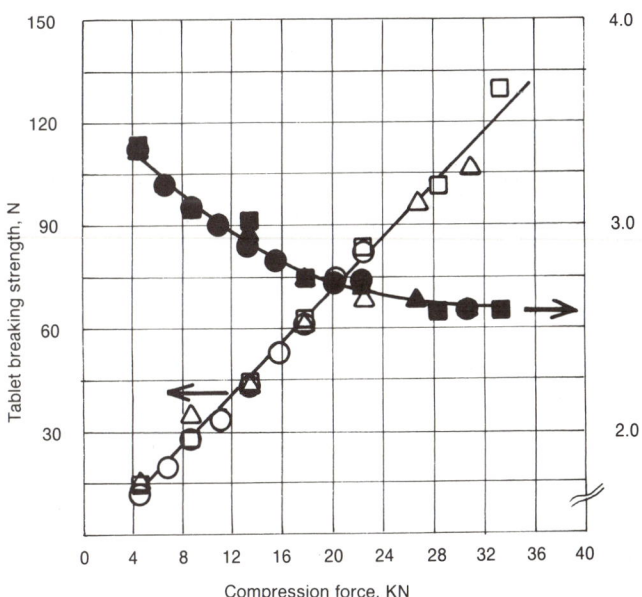

Dibasic Calcium Phosphate, *EmcomPress* (Mendell, Lot #B-392X)
O ● : Unlubricated, carver laboratory press (COM-5)
△ ▲ :Lubricated, carver laboratory press (COM-6)
□ ■ : Lubricated, instrumented stokes model f — single punch press (COM-4)
Figure: 29-COM-13   **Method:** COM-4, 5, 6

14. Safety

No cases of industrial illness have been documented due to exposure. Ingestion of large quantities may result in symptoms of gastro-intestinal irritation. Inhalation of high airborne concentrations may result in non-specific irritation of the upper respiratory tract. Contact with the eyes, mucous membranes or prolonged skin contact with strong aqueous slurries may result in local irritation.

15. Handling Precautions

Avoid ingestion, inhalation and contact with skin and mucous membranes.

16. Regulatory Acceptance

USP XVI; BP/EP 1980.

17. Applications in Pharmaceutical Formulation and Technology

Diluent for capsules and tablets. Adsorbent and thickening agent in creams and ointments. *EmcomPress* for direct compression formulations.

18. Related Substances

Monocalcium phosphate; tricalcium phosphate

19. Comments

Note: Stauffer Chemical Company's brand (*Ditab*) of unmilled dicalcium phosphate claims a maximum limit of 3 ppm of arsenic in their product.

20. Specific References

1. S. T. Horhota, J. Burgio, L. Loski and C. T. Rhodes, Effect of storage at specified temperature and humidity on properties of three directly compressible tablet formulations, *J. Pharm. Sci.*, 65 (12): 1746-1749 (1976).
2. M. H. Rubinstein and D. M. Bodey, Disaggregation of compressed tablets, *J. Pharm. Sci.*, 65 (12): 1749-1753 (1976).
3. Z. T. Chowhan, The effect of low and high humidity aging on hardness, disintegration time and dissolution rate of dibasic calcium phosphate - based tablets, *J. Pharm. Pharmacol.*, 32: 10-14 (1979).

USA: S. Weinstein*; P. Chemburkar*; J. W. Boenigk**
UK: K. A. Khan*; J. I. Wells*

Tribasic Calcium Phosphate

1. Nonproprietary Names
NF: Tribasic calcium phosphate
BP: Calcium phosphate

2. Functional Category
NF: Tablet and/or capsule diluent
BP: Pharmaceutical aid
Others: Filler for tablets and capsules; anti-caking agent.

3. Synonyms
Tricalcium orthophosphate; tertiary calcium phosphate; calcigenol simple; calcium orthophosphate; precipitated calcium phosphate; TCP

4. Chemical Name and CAS Registry Number
Calcium hydroxide phosphate [12167-74-7]

5. Empirical Formula   Molecular Weight
$Ca_5(OH)(PO_4)_3$ 502.32
$Ca_3(PO_4)_2Ca(OH)_2$

6. Structural Formula
—

7. Commercial Availability
USA
Baker Chemical Co., J.T.
Browning Chemical Corp.
Gallard-Schlesinger Chemical Mfg. Corp.
Mallinckrodt, Inc.
McKesson Chemical Co.
Mendell Co., Edward
Monsanto Co.
Pfaltz & Bauer, Inc.
Ruger Chemical Co.
Stauffer Chemical Co.
Thompson-Hayward Chemical Co.

UK
Albright & Wilson Ltd.
Charles Page and Co.

8. Method of Manufacture
Naturally occurring as minerals oxydapatit, voclicherite and whitlockite. Commercially prepared by treating phosphate-containing rock with sulfuric acid, then precipitated by addition of calcium hydroxide. Also obtained from calcined animal bones.

9. Description
A white, odorless, tasteless powder, stable in air.

10. Pharmacopeial Specifications

Test	NF	BP
Identification	+	+
Loss on ignition	≤8.0%	—
Water	—	≤2.5%
Water-soluble substances	≤0.5%	—
Chloride	≤0.14%	≤0.35%
Carbonate	+	+
Fluoride	≤0.0075%	≤50 ppm
Nitrate	+	—
Sulfate	≤0.8%	≤0.6%
Arsenic	≤3 ppm	≤4 ppm
Barium	+	—
Iron	—	≤400 ppm
Heavy metals	≤0.003%	≤30 ppm
Dibasic salt & Ca oxide	+	—
Acid-insoluble substances	≤0.2%	≤0.3%
Assay range	34.0-40.0% Ca^{++}	≥90.0% $Ca_3(PO_4)_2$

11. Typical Properties
Density: 3.14 g/cm^3
Bulk density: 0.32 g/cm^3
Melting point: 1670°C
Solubility: Soluble in dilute mineral acids; very slightly soluble in water; insoluble in alcohol.
Hygroscopicity: At relative humidities between about 15-65%, the equilibrium moisture content is about 2.0%, but at relative humidities above about 75%, tribasic calcium phosphate absorbs small amounts of moisture.

12. Stability and Storage Conditions
Store in a well-closed container. It is a stable compound, easily stored without caking problems.

13. Incompatibilities
Influences absorption of vitamin D. May form sparingly soluble phosphates with hormones. Forms calcium complex with tetracycline.

14. Safety
No documented cases of industrial illness from exposure have been observed. Ingestion or inhalation of excessive quantities may result in deposition of tricalcium phosphate crystals in the tissues. These crystals may lead to inflammation and cause tissue lesions in the areas of deposition.
Ingestion of large quantities may cause symptoms of gastrointestinal irritation, nausea, vomiting, cramps and diarrhea. Local irritation may result from eye contact with the solid material. Inhalation of high airborne concentrations of the dust may result in nonspecific irritation of the upper respiratory tract.

15. Handling Precautions
No restrictions specified.

16. Regulatory Acceptance
NF XVI; BP 1980

17. Applications in Pharmaceutical Formulation or Technology
Capsule diluent/filler
Tablet diluent/filler
Flow and non-caking agent

18. Related Substances
Dibasic calcium phosphate

19. Comments
Tricalcium phosphate provides a higher calcium load than dibasic calcium phosphate.

20. Specific References

1. A. M. Molokhia, M. A. Moustafa and M. W. Gouda, Effect of storage conditions on the hardness, disintegration and drug release from some tablet bases, *Drug Development And Industrial Pharmacy*, 8:(2), 283-292 (1982).

2. Z. T. Chowhan and A. A. Amaro, The effect of low and high humidity aging on the hardness, disintegration time and dissolution rate of tribasic calcium phosphate-based tablets, *Drug Development and Industrial Pharmacy*, 5:(6), 545-562 (1979).

USA: S. Weinstein*; A. Martino**; J. W. Boenigk**; J. Cooper**
UK: K. A. Khan*; J. Wells*

Calcium Stearate

1. Nonproprietary Name
NF: Calcium stearate

2. Functional Categories
USP: Tablet and capsule lubricant
Others: Stabilizing agent, suspending agent, viscosity controller, milling aid, emulsifier

3. Synonyms
Octadecanoic acid calcium salt; stearic acid calcium salt

4. Chemical Names and CAS Registry Number
Octadecanoic acid calcium salt
Calcium stearate [1592-23-0]

5. Empirical Formula   Molecular Weight
$C_{36}H_{70}CaO_4$ 607.00

6. Structural Formula
$[CH_3(CH_2)_{16}COO]_2Ca$

7. Commercial Availability
USA
Alba Chemical, Inc.
Browning Chemical Corp.
Conray Chemicals, Inc.
Emery Industries, Chemical Specialties Group
Fanning Corp., The
Goldschmidt Chemical Corp.
Harshaw Chemical Co.
Henkel KGaA
Ingredients International, Inc.
Inolex Chemical Co.
Mallinckrodt, Inc.
McKesson Chemical Co.
Personal Care Products Group, Emery Industries, Inc.
Pfaltz and Bauer, Inc.
Quad Chemical - Lonza Specialty Chemicals
Ruger Chemical Co.
SITCO (Shah International Trading Corp.)
Stepan Chemical Co.-Specialty Chemicals Dept.
Stoney-Mueller, Inc.
Tenneco Chemicals, Inc.
Thompson-Hayward Chemical Co.
Union Camp Corp., Terpene & Aromatics Div.
Van Dyk & Co.
Whittaker, Clark & Daniels, Inc.
Witco Chemical Corp., Organics Div.-NY

UK
Durham Chemicals Ltd.
Witco Chemical Ltd.

8. Method of Manufacture
Calcium stearate may be prepared by the reaction of calcium chloride and the sodium salts of the mixed fatty acids (stearic and palmitic). The calcium stearate is collected and washed with water to remove the sodium chloride.

9. Description
A fine, white to yellowish white, bulky powder having a slight, characteristic odor. It is unctuous and free from grittiness. It contains the equivalent of ≥ 9.0 and $\leq 10.5\%$ CaO (calcium oxide).

UK SEM: Calcium Stearate, Standard
Manufacturer: Durham Ltd. **Lot No.:** 0364

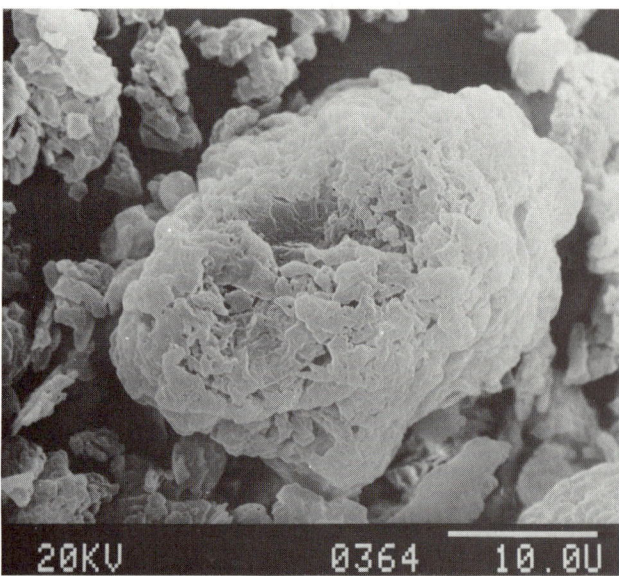

Calcium Stearate, Precipitated
Manufacturer: Witco Chemicals Ltd. **Lot No.:** 0438

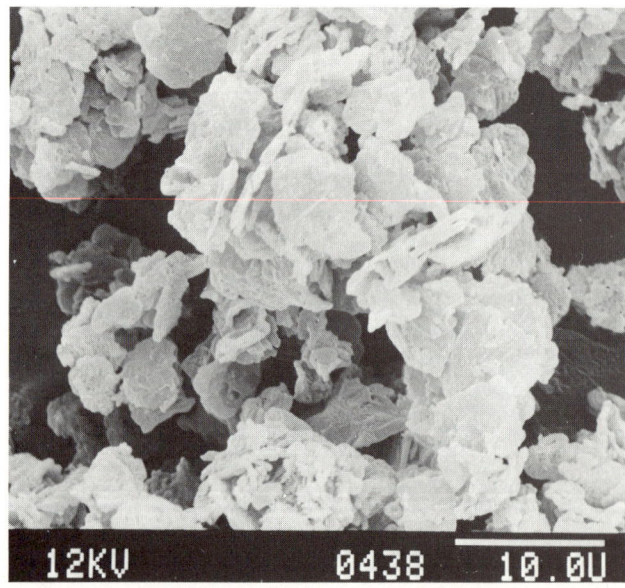

UK SEM: Witco "EA"
Manufacturer: Witco Chemicals, Ltd.

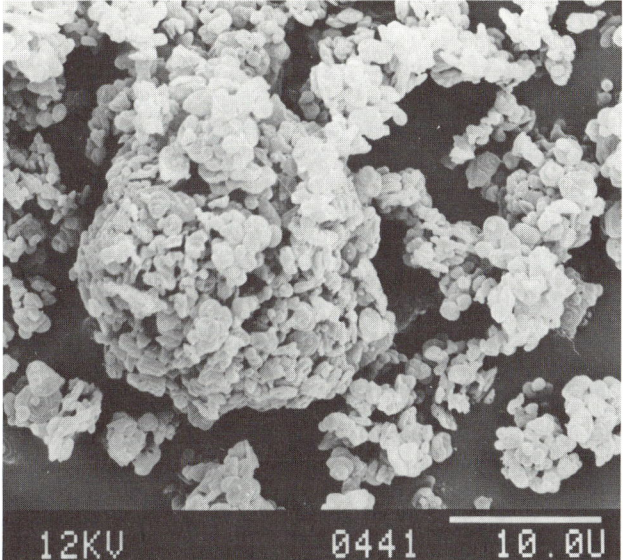

US: SEM:KY-7 Calcium Stearate, NF
Manufacturer: Mallinckrodt **Lot No.**: JMP

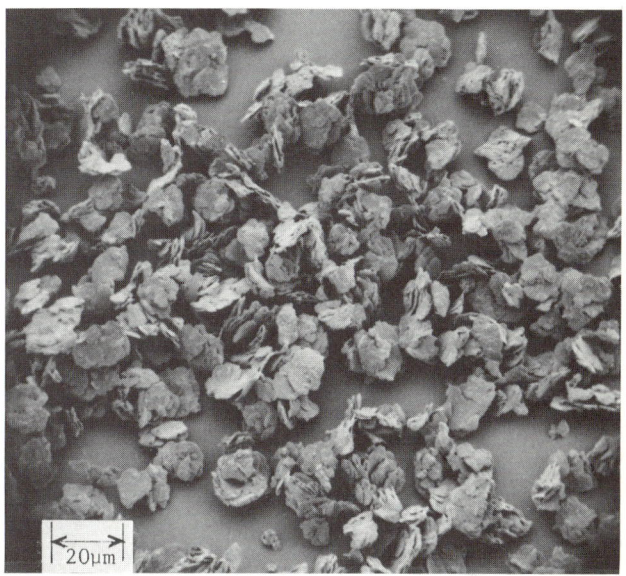

Magnification: 600× **Voltage**: 5 kV

UK SEM: Witco "Fused"
Manufacturer: Witco Chemicals, Ltd.

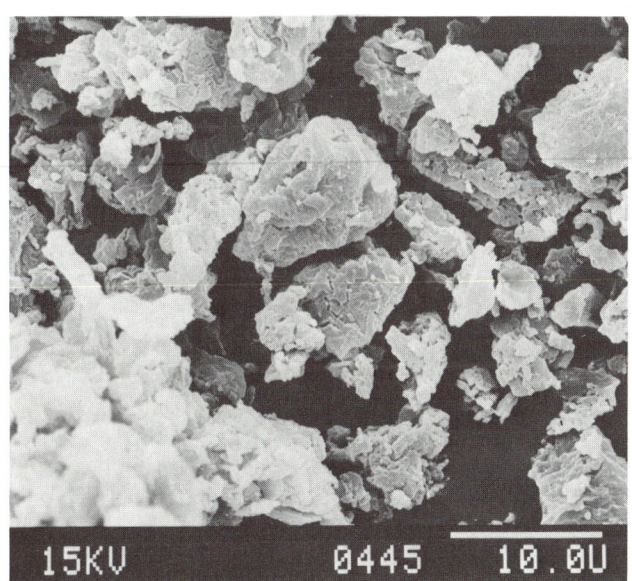

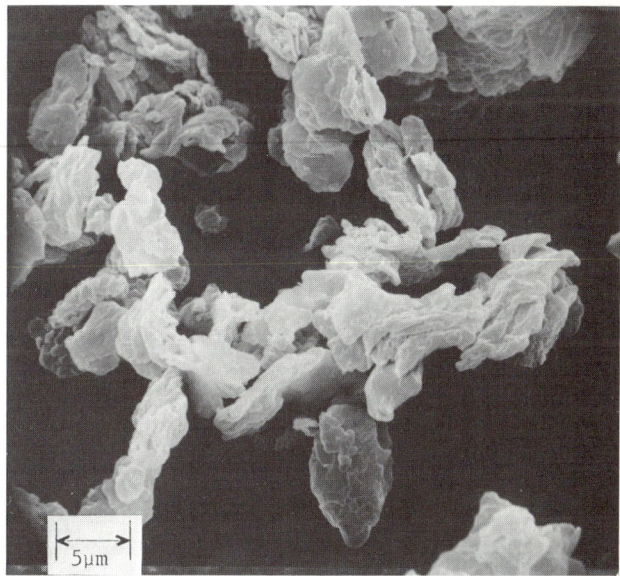

Magnification: 2400× **Voltage**: 5kV

10. Pharmacopeial Specifications

Test	NF
Identification	+
Loss on drying	≤4%
Arsenic content	≤3 ppm
Heavy metals	≤0.001%
Assay	9.0-10.5% CaO

11. Typical Properties

Academy HPE Laboratory Project Data

	Method	Lab #	Results
Moisture content	MC-23	21	2.96%[a]
Moisture content	MC-12	18	2.97%[b]
Compression	COM-7	12	Capping at 250 lb.[b]
Compression	COM-1	21	No compacts formed at 15.5-19.0 N/cm^2 [a]

Suppliers: [a]Witco, [b]Mallinckrodt

Solubility: Insoluble in water, lower alcohols, ether, ketones and other common solvents.
Ash: 9.9% - 10.3%
Water-soluble salts: 0.1%
Free fatty acid: 0.3 - 0.5%
Moisture: 2.5%
Softening point, °C: 160
Density, lbs/ft^3.: 7
Apparent Density, lbs/ft^3.: 26
Fineness through 200 mesh: 100% (99.5% through a 325 mesh screen)
Shear strength, kg/cm^2: 15.0
Typical value of lubrication: (using 2% of the lubricant): R = 0.94
Specific gravity: 1.035
Bulk, cc/10 g: 100/90
Melting point: 149° - 155°C
Particle size distribution (Coulter counter): 1.7-60μm
Polymorphism: No evidence by X-ray diffraction
Equilibrium moisture content: 3.06 - 3.47%
Specific surface area: 5.76 - 7.44 m^2
Flowability (Carr compressibility index): 21.2 - 22.6%
Compressibility: No compacts formed up to 90 N/cm^2
Friability: Not applicable
Acidity or alkalinity: pH 7.82 - 9.62
Chloride: <200 ppm
Sulfate: <0.25%
Acid value of fatty acid: 191-203

Bulk and Tapped Density

	Bulk Density g/cm^3	Tapped Density g/cm^3
Durham "Standard"	0.38	0.48
Witco "Precipitated"	0.16	0.20
Witco "EA"	0.21	0.27
Witco "Fused"	0.38	0.48

12. Stability and Storage

Preserve in a well-closed container.

13. Incompatibilities

—

14. Safety

Except for gastric irritation caused in part by osmotic disturbances, calcium *per se* has no significant oral toxicity.

15. Handling Precautions

No shipping regulations. Freight classification: Calcium stearate is classified as a metallic soap of fatty acid.

16. Regulatory Acceptance

NF XVI. FDA status: Calcium stearate is suitable for use in numerous indirect food-contact applications. Generally recognized as safe.

17. Applications in Pharmaceutical Formulation or Technology

Use	Concentration
Tablet lubricant	1% or less

18. Related Substance

Magnesium stearate

19. Comments

Calcium stearate has excellent lubricant properties, poor glidant properties and good anti-adherent properties. There have been relatively few articles concerning calcium stearate. It appears that the most recent investigations use magnesium stearate as a lubricating agent.

20. Specific References

1. Manufacturer's Literature: Mathe Division, The Norac Co. Inc., Lodi, N.J.
2. G. Busch and F. Neuwatt, metallic soaps as water-in-oil emulsifiers. I. communication, *J. Soc. Cosmetic Chemists,* 24:763-769 (1973).

USA: L. V. Allen*; J. W. Boenigk**
UK: J. A. Stead*

Calcium Sulfate

1. Nonproprietary Names

NF: Calcium sulfate, calcium sulfate dihydrate
BP: Dried calcium sulphate

2. Functional Category

NF: Tablet and/or capsule diluent; dessicant

3. Synonyms

Gypsum, alabaster, terra alba, satinite, satin spar, light spar, mineral white, native calcium sulfate, precipitated calcium sulfate
BP: Exsiccated calcium sulfate; plaster of paris

4. Chemical Names and CAS Registry Numbers

Calcium sulfate [7778-18-9]
Calcium sulfate dihydrate [10101-41-4]
Calcium sulfate hemihydrate [26499-65-0]

5. Empirical Formulae — Molecular Weights

Empirical Formulae	Molecular Weights
$CaSO_4$	136.14
$CaSO_4 \cdot 2H_2O$	172.17
$CaSO_4 \cdot \frac{1}{2} H_2O$	145.14

6. Structural Formulae

$CaSO_4$
$CaSO_4 \cdot 2H_2O$

7. Commercial Availability

USA

Calcium Carbonate Company
Hammil & Gillespie, Inc.
Jonas Chemical Corporation
Mallinckrodt, Inc.
Miles Laboratories, Inc.
U.S. Gypsum Company
Whittaker Clark & Daniels, Inc.
Woodward & Dickerson, Inc.

UK

British Gypsum
Frederick Allen & Sons, Ltd

8. Method of Manufacture

A powder containing about 95% by weight of calcium sulfate and 5% of water is made by carefully heating a purer variety of native gypsum until about three-fourths of the water has been expelled. A purer variety of calcium sulfate may also be made by reacting calcium carbonate with sulfuric acid.

9. Description

White to yellowish-white powder, odorless and tasteless.

10. Pharmacopeial Specifications

Test	NF	BP
Identification	+	+
Loss on drying	Anhydrous, ≤1.5%	—
	Dihydrate, 19.0-23.0%	—
Iron	≤0.01%	—
Heavy metals	≤0.001%	—
Assay range	98.0-101.0%	
Loss on ignition	—	4.5-8.0%
Acidity or alkalinity (pH of 20% slurry)	—	6.0-7.6
Setting properties	—	+

11. Typical Properties

(Dihydrate)
Density (KPH* Method): Bulk: 0.645 g/cm³; tapped: 1.250 g/cm³
Particle density (Pycnometry): 2.32 g/cm³
Moisture content: 19.8% (By Karl Fischer)
Polymorphic forms (X-ray diffraction): None found
Particle size distribution (Alpine air jet above 100 μm and Coulter Counter below 100 μm): Range: 0.100 μm - 2.5 μm
Specific surface area (Strohlein apparatus): 3154 cm²/g
Flowability (Carr Index): 48.4%
*Katalog Pharmazeutische Hilfsstoffe, Basel 1974

Academy HPE Laboratory Project Data		
Method	Lab #	Results
MC-27	18	2.085[a]
MC-24	21	19.80[c]
MC-23	21	18.86[c]
PSD-4	17[a]	

US sieve #	Particle Size (S, μm)	Weight % ± SD	
	S 1000	4.62 ±	2.18
18	590 S 1000	3.34 ±	1.51
30	297 S 590	2.57 ±	0.66
50	210 S 297	3.05 ±	0.62
70	149 S 210	3.22 ±	0.33
100	74 S 149	11.50 ±	0.33
200	S 74	71.70 ±	3.27
PAN			
FLO-2	3	NO FLOW	
PSD Plot	33	Fig. 33-PSD-1	
PSD Plot	3	Fig. 3-PSD-1	
COM Plot	2	Fig. 21-COM-27	
COM	3	NO COMPRESSION	

Suppliers: [a]J.T. Baker, [b]Fischer, [c]Canadian Lab Supply

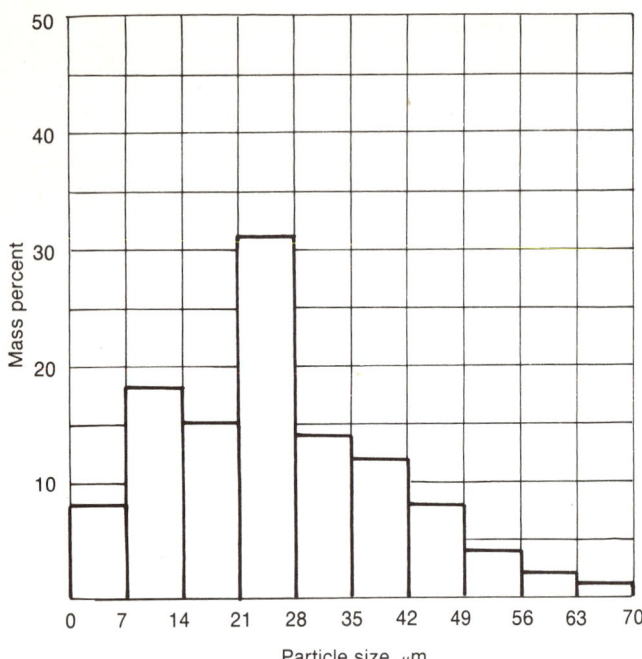

Calcium sulfate (Baker, Lot # 7314100)
Figure: 33-PSD-1   **Method:** PSD-8

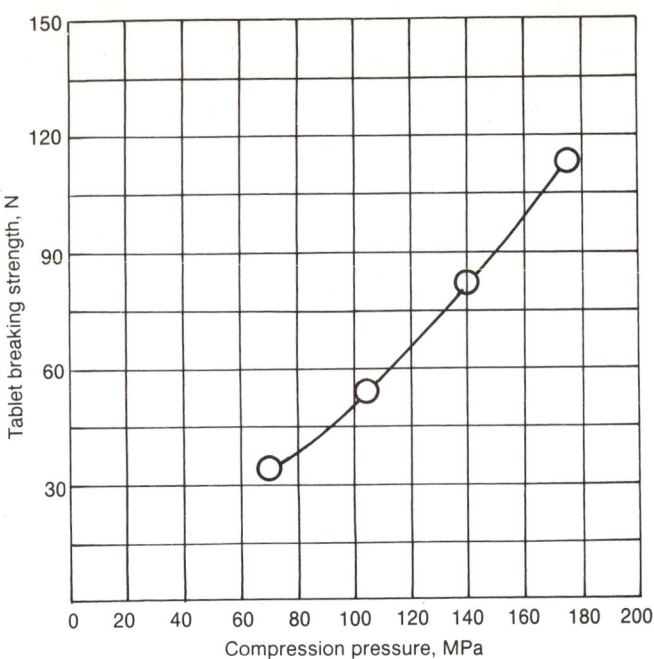

Calcium sulfate, dihydrate (Fisher, Lot #711313)
Tablet Weight: 700 mg

Figure: 21-COM-27   **Method:** COM-2

14. Safety

Because of limited intestinal absorption of calcium from its salts, hypercalcemia cannot be induced even when massive dosages are swallowed. Calcium salts are soluble in bronchial fluid; thus, pure salts do not precipitate pneumoconiosis. Calcium salts, when mixed with silicates, as in cement, may cause penumoconiosis, which is attributed to silicates.

15. Handling Precautions

Use a face mask to prevent excessive inhalation of the powder, which may saturate the bronchial fluid and lead to precipitation of calcium sulfate, causing blockage of air passages.

16. Regulatory Acceptance

NF XVI, BP 1980

17. Applications in Pharmaceutical Formulation

Diluent in compressed tablets and capsules. Dried calcium sulphate BP is used in plaster of Paris bandage and should not be used in tablets.

18. Related Substances

—

19. Comments

Calcium sulfate tends to absorb moisture, and therefore should be used with caution in the formulation of products containing drugs which easily decompose in the presence of moisture. Label calcium sulfate to indicate whether it is anhydrous or dihydrate.

20. Specific References

1. L. A. Bergman and F. J. Bandelin, *J. Pharm. Sci.*, 54: 445 (1965).
2. C. J. Schwartz and W. L. Suydam, *J. Pharm. Sci.*, 54: 1050 (1965).

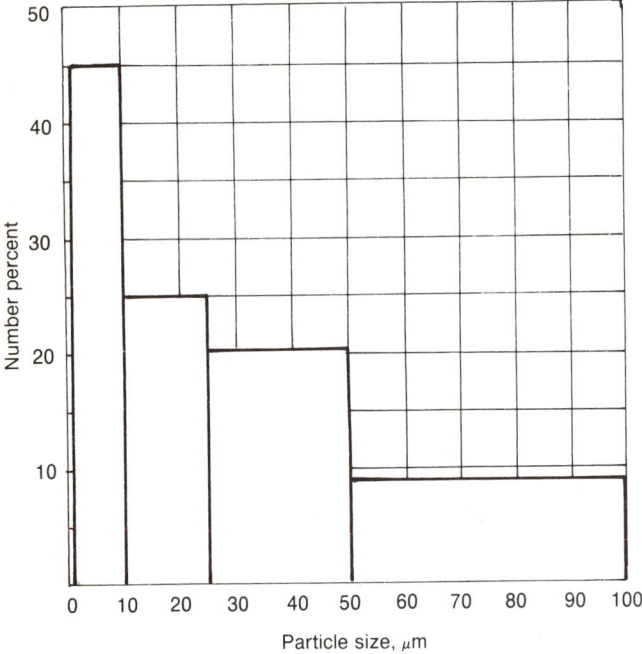

Calcium sulfate, anhydrous
Figure: 3-PSD-1   **Method:** PSD-9

12. Stability and Storage Conditions

Chemically stable, the powder may absorb moisture and cake. Store in a well-closed, moisture-resistant container.

13. Incompatibilities

Incompatibility in the solid state has not been reported. In the presence of moisture, the ionic calcium may be incompatible with amines, amino acids, peptides and proteins, which may form complexes.

USA: S. K. Malik*; A. Palmieri*; W. A. Vadino**
UK: A. B. Selkirk*

Carbomer

1. Nonproprietary Name

NF: Carbomer 934P
BP: Carbomer

2. Functional Category

NF: Suspending and/or viscosity-increasing agent
BP: Pharmaceutical aid

3. Synonyms

Carboxypolymethylene; carboxyvinyl polymer; acrylic acid polymer; *Carbopol*

4. Chemical Name and CAS Registry Number

Carboxypolymethylene [9007-20-9]

5. Empirical Formula   Molecular Weight

$-(C_3H_4O_2)_x \cdot (-C_3H_5-Sucrose)_y-$

Carbomer 934: 3×10^6
Carbomer 940: 4×10^6
Carbomer 941: 1×10^6

6. Structural Formula

7. Commercial Availability

USA

B. F. Goodrich Chemical Co.
San Mar Laboratories
Tanaco Products

UK

Honeywill & Stein Ltd.

8. Method of Manufacture

A synthetic, high molecular weight, cross-linked polymer of acrylic acid copolymerized with approximately 0.75-2% w/w of polyalkylsucrose. The end product contains 56-68% carboxylic acid groups.

9. Description

A white, fluffy, acidic, hygroscopic powder with a slight characteristic odor.

10. Pharmacopeial Specifications

Test	NF	BP
Identification	+	+
Loss on drying (at 80°C for 1 hr.)	≤2%	≤2.0%
Heavy metals	≤0.002%	—
Carboxylic acid group content	56-68%	56-68%
Sulfated ash	—	≤0.1%
Viscosity of 0.5% w/v carbomer 934 gel (neutralized)	2.94×10^4-3.94×10^4cps	—
Yield value	—	+

11. Typical Properties

The pH of a 1% dispersion of carbomer in water is approximately 3.0. Carbomer is soluble in water, alcohol and glycerin. Agents that can neutralize carbomer include sodium hydroxide; potassium hydroxide; sodium bicarbonate; borax; amino acids; polar organic amines, such as triethanolamine, and lauryl and stearyl amines, which are used as gelling agents in nonpolar systems. One gram of carbomer is neutralized by approximately 400 mg of sodium hydroxide. Neutralized aqueous gels of carbomer are more viscous between pH 6 and pH 11. The viscosity is considerably reduced if the pH is <3 or >12. The viscosity is also reduced in the presence of strong electrolytes. Gels rapidly lose viscosity on exposure to sunlight, but this reaction can be minimized by the addition of an antioxidant. Carbomer is hygroscopic.

Specific gravity: 1.4
Density, bulk: 5 g/cm³
Density, tapped: 1.4 g/cm³
Equilibrium moisture content (20°C and 40% RH): 8.0%
Viscosity (Brookfield, Model RVF or RVT at 20 rpm, using neutralized solutions at 25°C): 0.2% (spindle 4): 20.5-54.5 poise; 0.5% (spindle 6): 305-394 poise

Academy HPE Laboratory Project Data			
	Method	Lab #	Results
Bulk/tap density (934)	BTD-6	8	% consolidated Volume: 13.0% Weight: 11.0%
Bulk/tap density (941)	BTD-6	8	% consolidated Volume: 8.5% Weight: 8.0%

Supplier: Goodrich

12. Stability and Storage Conditions

Dry powder forms of carbomerdo not support the growth of molds and fungi; however, microorganisms grow well in unpreserved aqueous dispersions. Dispersions maintain their viscosity on storage during prolonged periods at room temperature or at elevated temperatures when stored away from light or with the addition of an antioxidant. Certain preservatives, such as benzoic acid, sodium benzoate and benzalkonium chloride, have been shown to cause a decrease in viscosity of the dispersion. Store in an airtight or well-closed container.

13. Incompatibilities

Carbomer is incompatible with phenol, cationic polymers, strong acids and high concentrations of electrolytes, and is discolored by resorcinol. Exposure to light causes oxidation, which is reflected in a decrease in viscosity.

14. Safety

Acute oral doses of carbomer 934P to rats, mice and guinea pigs produce LD_{50} values of 4.3, 4.6 and 2.5 g/kg, respectively. In dogs, no fatalities were noted with doses as high as 8 g/kg. No primary irritation or any evidence of sensitivity or allergic reaction in humans following topical application of dispersions containing carbomer has been observed. Carbomer in contact with the eye is very irritating. The material is difficult to remove with water, due to the gelatinous film that forms. When the eye comes into contact with carbomer, it should be irrigated with physiological saline, and not water.

15. Handling Precautions

Carbomer is very hygroscopic and should be kept as dry as possible to permit easy handling and processing and accurate weighing. Avoid contact with the eyes. Carbomer can also be irritating to the nose and throat.

16. Regulatory Acceptance

NF XXI; BP 1980

17. Applications in Pharmaceutical Formulation or Technology

Use	Concentration (%)
Emulsifying agent	0.1-0.5
Suspending agent	0.5-1.0
Gelling agent	0.5-2.0

Supplier: Goodrich
Other uses: Thickening agent in ointments and creams; tablet binder in sustained-release formulations.

18. Related Substances

None

19. Comments

Carbomer is more commonly used in pharmaceutical liquid and semisolid dosage forms than in tablets. Carbomer 934P is the only pharmaceutical grade of the resin that is approved for internal use.

20. Specific References

1. Literature issued by the B. F. Goodrich Co.
2. D. L. Secard, Carbopol Pharmaceuticals, *Drug and Cosmetic Industry*, 90: 28 (1962).

USA: J. W. McGinity*; M. R. Harris*; K. Patel*
UK: S. S. Davis*

Carbon Dioxide

1. Nonproprietary Names
USP: Carbon dioxide
BP/EP: Carbon dioxide

2. Functional Categories
USP: Air displacement
Other: Aerosol propellant

3. Synonyms
Carbonic acid gas; carbonic anhydride

4. Chemical Name and CAS Registry Number
Carbon dioxide [124-38-9]

5. Empirical Formula
CO_2

Molecular Weight
44.01

6. Structural Formula
O=C=O

7. Commercial Availability
USA

Air Products and Chemicals, Inc.
Liquid Carbonic Company
Roussel Corp.
Union Carbide Corp.

UK

Air Products, Ltd.
Distillers (Carbon Dioxide), Ltd.
Rhodia (UK), Ltd.

8. Method of Manufacture
By-product in the manufacture of lime. Incineration of coke or other carbonaceous material. Fermentation of glucose.

9. Description
Colorless, odorless, noncombustible gas with faint acid taste.

10. Pharmacopeial Specifications

Test	USP	BP/EP
Identification	+	+
Carbon monoxide	≤0.001%	≤10 ppm v/v
Hydrogen sulfide	≤1.0 ppm	—
Nitric oxide	≤2.5 ppm	—
Nitrogen dioxide	≤2.5 ppm	—
Ammonia	≤0.0025%	—
Sulfur dioxide	≤5 ppm	—
Water	≤150 mg/m³	—
Assay	≥99.0%	≥99.0% v/v
Acidity	—	≤20 ppm v/v
Phosphoric hydrides, hydrogen sulfide and organic reducing substances	—	+

11. Typical Properties
Density (liquid) at 25°C: 713.8 kg/m³
Density (vapor) at 25°C: 742.4 kg/m³
Solubility at 25°C (760mm g of CO_2/100 ml of water): 0.145
Miscibility at 25°C: ethanol 2.7*; isopropanol 2.5; acetone 6.5
Boiling point at 760 torr: −56.6°C
Vapor pressure (absolute) at 25°C: 64.36 × 10⁵ Pa
Viscosity at −17.8°C: 0.14 CCS
Flammability: Nonflammable
*Ostwald coefficient

12. Stability and Storage Conditions
Extremely stable and chemically nonreactive. Store in a tightlysealed cylinder. Avoid exposure to excessive heat.

13. Incompatibilities
Generally compatible.

14. Safety
Toxicity: UL rating—group 5.

15. Handling Precautions
Handle in accordance with procedures for handling metal cylinders or liquified gases. Use in well-ventilated rooms with safety devices for monitoring the vapor concentration in the room. Carbon dioxide does not support life, and only self-contained respirator systems should be used.

16. Regulatory Acceptance
USP XXI; BP/EP 1980

17. Applications in Pharmaceutical Formulation or Technology
Propellant for dispensing pharmaceutical aerosols.

18. Related Substances
Nitrogen; nitrous oxide

19. Comments
—

20. Specific References
1. M. A. Johnson and W. E. Dorland, "The Aerosol Handbook," W. E. Dorland Co., Caldwell, NJ, 1972.
2. H. Mintzer, Aerosols, in: "Dispensing of Medication," 7th ed., F. W. Martin, ed., Mack Publishing Co., Easton, PA, 1971.
3. P. A. Sanders, "Principles of Aerosol Technology," Van Nostrand Reinhold Company, New York, 1970.
4. I. Porush, Aerosols., in "Pharmaceutical Products: Science and Technology," Interscience Publishers, New York, 1961.
5. J. J. Sciarra, Pharmaceutical aerosols, in "The Theory and Practice of Industrial Pharmacy," 2nd ed., L. Lachman, H. A. Lieberman and J. L. Kanig, eds., Lea and Febiger, Philadelphia, PA, 1976.
6. J. J. Sciarra and L. Stoller, "The Science and Technology of Aerosol Packaging," John Wiley and Sons, New York, 1975.
7. J. J. Sciarra, Pharmaceutical and cosmetic aerosols, *J. Pharm. Sci.,* 63: 1815 (1974).
8. "The Physical Properties and Safety Books," The Distillers Company (Carbon Dioxide), Ltd., 1977.
9. Threshold limit values for 1979, Guidance note EH 15/79, *Health and Safety Executive,* Publ. HMSO ISBN 0-11-883193-3, London.

USA: J. Cooper*; K. Patel**
UK: P. J. Davies**

Carboxymethylcellulose Calcium

1. Nonproprietary Name
NF: Carboxymethylcellulose calcium

2. Functional Category
USP: Suspending and/or viscosity-increasing agent
Others: Disintegrating agent for granules, pills, and tablets; stabilizing agent for flavors

3. Synonym
Calcium carboxymethylcellulose; calcium CMC; CaCMC; carmellose calcium; *ECG 505*

4. Chemical Name and CAS Registry Number
Cellulose, carboxymethyl ether, calcium salt [9050-04-8]

5. Empirical Formula
$[C_6H_7O_2(OH)_{3-x} - 2(OCH_2-COOCa)_x]_n$

6. Structural Formula

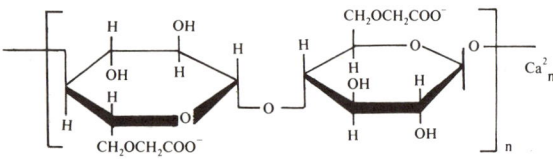

7. Commercial Availability

USA
Aceto Chemical Co., Inc.
BASF Wyandotte Corp.
Chugai International Co.
Conray Chemicals, Inc.
FMC Corp.

UK
Gotoku Pharmaceuticals Co., Ltd.
Kimpton Bros., Ltd.
Nippon CMC Co., Ltd.

8. Method of Manufacture
Cellulose, obtained as a pulp from plant tissue, is carboxymethylated, followed by its conversion into the calcium salt. It is graded on the basis of its degree of carboxymethylation and then pulverized.

9. Description
White to off-white fine powder

10. Pharmacopeial Specifications

Test	NF
Identification	+
Alkalinity	+
Loss on drying	≤10.0%
Residue on ignition	10.0-20.0%
Chloride	≤0.36%
Silicate	≤1.5%
Sulfate	≤0.96%
Arsenic	≤0.001%
Heavy metals	≤0.002%
Starch	+

11. Typical Properties
Apparent specific gravity (g/l): 450-550
Solubility: Insoluble in water, but swells to twice its volume. Insoluble in 0.1N HCl, but slightly soluble in 0.1N NaOH.
Equilibrium moisture content:

Relative humidity, 25°C (%)	Water uptake (% w/w)
15	3.0
40	5.5
65	7.1
84	8.0

Degree of polymerization: 300 ± 100
Degree of etherification: 0.6 ± 0.1
pH (1% dispersion): 4.5-6.0
Particle size: 95% through 200 mesh screen

12. Stability and Storage Conditions
Stable to heat and light. Must be protected from moisture. Preserve in a tightly sealed container.

13. Incompatibilities
—

14. Safety
Can be used as a food additive (≤2%) in Japan.

15. Handling Precautions
Low hazard. Adopt usual precautions for particulate solids.

16. Regulatory Acceptance
NF XVI

17. Applications in Pharmaceutical Formulations or Technology

Use	Concentration (%)
Tablet disintegrant	1-20
Tablet excipient/binder	5-20
Dispersant	1-2

Insoluble in water, but swells to several times its bulk. Although its primary use is as a disintegrant, it also functions as a binding agent and a dispersant. It can be used either inter- or intragranularly as a disintegrant.

18. Related Substances
Carboxymethylcellulose sodium

19. Comments
—

20. Specific References
1. "E.C.G. 505", Product Information Bulletin, Nichirin Kaguku Kogyo, Japan.
2. N. Kitamori and T. Makino, Improvement in pressure-dependent dissolution of trepibutone tablets by using intragranular disintegrants, *Drug Development and Industrial Pharmacy*, 8(1): 125-139 (1982).

USA: J. V. Boni*; P. Bernardo**
UK: J. F. Pickard*; J. N. Staniforth*

Carboxymethylcellulose Sodium

1. Nonproprietary Names
USP: Carboxymethylcellulose sodium
BP: Carmellose sodium; sodium carboxymethylcellulose

2. Functional Category
USP: Suspending and/or viscosity-increasing agent; tablet binder; coating agent
BP: Pharmaceutical aid
Others: Disintegrant; thickener; suspension stabilizer

3. Synonyms
Sodium cellulose glycolate; sodium CMC; CMC

4. Chemical Names and CAS Registry Number
Cellulose, carboxymethyl ether, sodium salt
Cellulose carboxymethyl ether sodium salt [9004-32-4]

5. Empirical Formula   Molecular Weight
$[C_6H_7O_2(OH)_{3-x}(OCH_2-COONa)_x]_n$ 90,000-700,000

6. Structural Formula

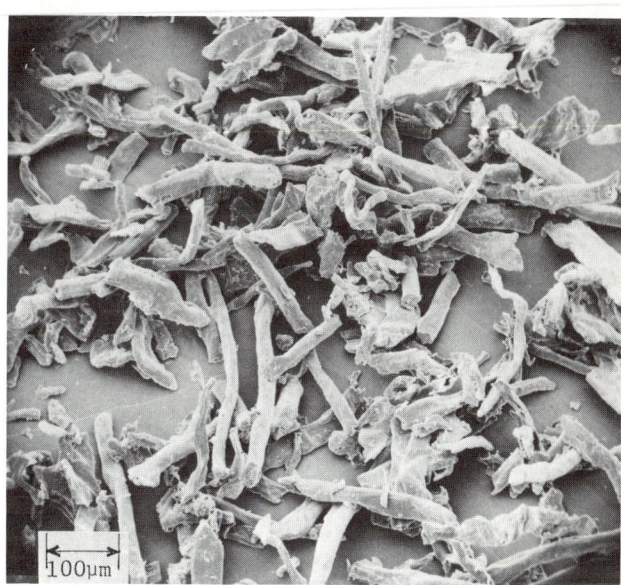

7. Commercial Availability
USA
Atomergic Chemetals Corp.
Buckeye Scientific Co., Inc.
Fallek Chemical Co.
FMC Corp./Food & Pharmaceutical Products Div.
Henkel Corporation
Hercules, Inc.
ICN/K & K Labs, Inc.
Pfaltz & Bauer, Inc.
Reisman Corp., H.
Robeco Chemicals, Inc.
Ruger Chemical Co.
SITCO (Shah International Trading Corp.)
United States Biochemicals Corp.

UK
British Celanese, Ltd.
Henkel KGaA
Hercules, Ltd.

8. Method of Manufacture
Carboxymethylcellulose sodium is prepared by the action of sodium monochloroacetate on alkalized cellulose. Sodium chloride and glycolate are obtained as by-products of this etherification.

9. Description
White to faintly yellow, odorless, hygroscopic powder or granular material having a faint paper-like taste.
The most frequently used Hercules grades have a degree of substitution (DS) of 0.7. This DS is defined as the average number of hydroxyl groups substituted per anhydroglucose unit. The Hercules product coding system identifies the degree of substitution, viscosity (H,M or L), maximum attainable viscosity (1% solution), solution characteristics, particle size (see Properties) and grade ("F" designating food, cosmetic, or pharmaceutical; "P" designating cosmetic or pharmaceutical; no designation indicating industrial grade). A typical product code would read as follows:
Hercules Cellulose Gum Type 7H3SCF
7   indicates a DS of 0.7
H   indicates high viscosity
3   indicates the maximum viscosity of 3,000 cps for a 1% solution
S   indicates smooth solution characteristics
C   indicates a coarse particle size
F   indicates food grade.

SEM:KY-12
Excipient: Carboxymethylcellulose sodium
Supplier: Buckeye Cellulose Corp.
Lot no.: 9247 AP

Magnification: 120× **Voltage:** 10kV

SEM:KY-12
Excipient: Carboxymethylcellulose sodium
Supplier: Buckeye Cellulose Corp.
Lot no.: 9247 AP

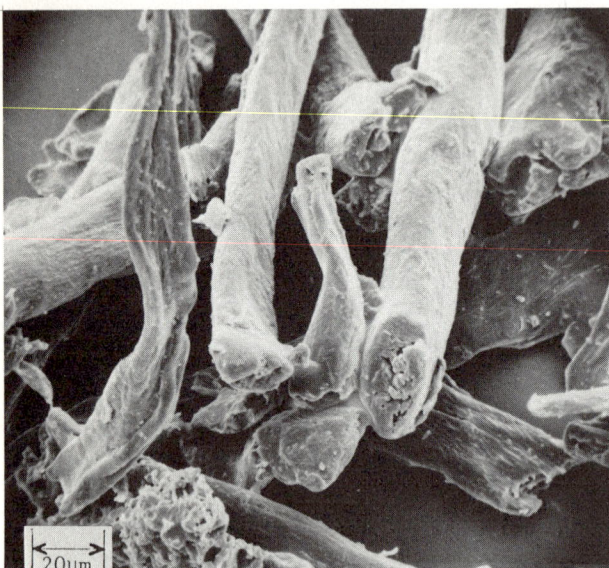

Magnification: 600× **Voltage**: 10kV

SEM:KY-13
Excipient: Carboxymethylcellulose sodium
Supplier: Hercules
Lot no.: 21 A-1 (44390)

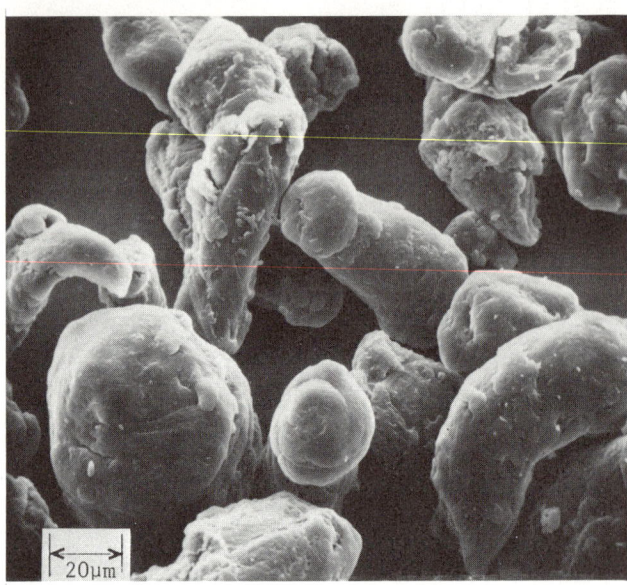

Magnification: 600× **Voltage**: 20kV

SEM:KY-13
Excipient: Carboxymethylcellulose sodium
Supplier: Hercules
Lot no.: 21 A-1 (44390)

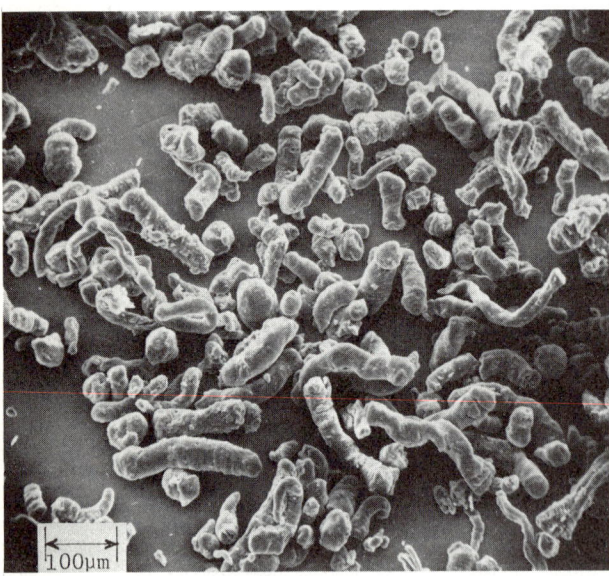

Magnification: 120× **Voltage**: 20kV

SEM:KY-14
Excipient: Carboxymethylcellulose sodium (CLD-2)
Supplier: Buckeye Cellulose Corp.
Lot no.: 21 A-2 (9247AD)

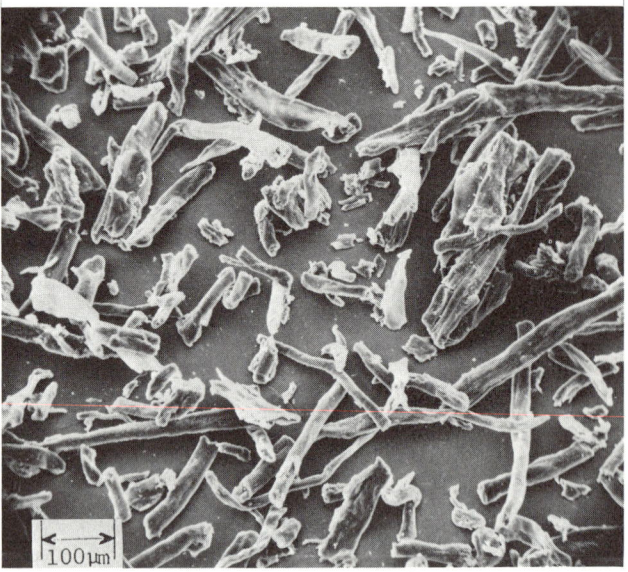

Magnification: 120× **Voltage**: 20kV

SEM:KY-14

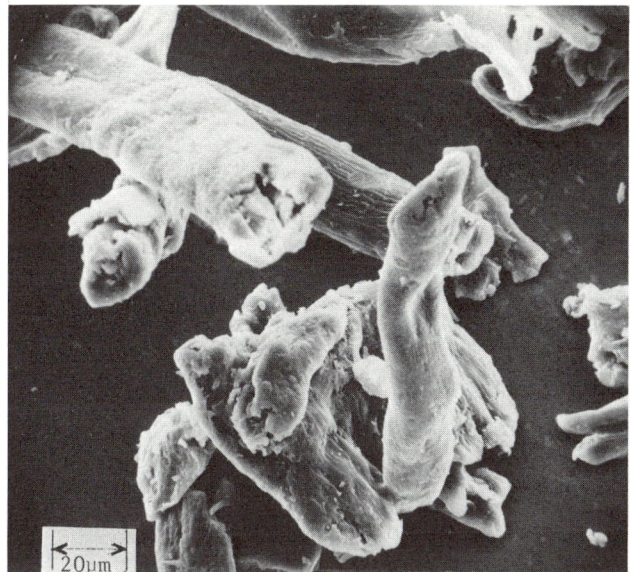

Magnification: 600× **Voltage:** 20kV

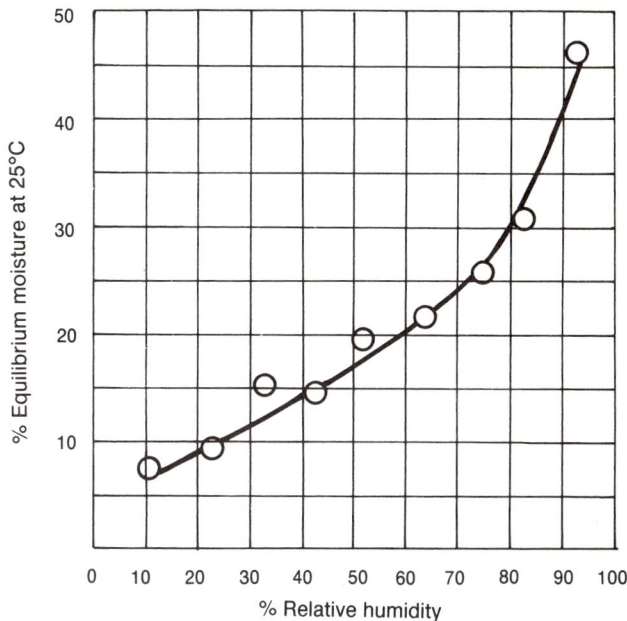

Carboxymethylcellulose sodium, USP (Hercules, Lot #76493)

Figure: 10-EMC-2 **Method:** EMC-1

10. Pharmacopeial Specifications

Test	USP	BP
Identification	+	+
pH (1 in 100 solution)	6.5-8.5	6.0-8.0
Loss on drying	≤10%	≤10%
Viscosity (2% solution)	≥80% and ≤120% of label statement	—
Viscosity (1% solution)	≥75% and ≤140% of label statement	—
Apparent viscosity	—	75-140%
Heavy metals	≤0.004%	≤20 ppm
Clarity and color of solution	—	+
Chloride	—	≤0.5%
Sulfated ash	—	20.0-33.3% (equiv. to 6.5 to 10.8% Na)
Assay	6.5 - 9.5% Na	6.5-10.8% Na

11. Typical Properties

Browning temperature: Approximately 227°C
Bulk density: 0.75 g/cm^3
Charring temperature: Approximately 252°C
Solubility: Soluble in water at all temperatures, giving a clear solution; practically insoluble in most organic solvents.
Viscosity: Aqueous solutions of sodium CMC exhibit pseudo-plastic flow behavior. The material is supplied in various viscosity grades (H, M, or L), the viscosity being directly proportional to the degree of polymerization.

Academy HPE Laboratory Project Data

	Method	Lab #	Results
Moisture Content	MC-10	10	8.5%[b]
Moisture Content	MC-7	5	6.5%[b]
EMC Plot	EMC-1	10	Fig.10-EMC-2[b]
SI Plot	SI-1	13	Fig.13-SI-3[a]
SI Plot	SI-1	13	Fig.13-SI-3[b]
SI Plot	SI-1	13	Fig.13-SI-3[b]
SI Plot	SI-1	13	Fig.13-SI-3[b]
SI Plot	SI-1	13	Fig.13-SI-3[a]

Supplier: [a]Buckeye; [b]Hercules

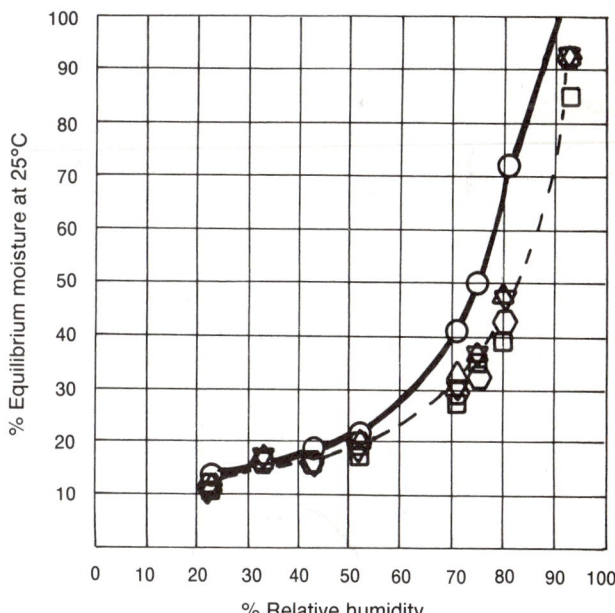

○ : Carboxymethyl cellulose sodium (Buckeye, Lot #9247AP)

△ : Carboxymethyl cellulose sodium, type 7LF (Hercules, Lot #21A-5)

▽ : Carboxymethyl cellulose sodium, type 7ML (Hercules, Lot #54816)

⬡ : Carboxymethyl cellulose sodium, type 7HF (Hercules, Lot #45515)

□ : Carboxymethyl cellulose sodium, type CLO-2 (Buckeye, Lot #9247AP)

Figure: 13-SI-3 **Method:** SI-1

12. Stability and Storage Conditions

Sterilization in both the dry state and in solution causes a decrease in viscosity. Irradiation of solutions will also cause a drop in viscosity. The bulk material is stable on storage. Preserve in tight containers.

13. Incompatibilities

Carboxymethylcellulose sodium is incompatible with strongly acidic solutions and with soluble salts of iron and some other metals, such as aluminum, mercury, and zinc.

14. Safety

Generally recognized as safe.

15. Handling Precautions

—

16. Regulatory Acceptance

USP XXI; BP 1980; GRAS List, FCC III

17. Applications in Pharmaceutical Formulations or Technology

Use	Concentration (%)
Emulsifying agent	0.25-1.0
Gel-forming agent	4.0 - 6.0
Binding agent	1%-6% in solution or as solid as required

18. Related Substances

Carboxymethylcellulose sodium 12 NF; its degree of substitution is not less than 1-15 and not more than 1.45, corresponding to an Na content of 10.5-12.0%. Cross carmellose.

19. Comments

—

20. References

—

USA: A. Bruno*; P. Bernardo**; J. Boylan*
UK: J. F. Pickard*

Hydrogenated Castor Oil

1. Nonproprietary Name
NF: Hydrogenated castor oil

2. Functional Category
NF: Stiffening agent
Others: Sustained-release coating material, hardening agent

3. Synonyms
Castorwax; Castorwax MP 70; Castorwax MP 80; Cenwachs G; Cerit SH; Opalwax; Sterotex K; Ceroxin; Cutina

4. Chemical Name and CAS Registry Number
Glyceryl-tris-12-hydroxystearate [8001-78-3]

5. Empirical Formula   Molecular Weight
$C_{57}O_9H_{110}$ 934 (approximately)

6. Structural Formula

7. Commercial Availability
USA

Capital City Products Company
Dura Commodities Corporation
W. C. Hardesty Company, Inc.
NL Industries, Inc.

8. Method of Manufacture
Hydrogenated castor oil is prepared by the hydrogenation of castor oil using a catalyst.

9. Description
Castorwax MP 70, MP 80
Cenwachs G: White, waxy flakes
Ceroxin: White to slightly yellow flakes or drops
Cerit SH: Hard, waxy consistency
Cutina: White to slightly yellow fine powder

10. Pharmacopeial Specifications

Test	NF
Melting range	85°–88°C
Heavy metals	0.001%
Free fatty acids	+
Hydroxyl value	154–162
Iodine value	≤5
Saponification value	176–182

11. Typical Properties
Acid value: Less than 5
Moisture content: Below 0.1%
Specific gravity: 1.023
Solubility: Insoluble in water; soluble in acetone, carbon tetrachloride and chloroform (10%).

Academy HPE Laboratory Project Data

	Method	Lab #	Results
Castorwax MP 70	BTD-6	8	Volume: 12.5%
Castorwax MP 70	BTD-6	8	Weight: 8.0%
Castorwax MP 80	BTD-6	8	Volume: 12.0%
Castorwax MP 80	BTD-6	8	Weight: 9.0%
Castorwax	BTD-6	8	Volume: 12.5%
Castorwax	BTD-6	8	Weight: 9.0%
Hydrogenated castor oil	PSD-4	17	

Sieve Size US Standard	Particle Size (S, μm)	Results Weight (%) ± sd
	S 1000	97.74 ± 1.34
18	590 S 1000	0.91 ± 0.63
30	297 S 590	0.23 ± 0.24
50	210 S 297	0.06 ± 0.05
70	149 S 210	0.78 ± 1.06
100	74 S 149	0.22 ± 0.08
200	S 74	0.06 ± 0.34
PAN		

	Method	Lab #	Results
Cerit SH	DE-1	7	1.07 ± 0.02[a]
Castorwax MP 70	DE-1	7	1.07 ± 0.02[b]
Castorwax MP 80	DE-1	7	0.985 ± 0.006[b]
Castorwax	DE-1	7	1.03 ± 0.01[b]

Suppliers: Durachem[a]; NL Industries, Inc.[b]

12. Stability and Storage Conditions
Store in a cool place; heat stable up to 150°C.

13. Incompatibilities
Hydrogenated castor oil is compatible with most natural vegetable and animal waxes.
No citations of known incompatibility occur in the literature.

14. Safety
Toxicity data in humans are lacking. The approximate acute oral LD_{50} in rats is greater than 5 g/kg of body weight. Preliminary topical study shows that hydrogenated castor oil does not elicit adverse dermal reactions in humans. Irritation tests on rabbits show that hydrogenated castor oil is a mild, transient irritant to the eye.

15. Handling Precautions
Keep away from fire and oxidizing materials.

16. Regulatory Acceptance
NF XVI; indirect food additive, Code of Federal Regulations: Title 21, Part 121, Subpart F, Sec. 121.2620.

17. Applications in Pharmaceutical Formulation or Technology

Use	Concentration (%)
Coating agent (delayed release)	5-20%
Delayed drug matrix	5-10%
Die lubricant	0.1-2%

18. Related Substances

Hydrogenated vegetable oil, NF

19. Comments

Products from different manufacturers may vary. *Sterotex K* is not hydrogenated castor oil, but hydrogenated cottonseed oil.

20. References

1. Charles H. Kline, Thixcin R-thixotrope, *Drug and Cosmetic Industry*, 95(6): 895-897, 960, 963, 973, 976 (Dec. 1964).
2. F. Q. Danish, E. L. Parrott, Effect of concentration and size of lubricant on flow rate of granules, *J. Pharm. Sci.*, 60: 752-754, (1971).
3. N. L. Industry Product Information Bulletins, DS-292, DS-401, TS-207, DS-400.
4. Dura Commodities Corporation: Technical Bulletin on Cerit SH.
5. F.D.A. Master Food File, No. 49.
6. J. C. Colbert, Controlled action drug forms, Noyes Data Corporation, Park Ridge, New Jersey, 1974, pp. 41 and 45.

USA: A. Yu*; J. Mullins**; P. Bernardo**
 UK: J. R. Nixon*

Cellulose Acetate Phthalate

1. Nonproprietary Names
NF: Cellulose acetate phthalate
BP/EP: Cellacephate

2. Functional Category
USP: Coating agent
BP: Pharmaceutical aid

3. Synonyms
Cellulose acetate phthalate; CAP; cellulose acetophthalate

4. Chemical Name and CAS Registry Number
Cellulose, acetate, 1,2-benzenedicarboxylate
Cellulose acetate phthalate [9004-38-0]

5. Empirical Formula   Molecular Weight
—   —

Cellulose is a polymer of glucose in which each glucose unit contains three hydroxyl groups. About half of the hydroxyl groups are acetylated and about one-fourth are esterified, with one of the two acid groups being phthalic acid. The other acid group is free.

6. Structural Formula

7. Commercial Availability
USA
Eastman Chemical Products, Inc.
Fallek Chemical Co.
ICN K & K Labs, Inc.
UK
Eastman Chemical International, AG

8. Method of Manufacture
The partial acetate ester of cellulose is reacted with phthalic anhydride in the presence of a tertiary organic base, such as pyridine.

9. Description
A white, free-flowing powder; tasteless; may have a slight odor of acetic acid.

10. Pharmacopeial Specifications

Test	NF	BP/EP
Identification	+	+
Apparent viscosity at 20°C	—	50-90 cps
Apparent viscosity at 25°C (15g+85g solvent)	50-90 cps	—
Loss on drying	≤5.0%	—
Residue on ignition	≤0.1%	—
Appearance of film	—	+
Solubility of film	—	+
Water	—	≤5.0%
Sulfated ash	—	≤0.1%
Free acid	≤6.0%	≤3.0%
Acetyl content	19.0-23.5%	17.0-23.0%
Phthalyl content	30.0-36.0%	30.0-40.0%

11. Typical Properties
Solubility: Insoluble in water, alcohols, hydrocarbons and chlorinated hydrocarbons. Soluble in a number of ketones, esters, ether alcohols, cyclic ethers and in certain solvent mixtures. The table below lists some of the solvents and solvent mixtures in which cellulose acetate phthalate has a solubility of 10% w/w or more:

Acetone	β-Methoxyethylene alcohol
Methyl ethyl ketone	Ethylene glycol monoacetate
Diacetone alcohol	Acetone:Ethanol 1:1
Dioxane	Acetone:Methanol 1:1
Methyl acetate	Acetone:Methanol 1:3
Ethoxyethyl acetate	Acetone:Methylene chloride 1:3
Ethyl lactate	Benzene:Methanol 1:1
Methoxyethyl acetate	Ethyl acetate:isopropanol 1:1

Soluble in certain buffered aqueous solutions as low as pH 6.0.
Viscosity: A 15% solution in acetone with a moisture content of 0.4% has a viscosity of 50-90 cps. This is a good coating solution with a honey-like consistency, but the viscosity is influenced by the purity of the solvent.
Hygroscopicity: Precautions are necessary to avoid excessive absorption of moisture.

Academy HPE Laboratory Project Data

	Method	Lab #	Results
Solubility (Water at 25°C)	SOL-8	30	0.08%
EMC Plot	EMC-1	5	Fig:5-EMC-1
SDI Plot	SDI-2	26	Fig:26-SDI-1
Moisture Content	MC-5	5	2.20%

Supplier: Eastman Chemical Products, Inc.

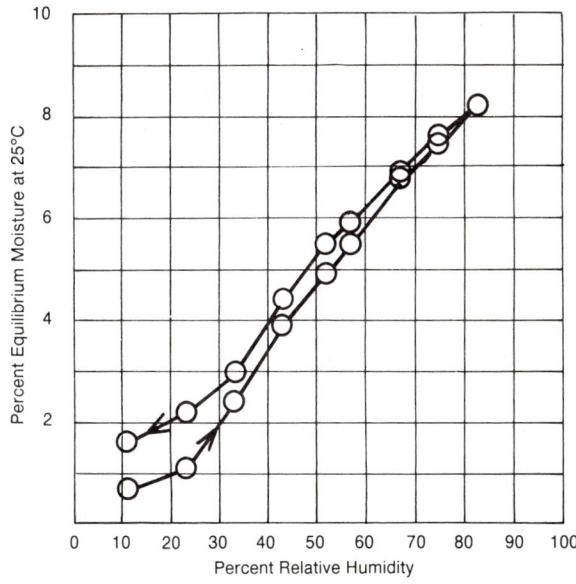

Cellulose Acetate Phthalate (Eastman, Lot #S-2090)

Figure: 26-SDI-1   Method: SDI-2

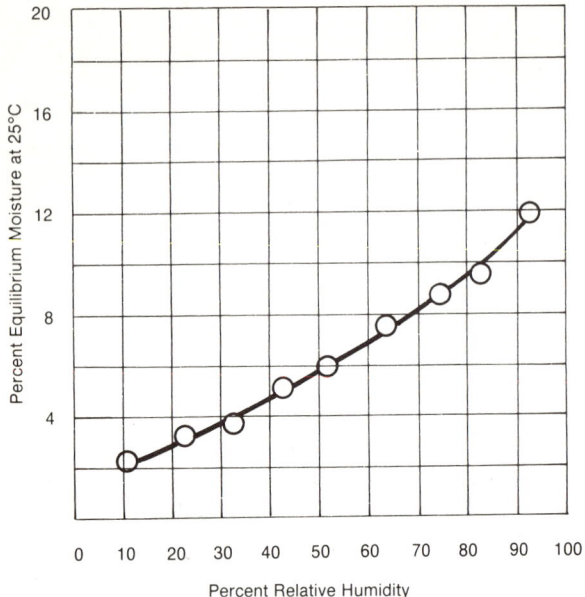

Cellulose Acetate Phthalate, NF (Eastman, Lot #C-2104)

Figure: 5-EMC-1   Method: EMC-1

12. Stability and Storage Conditions

Cellulose acetate phthalate is quite stable when properly stored. Slow hydrolysis will occur under prolonged adverse conditions (high temperatures and high humidity), with a resultant increase in free acid content, viscosity and odor of acetic acid.

Store in a tightly-sealed or well-closed container in a cool, dry environment.

13. Incompatibilities

Cellulose acetate phthalate is incompatible with ferrous sulfate, ferric chloride, silver nitrate, sodium citrate, aluminum sulfate, calcium chloride, mercuric chloride, barium nitrate, basic lead acetate, strong alkalis and acids.

14. Safety

Results of long term feeding in rats and dogs have indicated a low oral toxicity. Rats survived daily feedings of up to 30% in the diet for up to one year without showing a depression in growth. Dogs fed 16 grams daily in the diet for one year remained normal. Workmen exposed to dust where skin contact was unavoidable showed no dermal effects.

15. Handling Precautions

Avoid generation of excessive dust which, when fine, is capable of creating a dust explosion. When handling this material in large quantities, the guidelines established by NFPA No. 63 should be followed. Although a threshold limit value (TLV) has not been established, ventilation adequate for maintaining dust concentrations below the TLV for nuisance particulates (30 ppm/cf or 10 mg/m³) should be provided.

16. Regulatory Acceptance

NF XVI; BP/EP 1980

17. Applications in Pharmaceutical Formulation or Technology

Cellulose acetate phthalate (CAP) is used as an enteric coating material for tablets or capsules. Such coatings resist simulated gastric fluid, and dissolve in the intestinal fluid. Solutions of cellulose acetate phthalate are commonly applied to the tablets by a conventional "shot" process, as regularly used for sugar coating, or by one of the newer spray processes. Concentrations used are 0.5 to 9.0% of the core weight. The addition of plasticizers improves the water resistance of this coating material, and such plasticizers are more effective than when CAP is used alone. It is compatible with the following plasticizers: dimethylphthalate, diethyl phthalate, ethyl phthalylethyl glycolate, butyl phthalyl-butyl glycolate, tripropionin, dibutyl tartrate, glycerin, propylene glycol, polyethylene glycol and triacetin.

18. Related Substances

19. Comments

The plasticizer should be carefully chosen for improved performance on the basis of experimental evidence. The same plasticizer used in a different tablet base coating may not yield a satisfactory product.

In using mixed solvents, it is important to dissolve the CAP in the solvent with the greater dissolving power, and then to add the second solvent.

The CAP should always be added to the solvent; not the reverse.

Cellulose acetate phthalate films are permeable to certain ionic substances, such as potassium iodide and ammonium chloride. In such cases, an appropriate sealer subcoat should be used.

20. Specific References

1. J. Spitael, R. Kinget, and K. Naessen, Dissolution rate of cellulose acetate phthalate and Brönsted catalysis law, *Pharm. Ind.*, 42 (8), 846-849 (1980).
2. H. Takenaka, Y. Kawashima and S. Lin, Preparation of enteric-coated microcapsules for tabletting by spray drying technique and *in vitro* simulation of drug release from the tablet in GI tract, *J. Pharm. Sci.*, 69 (12), 1388-1392 (1980).
3. H. Takenaka, Y. Kawashima and S. Y. Lin, Polymorphism of spray-dried microencapsulated sulfamethoxazole with cellulose acetate phthalate and colloidal silica, montmorillonite or talc, *J. Pharm. Sci.*, 70 (11), 1256-1260 (1981).
4. H. Stricker and H. Kulke, Rate of disintegration and passage of enteric-coated tablets in gastrointestinal tract, *Pharm. Ind.*, 43 (10), 1018-1021 (1981).
5. J. C. Callahan, G. W. Cleary, M. Elefant, G. Kaplan, T. Kensler and R. Nash, Equilibrium moisture content of pharmaceutical excipients, *Drug Development and Industrial Pharmacy*, 8 (3), 355-369 (1982).

USA: E. Shek*, K. S. Alexander*; L. E. Small*
UK: J. S. Wilde*

Microcrystalline Cellulose

1. Nonproprietary Name

NF: Microcrystalline cellulose
BP: Microcrystalline cellulose

2. Functional Category

USP: Tablet and capsule diluent; tablet disintegrant; suspending and/or viscosity-increasing agent
BP: Pharmaceutical aid

3. Synonyms

Cellulose gel; crystalline cellulose; *Avicel* PH 101, 102

4. Chemical Name and CAS Registry Number

Cellulose [9004-34-6]

5. Empirical Formula/Molecular Weight

$(C_6H_{10}O_5)_n$
36,000 (approx.)
$n = 220$

6. Structural Formula

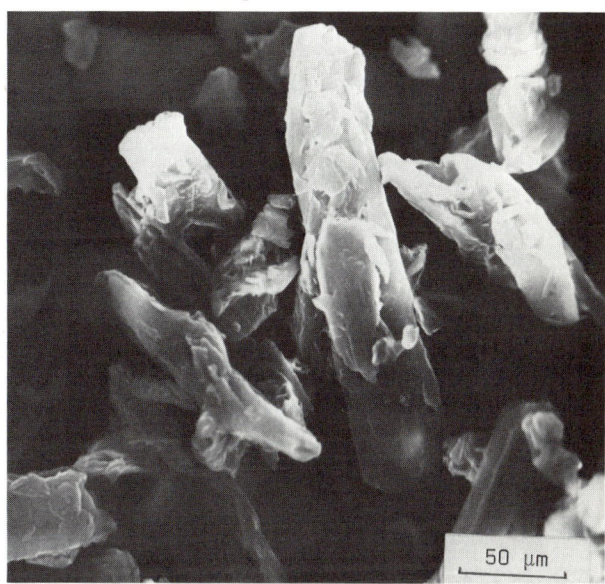

7. Commercial Availability

USA

Fallek Chemical Corp.
FMC Corp./Food & Pharmaceutical Products Div.
ICC Industries, Inc.
ICD Group, Inc.
Ingredients International, Inc.
Ruger Chemical Co.
Sitco (Shah International Trading Corp.)
United States Biochemicals Corp.

UK

Honeywell & Stein, Ltd.

8. Method of Manufacture

Microcrystalline cellulose is manufactured by the controlled hydrolysis of α-cellulose, obtained as a pulp from fibrous plant materials, with dilute mineral acid solutions. Following hydrolysis, the hydrocellulose is purified by filtration and the aqueous slurry is spray dried to form dry, porous particles of a broad size distribution.

9. Description

Purified, partially depolymerized cellulose occurs as a white, odorless, tasteless, crystalline powder composed of porous particles. Available in different particle size grades with different properties, i.e., 101 and 102.

SEM: UK-3
Excipient: *Avicel:* Grade PH 101
Supplier: Honeywell & Stein, Ltd.; lot #08345J
Manufacturer: FMC Corp., Ireland

50 µm

Magnification: 360 ×

10. Pharmacopeial Specifications

Test	NF	BP
Identification	+	+
pH (12.5% suspension)		(2% dispersion)
Grades with over 5% retained on a 37 µm screen	7.0	5.5-7.5
Grades with less than 5% retained on a 37 µm screen	5.0-7.0	
Loss on drying	≤5%	≤6.0%
Residue on ignition	≤0.05%	—
Water-soluble substances	≤10.2%	≤10 mg/5g
Grades with over 5% retained on a 37 µm screen	0.16%	
Grades with less than 5% retained on a 37 µm screen	0.24%	
Heavy metals	≤0.001%	≤10 ppm
Sulfated ash	—	≤0.1%
Starch	+	
Assay	97-102%	—
Ether-soluble substances	—	≤5 mg/10g
Solubility in copper	—	+
Starch and dextrins	—	+
Organic impurities	—	+

11. Typical Properties

Density: The average density of all types of commercially available microcrystalline cellulose is: Apparent density 0.28 g/cm³; tap density 0.43 g/cm³

Particle size: Commercial microcrystalline cellulose (*Avicel PH*) is available in four types:

Type	Average Particle Size, μm	Particle Size Analysis Mesh Size	Particle Size Analysis Percent Retained
PH-101	50	60	< 1.0
		200	<30.0
PH-102	100	60	< 8.0
		200	<45.0
PH-103	50	60	< 1.0
		200	<30.0
PH-105	20	60	< 0.1
		400	< 1.0

Refractive index: 1.55

Solubility: Insoluble in water, dilute acids and most organic solvents. Slightly soluble in sodium hydroxide solution (1 in 20).

Melting range: 260-270°C (Charring temp.)

Specific surface: Avicel (PH-101) 11.2 m²/g; Avicel (PH-102) 10.0 m²/g; Avicel (PH-103) 11.4 m²/g; Avicel (PH-105) 20.7 m²/g.

Academy HPE Laboratory Project Data			
Method	Grade	Lab #	Results
MC-3	PH101	31	3.745%
MC-3	PH105	31	4.655%
MC-3	PH103	31	3.065%
MC-3	PH102	31	3.315%
MC-8		5	3.600%
BTD-5	501	6	B: 0.622 g/cm³
BTD-5	509	6	T: 0.816 g/cm³
BTD-5	581	6	B: 0.614 g/cm³
BTD-5	581	6	T: 0.825 g/cm³
BTD-5	CL610	6	B: 0.630 g/cm³
BTD-5	CL611	6	T: 0.852 g/cm³
BTD-8	PH101	36	B: 0.320 g/cm³
BTD-8	PH101	36	T: 0.386 g/cm³
BTD-8	PH102	36	B: 0.307 g/cm³
BTD-8	PH102	36	T: 0.370 g/cm³
BTD-8	PH103	36	B: 0.301 g/cm³
BTD-8	PH103	36	T: 0.370 g/cm³
BTD-8	PH105	36	B: 0.260 g/cm³
BTD-8	PH105	36	T: 0.333 g/cm³
SOL-8 (Water-24°C)	PH101	30	0.10%
SOL-8	PH102	30	0.02%
DE-1	PH101	31	1.618
DE-1	PH102	31	1.554
DE-1	PH103	31	1.571
DE-1	PH105	31	1.573
EMC-1 Plot	PH101	5	Fig. 5-EMC-2
SI-1 Plot	PH102	13	Fig. 13-SI-4
SI-1 Plot	PH103	13	Fig. 13-SI-4
SI-1 Plot	PH105	13	Fig. 13-SI-4

Supplier: FMC Corp.

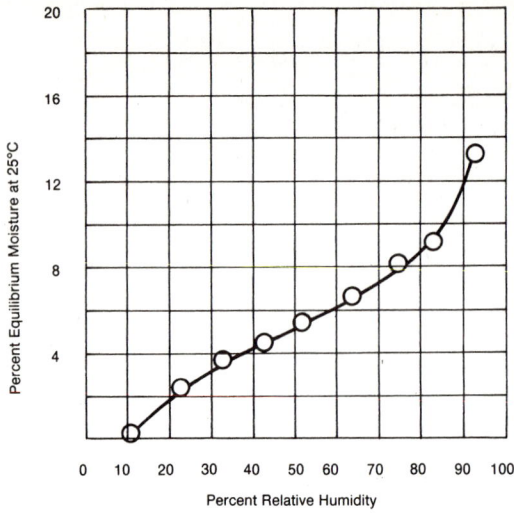

Microcrystalline cellulose, Avicel PH 101 (FMC Lot No. 1929)
Figure: 5-EMC-2   **Method:** EMC-1

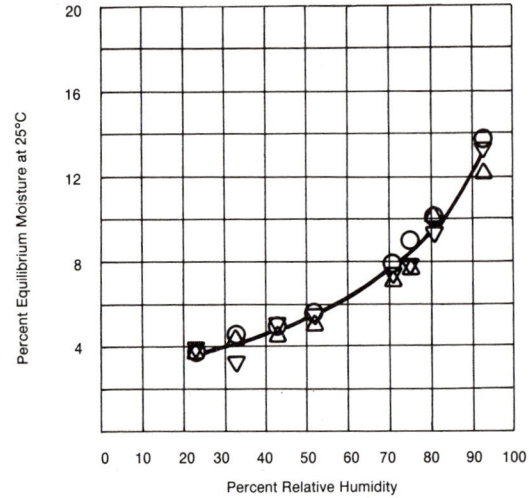

○ : Microcrystalline cellulose, Avicel PH 102 (FMC, Lot #2911-2904)

△ : Microcrystalline cellulose, Avicel PH 105 (FMC, Lot #5926)

▽ : Microcrystalline cellulose, Avicel PH 103 (FMC, Lot #3445)

Figure: 13-SI-4   **Method:** SI-1

12. Stability and Storage Conditions

Stable, hygroscopic.
Store in a well-closed container.

13. Incompatibilities

None cited in the literature.

14. Safety

Generally regarded as safe.

15. Handling Precautions

No restrictions.

16. Regulatory Acceptance

NF XVI; BP 1982

17. Applications in Pharmaceutical Formulation or Technology Use

Use	Concentration (%)
Tablet binder/diluent (wet granulation)	5-20
Tablet binder/diluent (direct compression)	5-20
Tablet disintegrant	5-15
Tablet glidant	5-15
Anti-adherent	5-20
Adsorbent	—
Capsule diluent	10-30

18. Related Substances

Microcrystalline cellulose and sodium carboxymethylcellulose sodium.

19. Comments

Two grades are available for pharmaceutical use, one colloidal and water-dispersible, containing 8.5-11% carboxymethylcellulose sodium; the other non-dispersible in water and used as a binder. Water-soluble chemicals can be adsorbed on the material prior to compression.

20. Specific References

1. J. C. Callahan, G. W. Cleary, M. Elefant, G. Kaplan, T. Kensler and R. A. Nash, Equilibrium moisture content of pharmaceutical excipients, *Drug Development and Industrial Pharmacy,* 8:(3), 355-369 (1982).
2. Z. T. Chowhan, A. A. Amaro and Y. P. Chow, Tablet to tablet dissolution variability and its relationship to the homogeneity of a water soluble drug, *Drug Development and Industrial Pharmacy,* 8:(2), 145-168 (1982).
3. R. W. Chlankurti, C. T. Rhodes and J. B. Schwartz, Some studies on compression properties of tablet mixtures using a computerized instrumented press, *Drug Development and Industrial Pharmacy,* 8:(1), 63-86 (1982).
4. R. L. Lamberson and G. E. Raynor, Jr., Tableting properties of Microcrystalline Cellulose, *Manufacturing Chemist and Aerosol News,* 47:(6), 55-61 (1976).
5. E. E. Enezian, "Direct compression of tablets using microcrystalline cellulose, *Pharm. Acta Helv.,* 47:(6/7), 321-363 (1972).
6. G. K. Bolhuis and C. F. Lerk, Comparative evaluation of excipients for direct compression, *Pharmaceutisch Weekblad,* 108:(22), 469-481 (1973).
7. C. F. Lerk, G. K. Bolhuis and A. H. de Boer, Comparative evaluation of excipients for direct compression II, *ibid.,* 109:(40), 945-955 (1974).
8. K. Marshall and D. Sixsmith, Some physical characteristics of microcrystalline cellulose, *Drug Development Communications,* 1:(1), 51-71 (1974-75).
9. C. F. Lerk, G. K. Bolhuis and A. H. de Boer, Effect of microcrystalline cellulose on liquid penetration and the disintegration of directly compressed tablets, *J. Pharm. Sci.,* 68:(2), 205-210 (1979).
10. R. G. Hollenbeck, G. E. Peck and D. O. Kildsig, Application of immersional calorimetry to investigation of solid-liquid interactions: Microcrystalline cellulose-water system, *J. Pharm. Sci.,* 67:(11), 1599-1606 (1978).
11. J. W. Wallace, J. J. Capozzi and R. F. Shangraw, Performance of pharmaceutical filler/binders as related to methods of powder characterization, *Pharm. Tech,* 7, Sept. 1983.

USA: D. Mufson*; A. Palmieri*; D. Sanvordeker*; Z. Chowhan**
UK: M. E. Aulton*

Powdered Cellulose

1. Nonproprietary Name
NF: Powdered cellulose

2. Functional Category
NF: Tablet and/or capsule diluent; sorbent
Others: Suspending agent

3. Synonym
Elcema; Solka-Floc

4. Chemical Name and CAS Registry Number
Cellulose — —

5. Empirical Formula
$(C_6H_{10}O_5)_n$ n = 1500

Molecular Weight
$\cong$ 243,000

6. Structural Formula

7. Commercial Availability

USA

Brown Company
Degussa, Inc.

UK

Degussa, Ltd.

8. Method of Manufacture
Powdered cellulose is manufactured by the mechanical processing of α-cellulose obtained as a pulp from fibrous plant materials.

9. Description
Powdered cellulose occurs as a white, odorless, tasteless powder of various finenesses, ranging from a free-flowing, dense powder to a coarse, fluffy, non-flowing material.

10. Pharmacopeial Specifications

Test	NF
Identification	+
pH (supernatant liquid of 10% w/w suspension)	5.0 - 7.5
Loss on drying	$\leq$7.0%
Residue on ignition	$\leq$0.3%
Water-soluble substances	$\leq$1.5%
Heavy metals	$\leq$0.001%
Starch	+
Assay	97-102%, calculated on dried basis

11. Typical Properties
Particle size and density: Commercial powdered cellulose is available in several types.

	Approximate Particle Size (μm)	Approximate Bulk Density, g/ml
***Elcema* Grade**		
P 050	1-50	0.300
P 100	1-100	0.250
P 150	1-150	0.200
G 250	1-250	0.400
***Solka-Floc* Grade**		
BW-20	80-120	0.14-0.34
BW-40	50-65	0.18-0.47
BW-100 Special	45-60	0.18-0.45
BW-100	35-45	0.29-0.56
BW-2030	30-45	0.27-0.59

Solubility: Insoluble in water, dilute acids and most organic solvents. Slightly soluble in sodium hydroxide solution (1 in 20). pH (aqueous dispersion): 1g in 8 ml. 5.5-7.0.

Academy HPE Laboratory Project Data		
Method	**Lab #**	**Results**
BTD-8	36	B: 0.287 g/ml[a]
BTD-8	36	T: 0.403 g/ml[a]
BTD-8	36	B: 0.208 g/ml[a]
BTD-8	36	T: 0.301 g/ml[a]
BTD-8	36	B: 0.139 g/ml[a]
BTD-8	36	T: 0.210 g/ml[a]
BTD-8	36	B: 0.176 g/ml[a]
BTD-8	36	B: 0.250 g/ml[a]
BTD-8	36	B: 0.302 g/ml[a]
BTD-8	36	T: 0.415 g/ml[a]
BTD-8	36	B: 0.391 g/ml[a]
BTD-8	36	T: 0.488 g/ml[a]
BTD-5	6	B: 0.372 g/ml[b]
BTD-5	6	T: 0.481 g/ml[b]
BTD-5	6	B: 0.197 g/ml[b]
BTD-5	6	T: 0.332 g/ml[b]
BTD-5	6	B: 0.211 g/ml[b]
BTD-5	6	T: 0.363 g/ml[b]
SOL-8 (Water 24°C)	30	0.06%[a]
DE-1	31	1.509[a]
EMC-1 Plot	18	Fig. 18-EMC-2[a]
SI-1 Plot	13	Fig. 13-SI-6[a]
SI-1 Plot	13	Fig. 13-SI-6[a]
SI-1 Plot	13	Fig. 13-SI-6[a]
SI-1 Plot	13	Fig. 13-SI-5[a]
SI-1 Plot	13	Fig. 13-SI-5[a]
SI-1 Plot	13	Fig. 13-SI-5[a]
COM-3 Plot	20	Fig. 20-COM-7[a]

Suppliers: Brown Co.[a]; Degussa[b]

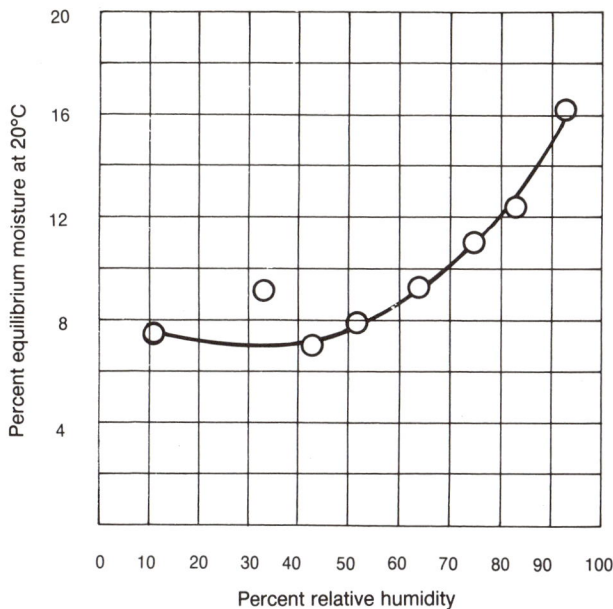

Powdered cellulose NF, *Solka-Floc* (Brown, Lot #30150)

Figure: 18-EMC-2   **Method:** EMC-1

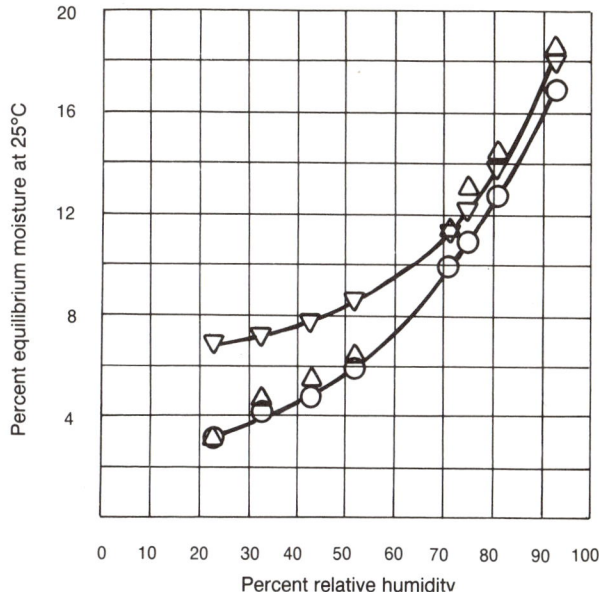

○ : Powdered cellulose, *Solka-Floc* BW 100
    (Brown, Lot #9-7-18B)
△ : Powdered cellulose, *Solka-Floc* BW 200
    (Brown, Lot #22A-20)
▽ : Powdered cellulose, *Solka-Floc* BW 2030
    (Brown, Lot #240)

Figure: 13-SI-5   **Method:** SI-1

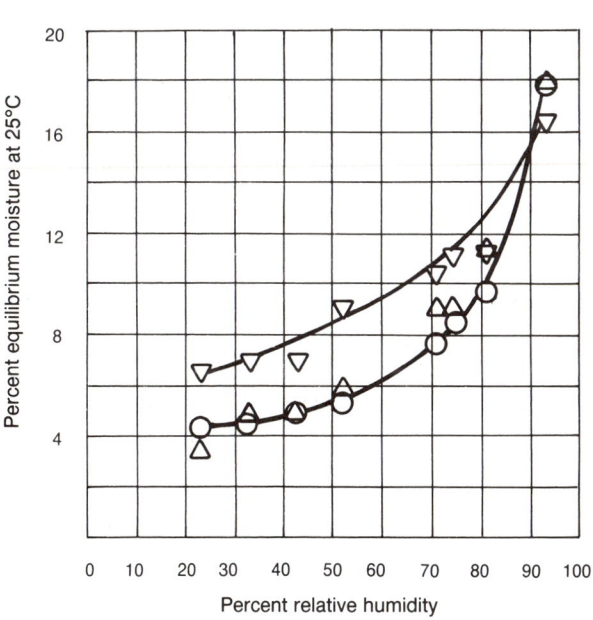

○ : Powdered cellulose, *Solka-Floc* BW 40
    (Brown, Lot #8-10-30A)
△ : Powdered cellulose, *Solka-Floc* BW 20
    (Brown, Lot #22A-19)
▽ : Powdered cellulose, *Solka-Floc* fine granular
    (Brown, Lot #9-10-8)

Figure: 13-SI-6   **Method:** SI-1

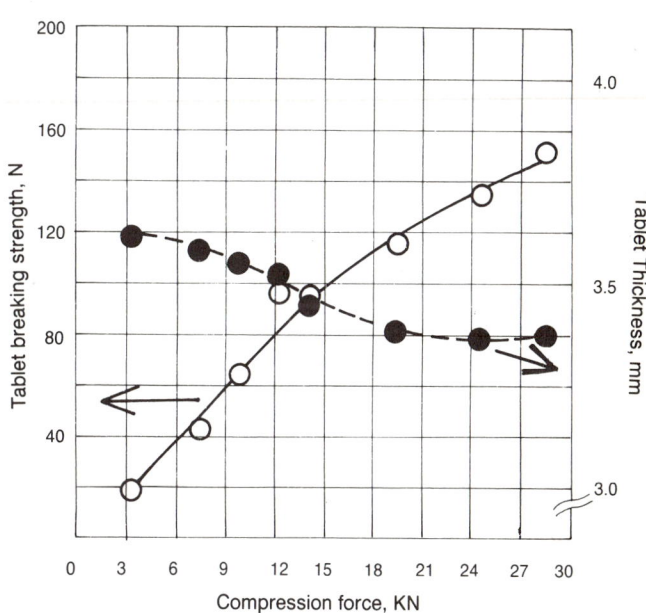

Solka-Floc, fine granular (Brown, Lot #9-10-8)

Mean tablet weight: 502 mg.
Minimum compressional force for compaction: 4.9 KN
Compressional force resulting in capping: >29.4 KN

Figure: 20-COM-7   **Method:** CCM-3

12. Stability and Storage
Stable. Store in a well-closed container.

13. Incompatibilities
No citations in the literature.

14. Safety
Safe

15. Handling Precautions
No restrictions specified.

16. Regulatory Acceptance
NF XVI

17. Applications in Pharmaceutical Formulation or Technology Use

Use	Concentration (%)
Binder	5-20
Filler	—
Disintegrant	5-15

18. Related Substances
Microcrystalline cellulose

19. Comments
None

20. Specific References

1. R. W. Chilamkurti, C. T. Rhodes and J. W. Schwartz, Some studies on compression properties of tablet mixtures using a computerized instrumented press, *Drug Development and Industrial Pharmacy*, 8:(1), 63-86 (1982).
2. A. M. Molokhia, M. A. Moustafa and M. W. Gouda, Effect of storage conditions on hardness, disintegration and drug release from some tablet bases, *Drug Development and Industrial Pharmacy*, 8:(2), 283-293 (1982).

USA: D. Mufson*; A. Palmieri*; D. Sanvordeker**; Z. Chowhan**
UK: M. E. Aulton*

Cetomacrogol Emulsifying Wax

1. Nonproprietary Name
BP: Cetomacrogol emulsifying wax

2. Functional Category
BP: Emulsifying agent (o/w)

3. Synonyms
Nonionic emulsifying wax; *Collone NI*; *Cyclogol Wax NI*; *Crodex N*

4. Chemical Names and CAS Registry Number

5. Empirical Formula   Molecular Weight
—   —

6. Structural Formula
—

7. Commercial Availability
UK
ABM Chemicals Ltd.
Croda Chemicals Ltd.
Witco Chemical Ltd.

8. Method of Manufacture
Cetostearyl alcohol /800 g and cetomacrogol 1000 /200 g are melted together and stirred until cold.

9. Description
White or off-white waxy solid or flakes which melt when heated to give a clear, almost white liquid; odor faint and characteristic of cetostearyl alcohol

10. Pharmacopeial Specifications

Test	BP
Identification	+
Acid value	≤ 0.5
Alkalinity	+
Hydroxyl value	175-192
Refractive index (at 60°C)	1.435-1.439
Saponification value	≤ 2.0
Solidifying point	45-53°C

11. Typical Properties
Density: 0.94 g/cm³
Iodine value: 0.15-0.16 (BP method)
Solubility:

Solvent	Solubility (20°C)
Water	Practically insoluble (forms an emulsion)
Alcohol (96%)	Moderately soluble
Ether	Partially soluble
Chloroform	Partially soluble
Fixed oils	Dissolves on warming
Liquid paraffin	Dissolves on warming

12. Stability and Storage
Stable

13. Incompatibilities
Tannin, phenol and phenolic materials, resorcinol, and benzocaine. Reduces antibacterial effect of quanternary ammonium compounds.

14. Safety
Submission under British Health and Safety at Work Act 1974 comments that it is not a toxicity risk, is not harmful to the skin, and is noncorrosive.

15. Handling Precautions
—

16. Regulatory Acceptance
BP 1980

17. Applications in Pharmaceutical Formulation and Technology
Used as an emulsifying agent in the production of o/w emulsions which are unaffected by moderate concentrations of electrolytes and are stable over a wide pH range. The concentration of wax used will alter the consistency of the product due to its "self-bodying action"; at concentrations up to about 5% the product is pourable. About 15% of cetomacrogol emulsifying wax is commonly used in creams, but concentrations as high as 25% are sometimes employed, e.g., in chlorhexidine cream BP. It is particularly recommended for use with salts of polyvalent metals and medicaments based on nitrogenous compounds. Creams are susceptible to microbial spoilage and should be adequately preserved. Additional uses are in a nonaqueous ointment base (cetomacrogol emulsifying ointment BP) and in barrier creams.

18. Related Substances
There are many similar preparations in the patent literature in which different nonionic surfactants are incorporated with different fatty alcohols.

19. Comments
—

20. Specific References
1. J. W. Hadgraft, *J. Pharm. Pharmacol.*, 6: 816 (1954).

USA: J Cooper**
UK: A. J. Winfield*

Cetostearyl Alcohol

1. Nonproprietary Name
NF: Cetostearyl alcohol
BP: Cetostearyl alcohol

2. Functional Category
USP: Stiffening agent
Others: Emollient; secondary emulsifying agent; viscosity-increasing agent

3. Synonym
Cetearyl alcohol; *Dehydag Wax O*; CO-1618

4. Chemical Name and CAS Registry Number
Cetostearyl alcohol [8005-44-5]

5. Empirical Formula   Molecular Weight

Cetyl alcohol—$C_{16}H_{34}O$ 242.43
Stearyl alcohol—$C_{18}H_{38}O$ 270.48
Myristyl alcohol—$C_{14}H_{30}O$ 214.38

6. Structural Formula
Cetyl alcohol: $CH_3-(CH_2)_{14}-CH_2OH$
Stearyl alcohol: $CH_3-(CH_2)_{16}-CH_2OH$
Myristyl alcohol: $CH_3-(CH_2)_{12}-CH_2OH$

7. Commercial Availability

USA

Croda, Inc.
Henkel Corp.
Proctor & Gamble Co.

UK

Albright & Wilson
Henkel Chemicals, Ltd.
Witco Chemical, Ltd.

8. Method of Manufacture
Cetostearyl alcohol is prepared by reduction of the appropriate fatty acids, or from sperm oils.

9. Description
Cetostearyl alcohol is a mixture of solid, aliphatic alcohols consisting mainly of stearyl and cetyl alcohols with small quantities of other alcohols, chiefly myristyl. The proportion of stearyl to cetyl alcohol varies considerably but usually consists of about 50-70% of stearyl alcohol and 20-35% of cetyl alcohol. White or cream-colored, unctuous masses, or almost-white flakes or granules. The odor is faint and characteristic, and the taste is bland. On heating, it melts to a clear, colorless or pale yellow liquid free of suspended matter.

10. Pharmacopeial Specifications

Test	NF	BP
Identification	+	—
Acidity	—	+
Acid value	≤2.0	—
Alcohols	—	+
Iodine value	≤4.0	≤3.0
Saponification value	—	≤2.0
Melting range	43°–53°C	—
Hydrocarbons	—	≤30.0 mg/g
Hydroxyl value	208-228	—
Assay	≥40% stearyl alcohol ≥90% combined alcohols	— —
Solidification range	—	45-53°C

11. Typical Properties
Density at 60°C: Approximately 0.816 g/cm^3
Initial boiling point: Not below 300°C
Solubility: Insoluble in water; soluble in solvent ether; less soluble in 95% alcohol and in light petroleum (boiling range 40°-60° C)
Water content: No more than traces of water are present.

12. Stability and Storage Conditions
Stable. Not liable to fatty ester hydrolysis, and does not become rancid. Store in a well-closed container.

13. Incompatibilities
No citations in the literature.

14. Safety
Negligible toxicity—not readily absorbed from the gastrointestinal tract.

15. Handling Precautions
No restrictions specified.

16. Regulatory Acceptance
NF XVI; BP 1980

17. Applications in Pharmaceutical Formulation or Technology
Cetostearyl alcohol is used as a consistency-imparting agent and emulsifier in both w/o and o/w emulsions. It acts as a stabilizer when mixed with more hyrophylic primary emulsifiers. It is also used in the preparation of nonaqueous creams and sticks.
It is an ingredient of emulsifying wax BP, paraffin ointment BP and simple ointment BP.

18. Related Substances
Cetyl alcohol NF; stearyl alcohol NF

19. Comments
Cetyl alcohol is usually 90-95% cetyl alcohol and 5-10% myristyl, stearyl and oleyl alcohols. Stearyl alcohol is about 96% pure, containing 1.5% cetyl and 2% arachidyl alcohols. Hydroxyl value determinations may not necessarily indicate these differences in composition, which may be sufficient to change emulsification behavior. Critical variables are the crystalline forms and the relative percentages of the four or five fatty acids present. These amounts may vary sufficiently in samples from different sources to effect changes in emulsion consistency or stability.

20. Specific References
None.

USA: F. Henry Markle*, J. Cooper**
UK: G. M. Eccleston*

Cetrimide

1. Nonproprietary Name

BP: Cetrimide

2. Functional Category

BP: Antiseptic detergent
Other: Antimicrobial preservative

3. Synonyms

Cetavlon, *Morphan CHSA*, *Silquat C100*, and *CTAB*. Synonyms formerly applied to the original cetrimide were cetrimonium bromide, cetyltrimethylammonium bromide.

4. Chemical Names and CAS Registry Number

The main component of cetrimide which conforms to the BP 1980 specification is:
Tetradecyltrimethylammonium bromide
N,N,N-Trimethyl-1-tetradecanaminium bromide [505-86-2]
In the original cetrimide specified in the BP 1953, the main component was:
Hexadecyltrimethylammonium bromide [8044-71-1] Technical grade
N,N,N-Trimethyl-1-hexadecanaminium bromide [57-09-0]
Pure grade

5. Empirical Formula   Molecular Weight

Cetrimide BP 1980 consists chiefly of tetradecyltrimethyl-ammonium bromide together with smaller amounts of dodecyl- and hexadecyl-trimethylammonium bromides:
Tetradecyltrimethylammonium bromide:
$C_{17}H_{38}BrN$ 336.4
For notes on original material see no. 18: *Related Substances*.

6. Structural Formula

Tetradecyltrimethylammonium bromide:

$$C_{14}H_{29} - \overset{\overset{\displaystyle CH_3}{|}}{\underset{\underset{\displaystyle CH_3}{|}}{N^+}} - CH_3 \; Br^-$$

7. Commercial Availability

USA

Cyclo Chemicals Corp.
Fallek Chemical Co.
Pfaltz & Bauer, Inc.

UK

A.B.M. Chemicals, Ltd.
Imperial Chemical Industries plc
Steetley Chemicals, Ltd.
Tenneco Organics, Ltd.

8. Method of Manufacture

Cetrimide is prepared by condensation of suitable alkyl bromides and trimethylamine.

9. Description

White to creamy white, free-flowing powder, having a faint but characteristic odor and a bitter, soapy taste.

SEM: **MF-5**
Excipient: Cetrimide
Supplier: Sigma Chemical Co.,

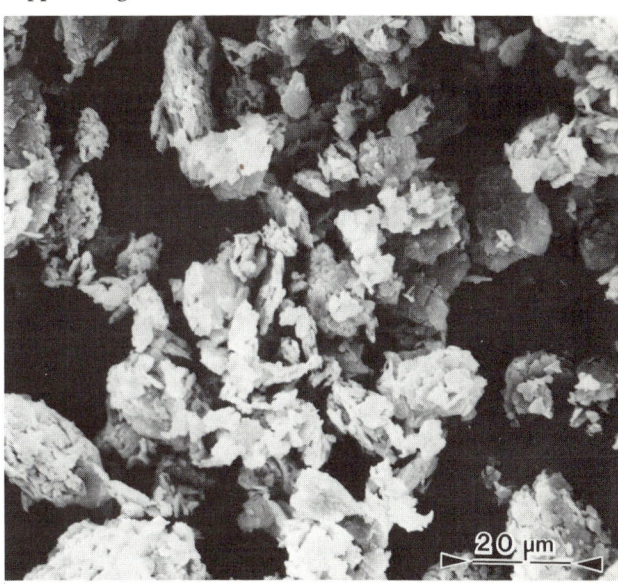

Magnification: 600×

SEM: **MF-5**
Excipient: Cetrimide
Supplier: Sigma Chemical Co.,

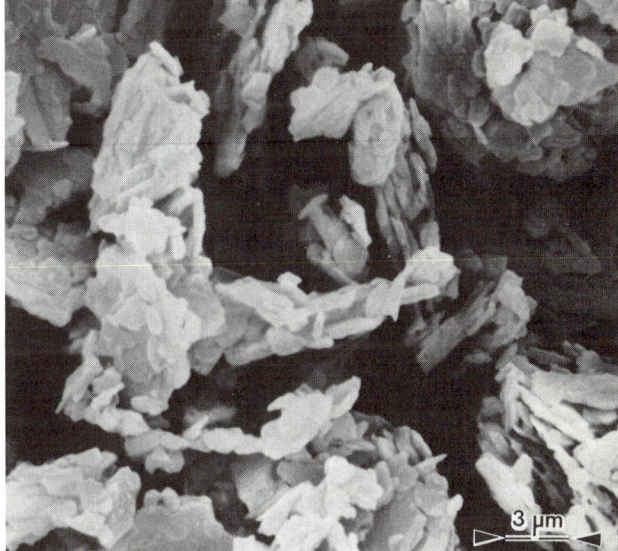

Magnification: 2,400×

10. Pharmacopeial Specifications

Test	BP
Identification	+
Acidity or alkalinity	+
Clarity of solution	+
Non-quaternary amines	+
Loss on drying	≤2.0%
Sulphated ash	≤0.5%
Assay	≥96.0% (calculated as $C_{17}H_{38}BrN$)

11. Typical Properties

Acidity/alkalinity: (1% w/v solution) pH 5-7.5

Antimicrobial activity: Bacteria: Gram positive species: Good bactericidal activity. Typical MIC for *Staphylococcus aureus:* 10 μg/ml; Gram negative species: Less active, in general, against gram negative species than against gram positive species. *Pseudomonas*—in particular *Pseudomonas aeruginosa*—may exhibit resistance. Typical MIC levels: *Escherichia coli:* 30 μg/ml; *Pseudomonas aeruginosa:* 300 μg/ml. Spores: Inactive against bacterial spores. Fungi: Relatively ineffective against fungi. Effect of pH: Most effective at neutral or slightly alkaline pH values; activity appreciably reduced in acidic media.

Critical micelle concentration: Approximately 0.01%.

Hygroscopicity: At 40-50% relative humidity and 20°C, flow properties are retarded.

Melting range: 232-247°C

Partition coefficients: Liquid paraffin—water: <1; vegetable oil—water: <1

Solubility: Soluble in water (1 in 2 at 25°C); very soluble in hot water and in ethanol; sparingly soluble in acetone; virtually insoluble in ether and benzene.

12. Stability and Storage Conditions

Solutions are stable at room temperature, and may be sterilized by autoclaving. Water containing metallic ions and organic matter may reduce potency. Store in an air-tight container.

13. Incompatibilities

Soaps, anionic surfactants, non-ionic surfactants in high concentration, bentonite, iodine, phenylmercuric nitrate, alkali hydroxides and acid dyes.

14. Safety

At concentrations used on the skin, solutions do not generally cause irritation, but some individuals have developed a hypersensitivity after repeated applications, usually exhibited as excessive dryness of the skin. Care should be taken to prevent strong solutions from entering the eyes. LD_{50} = about 50 mg/kg of body weight (intraperitoneally or intravenously in guinea pigs and rats). Fatal dose estimated to be 1-3 g in man. When ingested orally, the effects of cetrimide are similar to many other cationic detergents. Effects include nausea, vomiting, dyspnea and cyanosis due to paralysis of the respiratory muscles, possibly leading to asphyxia. One gram of the stearate salt of cetrimide ingested daily for three weeks by an adult male resulted in an inhibitory effect on intestinal absorption as shown by an increase in the bulk and softness of the feces. The man lost 15 lbs. in weight over the three week period. The effects were reversible.

15. Handling Precautions

Avoid inhalation, ingestion, skin and eye contact.

16. Regulatory Acceptance

BP/EP 1980

17. Applications in Pharmaceutical Formulation or Technology

Cetrimide has been used as a preservative in eye drops (0.005%) and as a cleanser for contact lenses.

As an ingredient of cetrimide emulsifying wax, it has been used in the production of o/w creams (e.g., cetrimide cream).

18. Related Substances

The original material supplied for medicinal use (cetrimide BP 1953; cetrimonium bromide, $C_{19}H_{42}BrN$, MW = 364.48) consisted largely of hexadecyltrimethylammonium bromide, with smaller amounts of analogous alkyltrimethyl-ammonium bromides. It contained a considerable proportion of inorganic salts (chiefly sodium bromide), and was less soluble than the present product.

19. Comments

As a precaution against contamination with *Pseudomonas* species resistant to cetrimide, stock solutions may be further protected by adding at least 7% v/v ethanol or 4% v/v isopropanol. In storage solutions for metal instruments, sodium nitrite may be added to reduce corrosion.

20. Specific References

1. I. R. Gucklhorn, *Manufacturing Chemist and Aerosol News*, 41: 28 (1970).
2. G. Sykes and R. Smart, *Amer. Perf. & Cosmet.*, 84: 45 (1969).
3. *Technical Data Sheet*, Aceto Chemical Co., Inc., Flushing, N.Y.
4. *Technical Data Sheet*, Hexcel Fine Organics, Lodi, N.J.

USA: H. Eisen*; A. Palmieri**
UK: M. C. Allwood*; J. Emerson*

Cetyl Alcohol

1. Nonproprietary Name
NF: Cetyl alcohol

2. Functional Category
NF: Stiffening agent
Other: Emulsifying and coating agent

3. Synonyms
n-Hexadecyl alcohol; cetanol; palmityl alcohol; *Adol-52*; *CO1695 CETYL*; *Laurex 16*

4. Chemical Names and CAS Registry Number
1-Hexadecanol
1-Hexadecanol [124-29-8; 36653-82-4]

5. Empirical Formula
$C_{16}H_{34}O$

Molecular Weight
242.44

6. Structural Formula
$CH_3(CH_2)_{14}CH_2OH$

7. Commercial Availability
USA

American Cyanamid
Marchon Products, Ltd.
Proctor and Gamble Distributing Co.
Sherex Chemical Co., Inc.

UK

Albright & Wilson Ltd.
Croda Chemicals Ltd.
Henkel Chemicals Ltd.
Sipon Products Ltd.
Witco Chemicals Ltd.

8. Method of Manufacture
Cetyl alcohol is manufactured by the saponification of spermaceti or by catalytic hydrogenation of the appropriate fatty acids.

SEM: KY-15
Excipient: Cetyl alcohol, C-50
Manufacturer: R.W. Greeff & Co.

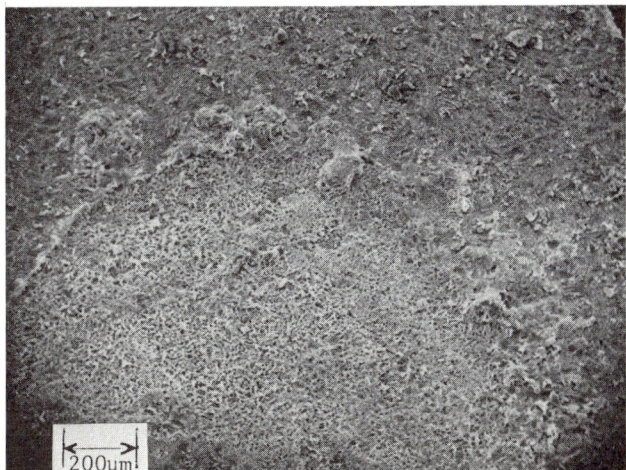

Magnification: 60× **Voltage:** 10 kV

9. Description
White flakes, granules, cubes or castings having a faint, characteristic odor and bland taste and having a waxy feel. Contains up to 10% of related fatty alcohols.

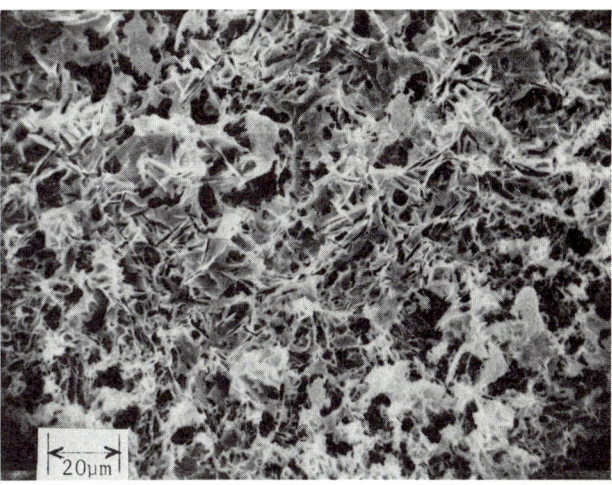

Magnification: 600× **Voltage:** 10 kV

SEM: KY-16
Excipient: Cetyl alcohol, N.F.
Manufacturer: Amend Drug & Chemical Co.
Lot no.: B11030F09

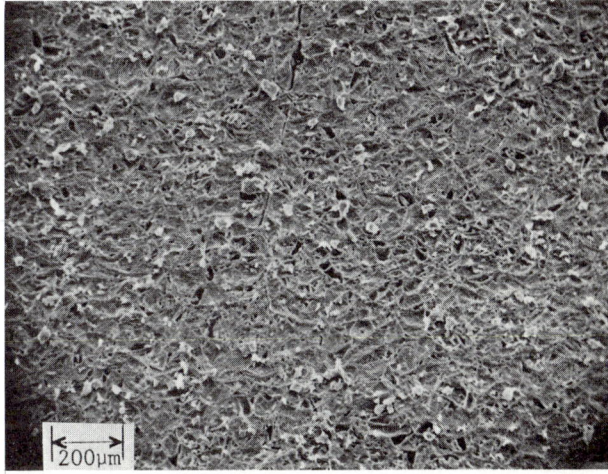

Magnification: 60× **Voltage:** 10 kV

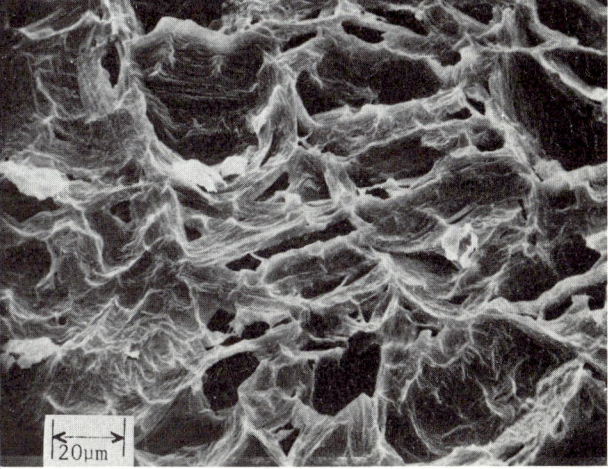

Magnification: 600× **Voltage:** 10 kV

SEM: KY-17
Excipient: Cetyl alcohol, N.F.
Manufacturer: Aceto Chemical Co.

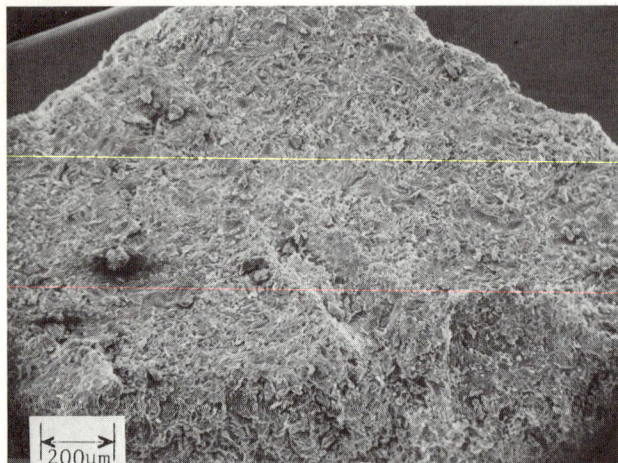

Magnification: 60× **Voltage:** 10 kV

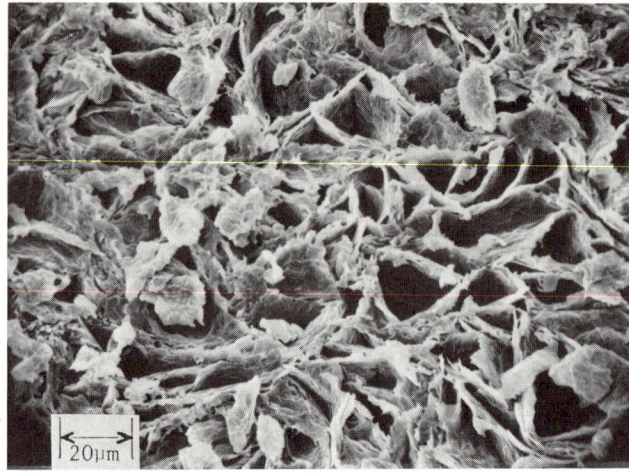

Magnification: 60× **Voltage:** 10 kV

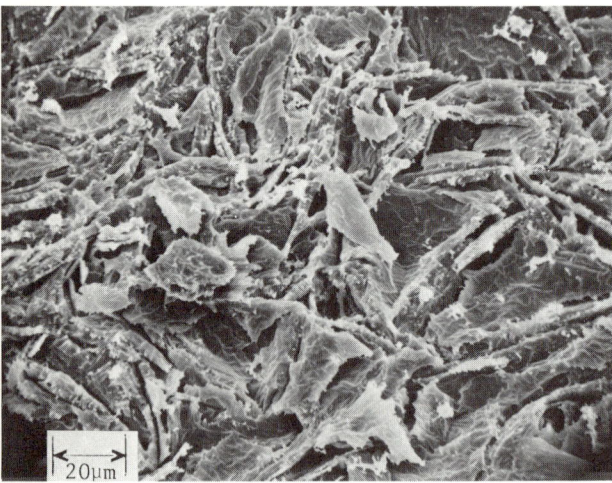

Magnification: 600× **Voltage:** 10 kV

SEM: KY-19
Excipient: Cetal-Cetyl alcohol
Manufacturer: Robinson-Wagner Co.   **Lot no.:** 9153

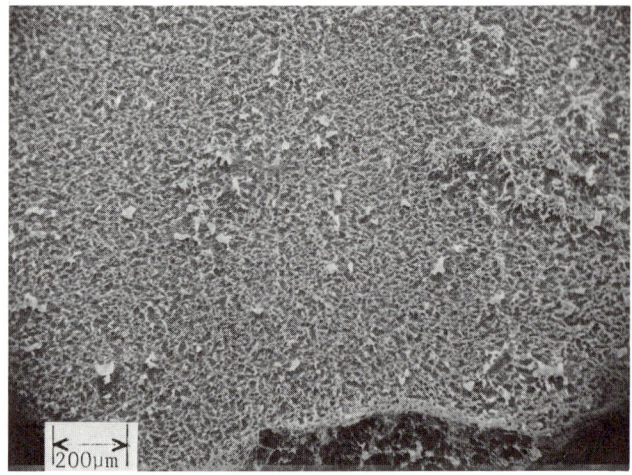

Magnification: 60× **Voltage:** 10 kV

SEM: KY-18
Excipient: Cetyl alcohol, N.F.
Manufacturer: Fallek Chemical Corp.   **Lot no.:** (9) #34

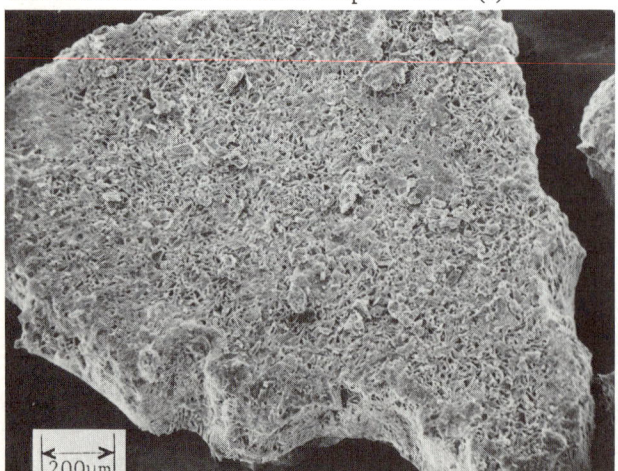

Magnification: 60× **Voltage:** 10 kV

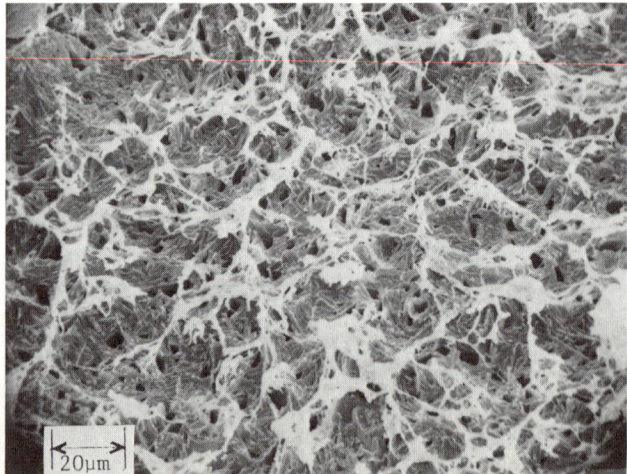

Magnification: 600× **Voltage:** 10 kV

SEM: KY-22
Excipient: Crodacol C(95)
Manufacturer: Croda Inc. **Lot no.:** 48020

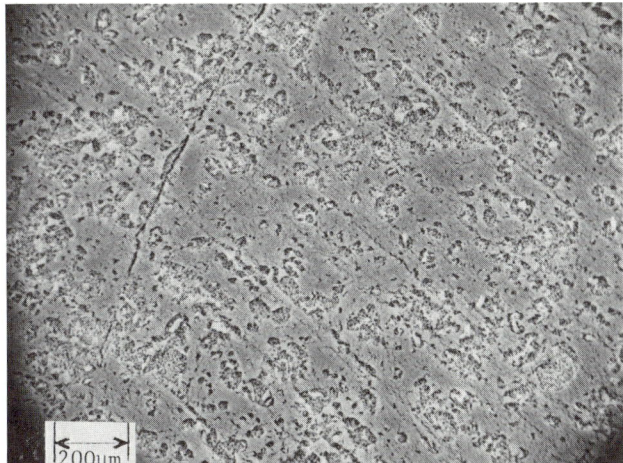

Magnification: 60× **Voltage:** 10 kV

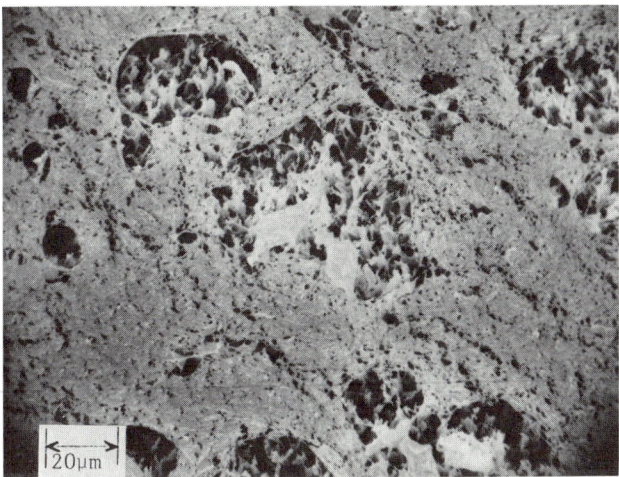

Magnification: 600× **Voltage:** 10 kV

10. Pharmacopeial Specifications

Test	NF
Identification	+
Melting range	45° C - 50° C
Acid value	≤2
Iodine value	≤5
Hydroxyl value	218-238
Assay	≥90% $C_{16}H_{34}O$

11. Typical Properties

Boiling point: 316° C - 344° C
Color, Lovibond (5¼"): 5Y/0.5R maximum
Density: 0.811-0.830 g/cm³
Solubility: Insoluble in water; soluble in alcohol, acetone, benzene, chloroform and ether. Miscible when melted with fats, liquid and solid paraffins and isopropyl myristate.
Refractive index (79° C): 1.4283
Saponification value: <1.0

Academy HPE Laboratory Project Data

Method	Lab #	Results
SOL-7 (Water 25° C)	32	<1.00%
SOL-7 (Water 37° C)	32	<1.00%
SOL-7 (Alcohol 25° C)	32	208 mg/ml
SOL-7 (Hexane 25° C)	32	76 mg/ml
SOL-7 (Prop. glycol)	32	<0.2 mg/ml
DE-1	7	0.907 ± 0.005[a]

Supplier: Am. Cyanamid[a]

12. Stability and Storage Conditions

Stable in the presence of acids and alkalis, light and air, and does not become rancid. Store in well-closed container.

13. Incompatibilities

No citations in the literature.

14. Safety

Non-toxic and non-irritating. Used in creams, ointments and suppositories.

15. Handling Precautions

No restrictions specified.

16. Regulatory Acceptance

NF XVI

17. Applications in Pharmaceutical Formulation or Technology

Use	Concentration (%)
Emulsifier	2-5
Stiffener	2-10
Emollient	2-5
Water absorption	5

Cetyl alcohol is used in the preparation of suppositories, delayed-release solid dosage forms, emulsions, lotions, creams and ointments. In suppositories, cetyl alcohol is used to raise the melting point. In prolonged action solid dosage forms, cetyl alcohol may be used to form a permeable barrier coating.

In lotions, creams and ointments, cetyl alcohol is used because of its emollient, water absorptive and emulsifying properties. It aids stability, improves texture and increases consistency. The emollient properties are due to cetyl alcohol being absorbed and retained by the epidermis, where it lubricates and softens the skin while imparting a characteristic velvety texture.

Cetyl alcohol is used for its water absorption properties in water-in-oil emulsions. For example, a mixture of 19 parts petrolatum and 1 part cetyl alcohol will absorb 40-50% of its weight of water. Cetyl alcohol is a weak emulsifier of the water-in-oil type emulsions. This allows a reduction in the amount of other emulsifying agents used in water-in-oil formulations. It may also increase consistency. Cetyl alcohol aids the stability of oil-in-water emulsions by combining with the water-soluble emulsifying agent. This mixed emulsifier produces a close packed, monomolecular barrier at the oil-globule water interface which forms a mechanical barrier against droplet coalescence. In semi-solid emulsions, excess cetyl alcohol combines with the aqueous emulsifier solution to form a visco-elastic continuous phase. This imparts semi-solid properties to the emulsions and also prevents droplet coalescence. Thus, cetyl alcohol is often referred to as a "consistency improver" or a "bodying agent," although it is emphasized that it may be coupled with a hydrophilic emulsifier to impart this property. Pure grades of cetyl alcohol do not form stable semi-solid emulsions. The technological uses and remarks refer mainly to commercial grades of cetyl alcohol. Pure cetyl alcohol may not show the same properties.

18. Related Substances

NF and cetostearyl alcohol (BP)—a blend of cetyl and stearyl alcohols. Alcohols containing 30-70% cetyl alcohol.

19. Comments

Cetyl alcohols of commerce have many grades available; they usually contain 60-70% cetyl alcohol and 20-30% stearyl alcohol, the remainder being related alcohols.

20. Specific References

—

USA: D. Pasquale*, E. S. Rattie**
UK: G. M. Eccleston*

Cetyl Esters Wax

1. Nonproprietary Name
NF: Cetyl esters wax

2. Functional Category
USP: Stiffening agent

3. Synonyms
Synthetic spermaceti; *Spermaceti Wax Replacement; Synaceti 116; Cyclochem SPS; Spermwax; Starfol Wax CG; Hywax 125; Kessco 653; Kessco 654*

4. Chemical Name and CAS Registry Number
—   [977067-67-6]

Cetyl Esters Wax is a mixture consisting primarily of esters of saturated fatty alcohols (C_{14} to C_{18}) and saturated fatty acids (C_{14} to C_{18}).

5. Empirical Formula   Molecular Weight
$C_xH_{2x}O_2$ Approximately 470 to 490
x = 26 to 38

6. Structural Formula

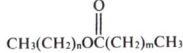

n = 13, 15, 17 primarily
m = 10, 12, 14, 16 primarily

7. Commercial Availability
USA
Armak Chemicals Div.
Ashland Chemical Co.
Cyclo Chemicals, Inc.
Frank B. Ross Co.
Robeco Chemicals, Inc.
Stevenson Bros. and Co.
Werner G. Smith, Inc.

UK
A&E Connock
A. F. Sutter & Co. Ltd.
Croda Chemicals Ltd.
Henkel Chemicals Ltd.
Highgate & Job Ltd.

8. Method of Manufacture
Cetyl esters wax is prepared by the direct esterification of the appropriate mixtures of fatty alcohols and fatty acids.

9. Description
White to off-white, somewhat translucent flakes (typically in the range of 5 µm to several millimeters in the largest dimension), having a crystalline structure and a pearly luster when caked. Has a faint odor (mild, aromatic, soap or tallow-like) and a bland, mild taste.

10. Pharmacopeial Specifications

Test	NF
Melting range	43-47°C
Acid value	≤5
Saponification value	109-120
Iodine value	≤1
Paraffin and free acids	+

11. Typical Properties
Cetyl esters wax is a mixture of esters of long-chain saturated fatty acids and fatty alcohols. It was developed as a synthetic replacement for spermaceti, which has been banned in the United States in order to protect the source of spermaceti, the sperm whale, as an endangered species. Several analyses of the ester mixture found in natural spermaceti have appeared in the literature. Different manufacturers of cetyl esters wax employ different mixtures of the various fatty acid or fatty alcohol esters in their products. These differences appear most obviously in the melting point, ranging from 43-47°C to 51-55°C, depending on the mixture. (Higher-melting material tends to be more purely cetyl and stearyl palmitates.)

Solubility*

Solvent	USP	(at 20°C unless otherwise noted)
Water	Insoluble	≪0.01 mg/ml
Absolute ethanol	—	0.6-1.2 mg/ml
95% ethanol	Practically insoluble	<0.1 mg/ml
95% ethanol (78°C)	Soluble	>400 mg/ml
Methylene chloride	—	300-400 mg/ml
Chloroform	Soluble	400-500 mg/ml
Hexane	Slightly soluble	125-150 mg/ml
Acetone	—	2-3 mg/ml
Ethyl acetate	—	12-15 mg/ml
Mineral oil (#35)	—	14-22 mg/ml
Fixed and volatile oils	Soluble	—
Ether	Soluble	—

*Measured on a range of representative products from various manufacturers; the higher-melting material tends to give the lower solubilities.

12. Stability and Storage Conditions
Store in a well-closed container in a cool, dry place. Avoid exposure to excessive heat (over 40°C).

13. Incompatibilities
Strongly acidic or strongly basic environments

14. Safety
Cetyl esters wax is a very innocuous material. It is neither a topical irritant nor a sensitizer, and exhibits an extremely low order of toxicity.

Acute oral LD_{50} (rat)	>16 g/kg
Draize eye irritation-FHSA (rabbit)	None to mild; short duration
Primary irritation-FHSA (rabbit)	None to very slight

15. Handling Precautions
—

16. Regulatory Acceptance

NF XVI

17. Applications in Pharmaceutical Formulation or Technology

Use	Concentration (%)
In cold cream	12.5 w/w
In rose water ointment	12.5 w/w
In spermaceti ointment	20 w/w
In topical creams/ointments	1-15

18. Related Substances

Natural spermaceti. Monographs for the naturally derived substance appear or have appeared in several pharmacopeias.

19. Comments

The use of natural spermaceti has been outlawed in the United States. The monograph for natural spermaceti appeared in BPC 1968, but was deleted from BPC 1973.

20. Specific References

These refer to natural spermaceti, but may be of general utility.

1. P. J. Holloway, The chromatographic analysis of spermaceti, *J. Pharm. Pharmac.* 20: 775-779 (1968), and references therein.
2. R. R. Egan and O. Portwood, Higher alcohols in skin lotions, *Cosmetics and Perfumery*, 89: (3), 39-42 (1974).
3. G. F. Spencer and R. Kleiman, Detection of spermaceti in a hand cream, *J. Am. Oil Chem. Soc.*, 55: 837-838 (1978).

USA: R. E. Jones*; J. Cooper**; B. Rasadi**

Chlorhexidine

1. Nonproprietary Names

BP: Chlorhexidine acetate
Chlorhexidine hydrochloride

2. Functional Category

BP: Chlorhexidine acetate: antibacterial
Chlorhexidine hydrochloride: antiseptic

3. Synonyms

Hibitane, Hibiclens

4. Chemical Names and CAS Registry Numbers

Chlorhexidine:

N,N''-Bis(4-chlorophenyl)-3,12-diimino-2,4,11,13-tetraazatetradecanediimidamide
1,1'-Hexamethylenebis [5-(4-chlorophenyl)biguanide]
1,6-Bis(N^5-p-chlorophenyl-N'-diguanido)hexane
1,6-Di(4'-chlorophenyldiguanido)hexane

Salts:

Diacetate
Dihydrochloride

CAS Registry Numbers:

Chlorhexidine [55-56-1]
Chlorhexidine acetate [56-95-1]
Chlorhexidine hydrochloride [3697-42-5]

5. Empirical Formula and Molecular Weight

	Molecular Weight
Chlorhexidine:	
$C_{22}H_{30}Cl_2N_{10}$	505.5
Chlorhexidine acetate:	
$C_{22}H_{30}Cl_2N_{10}, 2C_2H_4O_2$	625.6
Chlorhexidine hydrochloride:	
$C_{22}H_{30}Cl_2N_{10}, 2HCl$	578.4

6. Structural Formula

Cl—⟨benzene ring⟩—NHCNHCNH(CH₂)₆NHCNHCNH—⟨benzene ring⟩—Cl

7. Commercial Availability

USA

Lonza, Inc.
SST Corporation
Stuart Pharmaceuticals

UK

Imperial Chemical Industries, Ltd.
(Pharmaceuticals Division)
K & K-Greeff Chemicals, Ltd.

8. Method of Manufacture

Chlorhexidine is prepared by condensation of either poly-methylene bisdicyandiamide with parachloroaniline hydro-chloride or parachlorophenyldicyandiamine with hexa-methylenediamine dihydrochloride.
By synthesis from a series of biguanides.

9. Description

Chlorhexidine: White crystalline powder; odorless; bitter taste. Chlorhexidine acetate (BP 1980): White to pale cream, microcrystalline powder; odorless or almost odor-less. Chlorhexidine hydrochloride (BP 1980): White or almost white, crystalline powder; odorless; bitter taste.

SEM: MF-23
Excipient: Chlorhexidine base
Supplier: SST Corp.

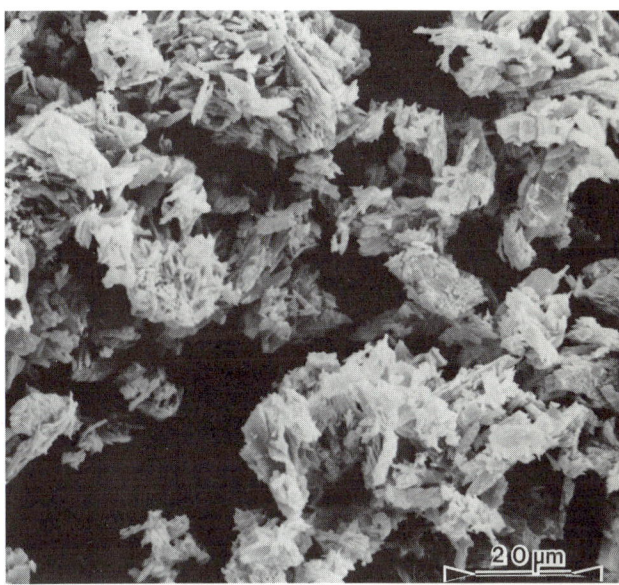

Magnification: 600×

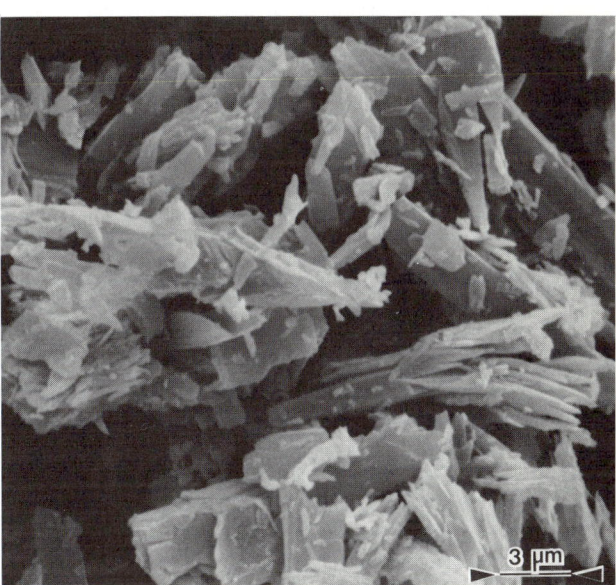

Magnification: 2,400×

10. Pharmacopeial Specifications

Test	Chlorhexidine Acetate BP	Chlorhexidine Hydrochloride BP
Identification	+	+
Acidity	−	−
Chloroaniline	+	+
Related substances	+	+
Loss on drying	≤3.5% (at 105°C)	≤2.0% (at 130°C)
Sulphated ash	≤0.2%	≤0.1%
Assay limits	97.5-101.0%	98.0-101.0%

11. Typical Properties

Antimicrobial activity:
Bacteria: Inhibitory at low concentrations; rapidly bactericidal at concentrations normally used for preservation and antisepsis.

Gram positive species: Active against most species; the MIC is normally in the range of 1-10 μg/ml.

e.g.:
Bacillus spp.	MIC 1.0-3	μg/ml
Clostridium spp.	MIC 1.8-70	μg/ml
Corynebacterium spp.	MIC 5.0-10	μg/ml
Staphylococcus spp.	MIC 0.5-6	μg/ml
Streptococcus spp.	MIC 0.1-7	μg/ml

Streptococcus faecalis is not inhibited by 1 mg/ml of chlorhexidine; a concentration of 2 to 5 mg/ml is necessary.
Acid-fast bacteria are resistant to chlorhexidine.
Gram negative species: Overall, somewhat less active against gram negative species than against gram positive species. Typical MICs are 1-15 μg/ml, but pseudomonads, particularly *Pseudomonas aeruginosa*, may be much more resistant. *Serratia marcescens* may also be resistant.

e.g.:
Escherichia coli	MIC 2.5-7.5	μg/ml
Klebsiella spp.	MIC 1.5-12.5	μg/ml
Proteus spp.	MIC 3-100	μg/ml
Pseudomonas spp.	MIC 3-60	μg/ml
Serratia marcescens	MIC 3-75	μg/ml
Salmonella spp.	MIC 1.6-15	μg/ml

Spores: Inactive against spores at normal room temperature. At 98-100°C there is activity against mesophilic spores.
Fungi: Slowly active against molds and yeasts, though generally less potent in its inhibitory activity against fungi than against bacteria.

e.g.:
Aspergillus spp.	MIC 75-500	μg/ml
Penicillium spp.	MIC 150-200	μg/ml
Microsporum spp.	MIC 12-18	μg/ml
Candida albicans	MIC 7-15	μg/ml
Saccharomyces spp.	MIC 50-125	μg/ml
Trichophyton spp.	MIC 2.5-14	μg/ml

Effect of pH: Activity is optimal at pH values of 5-7. Above pH 8, the chlorhexidine base may precipitate from aqueous solutions.
Critical micelle concentration: About 0.6% (depends on other ions in solution).
Melting point: Chlorhexidine: 132-134°C; chlorhexidine acetate: 154°C; chlorhexidine hydrochloride: 261°C, with decomposition.
Partition coefficient: Chlorhexidine acetate: liquid paraffin: water 0.075:1; arachis oil: water 0.04:1.

Solubility/miscibility (25°C):

Solvent	Chlorhexidine Acetate	Chlorhexidine Hydrochloride
Water	1 in 55	1 in 1700
Ethanol	1 in 15	1 in 450
Acetone	—	—
Propylene glycol	Very slightly soluble	1 in 50

Surface tension (0.6% solution): Approx. 50 mN/m (50 dyn/cm).

12. Stability and Storage Conditions

Chlorhexidine and its salts are stable at normal storage temperatures. Heating to 150°C will cause decomposition, yielding trace amounts of parachloroaniline. In this regard, the hydrochloride is more thermostable than the acetate. Aqueous solutions of chlorhexidine salts may undergo hydrolysis to form parachloroaniline. For example, after solutions of chlorhexidine gluconate (0.02%) of different pH values had been autoclaved at 120°C for 30 minutes, the following amounts of parachloroaniline were found by Jaminet (1970).

pH of solution	Parachloroaniline content
	(Per cent w/w of original chlorhexidine gluconate)
4.7	0.13
6.3	0.27
9.0	1.56

In buffered chlorhexidine acetate (0.05%) solutions, the pH of maximum stability was at 5.6. When solutions were autoclaved under various time-temperature combinations, the rate of hydrolysis increased markedly above 100°C and as pH increased or decreased from 5.6. At a given pH, chlorhexidine gluconate produced more parachloroaniline than did the acetate. It was found that chlorhexidine solutions containing parachloroaniline discolored in polypropylene or polyethylene bottles when exposed to direct sunlight. This discoloration was attributed to polymerization of parachloroaniline in solution.

It was predicted that in an autoclaved solution containing 0.01% chlorhexidine, the amount of parachloroaniline formed would be about 0.00003%. At these low concentrations there would be little likelihood of any toxic hazard as a result of the increase in parachloroaniline content in autoclaved solutions. Chlorhexidine salts and their solutions should be stored in tightly sealed containers, protected from light and at controlled temperatures (15-30°C). The hydrochloride salt absorbs significant amounts of moisture at temperatures up to 37°C and relative humidities up to 80%. Chlorhexidine solutions and aqueous based products may be packaged in glass, high-density polyethylene or polypropylene bottles provided that these are protected from light. Cork-based closures or liners should not be used.

As a precaution against contamination with *Pseudomonas* species resistant to chlorhexidine, stock solutions may be further protected by inclusion of at least 7% w/v ethanol or 4% w/v isopropanol.

13. Incompatibilities

Chlorhexidine salts are cationic in solution and, therefore, are incompatible with soaps and other anionic compounds. Salts are compatible with most cationic and non-ionic surface-active agents but, in high concentrations of surfactants, chlorhexidine activity can be substantially reduced due to micellar binding.
Salts of low aqueous solubility are formed and may precipitate from chlorhexidine solutions (of concentrations greater

than 0.05%) when in the presence of inorganic acids and certain organic acids and salts, e.g., benzoates, bicarbonates, borates, carbonates, chlorides, nitrates, phosphates and sulfates.

At chlorhexidine concentrations below 0.01%, precipitation is less likely. Insoluble salts may form in hard water due to interaction with calcium and magnesium cations. Solubility may be enhanced by the inclusion of surfactants, such as cetrimide or lissapol NX.

Other incompatible substances: Viscous materials—acacia, sodium alginate, sodium carboxymethylcellulose, starch and tragacanth. Also: brilliant green, chloramphenicol, copper sulfate, fluorescein sodium, formaldehyde, silver nitrate and zinc sulfate.

Interaction has been reported (Plaut, 1981) between chlorhexidine gluconate and the hydrogel poly (2-hydroxyethyl methacrylate), which is a component of some hydrophilic contact lenses.

14. Safety

The acute oral toxicity of chlorhexidine is low. It is poorly absorbed in the gastrointestinal tract. Humans have consumed 2 g daily for a week without untoward symptoms. There is minimal or no appreciable systemic absorption of chlorhexidine following extensive use in topical form.

In rats and mice the LD_{50} (oral) is 1.8 - 2 g per kg of body weight.

The incidence of skin sensitization is extremely low. Irritation to the conjunctiva occurs with solutions stronger than 0.1%, and the aqueous concentration normally recommended for contact with mucous surfaces is 0.05%. At this concentration there is no irritant effect on soft tissues, nor is healing delayed. The gluconate is frequently used at 1% strength in creams, lotions and disinfectant solutions. It is extremely dangerous to use chlorhexidine on the brain or meninges, and direct instillation into the middle ear can result in ototoxicity. When used in dental preparations, staining of teeth and oral lesions may result.

15. Handling Precautions

Avoid ingestion and inhalation.

16. Regulatory Acceptance

BP 1980: Chlorhexidine acetate; chlorhexidine hydrochloride

17. Applications in Pharmaceutical Formulation or Technology

Preservation of eye drops, usually as the acetate or gluconate salt at a concentration of 0.01%.

Solutions which contained between 0.002 and 0.006% chlorhexidine gluconate have been used for the disinfection of hydrophilic contact lenses.

Sterilization by heating with a bactericide. When autoclaving is not applicable, the BP 1980 allows the use of 0.01% w/v of chlorhexidine acetate and heating at 98° to 100°C for 30 minutes for certain eye drops and eye lotions.

For skin disinfection, chlorhexidine has been presented as an alcoholic solution (0.5% in 70% alcohol) and in conjunction (at 4%) with detergents as a surgical scrub. It is also a constituent of medicated dressings, dusting powders, sprays and creams. Aqueous solutions are used to reduce contamination in the humidifiers of ventilators and other respiratory apparati. In urology, chlorhexidine is used for catheter sterilization and in bladder irrigations.

18. Related Substances

Chlorhexidine gluconate solution, BP 1980.

19. Comments

Combinations of chlorhexidine acetate with the following substances have shown enhanced or more than additive activity towards *Pseudomonas aeruginosa*: benzyl alcohol, benzalkonium chloride, phenylethanol and phenylpropanol.

20. Specific References

1. H. C. Ansel, *J. Pharm. Sci.*, 56: 616 (1967).
2. G. E. Davies, J. Francis, A. R. Martin, F. L. Rose and G. Swain, *Brit. J. Pharmac.*, 9: 192 (1954).
3. J. Dolby, B. Gunnarsson, L. Kronberg, and H. Wikner, *Pharm. Acta Helv.*, 47: 615 (1972).
4. L. Flötra *et al*, *Scand. J. Dent. Res.*, 79: 119 (1971).
5. I. R. Gucklhorn, *Manuf. Chem.*, 41(1): 42 (1970).
6. D. D. Heard and R. W. Ashworth, *J. Pharm. Pharmac.*, 20, 505 (1968).
7. F. Jaminet, L. Delattre, J. P. Delporte, and A. Moes, *Pharm. Acta Helv.*, 45: 60 (1970).
8. B. Ljunggren and H. Moller, *Acta Derm.* (Stockholm), 52: 308 (1972).
9. W. Madsen, *Farm. Tidende*, 77: 1185 (1967).
10. J. A. Myers, *Lancet*, ii, 282 (1972).
11. B. S. Plaut, D. J. G. Davies, B. J. Meakin and N. E. Richardson, *J. Pharm. Pharmac.*, 33: 82 (1981).
12. H. N. Prince, W. S. Nomemaker, R. C. Norgard and D. L. Prince, *J. Pharm. Sci.*, 67: 1629 (1978).
13. R. Rose and G. Swain, *J. Chem. Soc.*, 4422 (1956).
14. N. Senior, *J. Soc. cosmet. Chem.*, 24: 259 (1973).
15. N. Senior, *Parf. & Kosmetik*, 57, 11 (1976).
16. J. E. Wahlberg and G. Wennersten, *Dermatologica* 143: 376 (1971).

USA: D. E. Auslander*; R. A. Nash*; K. W. Riebe
UK: M. C. Allwood*; J. Emerson*

Chlorobutanol

1. Nonproprietary Names
USP: Chlorobutanol
BP/EP: Chlorbutol

2. Functional Category
USP: Antimicrobial preservative
BP/EP. Antimicrobial preservative

3. Synonym
Chlorbutanol

4. Chemical Names and CAS Registry Numbers
2-Propanol,1,1,1-trichloro-2-methyl
1,1,1-Trichloro-2-methyl-2-propanol [57-15 8]
1,1,1-Trichloro-2-methyl-2-propanol hemihydrate [6001-64-5]

5. Empirical Formula   Molecular Weight
Anhydrous: $C_4H_7Cl_3O$ 177.46
Hemihydrate: $C_4H_7Cl_3O \cdot \frac{1}{2}H_2O$ 186.46

6. Structural Formula

$$CH_3 - \underset{\underset{CCl_3}{|}}{\overset{\overset{OH}{|}}{C}} - CH_3$$

7. Commercial Availability
USA
Eastern Chemicals Products
E. M. Laboratories, Inc.
R. W. Greeff Company, Inc.
McKesson Chemical Company
Stauffer Chemical Company

UK
Blagden Cambell Chemicals Ltd.

8. Method of Manufacture
Chlorobutanol is prepared by condensing acetone plus chloroform in the presence of solid potassium hydroxide.

9. Description
Colorless to white crystals with a musty, somewhat camphoraceous odor.

10. Pharmacopeial Specifications

Test	NF	BP/EP (Hemihydrate)	BP (Anhydrous)
Identification.	+	+	+
Reaction (litmus)	Neutral	Neutral	Neutral
Water	Anhydrous: ≤1% Hydrous: ≤6%	— —	≤1.0%
Chloride	≤0.07%	≤100 ppm	≤300 ppm
Assay range	Anhydrous basis: 98.0-100.5%	98.0-101.5%	98.0-101.5%
Melting point	—	~79°C	~95°C
Sulfated ash	—	≤ 0.1%	≤0.1%
Appearance of solution	—	+	+
Acidity	—	+	+

11. Typical Properties
Melting point or range: Anhydrous: 95-97°C; hemihydrate: 76-78°C.
Solubility: Ml required to dissolve 1 gram: water: 130; alcohol: 0.6; chloroform: 3; glycerol: 8; liquid paraffin (anhydrous form): 30; olive oil: 12; freely-soluble in ether and volatile oils. Very soluble in propylene glycol.
pH: Fresh aqueous solutions are neutral to litmus paper.
Volatility: chlorobutanol is volatile, and readily sublimes.
Microbiological properties: MIC values: gram positive: 650 μg/ml; gram negative: 1000 μg/ml; yeasts: 2500 μg/ml; fungi: 5000 μg/ml; above pH 5.5, activity is considerably reduced.
Chlorobutanol has antibacterial and antifungal properties. It has been shown to have activity against the following representative organisms: *Pseudomonas aeruginosa, Staphylococcus albus* and *Candida albicans*. It is considered to be effective against both gram-positive and gram-negative organisms and some fungi. Its activity is bacteriostatic and not bacteriocidal.

Academy HPE Laboratory Project Data

Method	Lab #	Results
MC-3	25	4.82[a]
MC-3	25	4.84[b]
MC-3	25	0.808[b]

Suppliers: Merck[a]; Stauffer Chemical Co.[b]

12. Stability and Storage Conditions
Storage conditions that are prescribed in the official compendia are as follows: USP: Tight container. BP/EP: Well-closed container. Chlorobutanol degradation is catalyzed by the hydroxide ion. The material has good stability with respect to pH at a pH value of 3. With an increase in pH, the stability becomes progressively worse. The room temperature half-life at pH 7.5 is about one-quarter of a year. Losses occur due to volatility. Appreciable losses occur during autoclaving. Porous containers result in losses from solutions. Polyethylene containers result in rapid loss. There is appreciable loss in and through stoppers in parenteral vials. Chlorobutanol will volatilize at higher temperatures and must be protected from light.

13. Incompatibilities
Chlorobutanol should be considered incompatible with plastic vials, rubber stoppers and magnesium trisilicate, due to adsorption. To a lesser extent, carboxymethylcellulose and polysorbate 80 reduce the activity of the compound (adsorption or complex formation). In aqueous solution at 0.5%, the compound is nearly saturated, and may crystallize at a cooler temperature.

14. Safety
Incubation of chlorobutanol with human conjunctival cells in culture demonstrated no toxicity at 0.2%. Cytotoxicity was evident, however, with concentrations of 0.3 and 0.4%. Chlorobutanol in a concentration of 0.1% shows epithelial toxicity when applied to isolated rabbit corneas. A partial loss of squamous cell layer of the corneal epithelium demonstrated by SEM and an associated increase in permeability were found. However chlorobutanol at a concentration of 0.5% applied topically to the intact eyes of rabbits did not produce corneal epithelial toxicity. Topical b.i.d. administration of 2% chlorobutanol for five days to intact rabbit eyes did not produce gross or microscopic evidence of toxic reaction of the corneal endothelium or epithelium. Single

doses of 0.03 or 0.10% epinephrine containing sodium bisulfite with either 0.1 or 0.5% chlorobutanol were injected into the aqueous humor of the eyes of cats. No adverse effects on the corneal endothelium were observed. Experiments on rabbits have established that after application of a drop of a standard local anesthetic such as 0.5% tetracaine or proparacaine hydrochloride, bathing the eyes continuously for twenty minutes with aqueous solutions containing 1.4% sodium chloride and 0.4% chlorobutanol produces definite keratitis epithelialis, which can be seen without magnification as a slight superficial haze in the cornea. The corneal epithelium becomes diffusely stainable with fluorescein, and under magnification has a ground-glass appearance. Freshly prepared solution at pH 5.5 has caused visible keratitis epithelialis after five to ten minutes of bathing. A solution which had been autoclaved and had pH 2.7 induced grossly evident disturbance of the corneal epithelium within three to five minutes. Control experiments in which rabbit eyes were anesthetized in the same way and were bathed for twenty minutes with a simple 1.4% solution of sodium chloride in water caused no disturbance of the cornea detectable grossly, under magnification, or by staining with fluorescein. The genotoxic potential of chlorobutanol has been evaluated in the Ames test (+), the drosophila test (−) and the micronucleus test (−). On the basis of these results chlorobutanol would not be considered to have genotoxic potential. Chlorobutanol has been widely employed as a very effective preservative in topical ophthalmic preparation without producing clinically recognized ocular distrubances even though applied several times a day for several years. However, when solutions containing 1.4% sodium chloride and 0.4% chlorobutanol have been employed in gonioscopy under the contact lens and this has been left on the eye for several minutes, in several patients an uncomfortable keratitis epithelialis has resulted, with fogging of vision, haloes around lights, and foreign-body type of discomfort beginning within the hour and becoming worse for several hours after the exposure. Fortunately, in all such instances the eyes have recovered spontaneously and completely in a day or two.

15. Handling Precautions

The compound is volatile, and should not be exposed to high temperatures. Avoid contact of material with skin, eyes or clothing. Wear gloves when handling. Avoid unnecessary inhalation of dust. In case of contact with skin, wash the affected areas with water and mild soap. Avoid exposure to heat and flame. Store in a tightly sealed container to avoid undue moisture absorption.

16. Regulatory Acceptance

NF XVI: Anhydrous or hemihydrate; BP 1980: anhydrous; BP/EP 1980: hemihydrate

17. Applications in Pharmaceutical Formulation or Technology

Chlorobutanol is primarily used in ophthalmic or parenteral dosage forms. The recommended concentration for use is 0.5%. It is commonly used as an antibacterial agent for epinephrine solutions, posterior pituitary solutions and ophthalmic preparations intended for the treatment of miosis. It is especially useful as an antibacterial agent in non-aqueous formulations.

18. Related Substances

Phenylethyl alcohol, USP, is used as a preservative at concentrations of 0.25 to 0.5%. It is frequently used in combination with other preservatives, including chlorobutanol. Phenoxyethanol is used as an antiseptic or preservative. It is used in a concentration range of 1 to 2.2%.

19. Comments

Chlorobutanol is considered to be compatible with most drugs and excipients. It has been reported that a combination of chlorobutanol and phenylethyl alcohol, both at a 0.5% concentration, has shown greater antibacterial activity than either compound alone. An advantage of the combination is that chlorobutanol dissolves in the other compound, and the ensuing liquid can then be dissolved in an aqueous pharmaceutical preparation without requiring heat.

20. Specific References

1. C. A. Lawrence and S. S. Block, *Disinfection, sterilization and preservation*, Lea and Febiger, Philadelphia, 1968, p. 568.
2. J. Klinefield and P. Ellis, Inhibition of microorganism by topical anesthetics, *Applied Microbiology*, 15: 1296 (1967).
3. L. Lachman *et al.*, Stability of antibacterial preservatives in parenteral solutions. I. Factors influencing the loss of antimicrobial agents from solutions in rubber-stoppered containers, *J. Pharm. Sci.*, 51: 224 (1962).
4. A. D. Nair and J. L. Lach, The kinetics of degradation of chlorobutanol, *J. Am. Pharm. Assoc.*, Sci. Ed., 48: 390 (1959).
5. H. D. Blackburn, A. E. Polack and M. S. Roberts, Preservation of ophthalmic solutions: Some observations on the use of chlorbutol in plastic containers, *J. Pharm. Pharmacol.*, 30: 666 (1978).

USA: I. Lippman*; J. Cooper*; W. H. Wong**
UK: M. C. Allwood**

Chlorocresol

1. Nonproprietary Name
BP: Chlorocresol

2. Functional Category
BP: Antiseptic and antimicrobial preservative

3. Synonyms
Parachlorometacresol; PCMC

4. Chemical Names and CAS Registry Number
4-Chloro-3-methylphenol [59-50-7]
3-Methyl-4-chlorophenol
6-Chloro-*m*-cresol
4-Chloro-*m*-cresol
6-Chloro-3-hydroxytoluene
2-Chloro-5-hydroxytoluene

5. Empirical Formula   Molecular Weight
C_7H_7ClO 142.6

6. Structural Formula

7. Commercial Availability

USA
Accurate Chemical & Scientific Corp.
Aceto Chemical Co.
Anachemia Chemicals, Inc.
Galard Schlesinger Chemical Manufacturing Co.
ICN/K & K Labs, Inc.
MC & B Manufacturing Chemists
Pfaltz & Bauer, Inc.

UK
BDH Chemicals, Ltd.
BTP Cocker Chemicals, Ltd.
Chas. Page and Co. Ltd.
Coalite Group, Ltd.
Diamond Shamrock Europe Ltd.
Koch-Light Laboratories, Ltd.
Peter Whiting (Chemicals), Ltd.
Wynmouth Lehr and Fatoils, Ltd.

8. Method of Manufacturing
Chlorocresol is prepared by chlorination of *m*-cresol.

9. Description
Colorless or almost colorless, dimorphous crystals with a characteristic phenolic odor.

10. Pharmacopeial Specifications

Test	BP
Identification	+
Melting point	64-66°C
Nonvolatile matter	≤0.1%

11. Typical Properties
Antimicrobial activity:

Bacteria: Similar bactericidal activities against both gram-positive and gram-negative species, including *Pseudomonas aeruginosa*. Concentrations in the region of 0.8 mg/ml, with a contact time of 10 minutes, are bactericidal. A typical MIC is 0.2 mg/ml.
Spores: At temperatures of 80°C or above and in concentrations greater than 0.012%, it is active against spores. It is much less active at room temperature. Heating at 98-100°C for 30 minutes in the presence of 0.2% chlorocresol has been used as a compendial method for the sterilization of solutions of substances which will not withstand autoclaving.
Fungi: Active against molds and yeasts. Fungicidal concentrations (after 24 hours of contact) range between 0.01 and 0.04%.
Effect of pH: Antimicrobial effectiveness decreases with increasing pH, to between pH 8 and 9. No activity above pH 9.
Boiling point: 235°C
Partition coefficients (at 25°C): Liquid paraffin-water: 1.53; arachis oil-water: 117.
pKa: 9.2
Solubility:

Solvent	(at 25°C unless otherwise stated)
Water	1 in 260*
Water (at 100°C)	1 in 50
Ethanol	1 in 0.4
Acetone	Soluble
Chloroform	Soluble
Ether	Soluble
Fixed oils	Soluble
Glycerol	Soluble
Terpenes	Soluble
Alkali hydroxide solutions	Soluble

* Aqueous solubility is decreased in the presence of electrolytes, particularly chlorides of sodium and potassium, and potassium sulfonate.
Melting point: Dimorphous crystals with a melting point of 55.5°C and 65°C.

12. Stability and Storage Conditions
Volatile at 100°C. Aqueous solutions may be autoclaved. Solutions in oil or glycerol may be sterilized by heating at 160°C for 1 hour. Aqueous solutions turn yellow on exposure to air and light. Store in a well-sealed container, protected from light.

13. Incompatibilities
Incompatible with solutions of calcium chloride, codeine phosphate, diamorphine hydrochloride and quinine hydrochloride. Other significant chemical interactions are few, but chlorocresol exhibits strong sorption or binding tendencies to organic materials such as rubber, certain plastics and nonionic surfactants. It has an affinity for oils.
It is lost from solutions to rubber closures, and in contact with polyethylene may initially be rapidly removed by sorption and then by permeation, the uptake being tempera-

ture dependent. Presoaking of components may reduce losses due to sorption, but not those by permeation. Chlorocresol may also be taken up by polymethyl methacrylate and by cellulose acetate. Losses to polypropylene or rigid polyvinyl chloride are usually small.

At a concentration of 0.1%, chlorocresol may be completely inactivated in the presence of nonionics, such as polysorbate 80, Nonex 99 and Lubrol W. Bactericidal activity is also reduced, due to binding, by cetomacrogol or methylcellulose. In emulsified or solubilized systems, chlorocresol readily partitions into the oil phase, particularly into vegetable oils.

14. Safety

It is less toxic than phenol: LD_{50} subcutaneously in rats is 0.4 mg/g. Sensitization reactions may follow the prolonged application of strong solutions to the skin; the sensitization index is 0.5%. Patch tests have shown that it is not a primary irritant at concentrations up to 0.2%. There have been reports of systemic reaction, delayed irritant reaction and hypersensitivity attributed to chlorocresol present in injections (notably in heparin injection preserved with chlorocresol 0.15%). At preservative concentrations, chlorocresol may be irritating to the eyes.

15. Handling Precautions

Protect against contact with the skin, eyes and mucous membranes.

16. Regulatory Acceptance

BP 1980; and the use of chlorocresol in foodstuffs is forbidden.

17. Application in Pharmaceutical Formulation or Technology

As an antimicrobial preservative for injections at 0.1% w/v. As an antimicrobial preservative in creams or lotions at 0.1 - 0.2%; may be less effective in the presence of anionic emulsifiers, cetomacrogol and other nonionic emulsifiers and vegetable oils.

For preservation, the French Codex suggests 0.3%, while the Swiss Pharmacopeia proposes 0.2%.

The BP 1980 describes sterilization by heating with a bactericide using chlorocresol 0.2%.

18. Related Substances

Chloroxylenol/parachlorometaxylenol. This compound is used similarly to chlorocresol. It is used in pharmaceutical creams in concentrations as high as 1.0%. It is reported to be effective in concentrations of 0.05 - 0.1%, and is considered to have a low order of toxicity.

19. Comments

Chlorocresol is described in the pharmacopeias of the following countries: Austria, Belgium, Brazil, Britain, India, Italy, Nordic countries, Switzerland and Yugoslavia.

This compound is more potent in acidic: pH than alkaline pH, and acts as a bactericidal agent when used in concentrations of 0.2% in solutions that are heat-sterilized. It has a characteristic odor which is difficult to mask, even at concentrations of 0.05% to 0.1%. It is considered dermatologically innocuous at these levels, but it is not suitable as a food perservative because of toxicity at higher levels.

20. Specific References

1. G. Sykes, *Disinfection and Sterilization*, 2nd ed., E. & F. N. Spon, London, 1965.
2. K. H. Wallhauser, *Pharm. Ind.*, 36: 10 (1974).
3. T. J. McCarthy, Dissolution of chlorocresol from various pharmaceutical formulations, *Pharm. Weekblad*, 110: 101 (1975).
4. S. J. A. Kazmi and A. G. Mitchell, Preservation of solubilized and emulsified systems I: Correlation of mathematically predicted preservation availability with antimicrobial activity, *J. Pharm. Sci.*, 67: 1260 (1978).
5. S. J. A. Kazmi and A. G. Mitchell, Preservation of solubilized and emulsified systems II: Theoretical development of capacity and its role in antimicrobial activity of chlorocresol in cetomacrogol-stabilized systems, *J. Pharm. Sci.*, 67: 1266 (1978).
6. M. S. Roberts, A. E. Polack, G. Martin and H. D. Blackburn, The storage of selected substances in aqueous solution in polyethylene containers: The effect of some physicochemical factors on the disappearance kinetics of the substances, *Inter. J. Pharm.*, 2: 295 (1979).
7. T. J. McCarthy, Interaction between aqueous preservative solutions and their plastic containers, *Pharm. Weekblad*, 105: 557 (1970).
8. T. J. McCarthy, Interaction between aqueous preservative solutions and their plastic containers, III, *Pharm. Weekblad*, 107: 1 (1972).
9. B. W. Hancock and A. Naysmith, Hypersensitivity to chlorocresol-preserved heparin, *B.M.J.*, 3: 746 (1975).
10. E. S. Ainley, I. G. Mackrie and D. Macarthur, Adverse reaction to chlorocresol-preserved heparin, *Lancet*, 1: 705 (1977).

USA: I. Lippman*; D. Walking*; G. W. Radebaugh**
UK: M. C. Allwood*; S. Malcolm**; J. Emerson**

Cholesterol

1. Nonproprietary Name
NF: Cholesterol

2. Functional Category
USP: Emulsifying and/or solubilizing agent

3. Synonym
Cholesterin

4. Chemical Names and CAS Registry Number
Cholest-5-en-3-ol, (3β) [57-88-5]
Cholest-5-en-3β-ol [57-88-5]

5. Empirical Formula   Molecular Weight
$C_{27}H_{46}O$ 386.67

6. Structural Formula

7. Commercial Availability
USA
Atomergic Chemetals Corp.
Bage, Inc.
Burlington Bio-Medical Corp.
Byron Chemical Co.
Canada Packers, Inc., Chemical Div.
Fanning Corp., The
ICN K & K Labs, Inc.
Lanaetex Products, Inc.
Organon, Inc.
Pfaltz & Bauer, Inc.
RITA Corp.
Robeco Chemicals, Inc.
Ruger Chemical Co.
Salsbury Laboratories, Inc., Chemical Dept.

UK
BDH Chemicals Ltd.
Croda Chemicals Ltd.
Koch-Light Labs, Ltd.
Sigma London Chemicals, Co., Ltd.

8. Method of Manufacture
The commercial product is normally obtained from the spinal cord of cattle by extraction with petroleum ethers (another natural source is as a component of wool lipids). Purification is normally accomplished by repeated bromination. Total synthesis has also been accomplished.

9. Description
A nearly odorless to faintly yellow solid which may become yellow to tan upon exposure to light and air.

SEM: MF-1
Excipient: Cholesterol
Manufacturer: Pfaltz & Bauer, Inc.

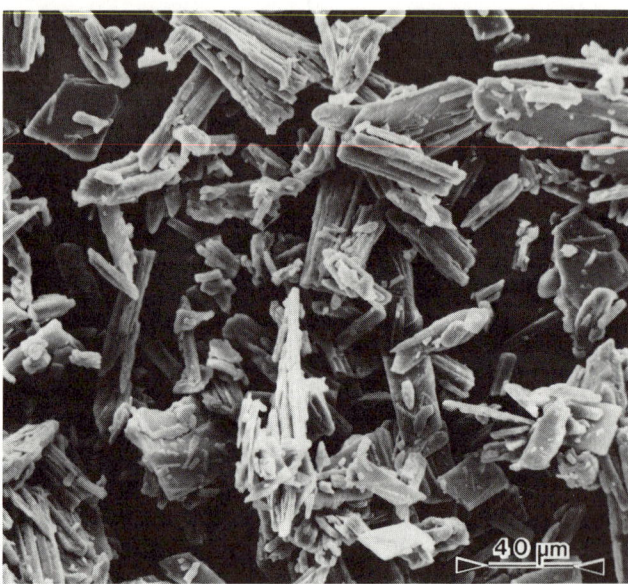

Magnification: 240×

SEM: MF-1
Excipient: Cholesterol

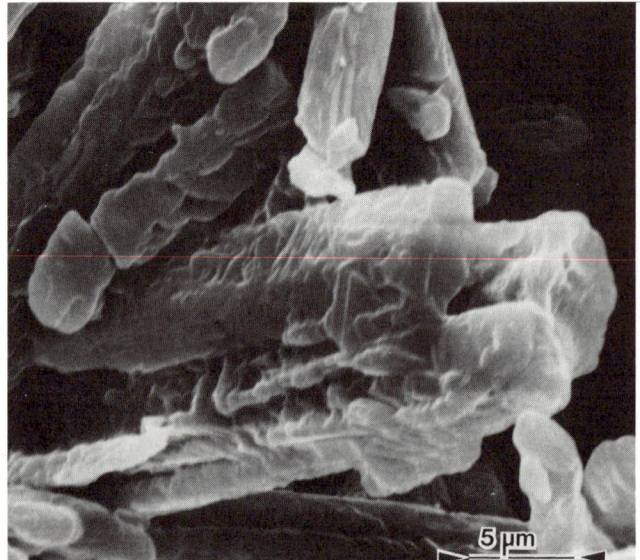

Magnification: 2,400×

10. Pharmacopeial Specifications

Test	NF
Identification	+
Acidity	≤0.3 ml 0.1N H_2SO_4 per 1.0 g sample
Loss on drying	≤0.3%
Residue on ignition	≤0.1%
Melting range	147° to 150° C
Specific rotation (2% w/v in dioxane)	−34° to −38°

11. Typical Properties

Solubility: Practically insoluble in water.

12. Stability and Storage Conditions

Stable. Store in a well-closed, light-resistant container.

13. Incompatibilities

Precipitated by digitonin.

14. Safety

—

15. Handling Precautions

None stated in literature but, due to alleged complicity of cholesterol in atherosclerosis and gallstones, inhalation or ingestion should probably be avoided.

16. Regulatory Acceptance

NF XVI

17. Applications in Pharmaceutical Formulation or Technology

Used in varying concentrations as an emulsifier in o/w emulsions or absorption ointment bases.

18. Related Substances

Cholesterol is a major component of lanolin alcohol (NF XVI), which is also used as an emulsifying agent in ointments and related dermatological products.

19. Comments

—

20. Specific References

1. J. B. Bogardus, Unusual cholesterol solubility in water/ glyceryl-1-monooctanoate solution, *J. Pharm. Sci.*, 71 (3): 370-372 (1982).
2. K. M. Feld, W. I. Higuchi and C-C Su, Influence of benzalkonium chloride on the dissolution behavior of several solid-phase preparations of cholesterol in bile acid solutions, *J. Pharm. Sci.*, 71(2): 182-188 (1982).

USA: A. Repta*; D. Walkling*

Citric Acid

1. Nonproprietary Names
USP: Citric acid anhydrous or monohydrate
BP/EP: Citric acid, citric acid monohydrate

2. Functional Category
USP: Acidifying agent, buffering agent
BP/EP: None
Others: Antioxidant, plasticizer; in film coatings; flavor enhancer

3. Synonyms
—

4. Chemical Names and CAS Registry Numbers
USP: 1,2,3-Propanetricarboxylic acid, 2-hydroxy-monohydrate [5949-29-1]
BP: 2-hydroxypropane-1,2,3-tricarboxylic acid [77-92-9]

5. Empirical Formula Molecular Weight
$C_6H_8O_7 \cdot H_2O$ 210.14
$C_6H_8O_7$ 192.12

6. Structural Formula

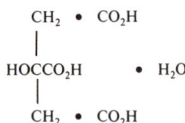

$$CH_2 \bullet CO_2H$$
$$|$$
$$HOCCO_2H \quad \bullet \quad H_2O$$
$$|$$
$$CH_2 \bullet CO_2H$$

7. Commercial Availability
USA
Ashland Chemical Co.
Bage, Inc.
Baker Chemical Co., J. T.
Browning Chemical Corp.
Continental Water Systems Corp.
Fallek Chemical Co.
Gallard-Schlesinger Chemical Mfg. Corp.
Hoffmann-LaRoche, Inc.
McKesson Chemical Co.
Miles Laboratories, Inc./Citro-tech Products/Industrial Mktg. Dept.
Neal & Co., M. F.
Pfaltz & Bauer, Inc.
Pfizer, Inc.-Chemical Div.
Ruger Chemical Co.
Sturge, Ltd., John & E.
Thompson-Hayward Chemical Co.
Uhe Co., George
United States Biochemicals Corp.

UK
Dinoval Ltd.
K & K-Greef
Pfizer Ltd.
Roche Products
Sturge, Ltd., John & E.

8. Method of Manufacture
Citric acid anhydrous is produced by mycological fermentation using crude sugars, such as, molasses and strains of aspergillus niger. It is also extracted from citrus fruit (lemon juice contains 5-8%) and pineapple waste.
Citric acid monohydrate crystals are formed from cold, aqueous solutions of citric acid, anhydrous.

9. Description
Colorless, translucent crystals, or white, granular to fine crystalline powder. It is odorless and has a strong acidic taste. It is effervescent in dry air.

SEM: MF-3
Excipient: Citric acid monohydrate
Supplier: Pfizer Co., Ltd.

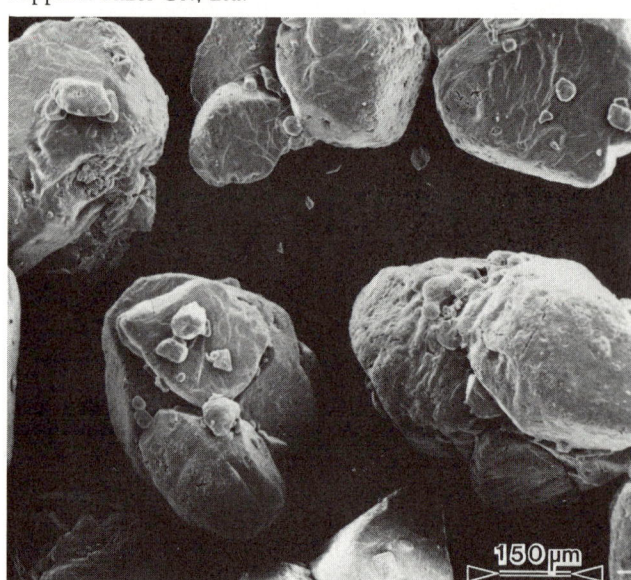

Magnification: 60×

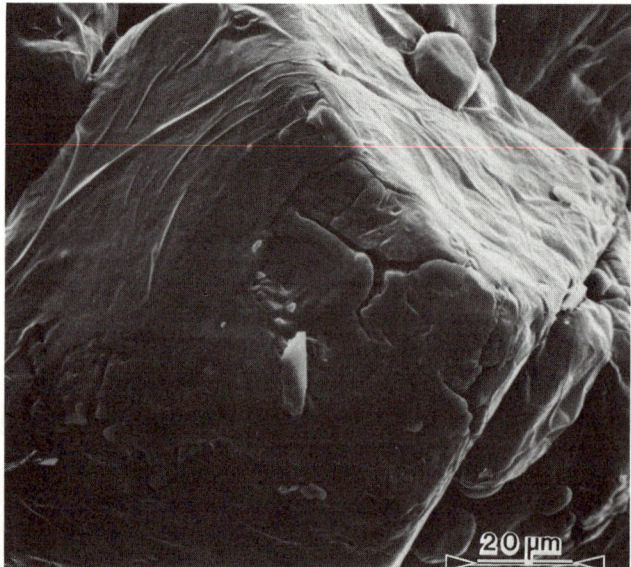

Magnification: 600×

SEM: MF-4
Excipient: Citric acid anhydrous
Supplier: Pfizer Co., Ltd.

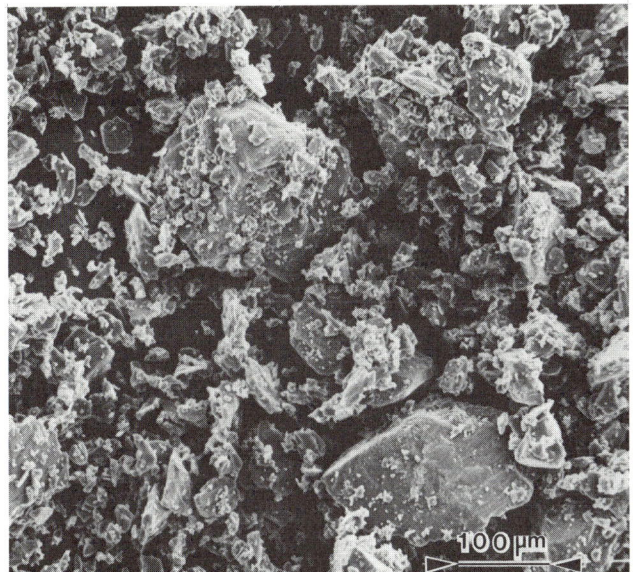

Magnification: 120×

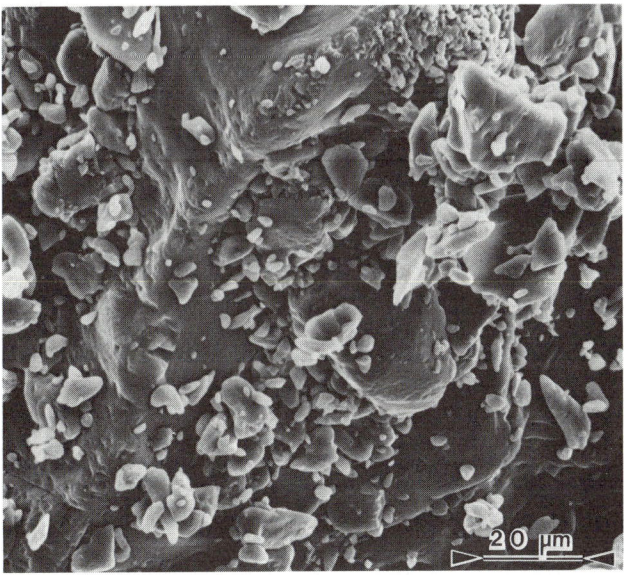

Magnification: 600×

10. Pharmacopeial Specifications

Test	NF	BP/EP
Assay	99.5-100.5% $C_6H_8O_7$ (anhydrous basis)	99.5-101.0% $C_6H_8O_7$ (anhydrous basis)
Identification	+	+
Water	≤0.5% (anhydrous) ≤8.8% (hydrous)	≤1.0% w/w (anhydrous) 7.5%-9.0% (mono-hydrate)
Residue on ignition	0.05%	—
Oxalate	+	≤500 ppm
Sulfate	+	+
Arsenic	3 ppm	—
Heavy metals	≤0.001%	≤10 ppm
Readily carbonizable substances	+	+
Clarity & color of solution	—	+
Barium	—	+
Calcium	—	+
Iron	—	≤50 ppm
Chloride	—	≤50 ppm
Sulphated ash	—	≤0.1%

11. Typical Properties

Solubility: Very soluble in water; freely soluble in alcohol; sparingly soluble in ether

Crystal structure: Orthohombic, monoclinic holohedra (anhydrous)

Melting point: 100° C (monobydrate); 153° C anhydrous

pH of 0.1 N Solution: 2.2; slightly deliquescent in moist air

pk_1: 3.128 at 25° C

pk_2: 4.761 at 25°C

pk_3: 6.396 at 25°C

Density: 1.665 g/cm^3

Academy HPE Laboratory Project Data		
Method	**Lab #**	**Results**
Citric acid, hydrous powder		
% Consolidation BTD-6	8	Volume: 23.3%
% Consolidation BTD-6	8	Weight: 23.0%
Hydrous, fine granular		
% Consolidation BTD-6	8	Volume: 5.0%
% Consolidation BTD-6	8	Weight: 7.0%
Hydrous, granular		
% Consolidation BTD-6	8	Volume: 7.5%
% Consolidation BTD-6	8	Weight: 6.0%

Method	Lab #	Results
Citric acid anhydrous powder		
% Consolidation BTD-6	8	Volume: 23.0%
% Consolidation BTD-6	8	Weight: 16.0%
Citric acid, fine granular anhydrous		
% Consolidation BTD-6	8	Volume: 8.5%
% Consolidation BTD-6	8	Weight: 7.0%
Citric acid, anhydrous, granular		
% Consolidation BTD-6	8	Volume: 6.0%
% Consolidation BTD-6	8	Weight: 6.0%

Supplier: Pfizer, Inc. Chemical Div.

12. Stability and Storage Conditions

Stable. Store in tight containers (USP) or well closed containers (BP/EP).

13. Incompatibilities

Citric acid is incompatible with potassium tartrate, alkali, alkaline earth carbonates and bicarbonates, acetates and sulfite. Dilute aqueous solutions may ferment on standing.

14. Safety

LD_{50} I.P. in rats: 975 mg/kg of body weight.

15. Handling Precautions

16. Regulatory Acceptance

USP XXI; BP/EP 1980

17. Applications in Pharmaceutical Formulation or Technology

Use	Concentration (%)
Improve flavor-liquid formulations	0.3-2.0
Buffer solution	>1M
Sequestering agent	0.3-2.0
Antioxidant	0.3-2.0

18. Related Substances

—

19. Comments

—

20. Specific References

1. N. R. Anderson, G. S. Banker, G. E. Peck, "Quantitative Evaluation of Pharmaceutical Effervescent Systems II: Stability Monitoring by Realitivity and Porosity Measurement," *J. Pharm Sci.*, 71(1): 7-13 (1982).

USA: T. Gillette*; G. E. Amidon**

Pharmaceutical Coloring Agents

Definition

A pharmaceutical coloring agent (colorant) is "any material that is a dye, pigment or other substance made by a process of synthesis, or extracted, isolated or otherwise derived from a vegetable, animal, mineral or other source that is employed solely in a pharmaceutical product to impart a color". (This quotation is an excerpt from a more detailed definition published in the Code of Federal Regulations).

Classification

According to their origin, colorants may be classified into three major groups: synthetic organic dyes, mineral pigments, and natural colorants. For technical and economic reasons, the application of natural colorants in pharmaceuticals is minimal. Therefore, this monograph concentrates on the properties of selected synthetic organic dyes and mineral pigments, but mention is also made of β-carotene and caramel. Colorants presently approved in the USA and in the UK are listed in Exhibit I and Exhibit II, respectively.

Purity

Table I summarizes the general purity requirements established in the USA, by the EEC (European Economic Community) and by the FAO/WHO (Food and Agriculture Organization and World Health Organization of the United Nations). These are valid unless otherwise specified in the individual monograph for any particular colorant.

Inorganic Impurities—The colorants should contain not more than 100 mg/kg of the following substances, taken separately: antimony, copper, chromium, zinc, barium sulphate, and not more than 200 mg/kg of these products taken together. They should not contain cadmium, mercury, selenium, tellurium, thallium, uranium or chromates, or soluble combinations of barium in detectable quantities.

Organic Impurities—The colorants should not contain (a) 2-naphthylamine, benzidine, amino-4-diphenyl (or xenylamine) or their derivatives; (b) polycyclic aromatic hydrocarbons; synthetic organic coloring matters should contain (c) not more than 0.01% of free aromatic amines; (d) sulphonated organic coloring matters should contain not more than 0.2% of substances extractable by diethyl ether.

Chemical and Physical Characteristics of Selected Colorants

In recent years, regulatory agencies in several countries restricted or eliminated the pharmaceutical use of many of the earlier permitted colorants because of carcinogenicity, intolerance, or for other reasons. The colorants selected as typical examples for this monograph are at this time approved not only in the United States and the United Kingdom, but also in a large number of other countries where the use of colorants in pharmaceuticals is regulated.

Erythrosine (FD&C Red No. 3)
Color Index No.: CI 45430
EEC No.: 127
Structure:

Chemical Name: Disodium salt of 3', 6'-Dihydroxy-2', 4', 5', 7'-tetraiodospiro [isobenzofuran-1 (3H) 9'-[9H]-xanthen]-3-one; 2', 4', 5', 7'-tetraiodofluorescein disodium salt
Molecular Weight: 879.92
Class: Xanthene
Preparation: Fluorescein is iodinated in aqueous or alcoholic solution and the product is converted to the disodium salt.
Description: Brown or reddish brown powder.
Absorption Maximum: In water, at 524 nm; in 95% ethanol, at 531 nm.
Color of Aqueous Solution: Cherry red; adding hydrochloric acid causes a yellowish brown precipitate.
Solubility: See Table II.
Stability: See Table III.
Compatibility: Compatible with 10% aqueous saccharose solution, saturated aqueous sodium bicarbonate solution, gelatin. Incompatible with aqueous solutions having a pH less than 4 (e.g., citric acid, ascorbic acid solutions); 10% glucose.

Purity, USA:
Volatile matter (at 135°C) and chlorides and sulfates (calculated as the sodium salts) total ≤13%
Water-insoluble matter ≤0.2%
Unhalogenated intermediates, total ≤0.1%

Table I. General Purity Requirements
(Specific purity requirements are listed in this monograph for the colorants selected as examples.)

	USA		EEC*	FAO/WHO
	FD&C	D&C		
Water insoluble matter				≤0.2%
Ether extracts				≤0.2%
Lead	≤10ppm[a]	≤20ppm[a]	≤20ppm	≤10ppm
Arsenic	≤1.4ppm[a]	≤2ppm[a]	≤5ppm	≤3ppm
Subsidiary colors			≤4%	≤4%
Volatile matter (135°C)				≤15%
Chlorides and sulfates (as Na salts)				≤15%
Inter-mediates			≤0.5% (except free aromatic amines)	≤0.5%
Miscellaneous	Heavy metals (except Pb and As) by pre-cipitation as sulfides			
	≤ trace	≤30 ppm		

[a] For provisionally listed colors only.
*Additional general EEC requirements:

NaI ≤0.4%
Triiodoresorcinol ≤0.2%
2(2′, 4′-Dihydroxy-3′, 5′-diiodo-benzoyl) benzoic acid ≤0.2%
Monoiodofluoresceins ≤1.0%
Other lower iodinated fluoresceins ≤9.0%
Pb ≤10 ppm
As ≤3 ppm
Total color ≥87%

Purity, EEC:
Products insoluble in water ≤0.2%
Mineral iodides ≤1000 mg/kg (assessed as NaI)
Accessory colorings ≤3%
Fluorescein: no detectable trace
General restrictions (Table I)

Application: Coloring foods and pharmaceuticals. Disclosing agent in dental tablets (showing plaques on teeth).

Tartrazine (FD&C Yellow No. 5)
Color Index No.: CI 19140
EEC No.: 102
Structure:

Chemical Name: 4, 5-Dihydro-5-oxo-(4-sulfophenyl) 4-[(4-sulfophenyl) azo]-1H-pyrazole-3-carboxylic acid trisodium salt
Class: Monoazo; pyrazolone
Preparation: Phenylhydrazine p-sulfonic acid is condensed with sodium ethyl oxalacetate; the obtained product is coupled wtih diazotized sulfanilic acid.
Description: Yellow or orange-yellow powder.
Absorption Maximum: At 425 nm
Color of Aqueous Solution: Yellow. It retains its color upon addition of hydrochloric acid; with sodium hydroxide, it turns reddish.
Solubility: See Table II.
Stability: See Table III.
Compatibility: Poorly compatible with citric acid solution. Incompatible with ascorbic acid, lactose, 10% glucose and saturated aqueous solution of sodium bicarbonate. Gelatin accelerates the fading of the color.
Applications: For product identity, and for improving appearance.

Purity, USA:
Volatile matter (at 135°C) and chlorides and sulfates (calculated as the sodium salts) ≤13.0%
Water insoluble matter ≤0.2%
Phenylhydrazine-p-sulfonic acid ≤0.1%
Other uncombined intermediates ≤0.2%
Subsidiary dyes ≤1.0%
Lead (as Pb) 10 ppm
Arsenic (as As) ≤3 ppm
Total color ≥87.0%
U.S. regulations require that prescription drugs for human use containing FD&C Yellow No. 5 bear the warning statement "This product contains FD&C Yellow No. 5 (tartrazine) which may cause allergic-type reactions (including bronchial asthma) in certain susceptible persons. Although the overall incidence of FD&C Yellow No. 5 (tartrazine) sensitivity in the general population is low, it is frequently seen in patients who also have aspirin hypersensitivity."

Purity, EEC:
Products insoluble in water ≤0.2%
Accessory colorings ≤1%
General restrictions (Table I)

Yellow Orange S (FD&C Yellow No. 6)
(Sunset Yellow FCF)
Color Index No.: CI 15985
EEC No.: 110
Structure:

Chemical Name: Disodium salt of 1-p-sulfophenylazo-2-naphthol-6-sulfonic acid
Molecular Weight: 452.37
Class: Monoazo
Preparation: Diazotized sulfanilic acid is coupled with Schaeffer's salt (sodium salt of beta-naphthol-6-sulfonic acid).
Description: Reddish yellow powder.
Absorption Maximum: 482 nm
Color of Aqueous Solution: Bright orange.
Solubility: See Table II.
Stability: See Table III.
Compatibility: Compatible with citric acid, glucose and saccharose solutions, and with the saturated solution of sodium bicarbonate. Incompatible with ascorbic acid, gelatin.

Purity, USA:
Volatile matter (at 135°C) ≤10.0%
Water-insoluble matter ≤0.5%
Ether extracts ≤0.2%
Chlorides and sulfates of sodium ≤5.0%
Mixed oxides ≤1.0%
Subsidiary dyes ≤5.0%
Pure dye (as determined by titration with titanium trichloride) ≥85.0%

Purity, EEC:
Products insoluble in water ≤0.2%
General restrictions (Table I)

Application: Pharmaceutical and food colorant.

Indigotine (FD&C Blue No. 2)
(Indigo Carmine)
Color Index No.: CI 73015
EEC No.: 132
Structure:

Chemical Name: Disodium salt of 5, 5′-indigotin-disulfonic acid
Molecular Weight: 466.37
Class: Indigoid
Preparation: Indigo is sulfonated with concentrated or fuming sulfuric acid
Description: Dark blue powder

Absorption Maximum: 604 nm
Color of Aqueous Solution: Blue or bluish purple
Solubility: See Table II
Stability: See Table III
Compatibility: Poorly compatible with citric acid and saccharose solution. Incompatible with ascorbic acid, glucose, lactose, sodium bicarbonate (saturated solution), gelatin.

Purity, USA:
Sum of volatile matter (at 135°C) and chlorides and sulfates (calculated as sodium salts) ≤15.0%
Water-insoluble matter ≤0.4%
Isatin-5-sulfonic acid ≤0.4%
5-Sulfoanthranilic acid ≤0.2%
Disodium salt of 2-(1, 3-dihydro-3-oxo-7-sulfo-2H-indol-2-ylidene)-2, 3-dihydro-3-oxo-1H-indole-5-sulfonic acid ≤18%.

Sodium salt of 2-(1, 3-dihydro-3-oxo-2H-indol-2-ylidene)-2, 3-dihydro-3-oxo-1H-indole-5-sulfonic acid ≤2%.
Lead (as Pb) ≤10 ppm
Arsenic (as As) ≤3 ppm
Mercury (as Hg) ≤1 ppm
Total color ≥85%

Purity, EEC:
Products insoluble in water ≤0.2%
Accessory colorings ≤1%
Isatinsulfonic acid ≤1%
General restrictions (Table 1)

Application: Coloring pharmaceutical preparations, including nylon surgical sutures.

Table II. Solubility Properties of Selected Dyes

| | SOLVENT (Solubility in g/liter; approximate values) | | | | | | | |
| | Water | | | Ethanol | Ace- | Glycerol | Propylene Glycol | |
	2°	25°	60°	75% (25°)	tone	100% (25°)	100% (25°)	50% (25°)
Erythrosine	90	90	170	6	1	200	200	68
Tartrazine	38	200	200	11	I*	180	70	200
Yellow Orange S	190	190	200	3	26	200	22	200
Indigotine	8	16	22	0.7	0.03	10	1	6

*I = Insoluble

Table III. Stability Properties of Selected Dyes

| | Heat Stability | | Light | pH | Oxi-dizing | Reduc-ing | Color Stability of Tablets (*) |
	105°	205°			Agents		
Erythrosine	G	A	P to G	(≥ 7)G (≤ 6)P	P	VP	<1 day
Tartrazine	O	VG	G to VG	(≤ 10)G			> 3 days
Yellow Orange S	VG	VG	G to VG	G		P	1-3 days
Indigotine	A	P	VP to P	P	VP	VP	> 3 days

(*) Measured on solid dosage forms (colored tablets), exposed to Xenotest of 200,00 lux irradiation.

A = Acceptable
G = Good
O = Outstanding

P = Poor
VG = Very good
VP = Very poor

Lakes

In manufacturing sugar coated and film coated tablets, as well as suppositories, the soluble synthetic organic dyes have been recently replaced by their lakes. These lakes are prepared by dissolving the soluble salt of the dye in water and precipitating it onto the surface of an aluminum hydrate substrate with the aid of aluminum sulfate. The excess water is removed by filtration or centrifugation, then the product is washed, dried and milled. If greater tinctorial strength is required, the particle size can be reduced to less than 1 μm.

The lakes owe their popularity to their limited solubility. In the case of coated tablets, this prevents color migration from the coating toward the core resulting in less surface variation in color on an individual table (mottling). Also, commercial lakes have a high purity, and therefore, conform with the stringent requirement affecting colorants for foods and drugs. The lakes' tinctorial strength, brightness and chemical resistance are less than the corresponding properties of the technical grade toner pigments,* but their light stability is better than that of soluble dyes.

Table IV summarizes data for selected aluminum lakes important to the pharmaceutical profession.

*An organic pigment containing no substratum or diluent.

Table IV. Characteristic Properties of Aluminum Lakes

		Erythrosine	Indigotine	Yellow Orange S	Tartrazine
Appearance		Rose red powder	Reddish blue powder	Reddish yellow powder	Greenish yellow powder
Pure dye content (%)		15–40	12–34	15–40	15–39
Solubility (% dye dissolved)	pH 1.3	0.4–0.5	84.2	93.8	97.2
	3	0.5–8.3	13.2	5.7	18.8
	5	77.3–88.2			
	7	75.7–86.5			
Chemical resistance Alkali		F	F	F	F
Acid		P	F	G	G

G = Good   F — Fair   P — Poor

Titanium Dioxide (TiO$_2$)
Color Index No.: CI 77891
EEC No.: 171
Molecular Weight: 79.90
Class: Inorganic pigment
Preparation: Ilmenite (FeTiO$_3$) is reacted with sulfuric acid, and the acidic solution is seeded with anatase or rutile crystals. The hydrolysate is calcinated and milled. Titanium may be also oxidized directly, or volatile inorganic titanium salts can be oxidized to titanium dioxide.
Description: White, odorless, tasteless powder.
Solubility: Insoluble in water, hydrochloric acid, nitric acid or diluted sulfuric acid. Soluble in hot concentrated sulfuric acid and in hydrofluoric acid. Also, it may be made soluble by fusion with potassium bisulfate, alkali hydroxides or carbonates.

Purity, USA:
Lead (as Pb) $\leq$ 10 ppm
Arsenic (as As) $\leq$ 1 ppm
Antimony (as Sb) $\leq$ 2 ppm
Mercury (as Hg) $\leq$ 1 ppm
Loss on ignition at 800° C (after drying for 3 hours at 105° C) $\leq$ 0.5%
Water soluble substances $\leq$ 0.3%
Acid soluble substances $\leq$ 0.5%
TiO$_2$ $\geq$ 99.0% (after drying for 3 hours at 105° C)
Lead, arsenic, and antimony shall be determined in the solution obtained by boiling 10 grams of the titanium dioxide for 15 minutes in 50 milliliters of 0.5N hydrochloric acid.

Purity, EEC:
Substances soluble in hydrochloric acid $\leq$ 0.0175 g/5 g (as the HC1 salt)
Pb $\leq$ 100 mg/kg
Zn $\leq$ 50 mg/kg
Soluble Ba compounds $\leq$ 5 mg/kg
General restrictions (except Pb) (Table I)

Application: Titanium dioxide is utilized to impart a white color on film coated tablets, sugar coated tablets, and gelatin capsules; in lakes, as an opacifier to ''extend'' the color. In addition to its use as a colorant, it is applied in topical preparations as a UV absorber.

Iron Oxides
Color Index No.: CI 77491 (red, brown)
CI 77492 (yellow)
CI 77499 (black)
EEC No.: 172
Formula: Yellow: Fe$_2$O$_3$.H$_2$O (97-98% monohydrate)
Red: Fe$_2$O$_3$
Black (or brown): FeO.Fe$_2$O$_3$
Manufacturing Process: Fe^{2+} salt solutions are precipitated and oxidized to black (or brown) iron oxide.
Description: Yellow, red, black or brown powder. Its color depends on the particle size, shape and the amount of the combined water.
Solubility: Insoluble in water, partially soluble in strong mineral acids.
Compatibility: It was reported that iron oxides make hard gelatin capsules brittle at higher temperatures when the residual moisture is 11-12%. This factor affects the use of iron oxides for coloring hard gelatin capsules and would limit the amount to be incorporated into the gelatin material.

Purity, USA:
As $\leq$ 3 ppm
Pb $\leq$ 10 ppm
Hg $\leq$ 3 ppm

Purity, EEC:
Se $\leq$ 2 mg/kg
Hg $\leq$ 1 mg/kg
General restrictions (Table I)

Applications: Iron oxides are gaining importance as mineral colorants as a result of recent limitations affecting many synthetic organic dyestuffs. Nevertheless, its use as a colorant is limited in the USA to a maximum ingestion of 5 mg of elemental iron per day. There are also some technical limitations (e.g., dullness of shade, weak tinctorial power, abrasiveness).

β-Carotene

Color Index No.: CI 75130 (natural)
CI 40800 (synthetic)
EEC No.: E160 (a)
Structure:

Molecular Weight: 536.89

Manufacturing Process: All industrial processes for carotinoids are based on β-ionone. This can be obtained by total synthesis from acetone and acetylene via dehydrolinalool. $β_{14}$-C-aldehyde and $β$-C_{19}-aldehyde are subsequent important intermediates. From two moles of $β$-C_{19}-aldehyde and acetylene, symmetrical β-carotene is synthesized.

Description: In the pure state it exists as red crystals (from light petroleum). β-Carotene is very susceptible to oxidation and commercially available material has to be stabilized by physical and chemical methods.

Solubility:

Water	insoluble
Ethanol	below 0.01%
Glycerol	insoluble
Fats, oils	0.05-0.08%
Chloroform	about 3%

Purity, USA:
1% solution in chloroform: clear
LOD ≤ 0.2%
Residue on ignition ≤ 0.2%
Pb ≤ 10 ppm
As ≤ 3 ppm
Assay (spectrophotometrically): 96-101%

Purity, EEC: Only general requirements.

Applications: β-Carotene is capable of producing shades varying from pale yellow to dark orange. It can be used as a color for sugar coated tablets prepared by the ladle process. Its instability toward light is a disadvantage and maximum use should be made of pack protection for the product. Spray coating techniques present even more of a light instability problem, probably due to atmosphere oxygen attack on the finely dispersed spray droplets.

Because of its water insolubility it cannot be used to color clear totally aqueous systems, and co-solvents such as ethanol must be used.

Suppository masses have been successfully colored with β-carotene in approximately 0.1% concentration.

Incompatibilities: Generally incompatible with oxidizing agents when decolorization will take place. Where light instability is a problem, consideration should be given to antioxidants, e.g., tocopherol or ascorbic acid.

Commercial β-carotene is usually available extended on a matrix such as acacia and malto-dextrin; tocopherol and sodium ascorbate are added as antioxidants. Individual containers are sealed under nitrogen. These forms of β-carotene are dispersible in aqueous systems.

β-Carotene is also available as micronized crystals suspended in an edible oil such as arachis oil.

Caramel

EEC No.: E150
Class: Processed substance derived from carbohydrate starting material.

Background: Caramel of commerce is produced almost exclusively for the food industry where this color constitutes, in weight terms, the vast majority of the total food color used by the industry. The number of different caramel products available is enormous but unfortunately they cannot be defined in chemical terms. Recently, moves have been made to restrict the number available so that caramel can be a much more closely defined product. Currently, the list stands at ten different types, the caramel in each case being defined by manufacturing process and product specification.

Description: A thick but free flowing dark reddish brown liquid with a slight odor.

Solubility and Stability: Generally soluble in aqueous media; compatible with dilute acids and alkalis. Pharmaceutical caramels are precipitated by high concentrations of alcohol (over approximately 60% v/v). Caramel types are available, however, which will tolerate high alcohol concentrations (caustic caramels).

Caramel is generally immiscible with organic solvents including acetone, ether, chloroform and light petroleum.

Manufacture: It is produced by heating a carbohydrate product in the presence of an accelerator. Caramel is not burnt sugar.

Purity, USA:
Pb≤10 ppm
As≤3 ppm
Hg≤0.1 ppm

Purity, EEC: General requirements must be met (Table I). Note that the BPC specification differs in the following aspects:
Cu≤300 ppm
Pb≤5 ppm
Fe≤100 ppm

Uses: Caramel is used to color liquid preparations. It gives clear solutions over a wide pH range. It is of course compatible with high sucrose concentration and can tolerate the alcohol levels encountered in internal preparations containing this solvent. Its stability towards light is good.

Caramel is not a neutral substance thus ammonia caramels are positively charged and ammonia sulphate caramels are negatively charged so that specific incompatibilities with large, charged molecules in a formula could exist.

Caramel is capable in aqueous solution of producing colors ranging from pale straw yellow to dark brown.

Analytical Methods

The chemical analysis of dyestuffs is as diversified as their chemical structure. During the manufacturing process several by-products and impurities may develop as well as unreacted intermediates. It is necessary to select an appropriate test method for each colorant, and determine the amount of impurities as a strict measure of quality control. The EEC directives specify the general and individual criteria for purity but usually fail to describe specific analytical procedures for determining either the pure dye content, or the amount of impurities. Therefore, it is left to the individual countries to set their own regulations regarding acceptable methods for colorant analysis. In the USA, the most generally used methods are those listed in the 9th and subsequent editions of the *Official Methods of Analysis*. In addition, a large number of papers have been published describing selective methods for the analysis of dyestuffs and pigments. Particularly helpful is the reference book by D.M. Marmion.

Color Measurements

Color is a physical phenomenon which is related to the radiant energy of the light that reaches the human eye after being reflected from and/or transmitted through an object. Obviously, the color perception varies with an individual's vision. Nevertheless, the reflected (or transmitted) light may be measured by optical instruments (such as a spectrophotometer). The instrument may be modified to measure the color, and this is done by comparing it to a standard such as barium sulfate or magnesium oxide. The photoelectric instruments measure the tristimulus values (the so-called color coordinates), and often with the aid of computers calculate the numerical values which can be used to define a color.

Pharmaceutical colorants are the best aids for identifying a product throughout the manufacturing and distribution process, and they are indispensable for the consumer. They certainly are "pharmaceutical necessities," and considerable efforts are made to reverse the current trend to eliminate the use of many colorants unless compelling and convincing scientific evidence would justify this action. Both in the USA and UK, government agencies and official committees supervise and regulate the use of colorants for pharmaceuticals.

Regulations: Historically, excipients, including colorants, were considered "inert" components with no or insignificant physiological effects. In the past decades, however, it has been recognized that excipients may chemically or physically interact with the drug substance, and influence its efficacy. Therefore, regulatory requirements for excipients are now established in many countries.

In the USA, the Food and Drug Administration is entrusted to regulate the manufacture and use of pharmaceuticals, and the 1960 Color Additive Amendments to the Food, Drug and Cosmetic Act define the responsibility of the Agency. The Act and its amendments require that colors for use in foods, drugs and cosmetics be shown to be safe for their intended uses. Exhibit I demonstrates the present status of the colorants application for drugs in the USA. While actually a fairly large selection of colors is available, many of the colorants are restricted to external use only, or otherwise. Regulations for individual colorants may impose specific restrictions, and usually permit their use only "in amounts consistent with good manufacturing practices." The major concern regarding the safety of colorants is their potential carcinogenicity, tolerance problems or lack of experimental evidence proving their safety. Expert committees of the World Health Organization have established and periodically update "Acceptable Daily Intake" (ADI) levels for the colorants. These are considered guidelines observed or approximated by many of the member nations. WHO also maintains an international monitoring system whose participants report adverse reactions observed on drugs or excipients including colorants.

The manufacture and analysis of dyestuffs is of a complex nature and many colorants approved permanently or provisionally for drug use need batch-to-batch certification by the FDA prior to their release to the user. (See Exhibit I.)

An effort has been made in recent years to reduce the number of dyes under provisional listing. Out of 84 colors on the list in 1976, only 11 remained in pending by May 1984. [Further details are available in the Code of Federal Regulations, Title 21.]

In the United Kingdom, the use of colors is regulated in compliance with EEC directives. Particularly important is directive 78/25/EEC (12 December 1977) which declares that "on health grounds, there is no reason why the Colouring Matters authorized for use in foodstuffs intended for human consumption should not also be authorized for use in medicinal products." The Colouring Matter in Food Regulations (1973) and its amendments include the coloring agents listed in Exhibit II. Unlike the United States, the EEC has no system for batch certification.

Exhibit I

List of Coloring Agents Permitted for Use in Drugs in the USA (as of April 1, 1984)

Permanently Listed	Restrictions	Subject to Certification
Alumina (Dried Aluminum Hydroxide)		No
Aluminum Powder	E*	No
Annatto Extract	(c)	No
Bismuth Oxychloride	E*	No
Bronze Powder	E*	No
Calcium Carbonate		No
Canthaxanthin	I	No
Caramel		No
β-Carotene	(c)	No
Chromium-Cobalt-Aluminum Oxide	S	No
Chromium Hydroxide Green	E*	No
Chromium Oxide Greens	E*	No
Cochineal Extract: Carmine		No
Copper Powder	E*	No
Dihydroxyacetone	E**	No
D&C Blue No. 4	E	Yes
D&C Blue No. 6	S-1	Yes
D&C Blue No. 9	S**	Yes
D&C Green No. 5	(a)	Yes
D&C Green No. 6	E, (b)	Yes
D&C Green No. 8	E (≤0.01%)	Yes
D&C Orange No. 4	E	Yes
D&C Orange No. 5	(d)	Yes
D&C Orange No. 10	E	Yes
D&C Red No. 6	(f)	Yes
D&C Red No. 7	(f)	Yes
D&C Red No. 17	E	Yes
D&C Red No. 21		Yes
D&C Red No. 22		Yes
D&C Red No. 27		Yes
D&C Red No. 28		Yes
D&C Red No. 30		Yes
D&C Red No. 31	E	Yes
D&C Red No. 34	E	Yes
D&C Red No. 39	E, (k)	Yes
D&C Violet No. 2	E, S-2	Yes
D&C Yellow No. 7	E	Yes
D&C Yellow No. 8	E	Yes
D&C Yellow No. 10		Yes
D&C Yellow No. 11	E	Yes
Ext. D&C Yellow No. 7	E	Yes
Ferric Ammonium Citrate	S-3	No
Ferric Ammonium Ferrocyanide	E*	No
Ferric Ferrocyanide	E*	No
FD&C Blue No. 1		Yes
FD&C Blue No. 2	S-4	Yes
FD&C Green No. 3		Yes
FD&C Red No. 3	(g)	Yes
FD&C Red No. 4	E	Yes
FD&C Red No. 40		Yes
FD&C Red No. 40 Lake		Yes
FD&C Yellow No. 5	(g)	Yes

List of Coloring Agents Permitted for Use in Drugs in the USA (as of April 1, 1984)

Permanently Listed	Restrictions	Subject to Certification
Guanine	E*	No
Iron Oxide, Synthetic	(1)	No
Logwood Extract	S-5	No
Mica	E*	No
Potassium Sodium Copper Chlorophyllin	(m)	No
Pyrogallol	S-6	No
Pyrophyllite	E	No
Talc		No
Titanium Dioxide		No
Zinc Oxide	E*	No

(a)   For Nylon 66 and/or Nylon 6 nonabsorbable surgical sutures, max. 0.6%. Permanent for drugs.

(b)   For polyethylene terephthalate surgical sutures, general and ophthalmic use, max. 0.75%; for polyglycolic acid surgical sutures, general and ophthalmic use, max. 0.1%; listed permanently for externally applied drugs.

(c)   Permitted in products intended for use in the area of the eyes.

I   Ingested drugs only.

E   External only.

E*   External, including products intended for use in the area of the eye.

E**   External only, intended solely or in part to impart a color on the human body.

S   Sutures only, special restrictions (ref. 1, page 255).

S-1   Sutures only, special restrictions (ref. 1, p. 286).

(d)   Internal use for drugs, mouthwashes and dentifrices; external not to exceed 5 mg/day.

(f)   Combined total of D&C Red No. 6 and D&C Red No. 7 not to exceed 5 mg/day.

S-2   Polygalactin 910 sutures, max. 0.2%; polydioxanone sutures, max. 0.3%.

(k)   Quaternary ammonium germicides, max. 0.1%.

S-3   Sutures, special restrictions (ref. 1, page 256).

S-4   Sutures, special restrictions (ref. 1, page 285); max. 1%. Provisional for ingested drugs.

(g)   For ingested use.

S-5   Sutures only; special restrictions (ref. 1, page 263).

(1)   Max. 5 mg Fe/day ingested. External use permitted.

(m)   Dentifrices, max. 0.1%.

(n)   0.75 mg/day ingested.

S-6   Sutures only; special restrictions (ref. 1, page 262).

List of Coloring Agents Permitted for Use in Drugs in the USA (as of April 1, 1984)

Provisionally Listed	Restrictions	Subject to Certification
D&C Orange No. 17	E	Yes
D&C Red No. 8	(a) (b)	Yes
D&C Red No. 9	(a) (b)	Yes
D&C Red No. 19	E	Yes
D&C Red No. 33	E; (m)	Yes
D&C Red No. 36	E; (o)	Yes
D&C Red No. 37	E	Yes
FD&C Blue No. 2	(p)	Yes
FD&C Red No. 3	E(*)	Yes
FD&C Yellow No. 5	E(*)	Yes
FD&C Yellow No. 6		Yes

E   External only.

(a)   For ingested use, max. 0.1 mg/day. In dentifrices and mouthwashes, see ref. 1, page 324.

(b)   Combined total of D&C Red No. 8 and D&C Red No. 9 for ingested use not to exceed 0.1 mg/day. External use permitted.

(m)   For ingested use, max. 0.75 mg/day. No restriction for dentifrices and mouthwashes.

(o)   For ingested use, max. 1.7 mg/day. No restriction for dentifrices and mouthwashes.

(p)   Provisional for ingested use. For sutures, see permanently listed colorants.

(*)   Permanent for ingested use. See also list for permanently listed colorants.

Exhibit II

List of Coloring Materials Authorized for Coloring Medicinal Products (In the United Kingdom and Other EEC Countries) up to June 1, 1985

(Annex I, Sections I and II of the Directive of October 23, 1962*)

No.	Common Name
E 100	Curcumin
E 101	Lactoflavin (Riboflavin)
E 102	Tartrazine
E 104	Quinoline Yellow
E 110	Orange Yellow S Sunset Yellow FCF
E 120	Cochineal Carminic Acid
E 122	Azorubine Carmoisine
E 123	Amaranth
E 124	Cochineal Red A Ponceau 4R
E 127	Erythrosine
E 131	Patent Blue V
E 132	Indigotin (Indigo Carmine)
E 140	Chlorophylls
E 141	Copper Complexes of Chlorophylls and Chlorophyllins
E 142	Acid Brilliant Green BS (Lissamine Green)
E 150	Caramel
E 151	Brilliant Black BN, Black PN
E 153	Carbo Medicinalis Vegetabilis (Charcoal)
E 160	Carotenoids:
	Alpha-, Beta-, Gamma-Carotene
	Bixin, Norbixin (Roucou Annatto)
	Capsanthin, Capsorubin
	Lycopene
	Beta-apo-8' Carotenal (C 30)
	Ethyl Ester of Beta-apo-8' Carotenoic Acid (C 30)
E 161	Xanthophylls:
	Flavoxanthin
	Lutein
	Kryptoxanthin
	Rubixanthin
	Violaxanthin
	Rhodoxant
	Canthaxanthin
E 162	Beetroot Red, Betanin
E 163	Anthocyanins
E 170**	Calcium Carbonate
E 171	Titanium Dioxide
E 172	Iron Oxides and Hydroxides

No.	Common Name
E 173**	Aluminum
E 174**	Silver
E 175**	Gold

* Council Directive of 23 October 1962 concerning the approximation of legislation of Member States concerning colouring materials which can be utilized in foodstuffs destined for human consumption OJ 115 of 11.11.1962, p. 2645/62.

Amended by:
— Directive 65/469/EEC of 25 October 1965—OJ 178 of 26.10.1965, p. 2793/65
— Directive 67/653/EEC of 24 October 1967—OJ 263 of 30.10.1967, p. 4
— Directive 68/419/EEC of 20 December 1968—OJ L 309 of 24.12.1968, p. 24
— Directive 70/358/EEC of 13 July 1970—OJ L 157 of 18.7.1970, p. 36
— Act of Accession—OJ L 73 of 27.3.1972, p. 14
— Directive 76/399/EEC of 4 April 1976—OJ L 108 of 26.4.1976, p. 19
— Directive 78/144/EEC of 3 January 1978—OJ L 44 of 15.2.1978
** For surface coloring only.

Comments to Exhibit II:
(1) Some Member States have further restrictions on the General EEC List. These are:

	Tartrazine	Amaranth	Lissamine Green
Belgium	F	F	
Denmark	N		
France	N	F	
Germany (FRG)**	N		F
Greece			F
Italy*	F	F	
Luxembourg***	N	N	
Netherlands	N	N	

F = Forbidden

N = Not advisable or legislation pending.

  * Ponceau 4R, Carmoisine, Sunset Yellow and Lissamine Green also 'N' category. Patent Blue V also 'F' category.

  ** Annatto E160B—Forbidden.

*** Vegetable Carbon Black E153—Forbidden.

(2) Also, many member states forbid azo colour, in particular tartrazine, for use in certain therapeutic categories.

Exhibit III

Color Manufacturers

This list is not exhaustive but does detail perhaps the major manufacturers of pharmaceutical color in the USA and Europe.

Water Soluble Dyes:

Bayer AG
Bayerwerk
D-5090 Leverkusen
West Germany

Buffalo Color Corporation
One Garret Mountain Plaza
West Paterson, NJ 07424
USA

Crompton and Knowles Corporation
Route 208
Fair Lawn, NJ 07410
USA

France Couleur S.A.
198-212 Route de Muaux
93410 Vaujours
France

Hilton Davis Chemical Co.
2235 Langdon Farm Road
Cincinnati, OH 45237
USA

Imperial Chemical Industries PLC
Organics Division
P.O. Box 42
Hexagon House
Blackley, Manchester, M9 3DH
England

H. Kohnstamm and Company Inc.
161 Avenue of the Americas
New York, NY 10013
USA

BV Nederlandse Kleursrof Industrie
Kliene Keppel
3940 Amersfoort
Holland

Riedel Arom
Van der Tann Strasse 34/38
Postfach 70
4600 Dortmund 1
West Germany

BASF—Siegle
Farben & Fasern AG
Sieglestr 25
PO Box 300620
D-7000 Stuttgart 30 (Feuerbach)
West Germany

McCormich-Stange Co.
342 North Western Avenue
Chicago, IL 60612
USA

Warner Jenkinson Company
2526 Baldwin Street
St. Louis, MO 63106
USA

Williams (Hounslow) Ltd.
Greville House
Hibernia Road
Hounslow, Middlesex TW3 3RX
England

Aluminum Lakes:

Colorcon Incorporated
904 West Point Pike
West Point, PA 19486
USA
(including F. G. Okie Division)

Crompton and Knowles Corporation
(as previously)

Hilton Davis Chemical Co.
(as previously)

H. Kohnstamm and Company Inc.
(as previously)

Warner Jenkinson Company
(as previously)

Williams (Hounslow) Ltd.
(as previously)

Titanium Dioxide:

BTP Tioxide Limited
Billingham, Cleveland TS23, 1PS
England

Du Pont de Nemours, and Co.
Wilmington, DE 19898
USA

Kronos Titan GmbH.
Postfach 100720
5090 Leverkusen 1
West Germany

β-Carotene:

F. Hoffmann-La Roche & Co., AG
Grenzacherstrasse 124
4058 Basel
Switzerland

Roche Products Ltd.
Fine Chemicals Division
318 High Street North
Dunstable, Beds. LU6 1BG
England

Caramel:

C.P.C. (UK) Ltd.
Industrial Division
Trafford Park
Manchester MI7 1PA
England.

References

1. Code of (USA) Federal Regulations, Title 21, Chapter I, Part 70 (Rev. April 1, 1984).
2. *Official Journal of the European Communities (OJ)*, No. 115, 11.11.62, Annex III.
3. Specifications for Identity and Purity and Toxicological Evaluation of Food Colours. FAO Nutrition Meetings Report Series, 1966, 38B;WHO/Food Add:66.25.
4. *OJ* No. 263/4, 30.10.67.
5. Turi, P., *Pharm. Ind. 39*, 5, 476-482 (1977).
6. Bidollet *et al.*, *R. Sci. Techn. Pharm. 2*, 117 (1973).
7. Spang-Brunner, B. and Schlumpf, M., *Schweiz. Apoth. Ztg. 111*, 37 (1973).
8. *Swiss Excipient Catalogue* (1974), Basel: Ciba-Geigy A.G., Hoffmann-La Roche & Co., and Sandoz, A.G.
9. Dunn, M.J. and Steinbach, S.P., "Food, Drug and Cosmetic Colors," in *Pigment Handbook* (Editor: Patton, T.C.), J. Wiley and Sons, New York (1973).
10. Hess, H. and Schrank, J., "Colouration of Pharmaceuticals—Possibilities and Technical Problems." (Presented at the International Symposium of Dyestuffs in Pharmaceuticals, Munich, June 1978.)
11. *Official Methods of Analysis of the Association of Official Analytical Chemists*, 9th Edition, 1960; 10th Edition, 1965; 11th Edition, 1970; 12th Edition, 1975; 13th Edition, 1980. Editor: Horwitz, Wm. Published by the AOAC, Washington, DC 20044.
12. Judd, D.B. and Wyszecki, G., *Color in Business, Science and Industry*, 2nd Edition. John Wiley and Sons, Inc., New York, 1963.
13. Resolution of the F.I.P. (Federation Internationale Pharmaceutique) on the "Use of Colourants in Pharmaceutical Preparations." 38th International Congress of Pharmaceutical Sciences, Cannes, 1978.
14. Cooper, J., *Australian J. of Pharm. Sciences*, 7, 9 (1978).
15. 8th Report of the Joint FAO/WHO Expert Committee on Food Additives (1965).
16. 18th Report of the Joint FAO/WHO Expert Committee on Food Additives (1974).
17. *Martindale: The Extra Pharmacopia*, 28th Edition (Editor: Reynolds, J.E.F.), Pharmaceutical Press, London (1982).
18. Steinbach, S.P., Personal Communication (Feb. 26, 1979), ref. 1, pp. 239-333.
19. Hogan, J.E., Personal Communication (June 10, 1985).
20. Marmion, D.M., *Handbook of U.S. Colorants for Foods, Drugs and Cosmetics*, 2nd Ed., John Wiley and Sons, Inc., New York 1984. (*Remark:* This Handbook is a comprehensive manual dealing with the regulations, analysis and applications of U.S. colorants.)

USA: P.G. Turi*

UK: T.M. Jones*; J.E. Hogan*

Corn Oil

1. Nonproprietary Name
NF: Corn oil

2. Functional Category
NF: Solvent and oleaginous vehicle

3. Synonyms
Maize oil; Maydol; Mazola oil

4. Chemical Name and CAS Registry Number
Corn oil

5. Empirical Formula and Molecular Weight
—

6. Structural Formula
Corn oil is composed of fatty acids, present as glycerides. A typical analysis of the fatty acids is oleic acid, 43.4%; linoleic acid, 39.1%; palmitic acid, 7.3%; stearic acid, 3.3%; arachidic acid, 0.4%; and lignoceric acid, 0.2%. Also present are small quantities of phosphatides, carbohydrates and coloring matter.

7. Commercial Availability
USA
A. E. Staley Mfg. Co.
Camilli, Albert & Laloue
Dormar Chemicals, Inc.
Durkee Industrial Foods/SCM Corp.
Ingredients International, Inc.
Ruger Chemical Co.
Tri-K Industries, Inc.
United States Biochemicals Corp.
Welch, Holme & Clark Co.

UK
J. Bibby & Sons
M. Hamburger & Sons
E.J.R. Lovelock

8. Method of Manufacture
The germ or embryo of *Zea mays* contains nearly 50% fixed oil, compared with 3.0-6.5% in the whole kernel. The oil is obtained from the embryo by expression. Refining involves treatment in dilute alkali to neutralize the acids, decolorizing with fuller's earth or activated carbon, removing odor with steam under pressure and chilling to remove waxy components.

9. Description
Clear, light yellow, oily liquid having a faint characteristic odor and taste.

10. Pharmacopeial Specifications

Test	NF
Specific gravity	0.914 to 0.921
Heavy metals	$\leq$0.001%
Cottonseed oil	+
Solidification range of the fatty acids	14.0-21.5°C
Free fatty acids	+
Iodine value	102-130
Saponification value	187-193
Unsaponifiable matter	$\leq$1.5%

11. Typical Properties
Refractive index: $n_D^{40} = 1.464\text{-}1.468$
$n_D^{25} = 1.470\text{-}1.474$
Solubility: Slightly soluble in alcohol; miscible with ether, chloroform, benzene and solvent hexane.

Academy HPE Laboratory Project Data

Method	Lab #	Results
		Viscosity
VIS-2	30	37.36 cps[b]
VIS-2	30	38.83 cps[a]
		Specific Gravity
DE-5	30	0.918[a]
DE-5	30	0.915[b]

Supplier: [a]Welch, Holme & Clark Co., [b]Capital

12. Stability and Storage
Stable: the oil should be preserved in a tightly sealed, light-resistant container. Avoid exposure to excessive heat.

13. Incompatibilities
No citations in the literature.

14. Safety
No serious toxic manifestations after oral ingestion have been cited in the literature.

15. Handling Precautions
No restrictions specified.

16. Regulatory Acceptance
NF XVI

17. Applications in Pharmaceutical Formulation or Technology

Use	Concentration
Oral nutritional supplement	67% as emulsion
Emulsion	as required
Cholecystography	as required
Solvent or vehicle for parenteral products	as required

18. Related Substances
Cottonseed oil, peanut oil, sesame oil

19. Comments
None

20. Specific References
None

USA: A. Rahman*; D. Sanvordeker**; F. A. Chrzanowski**

Cottonseed Oil

1. Nonproprietary Name
NF: Cottonseed oil

2. Functional Category
NF: Solvent and oleaginous vehicle

3. Synonym
Cotton oil

4. Chemical Name and CAS Registry Number
Cottonseed oil

5. Empirical Formula   Molecular Weight
—   —

6. Structural Formula
A typical analysis of refined cottonseed oil indicates the composition of the acids, present as glycerides, to be: linoleic acid, 39.3%; oleic acid, 33.1%; palmitic acid, 19.1%; stearic acid, 1.9%; arachidic acid, 0.6%; and myristic acid, 0.3%. Also present are small quantities of phospholipid, phytosterols and pigments. The toxic polyphenolic pigment gossypol is present in raw cottonseed and in the oil cake remaining after expression of oil. It is not found in refined oil.

7. Commercial Availability
USA

Durkee Industrial Foods/SCM Corp.
Ruger Chemical Co.
Tri-K Industries, Inc.
United States Biochemicals Corp.
Welch, Holme & Clark Co.

UK

E.J.R. Lovelock, Ltd.
Forum Chemicals
J. Bibby & Sons, Ltd.

8. Method of Manufacture
The seeds contain about 15% oil. The testae of the seeds are first separated, and the kernels are then exposed to powerful expression in hydraulic presses. The crude oil thus obtained has a bright red or blackish-red color. It requires purification before it is suitable for food or medicinal purposes.

9. Description
Pale yellow or yellow, oily liquid, odorless, or nearly so, with a bland, nutty taste. At temperatures below 10°C, particles of solid fat may separate from the oil; and at about 0° to −5°C, the oil becomes solid or nearly so. If it solidifies, the oil should be remelted and thoroughly mixed before any of it is used.

10. Pharmacopeial Specifications

Test	NF
Identification	+
Specific gravity	0.915 - 0.921
Heavy metals	$\leq$0.001%
Trichloroethylene	+
Solidification range of fatty acids	31° - 35°
Free fatty acids	+
Iodine value	109 - 120
Saponification value	190 - 198

11. Typical Properties
Refractive index: n_D^{40} = 1.4645 to 1.4655
Solubility: Slightly soluble in alcohol; miscible with carbon disulfide, chloroform and petroleum ether.
Viscosity: Up to 70.4 cps (20°C).
Surface Tension: 35.4 dynes/cm (20°C)
31.3 dynes/cm (80°C)

Academy HPE Laboratory Project Data

Method	Lab #	Results
VIS-2	30	Viscosity 39.19 cps
DE-5	30	Specific gravity 0.916

Supplier: Welch, Home & Clark Co.

12. Stability and Storage Conditions
Stable: Store in an airtight, lightresistant container and avoid excessive exposure to heat.

13. Incompatibilities
No citations in the literature.

14. Safety
Intravenous infusion of cottonseed oil emulsions may cause moderate sinus bradycardia and a slight rise in blood pressure. If reactions characterized by dyspnea, cyanosis, myalgia, nausea, vomiting, headache, lumbar pains, flushing, or hypotension develop, the infusion should be stopped. Toxic effects of the emulsion may be treated by intravenous administration of a corticosteroid and an antihistamine. The treatment with epinephrine, 0.5 to 1 ml of a 1 in 1,000 solution by subcutaneous or intramuscular injection, may be necessary. Heparin may be given, if needed, to aid the clearance of fat from the circulation.

15. Handling Precautions
No restrictions specified.

16. Regulatory Acceptance
NF XVI

17. Applications in Pharmaceutical Formulation or Technology

Use	Concentration
IV emulsions	10-15% w/v
Vehicle for IM dosage forms	As required

18. Related Substances
Peanut oil; corn oil; sesame oil

19. Comments
None

20. Specific References:
1. W. H. Cole, Fat emulsion for intravenous use, *J. Am. Med. Assoc.*, 166: 1042 (1958).

USA: A. Rahman*; D. Sanvordeker*; F. A. Chrzanowski**

Dextrin

1. Nonproprietary Name
BP: Dextrin

2. Functional Categories
Binder; thickening agent; emulsion stabilizer

3. Synonyms
British gum; starch gum; gommelin

4. Chemical Name and CAS Registry Number
Dextrin [9004-53-9]

5. Empirical Formula
$(C_6H_{10}O_5)_n \cdot XH_2O$

Molecular Weight
$(162.14)_n$
Mol. wt. depends on the number of $[C_6H_{10}O_5]$ units; an average value is 4500.

6. Structural Formula

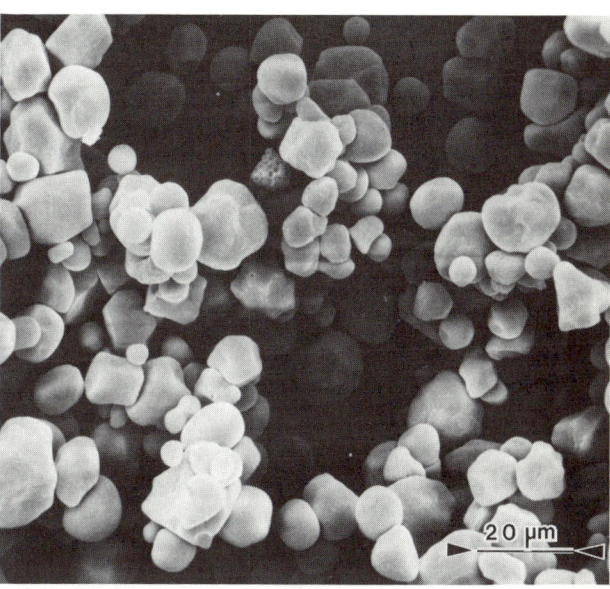

7. Commerical Availability

USA

American Maize Products Company
Borden Chemical
CPC International, Inc.

UK

Laing-National Ltd.
L. J. Rickards & Co. Ltd.

8. Method of Manufacture
Dextrin is produced by the incomplete hydrolysis of starch with dilute acids, or by heating dry starch.

9. Description
White or yellowish amorphous powder or granules with a slight, charactertistic odor and a sweet taste.

SEM-MF-24
Excipient: Dextrin (white corn, powder)
Supplier: Matheson Colleman & Bell

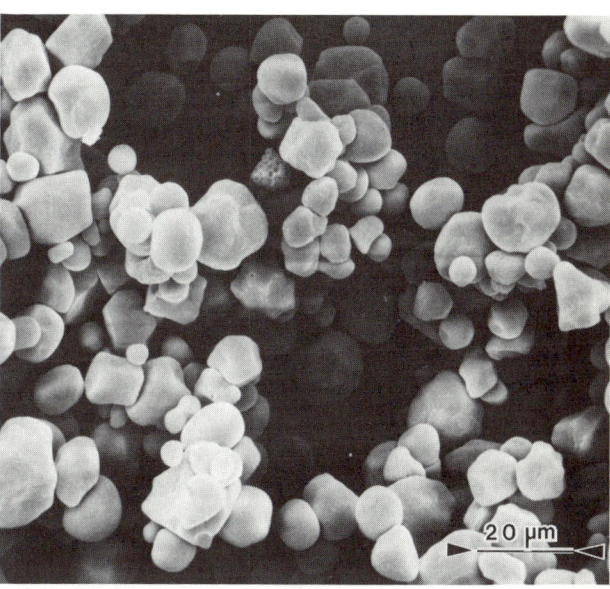

Magnification: 600×

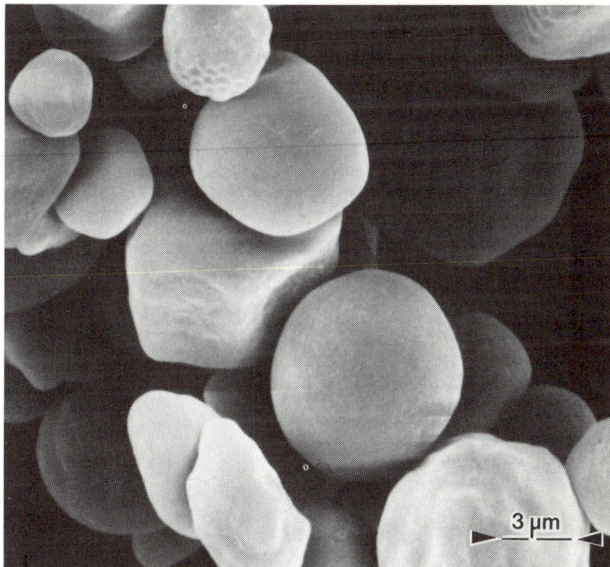

Magnification: 2,400×

10. Pharmacopeial Specifications

Test	BP
Identification	+
Acidity	+
Heavy metals	≤40 ppm
Chloride	≤0.2%
Protein	≤0.5%
Reducing substances	≤10% (calculated as $C_6H_{12}O_6$)
Loss on drying	≤11%
Ash	≤0.5%

11. Typical Properties

Density: Bulk-0.80 g/cm^3; tapped-0.91 g/cm^3
Melting point: 178°C (with decomposition)
Moisture content: 5% (Karl Fischer)
Particle size distribution: (Alpine air jet sieve)

Sieve Aperture (μm)	Weight Retained (%)
500	0.4
355	1.4
180	13.8
106	18.7
75	21.1
56.25	54.8
37.5	60.1

Solubility:

Solvent	
Water	Slowly soluble in cold water; readily soluble in boiling water to form a mucilage.
Ethanol (100%)	Insoluble
Propan-2-ol	Insoluble
Ether	Insoluble

Specific surface area: 0.14 m^2/g (Quantasorb)

12. Stability and Storage Conditions

In aqueous solutions, dextrin molecules tend to aggregate as density, temperature, pH, or other characteristics change. An increase in viscosity is caused by gelation or retrogradation as dextrin solutions age, and is particularly noticeable in the less soluble corn-starch dextrins. Dextrin solutions are thixotropic, i.e., fluidized under pressure or motion but changed to a soft paste or a gel when allowed to stand. Conversely, acids present in dextrin as residues from manufacturing can cause its further hydrolysis and result in a gradual thinning of the solution. Residual acid will also cause a reduction in viscosity of dextrin during dry storage. Residual acid is often found in the less-soluble dextrin as pyrodextrins. To eliminate these problems, dextrin manufacturers neutralize dextrins of low solubility with ammonia or sodium carbonate in the cooling vessel. Store in an air-tight container.

13. Incompatibilities

—

14. Safety

LD$_{50}$ in the mouse, by intravenous administration, is 350 mg/kg of body weight.

15. Handling Precautions

—

16. Regulatory Acceptance

BP 1980; USP XXI (as a reagent); generally accepted in Europe as a constituent of some infant foods.

17. Applications in Pharmaceutical Formulation or Technology

An adhesive and stiffening agent for surgical dressings; a granulating binder for tableting; a sugar-coating ingredient which serves as a plasticizer and adhesive; a thickening agent for suspensions.

18. Related Substances

Crystal Gums (Laing National): A brand of dextrin containing carbohydrate not less than 98% of dry weight.
Caloreen (Roussel): A water-soluble mixture of dextrins which consists predominantly of polysaccharides containing an average of 5 glucose molecules, with energy content 400 K cal, sodium and potassium less than 1.8 mmol (1.8 mEq) per 100 g. *Caloreen* has a mean molecular weight of about 840, which does not change after heating. No increase in the reducing sugar content occurs after 4 hours at 115° to 116°C. A 22% solution is iso-osmotic with serum.
Dextri-Maltose: A mixture of maltose and dextrins obtained by enzymic action of barley malt on corn flour. Light, amorphous powder. Readily soluble in water or milk.

19. Comments

Dextrin is acceptable to the Food and Drug Administration for use in foods, cosmetics and surgical dressings.

20. Specific References

1. D. French, Chemical and physical properties of starch, *J. Animal Science*, 37: 1048, 1061 (1973).
2. R. W. Satterthwaite and D. J. Iwinski; Starch Dextrins. In: *Industrial Gums*, R. L. Whistler and J. N. Bemiller, Eds., Academic Press, New York, 1973, 577-599.
3. *The Toxic Substances List*, H. E. Christensen, T. T. Luginbyhl and B. S. Carroll, Eds., U.S. Dept. of Health, Education and Welfare, Public Health Service, Rockville, Maryland, 1974, 249.

USA: P. Tsai*; P. Bernardo**
UK: P. C. Record*

Dextrose

1. Nonproprietary Names

USP: Dextrose anhydrous and monohydrate
BP: Anhydrous glucose, glucose, glucose for parenteral use

2. Functional Categories

USP: Sweetening agent; tonicity agent
Others: Direct compression diluent; flavor or color carrier

3. Synonyms

D-Glucose monohydrate; corn sugar; grape sugar; anhydrous dextrose; dextrose monohydrate; glucose; medicinal glucose; purified glucose; cerelose; starch sugar; dextrosol; *Staleydex*; *Clintose*

4. Chemical Names and CAS Registry Number

D-Glucose monohydrate
D-Glucose monohydrate [5996-10-1]
D-Glucose anhydrous [50-99-7]

5. Empirical Formula   Molecular Weight

$C_6H_{12}O_6$ Dextrose, anhydrous   180.16
$C_6H_{12}O_6 \cdot H_2O$ Dextrose, mono-   198.17
hydrate

6. Structural Formula

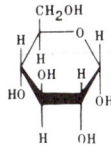

7. Commercial Availability

USA

A. E. Staley Manufacturing Co.
Clinton Corn Processing Co.
Corn Products Co.
Mallinckrodt, Inc.

UK

CPC (UK) Ltd.
K&K-Greef Chemicals
Roquette (UK) Ltd.
Tunnel Avebe Starches Ltd.
Tunnel Refineries Ltd.

8. Method of Manufacture

Dextrose, a monosaccharide sugar, is widely distributed in the plant kingdom and is manufactured on a large scale by the acid hydrolysis of starch, usually cornstarch.

9. Description

Colorless crystals or a white or cream-colored crystalline or granular powder; odorless; sweet

SEM: MF-22
Excipient: D-Glucose, anhydrous (granular)
Supplier: Mallinckrodt/**Lot No.:** KLKZ

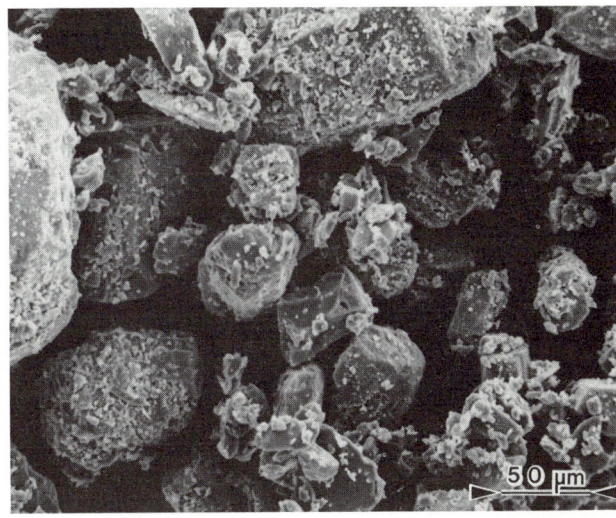

Magnification: 180✕

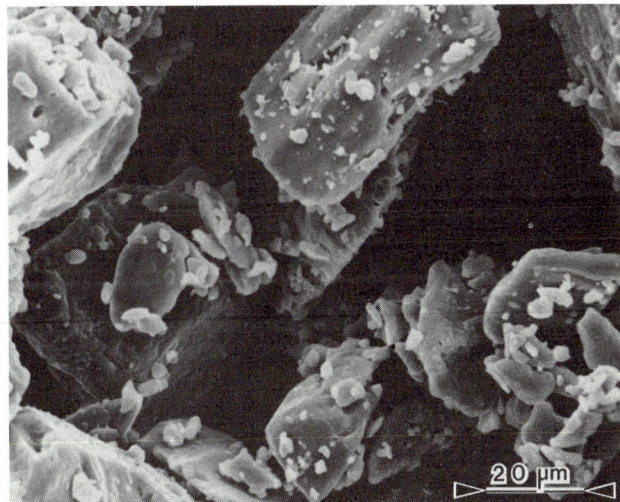

Magnification: 600✕

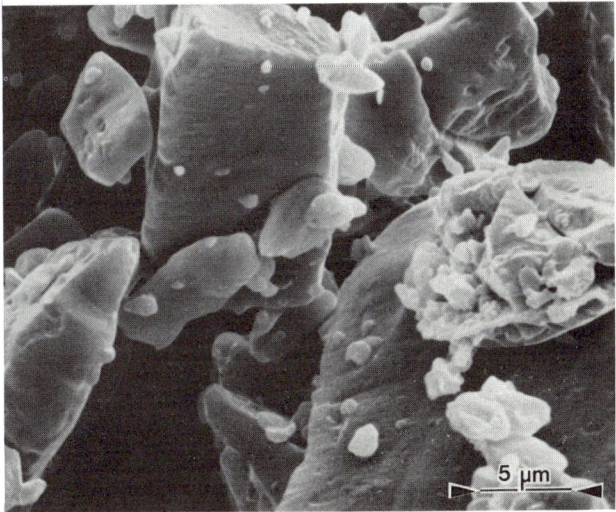

Magnification: 1800✕

10. Pharmacopeial Specifications

Test	USP
Identification	+
Acidity	+
Specific rotation	+52.6° – +53.2°
Color of solution	+
Water (anhydrous dextrose)	≤0.5%
Water (hydrous dextrose)	7.5–9.5%
Residue on ignition	≤0.1%
Chloride	≤0.018%
Sulfate	≤0.025%
Arsenic	≤1 ppm
Heavy metals	≤5 ppm
Dextrin	+
Soluble starch, sulfites	+

Test	Anhydrous BP/EP	Monohydrate BP	Monohydrate parenteral BP/EP
Identification	+	+	+
Clarity, odor and color of solution	+	+	+
Specific optical rotation	+52.5° to 53.0°	+52.5° to 53.0°	+52.5° to 53.0°
Acidity or alkalinity	+	+	+
Arsenic	≤1 ppm	≤1 ppm	≤1 ppm
Barium	+	+	+
Calcium	≤200 ppm	≤200 ppm	≤200 ppm
Lead	≤0.5 ppm	≤0.5 ppm	≤0.5 ppm
Chloride	≤125 ppm	≤125 ppm	≤125 ppm
Sulfate	≤200 ppm	≤200 ppm	≤200 ppm
Sulfite	+	+	+
Foreign sugars, soluble starch and dextrins	+	+	+
Water	≤1.0%	–	7.0–9.5%
Loss on drying	–	7.0–10.0%	–
Sulfated ash	≤0.1%	≤0.1%	≤0.1%

11. Typical Properties

Density (bulk): 1.3–1.4 g/ml (anhydrous)
Density (He): 1.54 g/ml (anhydrous and α-monohydrate)
Density (tapped): 1.1–1.2 g/ml (anhydrous)
Heat of solution: 25.2 cal/g
Hygroscopicity: At relative humidities between approximately 35 and 85% at 25°C, dextrose (anhydrous dextrose) absorbs significant amounts of moisture, and the monohydrate is formed at the higher humidities. At relative humidities below 35% and above 85%, insignificant and substantial amounts of moisture are absorbed, respectively.
Melting point: 146°C (anhydrous); 118–120°C (monohydrate); 146°C (α-form, anhydrous); 83°C (α-form, monohydrate); 148–155°C (β-form, monohydrate)
pH value: 5.9 (0.5 M aqueous solution)
Refractive index: $n_D^{20} = 1.3479$ (10% aqueous solution)
Solubility: Freely soluble in water (1 g in about 1 ml). Very soluble in boiling water. Sparingly soluble in boiling alcohol. Slightly soluble in alcohol. Soluble in glycerin. Insoluble in ether, acetone, and chloroform.
Solubility at equilibrium:
At 25°C   56 g/100 g of solution
At 45°C   72 g/100 g of solution
At 75°C   87 g/100 g of solution
Tonicity: A 5.51% solution in water is iso-osmotic with serum.

Academy HPE Laboratory Project Data

	Method	Lab #	Results
Moisture content	MC-30	14	0.22%[b]
Moisture content	MC-30	14	0.31%[a]
Moisture content	MC-10	28	0.039%
Moisture content	MC-10	28	8.73%[c]
Moisture content	MC-10	10	8.30%[a]
Density (anhydrous USP)	DE-1	31	1.556 g/cm³ [a]
Density (granular USP)	DE-1	31	1.557
Particle size distribution	PSD-4	17[a]	

USS sieve size	Particle size (S, µm)	Lab #	Weight (%)±SD
	S>590		2.07±0.30
30	297<S<590		2.25±0.41
50	210<S<297		18.57±1.94
70	149<S<210		28.41±0.56
100	125<S<149		20.97±0.94
120	74<S<125		15.68±1.50
200	S<74		12.03±0.85
Particle size distribution	PSD-4	17	

USS sieve size	Particle size (S, µm)	Weight (%)±SD
	S>590	0.98±0.44
30	297<S<590	5.06±0.56
50	210<S<297	34.58±0.75
70	149<S<210	25.74±0.24
100	125<S<149	14.58±0.45
120	74<S<125	14.01±0.55
200	S<74	5.05±1.68

	Method	Lab #	Results
Flowability (anhydrous)	FLO-1	14	No flow[a]
Flowability (anhydrous, granular)	FLO-1	14	Bridging[b]
Flowability (hydrous USP)	FLO-1	14	35 g/sec.[a]
EMC plot	EMC-1	10	Fig. 10-EMC-3[b]
SDI plot	SDI-1	14	Fig. 14-SDI-1[b]
SDI plot	SDI-1	14	Fig. 14-SDI-2[a]
SDI plot	SDI-1	14	Fig. 14-SDI-2[b]
COM plot	COM-3	20	Fig. 20-COM-3[c]
COM plot	COM-3	20	Fig. 20-COM-6[a]

Suppliers: Corn Products Co.[a]; Mallinckrodt, Inc.[b]; A. E. Staley Manufacturing Co.[c]

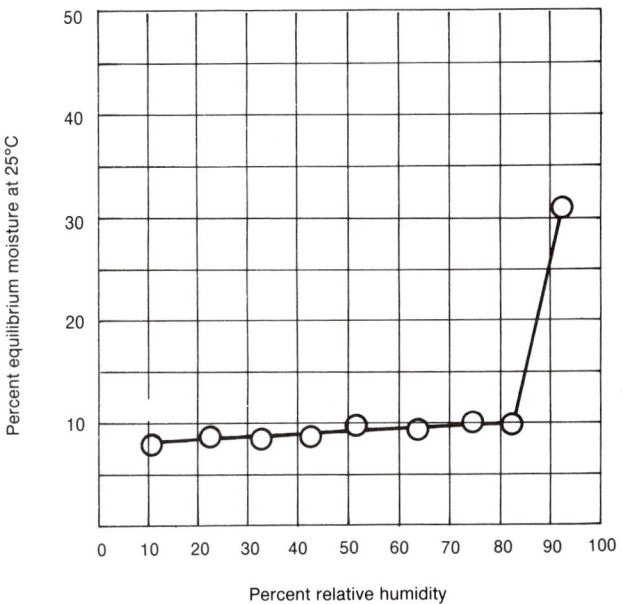

Dextrose USP, cerelose (CPC, Lot #CP44)

Figure: 10-EMC-3   **Method:** EMC-1

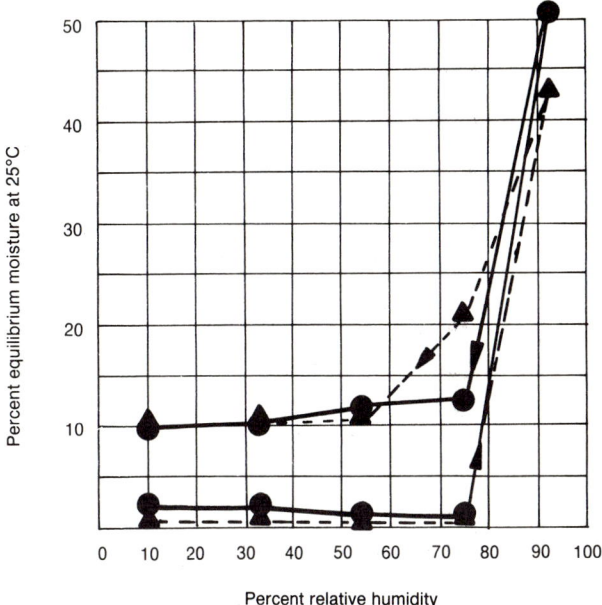

●: Dextrose USP, anhydrous (Corn Products, Lot #2502)
▲: Detrose, anhydrous (Mallinckrodt, Lot #4908)

Figure: 14-SDI-2   **Method:** SDI-1

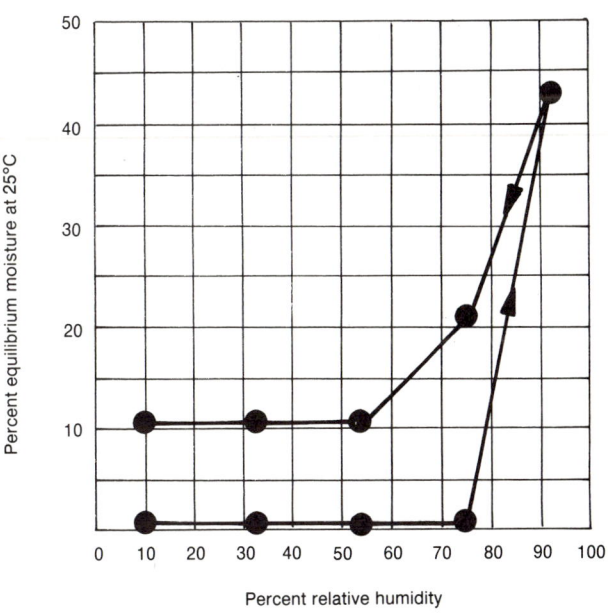

Dextrose, anhydrous, (Mallinckrodt, Lot #4905)

Figure: 14-SDI-1   **Method:** SDI-1

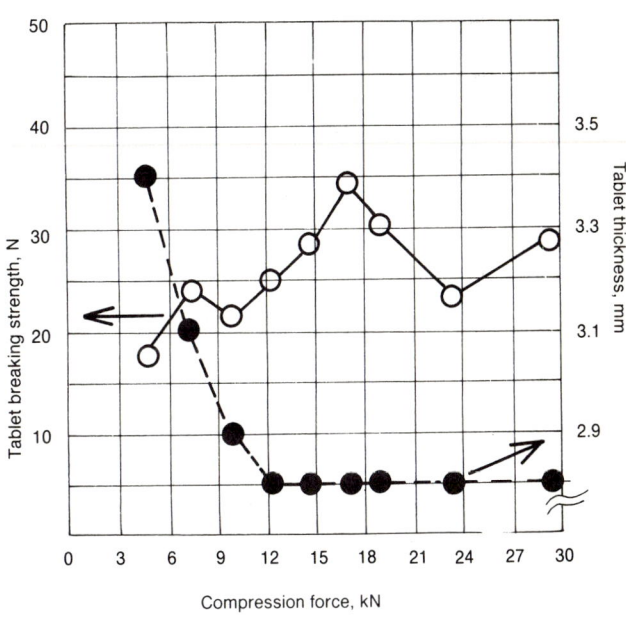

Dextrose, Staleydex (Staley, Lot #0F04Y)

Mean tablet weight: 502 mg
Minimum compressional force for compaction: 4.9 kN
Compressional force resulting in capping: 7.35 kN
0.5% magnesium stearate required as lubricant

Figure: 20-COM-3   **Method:** COM-3

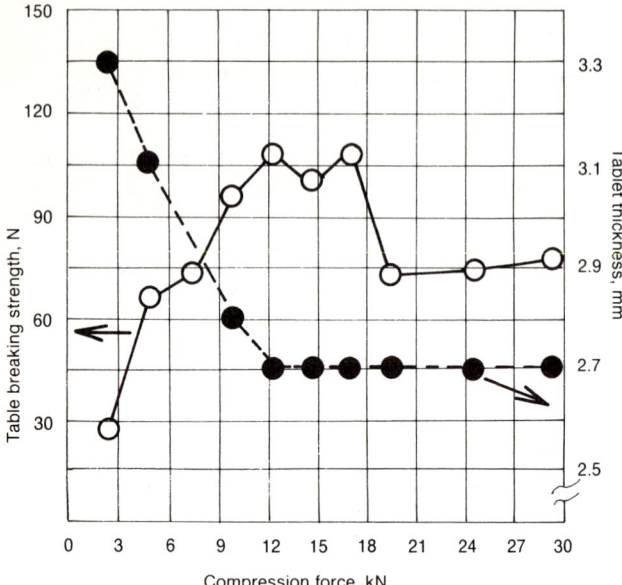

Dextrose, cerelose (Corn Products, Lot #37A-1)

Mean tablet weight: 508.3 mg
Minimum compressional force for compaction: 2.45 kN
Compressional force resulting in capping: 14.7 kN
0.5% magnesium stearate required as lubricant

Figure: 20-COM-6   Method: COM-3

12. Stability and Storage Conditions

Good stability under dry storage conditions. Store in a well-closed container. Dextrose absorbs insignificant amounts of moisture at 25° C and relative humidities of up to 85% and substantial amounts at higher relative humidities.

13. Incompatibilities

Brown coloration and decomposition with strong alkali. There was a loss of clarity when intravenous solutions of dextrose were mixed with those of cyanocobalamin, kanamycin sulfate, novobiocin sodium, and warfarin sodium. Decomposition of B-complex vitamins occurs when they are warmed with dextrose. In the aldehyde form, dextrose can react with amines, amides, amino acids, peptides, and proteins. Stability of erythromycin glucectate in dextrose injection could be assured only if the pH of the dextrose injection was greater than 5.05. Dextrose may cause browning of tablets containing amines.

14. Safety

LD_{50} (intravenous) in rabbits: 35 g/kg. Concentrated dextrose solutions given by mouth may cause nausea and vomiting. Intravenous infusions of concentrated dextrose injections are liable to cause local vein irritation. Thrombophlebitis has been observed following the intravenous infusion of iso-osmotic dextrose injections with low pH (due to overheating during sterilization). The incidence of phlebitis may be reduced by adding sufficient sodium bicarbonate to raise the pH of the infusion above 7.

15. Handling Precautions

No restrictions specified except to store in a well-closed container.

16. Regulatory Acceptance

USP XXI; BP/EP 1980

17. Applications in Pharmaceutical Formulation or Technology

Sweetening agent; tonicity agent; tablet binder/diluent (direct compression); tablet binder (liquid glucose). The use of commercial food-grade dextrose (monohydrate) was compared with spray-dried lactose as a tablet excipient in the preparation by direct compression of tablets of phenobarbitone, amphetamine sulfate and methylamphetamine hydrochloride. Tableting results were comparable with those obtained with lactose. However, more lubrication was required with dextrose. Tablets prepared with dextrose had a greater tendency to harden and were less friable. In the presence of amines, dextrose may cause browning of tablets. The addition of starch or microcrystalline cellulose is not recommended. Dextrose was found to be a suitable agent for direct compression tablet making. The monohydrate dextrose is used as a filler and binder, especially for chewable tablets.

18. Related Substances

Liquid glucose (corn syrup). It is a colorless or almost colorless, odorless, very viscous syrup with a sweet taste. It consists of a mixture of dextrose, maltose, dextrins, and water (dextrose content, 10-20%). It is used as a pill excipient, either alone or as liquid glucose syrup. Liquid glucose is sometimes used instead of dextrose for oral administration. Liquid glucose must not be used in the place of dextrose for intravenous injection. It is a pharmaceutical necessity for cocoa syrup.
Dextrates NF

19. Comments

The preparation of dextrose-containing solutions for injection or infusion must be related to the content of the anhydrous substance.

20. Specific References

1. W. T. Wing, *J. Pharm. Pharmacol.*, 12: 191 T (1960).
2. J. A. Patel and G. L. Phillips, *Am. J. Hosp. Pharm.*, 23: 409 (1966).
3. M. Edward, *Am. J. Hosp. Pharm.*, 24: 440 (1967).
4. R. N. DuVall, K. T. Koshy and R. E. Dashiell, *J. Pharm. Sci.*, 54: 1196 (1965).
5. A. J. Bruno, *J. Pharm. Sci.*, 59: 1336 (1970).

USA: D. Popli*; J. Cooper*; F. D. L. Masilungan**

Dichlorodifluoromethane

1. Nonproprietary Names

NF: Dichlorodifluoromethane
BP: Dichlorodifluoromethane

2. Functional Category

USP: Aerosol propellant
BP: Aerosol propellant

3. Synonyms

Propellant 12, refrigerant 12, *Freon*, *Genetron*, *Ucon*

4. Chemical Names and CAS Registry Number

Methane, dichlorodifluoro, dichlorodifluoromethane
[75-71-8]

5. Empirical Formula   Molecular Weight

CCl_2F_2 120.91

6. Structural Formula

—

7. Commercial Availability

USA

Allied Chemical Corp.
E. I. DuPont De Nemours & Co.
Union Carbide Corp.

UK

Imperial Chemical Industries plc
ISC Chemicals Ltd.

8. Method of Manufacture

Dichlorodifluoromethane is prepared by the addition of fluorine to carbon tetrachloride in the presence of a suitable catalyst, such as polyvalent antimony.

$$2\ CCl_4 + 3HF \rightarrow CCl_3F + CCl_2F_2 + 3HCl$$

It is further purified to remove all traces of water and hydrochloric acid as well as traces of the starting and intermediate materials.

9. Description

Dichlorodifluoromethane is a liquefied gas and exists as a liquid at room temperature when contained under its own vapor pressure or as a gas when exposed to room temperature and atmospheric pressure. It is practically odorless and colorless and an essentially clear liquid. The gas in high concentrations has a faint ether-like odor. It is noncorrosive, nonirritating and nonflammable.

10. Pharmacopeial Specifications

Test	NF	BP
Identification	+	+
Boiling temperature	−30°C approx.	−29.8°C
Water	≤0.001%	≤0.001% w/w
High boiling residues	≤0.01%	≤0.01%
Inorganic chlorides	+	+
Distillation range	—	0.2°C
Acidity	—	≤2 ppm
Solubility	—	Immiscible with water

11. Typical Properties

Boiling point: −21.6°F; −29.8°C
Freezing point: −252°F; −158°C
Vapor pressure (psia)*: 84.9 at 70°F; 196.0 at 130°F
Liquid density (g/ml): 1.325 at 70°F; 1.191 at 130°F
Liquid viscosity (centipoise): 0.262 at 70°F; 0.227 at 130°F
Surface tension (dyne/cm): 9 at 77°F
Solubility of propellant in water (w/w %): 0.028 at 77°F
Limits of inflammability: nonflammable

* psia = psig + 14.7

12. Stability and Storage Conditions

Dichlorodifluoromethane is a nonreactive and stable compound. The compressed gas is also stable when used as a propellant, and does not present any stability problems. It should be stored in a cool place.

13. Incompatibilities

Other than the lack of miscibility of the fluorocarbon propellant with water, there are no practical incompatibilities with the usual ingredients used in the formulation of pharmaceutical aerosols. The propellant is generally miscible with nonpolar materials and some semipolar materials. For pharmaceutical aerosols, ethyl alcohol is the most useful cosolvent, and finds widespread use in the formulation of pharamceutical aerosols. Glycols, oils and other similar materials exhibit varying miscibility with the propellant.

14. Safety

The safety of the fluorocarbon has been established. The propellants used for oral aerosol products generally vaporize quickly, and most of the vapors escape and are not inhaled. A small amount of the propellant may be inhaled with the active ingredient and be carried to the respiratory system. However, these amounts of propellant do not present a toxicological problem. They are quickly cleared from the lungs. Deliberate inhalation of excessive quantities of fluorocarbon propellant may result in death, and the following ''warning'' statement must appear on the label of all aerosols:

WARNING: Avoid inhaling. Keep away from eyes or other mucous membranes. (Aerosols designed specifically for oral inhalation need not contain this statement).

WARNING: Do not inhale directly; deliberate inhalation of contents can cause death.

OR

WARNING: Use only as directed; intentional misuse by deliberately concentrating and inhaling the contents can be harmful or fatal.

Additionally, the label should contain the following information:

WARNING: Contents under pressure. Do not puncture or incinerate container. Do not expose to heat or store at room temperature above 120°F (49°C). Keep out of the reach of children.

The Environmental Protection Agency (EPA) requires the following on all aerosols containing fluorocarbons as the propellant:

WARNING: Contains a chlorofluorocarbon that may harm the public health and environment by reducing ozone in the upper atmosphere.

When the fluorocarbon propellants are used for topical aerosols they may cause a chilling effect on the skin. The effect has been somewhat overcome by the use of vapor tap valves. The propellants quickly vaporize from the skin, and are nonirritating when used as directed.

15. Handling Precautions

These materials are liquefied gases and should be handled accordingly. They should be used in a well-ventilated room. It should be noted that fluorocarbon vapors are heavier than air and do not support life. Therefore, when cleaning large tanks which may have contained fluorocarbons, adequate provisions for oxygen in the tanks must be made in order to protect the worker cleaning the tanks.

16. Regulatory Acceptance

NF XVI; BP 1980

17. Applications in Pharmaceutical Formulation or Technology

The use of fluorocarbon propellants has been seriously curtailed by the regulatory action on the part of the FDA, EPA and CPA. Based on these regulations, fluorocarbons can be used as a propellant for oral inhalant aerosols (on an NDA), contraceptive foams and cytology sprays.

18. Related Substances

Trichloromonofluoromethane; dichlorotetrafluoroethane

19. Comments

Due to recent changes in regulations, most pharmaceutical aerosols are currently being reformulated from a fluorocarbon system to a hydrocarbon system. Where this is not possible or practical, other mechanical means for the dispensing of the product as a spray are being investigated, such as pumps.

20. Specific References

1. J. J. Sciarra, Pharmaceutical and cosmetic aerosols, *J. Pharm. Sci.,* 63:1815-1836 (1974).
2. S. Niazi and W. L. Chiou, Fluorocarbon aerosol propellants XI: pharmacokinetics of dichlorodifluoromethane in dogs following single dose and multiple dosing, *J. Pharm. Sci.,* 66(1): 49-53 (1977).

USA: J. J. Sciarra*; Z. Chowan**
UK: P. J. Davies

Dichlorotetrafluoroethane

Surface tension (dyne/cm): 13 at 77°F
Solubility in water (w/w %): 0.013 at 77°F
* psia = psig + 14.7

1. Nonproprietary Name
NF: Dichlorotetrafluoroethane
BP: Dichlorotetrafluoroethane

2. Functional Category
USP: Aerosol propellant
BP: Aerosol propellant

3. Synonyms
Propellant 114, refrigerant 114, *Freon, Gentron, Ucon*

4. Chemical Name and CAS Registry Number
Ethane-1,2-dichloro-1,1,2,2-tetrafluoro-.
1,2-Dichlorotetrafluoroethane [76-14-2]

5. Empirical Formula   Molecular Weight
$C_2Cl_2F_4$ 170.92

6. Structural Formula
—

7. Commercial Availability
USA
Allied Chemical Corp.
E. I. DuPont De Nemours Co.
Union Carbide Corp.

UK
Imperial Chemical Industries plc
ISC Chemicals Ltd.

8. Method of Manufacture
This fluorinated hydrocarbon is generally prepared by the addition of fluorine to a suitable chlorinated hydrocarbon in the presence of a suitable catalyst, such as polyvalent antimony.
$$CCl_2 = CCl_2 + Cl_2 + 4HF \rightarrow$$
$$CClF_2CClF_2 + 4HCl$$

9. Description
A colorless, nonflammable gas; odor faintly ethereal.

10. Pharmacopeial Specifications

Test	NF	BP
Identification	+	+
Boiling temperature	4°C approx.	about 3.5°C
Water	≤0.001%	≤0.001%
High boiling residues (matter)	≤0.01%	≤0.01%
Chlorides	+	+
Acidity	—	+

11. Typical Properties
Boiling point (1 atm): 39.4°F; 3.55°C
Freezing point: −137°F; −94°C
Vapor pressure (psia):* 27.6 at 70°F; 73.5 at 130°F
Liquid density (g/ml): 1.468 at 70°F; 1.360 at 130°F
Liquid viscosity (centipoise): 0.386 at 70°F; 0.296 at 130°F

12. Stability and Storage Conditions
Dichlorotetrafluoroethane is a non-reactive and stable compound. The compressed gas is also stable when used as a propellant and does not present any stability problems. It should be stored in a cool place.

13. Incompatibilities
Other than the lack of miscibility of the fluorocarbon propellant with water, there are no practical incompatibilities with the usual ingredients used in formulation of pharmaceutical aerosols. The propellant is generally miscible with nonpolar materials and some semipolar materials. For pharmaceutical aerosols, ethyl alcohol is the most useful cosolvent, and finds widespread use in the formulation of pharmaceutical aerosols. Glycols, oils and other similar materials exhibit varying miscibility with the propellant.

14. Safety
The safety of the fluorocarbon has been established. The propellants used for oral aerosol products generally vaporize quickly, and most of the vapors escape and are not inhaled. A small amount of the propellant may be inhaled with the active ingredient and carried to the respiratory system. However, these amounts of propellant do not present a toxicological problem. They are quickly cleared from the lungs. Deliberate inhalation of excessive quantities of fluorocabon propellant may result in death, and the following "warning" statement must appear on the label of all aerosols:

WARNING: Avoid inhaling. Keep away from eyes or other mucous membranes. (Aerosols designed specifically for oral inhalation need not contain this statement).

WARNING: Do not inhale directly; deliberate inhalation of contents can cause death.
OR
WARNING: Use only as directed; intentional misuse by deliberately concentrating and inhaling the contents can be harmful or fatal.

Additionally, the label should contain the following information:
WARNING: Contents under pressure. Do not puncture or incinerate container. Do not expose to heat or store at room temperature above 120°F (49°C). Keep out of the reach of children.

The Environmental Protection Agency (EPA) requires the following on all aerosols containing fluorocarbons as the propellant:
WARNING: Contains a chlorofluorocarbon that may harm the public health and environment by reducing ozone in the upper atmosphere.

When the fluorocarbon propellants are used for topical aerosols they may cause a chilling effect on the skin. The effect has been somewhat overcome by the use of vapor tap valves. The propellants quickly vaporize from the skin and are nonirritating when used as directed.

15. Handling Precautions

These materials are liquefied gases and should be handled accordingly. They should be used in a well-ventilated room. It should be noted that fluorocarbon vapors are heavier than air and do not support life; therefore, when cleaning large tanks which may have contained fluorocarbons, adequate provisions for oxygen in the tanks must be made in order to protect the worker cleaning the tanks.

16. Regulatory Acceptance

NF XVI; BP 1980

17. Applications in Pharmaceutical Formulation or Technology

The use of fluorocarbon propellants has been seriously curtailed by the regulatory action on the part of the FDA, EPA and CPA. Based on these regulations, fluorocarbons can be used as propellants for oral inhalant aerosols (on an NDA), contraceptive foams and cytology sprays.

18. Related Substances

Dichlorodifluoromethane; trichloromonofluoromethane

19. Comments

This propellant overcame the disadvantage of a distinct carbon tetrachloride-like odor which is found in propellant 11 and is useful in formulating oral products. Since it is highly fluorinated, it possesses limited solubility characteristics not only in water but also in many medicinal substances, and, in addition, is more expensive than propellant 11. Propellant 114 in combination with propellant 12 is generally used for oral aerosols.

20. Specific References

1. J. J. Sciarra, Pharmaceutical and cosmetic aerosols, *J. Pharm. Sci.*, 63: 1815-1836 (1974).
2. S. Niazi and W. L. Chiou, Fluorocarbon aerosol propellants XI: pharmacokinetics of dichlorotetrafluoroethane in dogs, *J. Pharm. Sci.*, 65 (1): 60-64 (1976).

USA: J. J. Sciarra*; Z. Chowhan*
UK: P. J. Davies

Diethanolamine

1. Nonproprietary Name
NF: Diethanolamine

2. Functional Category
USP: Alkalinizing agent; emulsifying agent (adjunct)

3. Synonyms
Diethylolamine; bis(hydroxyethyl)amine; 2,2'-dihydroxydiethylamine; diolamine; *Alkanolamines; Ethanolamines*

4. Chemical Name and CAS Registry Number
Ethanol, 2,2,'-iminobis-
2,2'-Iminodiethanol [111-42-2]

5 Empirical Formula   Molecular Weight
$C_4H_{11}NO_2$ 105.14

6. Structural Formula
$(HOCH_2CH_2)_2NH$

7. Commercial Availability
USA
BASF Wyandotte Corp.
Dow Chemical Company
Olin Corp.

UK
Shell Chemicals (UK) Ltd.
Unalco Ltd.

8. Method of Manufacture
Production of the ethanolamines is accomplished by reacting ethylene oxide with ammonia to yield a mixture of the three compounds. By a series of separation procedures, monoethanolamine, diethanolamine and triethanolamine are obtained.

9. Description
At room temperature it is a white solid. Above room temperature it is a clear, water-white, viscous liquid with a mildly ammoniacal odor.

10. Pharmacopeial Specifications

Test	NF
Identification	+
Refractive index (30°C)	1.473-1.476
Water	$\leq 0.15\%$
Triethanolamine	$\leq 1.0\%$
Assay range	98.5-101.0%

11. Typical Properties
Melting point, °C: 28.0
Boiling point, °C at 760 mm: 268.8
Flash point (open cup), °C: 138
Refractive index, 30°C: 1.4753
Solubility, 20°C, % by wt. in water: 96.4
Specific gravity, 30°C: 1.0881
Vapor pressure, 20°C, mm Hg: 0.01
Viscosity (absolute), 30°C, cps: 380
Surface tension, 20°C, dynes/cm: 49.0

pH (0.1N solution): 11.0
Dipole moment: 2.81
Solubility: Miscible with water, methanol and acetone. Solubility at 25°C in benzene: 4.2%; in ether: 0.8%; in carbon tetrachloride: <0.1%; in n-heptane: <0.1%.
Hygroscopicity: Very hygroscopic.
Chemical properties: The ethanolamines are characterized by the presence of a basic nitrogen atom and hydroxyl group(s). Thus, they are capable of undergoing reactions typical for both amines and alcohols. The amine group usually exhibits the greater activity whenever it is possible for a reaction to take place at either the amine or hydroxyl group. Diethanolamine is a secondary amine, and displays the usual properties of this class of nitrogen bases.

12. Stability and Storage Conditions
The ethanolamines present no unusual problems in handling under ordinary conditions. In general, it is advisable to store them in air-tight containers protected from light, and the storage temperature should not exceed 50°C. Stainless steel should be used for prolonged storage. This will prevent color changes. The color may develop due to the absorption of atmospheric oxygen. Thus, storage tanks should also be gas-padded, if color is important. Ethanolamines are hygroscopic. If water content is to be minimized, a dry, inert gas pad under pressure should also be used when stored in tanks.

13. Incompatibilities
Ethanolamines will react with acids to form salts and esters. Diethanolamine will react with acids, acid anhydrides, acid chlorides and esters to form amide derivatives, and with propylene carbonate or other cyclic carbonates to give the correponding carbonates. As a secondary amine, diethanolamine reacts with aldehydes and ketones to yield aldimines and ketimines. Diethanolamine reacts with copper to form complex salts. Discoloration and precipitation will take place in the presence of heavy metal salts.

14. Safety
All of the ethanolamines are capable of producing severe eye injuries. They may be health hazards primarily because of their instant action on the skin and in eyes. The mono- and diethanolamines are also considered to be slightly hazardous from the standpoint of oral administration. Insofar as absorption through the skin is concerned, only pure monoethanolamine has a definite toxicity. In this respect, di- and triethanolamine are much less toxic. The table below summarizes the acute toxicity of diethanolamine.

Acute oral LD_{50}, g/kg	1.5
Acute dermal toxicity LD_{50}, g/kg	Low toxicity

15. Handling Precautions
Personal protective equipment should be used by personnel handling concentrated solutions of ethanolamines.

16. Regulatory Acceptance
NF XVI

17. Applications in Pharmaceutical Formulation or Technology
Diethanolamine and its fatty acid amides are used for various buffering purposes, including the preparation of emulsions. Diethanolamine has been utilized to form the soluble salts of active compounds. It was reported to solubilize by salt

formation slightly soluble iodinated organic acids used as contrast media.

Diethanolamine was reported to inhibit the discoloration of aqueous compositions containing hexamethylene-tetra-mine-1,3-dichloropropene salts. (C. S. Polemenakos and H. G. Langer, *C.A. 83:* 197840s, 1975).

18. Related Substances

—

19. Comments

—

20. Specific References

1. *Ethanolamines, Technical Brochure,* Jefferson Chemical Company, Inc. 1972.
2. *Ethanolamines, Product Data,* Olin Chemicals; *Diethanolamine. Material Safety Data,* Olin Chemicals, 1977.
3. *Diethanolamine, Technical Leaflet,* BASF AG, 1971; *Alkanolamines,* BASF AG, 1972.

USA: E. Shek*, G. S. Brenner**

Diethyl Phthalate

1. Nonproprietary Name
NF: Diethyl phthalate
BP: Diethyl phthalate

2. Functional Categories
NF: Plasticizer
Others: Fixative for perfumes; alcohol denaturant

3. Synonyms
Ethyl phthalate; *Kodaflex DEP*

4. Chemical Names and CAS Registry Number
1,2-Benzenedicarboxylic acid, diethyl ester   [84-66-2]
Ethyl-O-benzene-1,2-dicarboxylate

5. Empirical Formula   Molecular Weight
$C_{12}H_{14}O_4$ 222.24

6. Structural Formula

7. Commercial Availability
USA

Berje Chemical Products, Inc.
Eastman Chemical Products, Inc.,
Kay-Fries, Inc.
Pfizer Chemicals Division
Stoney-Mueller, Incorporated
Technical Petrolatum Company

UK

BP Chemicals Ltd.
Bush, Boake, Allen Ltd.

8. Method of Manufacture
Diethyl phthalate is produced by the reaction of ethyl alcohol and phthalic acid.

9. Description
Clear, colorless, oily liquid. Practically odorless, or with a very slight aromatic odor. Bitter, disagreeable in taste.

10. Pharmacopeial Specifications

Test	NF	BP
Weight per ml	—	1.115-1.119
Refractive index (20°C)	1.500-1.505	1.500-1.505
Identification	+	+
Specific gravity (20°C)	1.118-1.122	—
Acidity	+	+
Water	≤0.2%	≤0.2%
Residue on ignition	≤0.02%	—
Assay (anhydrous basis)	98.0-102.0%	99.0-100.5%
Related substances	—	+
Sulphated ash	—	≤0.02%

USP reference standard available (do not dry before using)

11. Typical Properties
Boiling point: 295°C
Flash point: 140°C
Refractive index: 1.5049 (at 14°C, sodium light)
Solubility: Insoluble in water; miscible with alcohol, ether, and many other organic solvents
Specific gravity: 1.232 at 14°C

12. Stability and Storage Conditions
Stable to light and high temperatures. However, when exposed to heat or flame, there is a slight danger of fire since diethyl phthalate can react with oxidizing materials. It should be stored in tight containers in a cool location.

13. Incompatibilities
Diethyl phthalate can react with oxidizing materials.

14. Safety
Diethyl phthalate has an oral LD_{50} of 1.0 g/kg in rabbits, an intraperitoneal LD_{50} of 2.8 g/kg in mice and a subcutaneous LD_{50} of 3.0 g/kg in guinea pigs. The oral LD_{50} in rats has been reported variously as 8.2 ml/kg and 9.5-31 g/kg. Skin irritation is slight in experimental animals. Rats survived a six-hour exposure to atmospheric concentrations of 511 ppm generated at 150°C. It is irritating to mucous membranes. Exposure to heated vapor may result in some transient irritation of the nose and throat. Taken orally in large amounts, diethyl phthalate causes paralysis of the central nervous system.

15. Handling Precautions
Avoid contact. Use with ventilation adequate to maintain vapor concentrations below the threshold limit value of 5 mg/m³. No adverse effects of over-exposure expected other than possible transient irritation of the nose and throat. In case of a spill, remove all ignition sources. Soak up the spill with an absorbent material and incinerate.

16. Regulatory Acceptance
NF XVI; BP 1980

17. Applications in Pharmaceutical Formulation or Technology
Used as a plasticizer for film coatings on tablets, beads and granules at concentrations of 10-30%

18. Related Substances
—

19. Comments
Diethyl phthalate is used as a perfume fixative at a concentration of 0.1 to 0.5% the weight of the perfume used. It is also used as a denaturant in alcohol.

20. Specific Reference
1. G. S. Banker, *J. Pharm. Sci.*, 55:81 (1966).

USA: T. A. Wheatley*, G. E. Reier*, P. Bernardo**, J. Cooper**

Docusate Sodium

1. Nonproprietary Name
USP: Docusate sodium
BPC: Dioctyl sodium sulphosuccinate

2. Functional Categories
USP: Wetting and/or solubilizing agent
Others: Anionic surface-active agent

3. Synonyms
Sodium dioctyl sulfosuccinate; sodium dioctyl sulphosucci-nate; dioctyl sodium sulfosuccinate; *Doss aerosol OT*; *Alphasol OT*; *Colace*; *Condanol SB-DO 60%*; *Coprol*; *Defilin*; *Dioctylal*; *Dioctyl-medo*; *Diomedicone*; *Diovac*; *Disonate*; *Doxinate*; *Doxol*; *DSS*; *Ilozoft*; *Manoxol OT/P*; *Milkinol*; *Molcer*; *Molofac*; *Nevax*; *Obston*; *Physiolax*; *Siponol O*; *Soffecine*; *Softil*; *Soliwax*; *Vatsol OT*; *Velmol*; *Waxol*.

4. Chemical Names and CAS Registry Number
Butanedioic acid, sulfo-, 1,4-bis(2-ethylhexyl) ester, sodium salt
Sodium 1,4-bis-(2-ethylhexyl) sulfosuccinate [577-11-7]

5. Empirical Formula   Molecular Weight
$C_{20}H_{37}NaO_7S$ 444.56

6. Structural Formula

$$CH_2COOCH_2CH(CH_2)_3CH_3$$
$$NaO_3S-CHCOOCH_2CH(CH_2)_3CH_3$$
(with C_2H_5 side chains)

7. Commercial Availability
USA

American Cyanamid Co.
EM Laboratories, Inc.
Finetex, Inc.

UK

Allied Colloids, Ltd.
Cynamid of Great Britain, Ltd.
Manchem, Ltd.

8. Method of Manufacture
Maleic anhydride is treated with 2-ethylhexanol to produce dioctyl maleate, which is then reacted with sodium bisulfite.

9. Description
White, wax-like, bitter tasting, hygroscopic, plastic solid with a characteristic octanol-like odor; usually available in the form of pellets or flakes.

10. Pharmacopeial Specifications

Test	USP	BP
Identification	+	+
Assay	99.0-100.5%	≥98.5%
Clarity of solution	+	—
Water content	≤2.0%	—
Residue on ignition	15.5-16.2%	—
Arsenic	≤3 ppm	—
Heavy metals	≤0.001%	—
Bis(2-ethylhexyl) maleate	≤0.4%	—
Loss on drying	—	≤3.0%
Sulfated ash	—	15.5-16.3%

11. Typical Properties
Density: 1.1 g/ml
Melting point: 153-157°C
pH: pH of a 1% solution is between 5.8 and 6.9.
Solubility: Water (g/l): 15 (25°), 18 (30°), 23 (40°), 30 (50°), 40 (60°), 55 (70°); higher concentrations form a thick gel. Soluble in 1 part of chloroform; in 1 part of ether; and in 3 parts of alcohol. Also soluble in carbon tetrachloride, petroleum ether, naptha, xylene, dibutyl phthalate, liquid petrolatum, acetone and vegetable oils.
Solution preparation: A convenient way of making a 1% aqueous solution is to add 1 g of solid docusate sodium to about 50 ml of water and to apply gentle heat. It dissolves in a short time, and the resulting solution can be made up to 100 ml with water. Alternatively, 1 g may be soaked overnight in 50 ml of water; the additional water may then be added with gentle heating and stirring.
Surface activity: Surface tension (dynes/cm) in water at 25°C: 62.8 (0.001%); 28.7 (0.1%); 26.0 (1.0%). Interfacial tension (dynes/cm) in water versus mineral oil at 25°C: 20.7 (0.01%); 5.9 (0.1%); 1.84 (1.0%). Critical micelle concentration (CMC) in water at 25°C: 2.5×10^{-3}M (0.11 g/100 ml).
Acid number: Max. 2.5
Saponification number: 240-253
Iodine number: Max. 0.25
Hydroxyl number: 6-8 (using 5.0 g DSS)

Academy HPE Laboratory Project Data		
Method	Lab #	Results
DE-1	7	1.16 + 0.03
MC-29	23	1.51%
SOL-6		
Water (25°C)	23	0.028
Water (37°C)	23	0.107-0.111g/ml
Alcohol (25°C)	23	>1.0 g/ml
Alcohol (37°C)	23	>1.0 g/ml
Propy. glycol (25°C)	23	0.80 - 1.25 g/ml
Propy. glycol (37°C)	23	0.80 - 1.25 g/ml
Hexane (25°C)	23	>2.5 g/ml
Hexane (37°C)	23	>2.5 g/ml

Supplier: American Cynamid

12. Stability and Storage Conditions
Preserve in a well-closed container. At room temperature, docusate sodium is stable in acid solution, but hydrolyzes slowly in weak alkaline solutions and rapidly in solutions above pH 10. For all practical purposes the compound is stable at room temperature between pH 1 and pH 10. The addition of electrolytes to aqueous solutions may cause turbidity.

13. Incompatibilities
Electrolytes added to aqueous solutions of docusate sodium can cause turbidity. However, it possesses greater tolerance to calcium, magnesium and other polyvalent ions as compared to other surface-active agents. Incompatible with alkali at pH greater than 10.

14. Safety
LD_{50} (oral—mice); 1.5 to 4.8 g/kg; (subcutaneous—mice): 4.07 g/kg; (oral—guinea pig): 0.65 g/kg; (oral—rat): 1.9-4.06 g/kg. Formulations containing very large quantities of docusate sodium as an excipient could cause unintended effects. It has the potential for oral absorption and for the

alteration of the gastro-intestinal epithelium. The GI or hepatic absorption of other drugs might be facilitated, leading to potentiation. Docusate sodium should not be administered with liquid paraffin, as it may increase the absorption of the oil. Solutions with concentrations greater than 0.1% can cause inflammation. Contact with the eyes should be avoided. When heated to decomposition, docusate sodium emits toxic fumes, and is moderately dangerous.

15. Handling Precautions

Because of hygroscopicity, it should be stored in a tight container. Contact with the eyes should be avoided. Avoid ingestion, inhalation and skin contact.

16. Regulatory Acceptance

USP XXI; BPC 1973.

17. Applications in Pharmaceutical Formulation and Technology

Use	Concentration/Dose (%)
Surfactant (wetting/dispersing/emulsifying agent)	0.01 - 1
Tablet disintegrant	~0.5
Tablet coating agent	E.g., coating solution - 20% docusate sodium, 2-15% sodium benzoate, 0.5% propylene glycol; solution made in 70% ethyl alcohol.

Docusate sodium may be used in capsule and direct compression tablet formulations to assist in wetting and dissolution.

18. Related Substances

Docusate calcium USP. This white, amorphous solid is used as an emulsifying, wetting and dispersing agent for external preparations. Its oral use may occasionally be accompanied by mild cramping pains.
Docusate potassium USP.

19. Comments

This excipient can alter the dissolution and bioavailability of some drugs.

20. Specific References

1. D.N. Shah, J.R. Feldkamp, J.L. White and S.L. Hem, Effect of the pH-zero point of charge relationship on the interaction of ionic compounds and polyols with aluminum hydroxide gel, *J. Pharm. Sci.*, 71: (2), 266-268 (1982).
2. W.G. Chambliss, R.W. Cleary, R. Fischer, A.B. Jones, P. Skierkowski, W. Nicholes and A.H. Kibbe, Effect of docusate sodium on drug release from a controlled release dosage form, *J. Pharm. Sci.*, 70: (11), 1248-1251 (1981).

USA: J. Lach*; S.K. Mallick*; P. Bernardo**
UK: G.G. Liversidge*

Edetic Acid and Edetates

1. Nonproprietary Name

NF: Edetic acid
USP: Edetate disodium, edetate calcium disodium
BP: Disodium edetate, sodium calciumedetate

2. Functional Category

USP: Edetic acid: Chelating agent
USP: Edetate disodium: Chelating agent
BP: Edetate calcium disodium: Chelating substance used in the treatment of lead poisoning.

3. Synonyms

Edetic acid:Ethylenediaminetetraacetic acid; EDTA; *Versene*; *Questrex*; *Sequestrene*; *Detaric Acid*; *Nuilapon*.
Edetate disodium: disodium edathamil, disodium tetracemate, tetracemindinatrium.
Edetate calcium disodium: ethylenediaminetetraacetic acid calcium disodium chelate, calcium EDTA, edathamil calcium-disodium, *Endrate, Sequestrene, Nullapons, Detaric acid, Detarex, Versenate*

4. Chemical Names and CAS Registry Numbers

Edetic acid: Glycine,N,N'-1,2-ethanediylbis [N-(carboxymethyl)-(ethylenedinitrilo)tetraacetic acid [60-00-4]
Edetate disodium: Glycine,N,N'-1,2-ethanediylbis [N-(carboxymethyl)-disodium salt-disodium (ethylenedinitrilo)tetraacetate, dihydrate [6381-92-6], anhydrous [139-33-3]
Edetate calcium disodium: Calciate(2-), [[N,N'-1,2-ethanediylbis[N-(carboxymethyl)-glycinato]](4-)-N,N', $O, O' O^N$, O^{N1}]-disodium, hydrate, (OC-6-21)-disodium[(ethylenedinitrilo) tetraacetato]calciate(2-), hydrate [23411-34-9], anhydrous [62-33-9]

5. Empirical Formulas

	Molecular Weights
Edetic acid:	
$C_{10}H_{16}N_2O_8$	292.2
Edetate disodium:	
$C_{10}H_{14}N_2Na_2O_8 \cdot 2H_2O$	372.2
$C_{10}H_{14}N_2Na_2O_8$	336.2
Edetate calcium disodium:	
$C_{10}H_{12}CaN_2Na_2O_8 \cdot 2H_2O$	410.3
$C_{10}H_{12}CaN_2Na_2O_8$	374.3

Edetate calcium disodium USP is described as a mixture of the dihydrate and the trihydrate, predominantly the dihydrate. Sodium calciumedetate BP is described as the dihydrate.

6. Structural Formulas

Edetic acid:
$(HOOCCH_2)_2NCH_2CH_2N(CH_2COOH)_2$

Edetate disodium:

Edetate calcium disodium:

7. Commercial Availability

USA

Akzo Chernio, Armak Co., Agent
Atomergic Chemetals Corp.
Ciba Geigy Corp., Dyestuffs & Chemicals Div.
Dogussa Corp.
Grace & Co., W.R., Organic Chemicals Div.
Jordan Chemical Co.
Lowenstein Dyes & Cosmetics, Inc.
Onyx Chemical Co.
Pfaltz & Bauer, Inc.
Surfactants, Inc.
Thompson-Hayward Chemical Co.
Tri-K Industries, Inc.
United States Biochemicals Corp.

UK

Abbott Laboratories, Ltd.
ABM Chemicals, Ltd.
Allied Colloids (Mfg.), Ltd.
Ciba-Geigy (UK) Ltd.
Croda Food Ingredients, Ltd.
Fisons Scientific Apparatus, Ltd.
GAF (Great Britain), Ltd.
W.R. Grace Co., Ltd.
Hopkin and Williams
Riker Laboratories
Sigma London Chemical Co., Ltd.

8. Method of Manufacture

Edetic acid is prepared by the condensation of ethylene diamine with sodium monochloroacetate in the presence of sodium carbonate. An aqueous solution of the reactants is heated to about 90°C for ten hours, then cooled, and hydrochloric acid is added to precipitate the edetic acid. (U.S. Pat. 2, 130, 505). It is also prepared by the reaction of ethylene diamine with hydrogen cyanide and formaldehyde: with subsequent hydrolysis of the tetranitrile, or under alkaline conditions with continuous extraction of ammonia. The disodium salt is formed from edetic acid by the addition of sodium hydroxide. Edetate calcium disodium is prepared by the addition of calcium carbonate to a solution of edetate disodium.

9. Description

Edetic acid: White crystalline powder. Edetate disodium: White crystalline powder; odorless; slightly acid taste. Edetate calcium disodium: White or creamy-white crystalline powder or granules; odorless, or with a slight odor; tasteless, or with a faint saline taste. Slightly hygroscopic.

10. Pharmacopeial Specifications

Edetic acid:

Test	NF
Identification	+
Residue on ignition	≤0.2%
Heavy metals	≤0.003%
Nitrilotriacetic acid	≤0.3%
Iron	≤0.005%
Assay limits	98.0 - 100.5%

Edetate disodium:

Test	USP	BP
Identification	+	+
pH (acidity)	4.0 - 6.0	4.0 - 5.5
	(1 in 20 solution)	(5% solution)
Loss on drying	8.7 - 11.4%	—
Calcium	+	—
Heavy metals	0.005%	≤20 ppm
Iron	—	≤80 ppm
Nitrilotriacetic acid	0.1%	—
Cyanide	—	+
Assay limits	99.0 - 101.0%	≥98.0%
	(calculated on	(dihydrate)
	(dried basis)	

Edetate calcium disodium:

Test	USP	BP
Identification	+	+
pH (acidity or alkalinity)	6.5 - 8.0	6.5 - 8.0
	(1 in 5 solution)	(20% solution)
Water	≤13.0%	—
Iron	—	≤80 ppm
Heavy metals	≤0.002%	≤20 ppm
Magnesium-chelating substances	+	—
Chloride	—	≤0.07%
Cyanide	—	+
Sulfate	—	≤0.24%
Disodium edetate	—	+
Loss on drying	—	8.0 - 11.0%
Assay limits (calculated on anhydrous basis)	97.0 - 102.0%	97.0 - 103.0%

11. Typical Properties

Freezing point depression: Edetate disodium: 0.14°C (1% solution)

Melting point: Edetic acid: >220°C with decomposition

pH: Edetic acid: 2.2 (0.2% solution)

      Edetate disodium: 4.3 - 4.7 (1% solution in CO_2-free water)

pK: Edetic acid: pK_{a1} 2.00
             pK_{a2} 2.67
             pK_{a3} 6.16
             pK_{a4} 10.26

Refractive index: Edetate disodium: 1.335 (1% solution)

Relative density: Edetate disodium: 1.004 (1% solution)

Solubility:

Solvent	Solubility
Edetic acid:	
Water	2 g/L*
Solutions of alkali hydroxides	Soluble
Edetate disodium:	
Water	1 in 11
Ethanol (96%)	Slightly soluble
Chloroform	Practically insoluble
Ether	Practically insoluble
Edetate calcium disodium:	
Water	1 in 2
Ethanol (96%)	Very slightly soluble
Chloroform	Practically insoluble
Ether	Practically insoluble

Viscosity: Edetate disodium: 1.03 mm²/s (1% solution)

* 0.5 g/L given in the Merck Index

12. Stability and Storage Conditions

Fairly stable in the solid state. Store in tight containers. The edetate salts are more stable than the free acid, which decarboxylates if heated above 150°C. Edetate disodium loses water on crystallization when heated to 120°C. Edetate calcium disodium is slightly hygroscopic and should be protected from moisture. Solutions may be sterilized by autoclaving, and should be stored in an alkali-free container.

13. Incompatibilities

Polyvalent metal ions. Edetic acid and edetate disodium behave as weak acids, displacing carbon dioxide from carbonates and reacting with metals to form hydrogen. Insulin may be inactivated due to the chelation of zinc. When a calcium gluconate injection which was stabilized with edetate disodium was mixed with a solution for total parenteral nutrition, chelation of trace metals in the TPN solution occurred. Edetate calcium disodium was incompatible with amphotericin and with hydralazine hydrochloride in infusion fluids.

14. Safety

Edetate disodium is poorly absorbed from the gastrointestinal tract. The LD_{50} (oral) in rats is 2 g/kg of body weight. Edetic acid and the disodium salt chelate calcium can, in large doses, cause calcium depletion. If used in preparations for the mouth, they can leach calcium from the teeth. Edetate calcium disodium does not chelate calcium. A study of the carcinogenic potential of edetate trisodium has reported that the incidence of tumors in laboratory animals fed this material was essentially the same as found in the control group. The estimated acceptable daily intake of edetate in food is up to 2.5 mg/kg of body weight.

15. Handling Precautions

Solutions of edetates should not be allowed to come into contact with metal items (e.g., filters). Avoid ingestion, inhalation and contact with skin, eyes and nose.

16. Regulatory Acceptance

Edetic acid: NF XVI
Edetate disodium: USP XXI; BP 1980
Edetate calcium disodium: USP XXI; BP 1980
Disodium edetate and sodium calcium edetate are permitted in certain foods and drinks in the U.K. under the Miscellaneous Additives in Food Regulations, 1974 and the Miscellaneous Additives in Food (Scotland) Regulations, 1974.

17. Applications in Pharmaceutical Formulation or Technology

The edetates are chelating agents; that is, they form stable water-soluble complexes (chelates) with alkaline earth and heavy metal ions. The chelated form has few of the properties of the free ion, and for this reason chelating agents are often described as "removing" ions from solution (also called sequestering). The stability of the metal-edetate complex depends on the metal ion involved and also on the pH. The calcium chelate is relatively weak and will preferentially chelate heavy metals, such as iron, copper and lead, releasing calcium ions.

Uses:

Water softener—Edetic acid and edetate disodium will chelate calcium and magnesium ions in hard water; edetate calcium disodium is not effective. Many cosmetic and toiletry products (e.g., soaps) contain edetic acid as a water softener.

Antioxidant synergists—Edetates have been used to sequester traces of metal ions, particularly copper, iron and manganese, which might otherwise catalyze autooxidation reactions. They have been used both alone and in combination with true antioxidants. Concentrations in the range 0.005 - 0.1% have been employed. Edetates have been used to stabilize epinephrine, ascorbic acid, folic acid, formaldehyde, gums and resins, hyaluronidase, corticoids, hydrogen peroxide, oxytetracycline, penicillin, salicylic acid and unsaturated fatty acids. Essential oils can be washed with a 2% solution of edetate to remove trace metals.

Antibacterial synergist—Although the edetates have no bactericidal activity, they may exert a bacteriostatic effect by chelating trace metals necessary for growth (e.g., magnesium). Edetate disodium has also been found to enhance the activity of several preservatives, particularly benzalkonium chloride, against *Pseudomonas aeruginosa*. The concentrations usually employed are 0.1% of edetate disodium with 0.01% benzalkonium chloride. Many solutions used for the cleaning, storage and wetting of contact lenses contain edetate disodium. The concentration most commonly used is 0.1%.

Anticoagulant—By chelating calcium, edetate disodium prevents the coagulation of blood *in vitro*. Concentrations of 0.1% (in small samples for hematological testing) to 0.3% (in transfusions) have been used.

18. Related Substances

The tri- and tetrasodium salts of edetic acid are readily available and have similar uses. The trisodium salt can be formed by adding a solution of sodium hydroxide to edetate disodium (as in the preparation of trisodium edetate injection BP). In the U.S.A., the name "sodium edetate" is used to refer to the tetrasodium salt. Other salts of edetic acid which are commercially available include diammonium-, dimagnesium-, dipotassium-, ferric sodium- and magnesium disodium edetates. Disodium copper edetate is used as an intramuscular injection to treat copper deficiency in cattle. Edetic acid and iodine form a colorless addition compound which is bactericidal.

19. Comments

None

20. References

1. J. R. Hart, Chelating agents in cosmetic and toiletry products, *Cosmet. Toilet.*, 93: 28 (1978).
2. R. M. E. Richards and R. H. Cavill, Electron microscope study of the effect of benzalkonium chloride and edetate disodium on the cell envelope of *Ps. aeruginosa*, *J. Pharm. Sci.*, 65: 76 (1976).
3. L. Chalmers, The uses of EDTA and other chelates in industry, *Man. Chem.*, 49: (March), 79 (1978).
4. L. Lachman, Uses of edetates as chelating agents in the formulation of liquid pharmaceuticals, *Drug Cosmet. Ind.*, 102: (Feb.), 43 (1968).
5. "Bioassay of trisodium ethylenediaminetetraacetate trihydrate (EDTA) for possible carcinogenicity," *National Cancer Institute Carcinogenesis Technical Report Series*, No. 11 (1977).
6. "Review of edetates as antioxidant synergists", *Fd. Add. Ser. Wld. Hlth. Org.*, No. 3 (1972).

USA: J. C. Cradock*; D. C. Kriesel**
UK: R. C. F. Baker*; S. B. Williamson**

Ethyl Oleate

1. Nonproprietary Name
NF: Ethyl oleate
BP: Ethyl oleate

2. Functional Category
NF: Oleaginous vehicle

3. Synonyms
Oleic acid, ethyl ester; aethylis oleas

4. Chemical Name and CAS Registry Number
9-Octadecenoic acid, (Z)-, ethyl ester
Ethyl oleate [111-62-6]

5. Empirical Formula   Molecular Weight
$C_{20}H_{38}O_2$ 310.52

6. Structural Formula
HC CH$_2$(CH$_2$)$_6$COOC$_2$H$_5$
‖
HC CH$_2$(CH$_2$)$_6$CH$_3$

7. Commercial Availability
USA
Aceto Chemical Co., Inc.
Chemical Service Inc.
Eastman Organic Chemical
Fisher Scientific Co.
ICN-K&K Laboratories, Inc.
J. T. Baker Chemical Co.
Lachat Chemicals, Inc.
Pfaltz & Bauer, Inc.

UK
Croda Chemicals, Ltd.
Leek Chemicals, Ltd.
Unichema International

8. Method of Manufacture
Ethyl oleate is prepared by the reaction of ethanol with oleoyl chloride in the presence of a suitable hydrogen chloride acceptor.

9. Description
A pale yellow to almost colorless, mobile, oily liquid with a taste resembling that of olive oil. It has a slight but not rancid odor.

10. Pharmacopeial Specifications

Test	NF	BP
Specific gravity (at 20°C)	0.866-0.874	—
Weight per ml (at 20°C)	—	0.869-0.874 g.
Viscosity	≥5.15 cps	—
Refractive index	1.443-1.450	—
Acid value	≤0.5	≤0.5
Iodine value	75-85	75-84
Saponification value	177-188	—
Peroxides	—	+
Assay	—	100-105% w/w

11. Typical Properties
Boiling point: 205-208°C (some decomposition)
Flash point: 175.3°C
Moisture content: Equilibrium moisture content: 0.08% (at 20°C and 52% RH); Moisture sorption isotherm: Values determined by Karl Fischer titration of samples at equilibrium after storage for five days in desiccators over saturated solutions of appropriate salts. (Fig. 1)

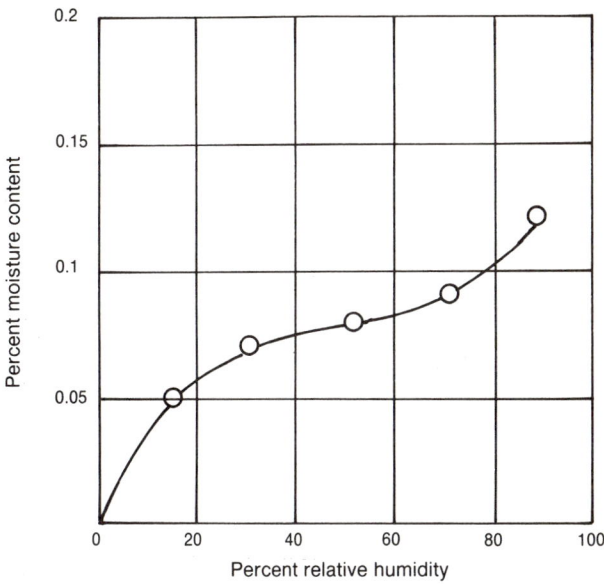

Fig. 1: Moisture sorption isotherm of ethyl oleate.

Miscibility:

Solvent	Miscibility (at 20°C)
Water	Immiscible
Ethanol (100% and 96%)	Miscible in all proportions
Propylene glycol	Immiscible
Propan-2-ol	Miscible in all proportions
Glycerol	Immiscible
Acetone	Miscible in all proportions
Chloroform	Miscible in all proportions
Ether	Miscible in all proportions
Fixed oils and fats	Miscible

Solidification point: −32°C (approximately)

12. Stability and Storage Conditions
Ethyl oleate should be stored in a cool place in a small, well-filled, air-tight container, protected from light. When a partially filled container is used, the air should be replaced by Nitrogen or another inert gas. Ethyl oleate oxidizes on exposure to air, resulting in an increase in the peroxide value. It remains clear at 5°C, but discolors on standing. Anti-oxidants are frequently used to extend the shelf life of ethyl oleate. Protection from oxidation for over two years has been achieved by storing it in amber glass bottles and the addition of a double or triple mixture of propyl gallate, butylated hydroxyanisole, butylated hydroxytoluene and citric or ascorbic acid. A concentration of 0.03% w/v of a mixture of propyl gallate (37.5%), butylated hydroxytoluene (37.5%) and butylated hydroxyanisole (25%) was found to be the best anti-oxidant for ethyl oleate. Ethyl oleate may be sterilized by heating at 150°C for 1 hour.

13. Incompatibilities

Ethyl oleate dissolves some kinds of rubber and causes others to swell. Ethyl oleate may react with oxidizing agents.

14. Safety

No toxicity data available in the literature. Generally considered to be of low toxicity, but ingestion should be avoided. Ethyl oleate has been found to cause minimal tissue irritation. No reports of intramuscular irritation during use have been recorded.

15. Handling Precautions

During sterilization by dry heat, a slight fire hazard exists, as ethyl oleate can react with oxidizing agents.

16. Regulatory Acceptance

NF XVI; BP 1980

17. Applications in Pharmaceutical Formulation or Technology

Ethyl oleate is used as a vehicle for certain parenteral preparations which are to be administered by the intramuscular route. It is a good solvent for steroid and other oil-soluble medications. It is a superior solvent for fixed oils and is therefore sometimes used instead of them as a vehicle for injections. It has properties very similar to those of almond oil and arachis oil, but has the advantage over fixed oils in that it is less viscous and more rapidly absorbed by the tissues.

18. Related Substances

—

19. Comments

—

20. Specific References

1. S. L. Hem, D. R. Brigh, G. S. Banker and J. P. Pogue, *Drug Development Communications*, 1: (5), 471 (1974-75).
2. A. J. Spiegel and M. M. Noseworthy, Review article, Use of nonaqueous solvents in parenteral products, *J. Pharm. Sci*, 52: (10), 917 (1963).
3. N. M. Nikolayeve and M. H. Glyzman, *Farmatsiya (Moscov)*, 26: 25 (1977).
4. P. Alemany and A. Del Pozo, *Galenica Acta*, 16: 335 (1963).

USA: J. C. Cradock*; A. Palmieri**
UK: F. S. S. Morton*; W. Lund**

Ethylcellulose

1. Nonproprietary Name
NF: Ethylcellulose

2. Functional Category
NF: Tablet binder; coating agent

3. Synonyms
Ethyl cellulose; *Ethocel*

4. Chemical Names and CAS Registry Number
Cellulose, ethyl ether
Cellulose ethyl ether [9004-57-3]

5. Empirical Formula   Molecular Weight

$C_{12}H_{23}O_6 (C_{12}H_{22}O_5)_{n-2} C_{12}H_{23}O_5$ N.A.

Ethylcellulose with complete ethoxyl substitution.
The cellulose molecule is a chain of β-anhydroglucose units joined together by acetal linkages. Each anhydroglucose unit has three replaceable hydroxyl groups which are substituted to the extent of 2.25 to 2.60 ethoxyl groups per unit (or 44 to 50 percent ethoxyl content).

6. Structural Formula

a

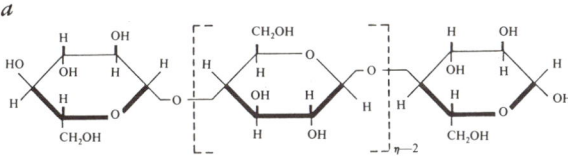

b

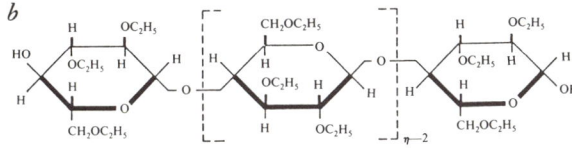

a. Structural formula of cellulose
b. Structural formula of ethylcellulose with complete (54.88%) ethoxyl substitution.

7. Commercial Availability
USA

The Dow Chemical Company
Hercules, Inc.

UK

Hercules, Ltd.
K&K-Greeff Chemicals, Ltd.

8. Method of Manufacture
Alkali cellulose is reacted with ethyl chloride, as expressed by the following type reaction:
$RONa + C_2H_5Cl \rightarrow ROC_2H_5 + NaCl$
where R represents the cellulose radical.

9. Description
A tasteless, free-flowing, white to light tan powder.

SEM: KY-23
Excipient: Ethylcellulose N-100 NF
Manufacturer: Hercules   **Lot no.:** 57911

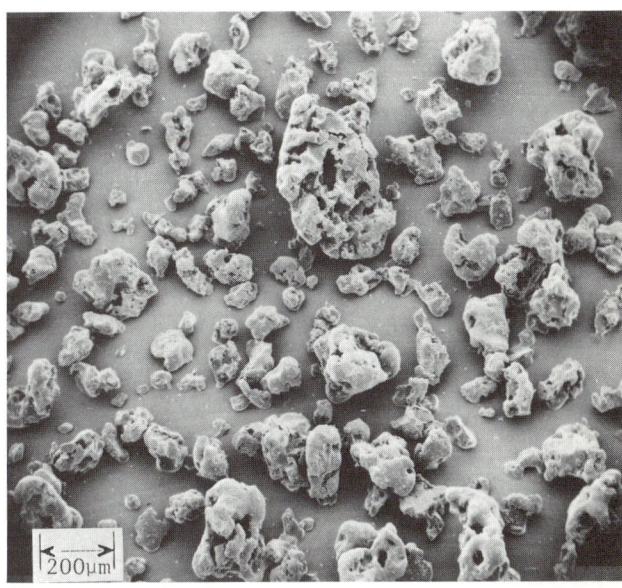

Magnification: 60×   **Voltage:** 10 kV

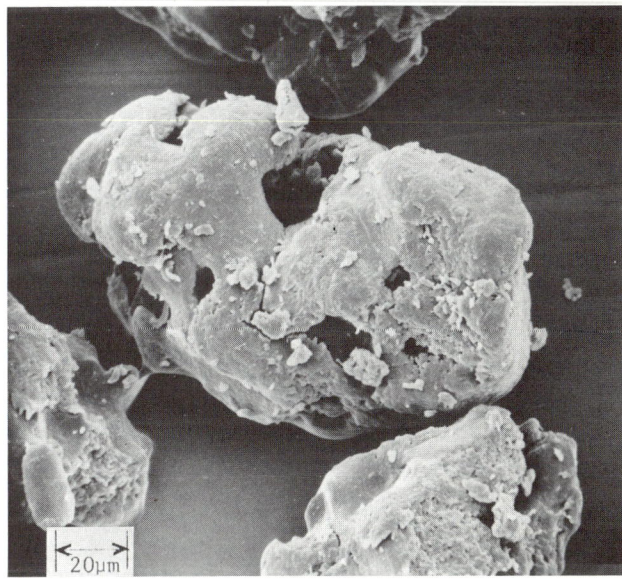

Magnification: 600×   **Voltage:** 10KV

SEM: KY-24
Excipient: *Ethocel* ethylcellulose
Manufacturer: Dow   **Lot no.:** 103051

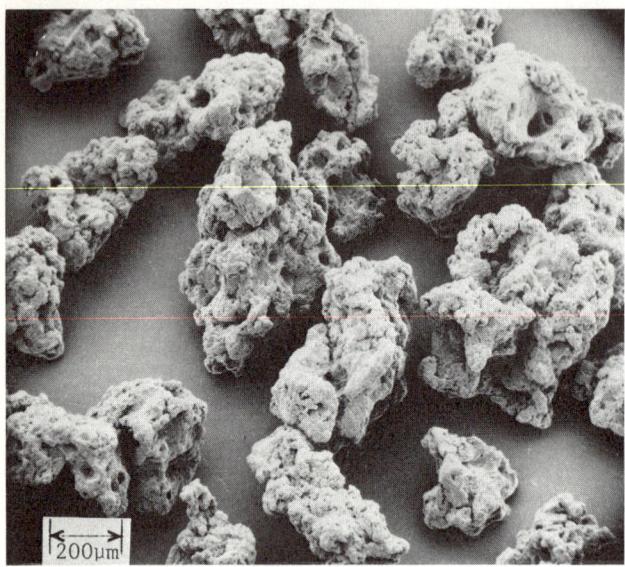

Magnification: 60×   **Voltage:** 10 kV

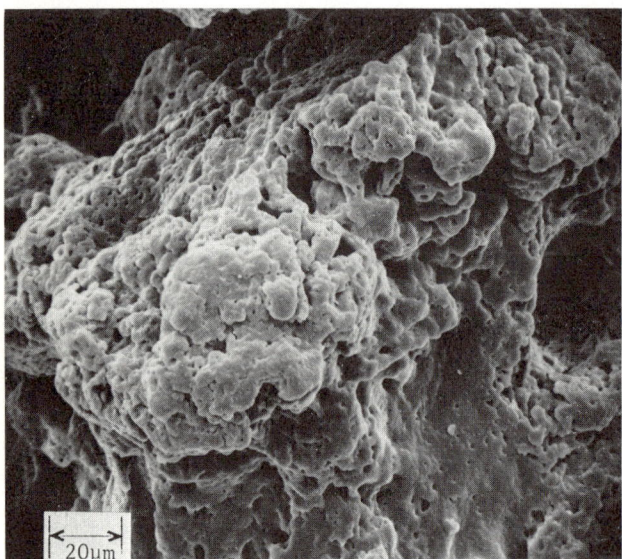

Magnification: 600×   **Voltage:** 10kV

10. Pharmacopeial Specifications

Test	NF
Identification	+
Viscosity	+
Loss on drying	≤3.0%
Residue on ignition	≤0.4%
Assay for ethoxyl groups	44.0–51.0
Arsenic	≤3ppm
Lead	≤10ppm
Heavy metals	≤40ppm

11. Typical Properties

Specific gravity: 1.14
Specific volume in solution: (in³/lb): 23.9
Hygroscopicity: The various types of ethylcellulose are not affected by water. They take up very little water from humid air or during immersion, and that small amount evaporates readily.
Film properties, 3 mil film: Tensile strength, lb/in², 6,800-10,500; % elongation at rupture, 7-30; flexibility, MIT folds (a) 160-2,000; hardness index, sward (b) 52-61.
Light transmission, practically complete, Å: 3,100-4,000; *water vapor transmission, 3 mil film* (g/m²/24 hours), 890
Dielectric constant at 25° C, 1 kc: 3.0-4.1
Power factor at 25° C, 1 kg: 0.002-0.02
Moisture absorption* by film in 24 hours. At 80% R.H.: 2%
Odor*: None
Refractive index*: 1.47
Solubility: Insoluble in water, glycerin and propylene glycol, but soluble in varying degrees in certain organic solvents, depending upon the ethoxyl content. The addition of 10-20% of a lower aliphatic alcohol to solvents, such as ketones, esters and hydrocarbons, can improve the solubility.
Softening point*, ° C: 152-162
Taste: None
Viscosity: Properties of ethylcellulose, such as tensile strength, elongation, and flexibility, depend largely upon the degree of polymerization, which can be measured by viscosity. Therefore, within each type based on ethoxyl content there exist low to high viscosity types, based on degree of polymerization.

(a) See ASTM D-643-43
(b) See H. A. Gardner and G. G. Sward, Point Testing Manual, 12th ed., Gardner Lab., Inc., Bethesda, MD

Academy HPE Laboratory Project Data

	Method	Lab #	Results
Moisture content[a]	MC-29	23	1.853%
Moisture content[a]	MC-20	15	0.700%
Moisture content[b]	MC-29	23	1.020%
Particle size dist.[a]	PSD-6	23	% Retained
			35 Mesh: 7.95
			48 Mesh: 11.24
			60 Mesh: 11.90
			80 Mesh: 14.80
			100 Mesh: 20.45
			150 Mesh: 12.26
			200 Mesh: 9.86
			PAN 11.25
Particle size dist.[b]	PSD-6	23	% Retained
			35 Mesh: 10.40
			48 Mesh: 43.13
			60 Mesh: 16.93
			80 Mesh: 12.62
			100 Mesh: 3.42
			150 Mesh: 1.40
			200 Mesh: 0.50
			PAN 1.60
Solubility[b]	SOL-6	23	
Water (25° C)			0.010 g/ml
Water (37° C)			0.012 g/ml
Alcohol (25° C)			0.015 g/ml
Alcohol (37° C)			0.025 g/ml
Prop. glycol (25° C)			0.025 g/ml
Prop. glycol (37° C)			0.025 g/ml
Hexane (25° C)			<0.002 g/ml
Hexane (37° C)			<0.006 g/ml
Solubility[a]	SOL-6	23	
Water (25° C)			<0.001 g/ml
Water (37° C)			<0.001 g/ml
Alcohol (25° C)			0.053 g/ml

Academy HPE Laboratory Project Data

	Method	Lab #	Results
Alcohol (37° C)			0.066 g/ml
Prop. glycol (25° C)			0.025 g/ml
Prop. glycol (37° C)			0.025 g/ml
Hexane (25° C)			<0.002 g/ml
Hexane (37° C)			<0.006 g/ml
Average flow rate[b]	FLO-3	24	1.66266g/sec
Particle friability[b]	PF-1	36	0.068
EMC plot[a]	EMC-1	15	Fig: 15-EMC-2

Suppliers: Hercules Ltd.[a]; Dow Chemical Co.[b]

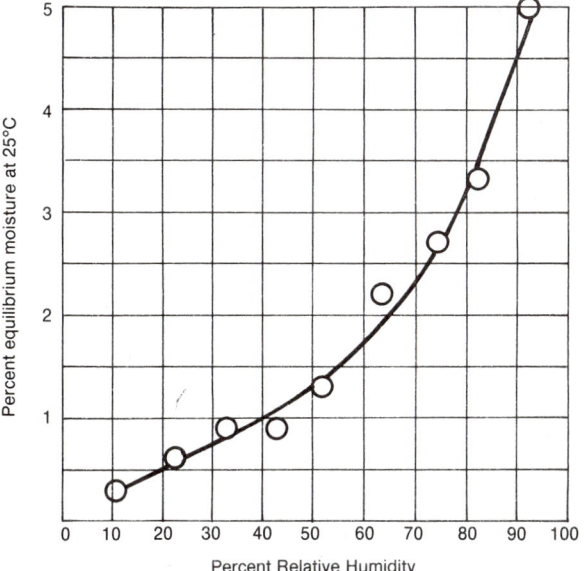

Ethycellulose NF (Hercules Ltd., Lot #58587)

Figure: 15-EMC-2   Method: EMC-1

12. Stability and Storage Conditions

It is resistant to alkalis, both dilute and concentrated, and to salt solutions. It is more sensitive to acidic materials than are cellulose esters. However, the material can withstand dilute acids for a limited period of exposure. Ethylcellulose is subject to oxidative degradation in the presence of sunlight or UV light at elevated temperatures. This may be prevented by use of an antioxidant and a compound with light absorption properties between 230-340 nm. Ethylcellulose should be stored between 7° and 32°C in a dry area away from all sources of heat. Store in a well-closed container.

13. Incompatibilities

Incompatible with paraffin wax and microcrystalline wax.

14. Safety

Essentially non-toxic.

15. Handling Precautions

In storage or in use, it is important to prevent dusts or fines from ethylcellulose from reaching potentially explosive levels in the air. Ethylcellulose products are considered not to present a health hazard to personnel handling the polymer.

16. Regulatory Acceptance

NF XVI

17. Applications in Pharmaceutical Formulation or Technology

Binder in tablets. Ethylcellulose may be blended dry and wet-granulated with a solvent such as alcohol. Tablets made with ethylcellulose as a binder tend to exhibit poor dissolution and poor drug absorption.

Coating material for tablets. Ethylcellulose by itself forms a water-insoluble film coating. It is commonly used with hydroxypropylmethylcellulose to alter the solubility of the film. Other materials may be used for this as well.

Coating material for stabilization. Ethylcellulose dissolved in isopropanol is used to coat ascorbic acid granules to prevent oxidation.

Coating to prevent unpleasant taste. Ethylcellulose may be used to coat drugs that have an unpleasant taste.

Slow drug release from films. Caffeine and salicylic acid incorporated into ethylcellulose films have been shown to exhibit diffusion-controlled release.

Coating for drug microcapsules. Ethylcellulose has been used to coat particles of drugs to form microcapsules. This type of microcapsule slows dissolution of the drug as a function of microcapsule wall thickness.

Thickening agent in creams, lotions or gels. Ethylcellulose may be used in these types of formulations, provided an appropriate solvent is used.

18. Related Substances

—

19. Comments

Plasticizer compatibility. Dibutyl phthalate, diethyl phthalate, dimethyl phthalate, benzyl benzoate, butyl and glycol esters of fatty acids, refined mineral oils, oleic acid, stearic acid, cetyl alcohol, stearyl alcohol, castor oil, corn oil, camphor and numerous others. Ethyl cellulose is available as an aqueous polymer dispersion (latex) for use in film coatings (*Aquacoat*) that allows for high solid content liquids with relatively low viscosity.

20. Specific References

1. "Ethylcellulose, Properties and Uses," Hercules, Inc. (1974).
2. "Solubility Parameter Maps of Hercules Film-Formers," CSL-204, Hercules, Inc.
3. "Tough Ethocel Ethylcellulose Resins," The Dow Chemical Company (1975).
4. J. D. Wellons and V. Stannett, *J. Polymer Sci.*, Pt. A-1, 4:593 (1966).
5. L. Tomasini, K. Radeva and M. Goshkaryan, *Tr., Nauchnoizsled. Khim-Farm. Inst.*, 9:401 (1974).
6. "Coating News: Market and Product Facts," M-341B, Hercules Inc., Wilmington, Delaware (1980).
7. J. Morel, French Patent No. 1,462, 193.
8. M. Donbrow, M. Friedman, *J. Pharm. Sci.*, 64: 76 (1975).
9. I. Jalsenjak, C. F. Nicolaidou and J. R. Nixon, *J. Pharm. Pharmac.*, 28: 912 (1976).
10. H. Oya Alpar and V. Walters, The prolongation of the *in vitro* dissolution of a soluble drug (Phenethicillin Potassium) by microencapsulation with ethylcellulose, *J. Pharm. Pharmacol.*, 33: 419-422 (1981).
11. S. Benita and M. Donbrow, Effect of polyisobutylene on ethylcellulose-walled microcapsules wall structure and thickness of salicylamide and theophylline microcapsules, *J. Pharm. Sci.*, 71 (2): 205-210 (1982).

USA: J. S. Kent*; Z. Chowhan**
UK: R. C. Rowe*

Ethylparaben

1. Nonproprietary Names

NF: Ethylparaben
BP: Ethyl hydroxybenzoate

2. Functional Category

USP: Antimicrobial preservative
BP: Antimicrobial preservative

3. Synonyms

Ethyl chemosept; ethyl parasept; *Betacide E*; *Ethylparaben*; *Nipabutyl A*; *Protaben E*; *Tegosept M*

4. Chemical Names and CAS Registry Number

4-Hydroxybenzoic acid ethyl ester
Ethyl *p*-hydroxybenzoate [120-47-8]
Ethyl 4-hydroxybenzoate

5. Empirical Formula

$C_9H_{10}O_3$

Molecular Weight

166.18

6. Structural Formula

7. Commercial Availability

USA

Beta Chemical Corporation
Inolex Personal Care Division
Mallinckrodt, Inc.
Napp Chemicals
Nipa Laboratories, Inc.
Protameen Chemicals, Inc.
Tenneco Chemical, Inc.

UK

BDH Chemicals
Bofors (Great Britain) Co., Ltd.
Bush, Boake, Allen, Ltd.
Nipa Laboratories, Ltd.

8. Method of Manufacture

Ethylparaben is prepared by the esterification of *p*-hydroxybenzoic acid with ethanol.

9. Description

White, crystalline, almost odorless powder.

SEM-MF-10
Excipient: Ethylparaben

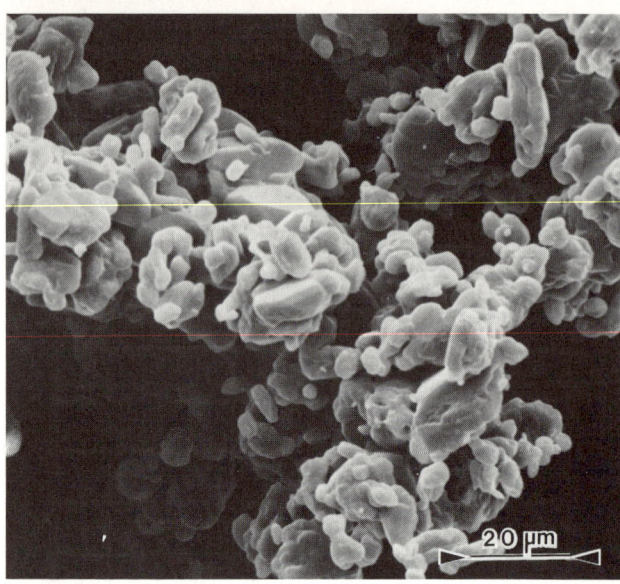

Magnification: 600×

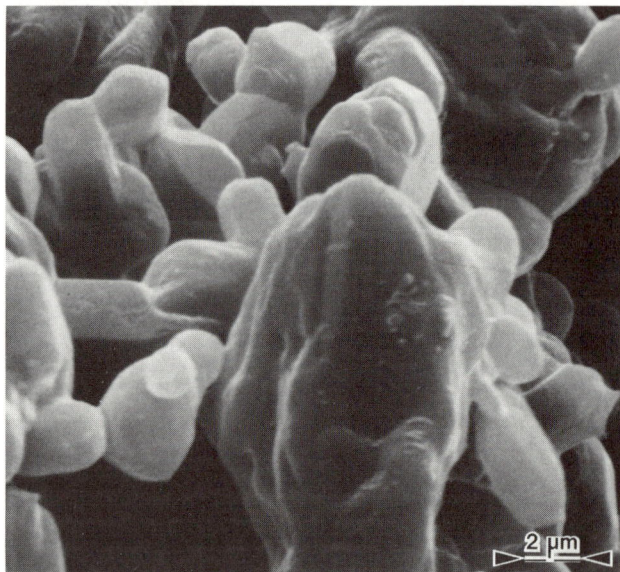

Magnification: 3,000×

10. Pharmacopeial Specifications

Test	NF	BP
Identification	+	+
Melting range	115°-118°C	~117°C
Acidity	+	+
Loss on drying	≤0.5%	—
Residue on ignition	≤0.05%	—
Assay	99.0-100.5%	99.0-101.0%
Sulfated ash	—	≤0.1%

11. Typical Properties

Solubility: Almost insoluble in cold water (0.17% w/v at 25°C; 0.86% w/v at 80°C); readily soluble in ethanol (50% w/v), acetone or propylene glycol.

Academy HPE Laboratory Project Data			
	Method	Lab #	Results
Solubility (water)	SOL-8	30	0.085%

12. Stability and Storage Conditions

Ethylparaben should be stored in a well-closed container. Aqueous solutions at pH 3-6 can be sterilized at 120°C for 20 minutes without decomposition. Aqueous solutions at pH 3-6 are relatively stable at room temperature. Aqueous solutions at pH 8 or higher are subject to hydrolysis.

13. Incompatibilities

The antimicrobial properties of ethylparaben are reduced in the presence of non-ionic surfactants. Adsorption to plastics is greater than that observed with methylparaben. Ethylparaben is discolored in the presence of iron and is subject to hydrolysis by weak alkalis and strong acids.

14. Safety

Ethylparaben may cause occasional hypersensitivity, which is usually manifested as dermatitis. The acute and chronic toxicity of ethylparaben is low.

15. Handling Precautions

—

16. Regulatory Acceptance

NF XVI; BP 1980

17. Applications in Pharmaceutical Formulation or Technology

Ethylparaben alone or in combination with other esters of *p*-hydroxybenzoic acid or with other antimicrobial agents is used as a preservative in cosmetic and pharmaceutical preparations.

18. Related Substances

Butylparaben; methylparaben; propylparaben

19. Comments

The following tabulation lists the minimal concentration (% in water) of ethylparaben required to inhibit growth.

Aerobacter aerogenes ATCC 8308	0.1
Aspergillus niger ATCC 10254	0.04
Bacillus cereus var. *mycoides* ATCC 6462	0.1
Bacillus subtilis ATCC 6633	0.1
Candida albicans ATCC 10231	0.1
Escherichia coli ATCC 9637	0.1
Klebsiella pneumoniae ATCC 10031	0.05
Penicillium digitatum ATC 10030	0.025
Rhizopus nigricans ATCC 6227A	0.025
Saccharomyces cerevisiae ATCC 9763	0.05
Staphylococcus aureus ATCC 6538P	0.1

The antimicrobial effectiveness decreases with increasing pH due to the formation of phenolate anion.

20. Specific References

1. "S. M. Blaug and D. E. Grant, Kinetics of degradation of parabens, *J. Soc. Cosmet. Chem.*, 25:495 (1974).
2. J. Schimmel and M. N. Slotsky, Preservation of cosmetics. In: "Cosmetics, Science and Technology," 2nd Ed., Vol. III, M. S. Balsam and E. Sagarin, Eds., Wiley–Interscience, New York, 1974, pp. 391-470.
3. T. R. Aalto *et al.*, *p*-Hydroxybenzoic acid esters as preservatives, *J. Am. Pharm. Assoc. Sci. Ed.*, 42:449 (1953).
4. E. L. Richardson, Preservatives: Frequency of use in cosmetic formulas as disclosed to FDA, *Cosmetic and Toiletries*, 92:85-88 (1977).
5. K. Kakemi, H. Sezaki, E. Arakawa, K. Kimura and K. Ikeda, Interactions of parabens and other pharmaceutical adjuvants with plastic containers, *Chem. Pharm. Bull.*, 19:2523-29 (1971).

USA: M. Rieger*, P. Kotwal**, Z. Chowhan**
U.K.: M. C. Allwood*

Fumaric Acid

1. Nonproprietary Name
NF: Fumaric acid

2. Functional Categories
USP: Acidifying agent
Other: Flavoring agent

3. Synonyms
Allomaleic acid; boletic acid

4. Chemical Names and CAS Registry Number
2 - Butenedioic acid
trans -1,2-ethylenedicarboxylic acid [110-17-8]

5. Empirical Formula   Molecular Weight
$C_4H_4O_4$ 116.07

6. Structural Formula

    HOC-COOH
       ‖
 HOOC-COH

7. Commercial Availability
USA
American International Chemical, Inc.
Atomergic Chemetals Corp.
Chemical Dynamics Corp.
Fallek Chemical Co.
Gallard-Schlesinger Chemical Mfg. Corp.
ICN K & K Labs, Inc.
Monsanto Co.
Pfaltz & Bauer, Inc.
Pfizer, Inc.-Chemical Div.
Tenneco Chemicals, Inc.
Unites States Biochemicals Corp.

UK
BDH Chemicals, Ltd.
Croda Food Ingredients, Ltd.
Fisons, Ltd.

8. Method of Manufacture
From glucose by the action of fungi such as *Rhizopus nigricans;* as a by-product in the manufacture of maleic and phthalic anhydrides; by the isomerization of maleic acid using heat or a catalyst.

9. Description
White, odorless or nearly odorless, crystalline powder.

10. Pharmacopeial Specifications

Test	NF
Identification	+
Water (by Karl Fischer)	≤ 0.5%
Residue on ignition	≤ 0.1%
Heavy metals	≤ 0.001%
Maleic acid	≤ 0.1%
Assay (anhydrous)	99.5-100.5%

11. Typical Properties
Sublimes at 200°C: Melts at 287°C (closed capillary)
Density at 20°C: 1.63 g/cm^3 (particle); 0.77 g/cm^3 (bulk); 0.93 g/cm^3 (tapped).
pH (saturated, aqueous at 20°C): 2.45
pKa_1: 3.03, *pKa_2:* 4.54, at 25°C
Solubility (g/L at 20°C): Water: 4.5, ethanol (100%): 36, propylene glycol: 30. Almost insoluble in olive oil, chloroform, carbon tetrachloride and benzene.

12. Stability and Storage Conditions
Subject to degradation by both aerobic and anaerobic organisms. Store in a well-closed container.

13. Incompatibilities
Incompatabilities are the same as those usually associated with organic acids.

14. Safety
Intraperitoneal LD_{50} (mouse): 200 mg/kg.
Acute toxic hazard is slight: (a) as a local irritant; and (b) by systemic ingestion.

15. Handling Precautions
Slight fire hazard—explosion hazard with heavy dust collection. Avoid contact with eyes or mucous membranes. Flush with water on contact.

16. Regulatory Status
NF XVI. In the UK, fumaric acid has been permitted for general food use under the Miscellaneous Additives in Food Regulations (1980).

17. Applications in Pharmaceutical Formulation or Technology
An acidulant and flavoring agent in pharmaceutical liquid preparations. An alternative to tartaric acid. Used in combination with antioxidants due to its ability to act as a chelating agent.

18. Related Substances
Tartaric acid

19. Comments
—

20. Specific References
1. *Fumaric Acid*—Technical Bulletin 1c/F1-S, Monsanto Corp.
2. *Food Acidulants*—Technical Bulletin, Pfizer Corp.
3. Malic and Fumaric Acids, *Manufacturing Chemist and Aerosol News*, 35: 56, Dec. (1964).

USA: L. E. Small*; K. R. Heimlich**
UK: S. Williamson*; W. Lund**

Gelatin

1. Nonproprietary Name

NF: Gelatin
BP: Gelatin

2. Functional Categories

USP: Coating agent; suspending and/or viscosity-increasing agent; tablet binder

3. Synonyms

Gelfoam, Puragel, Pharmagel A, Pharmagel B

4. Chemical Name

Gelatin

5. Empirical Formula and Molecular Weight

Gelatin is a generic term used to describe a mixture of fractions differing principally in molecular size. These fractions are composed entirely of amino acid radicals joined together by peptide linkages to form linear polymers, varying in molecular weight from 15,000 to 250,000.
Elemental analyses are as follows: carbon 50.5%; hydrogen 6.8%; nitrogen 17.0%; and oxygen 25.2%. Since it is derived from collagen, it is properly classified as a derived protein. It gives typical protein reactions and is hydrolyzed by most of the proteolytic systems to yield its peptide or amino acid components.

6. Structural Formula

—

7. Commercial Availability

USA

Atlantic Gelatin, General Foods Corp.
Burtonite Co., Inc.
Comerican Int'l., Inc.
Peter Cooper Corp.
Desno Chemical Corp.
Gelatin Mfg. Inst. of Amer.
Grayslake Gelatin Co.
Keystone Gelatin Co.
Kind & Knox Gelatin Co.
P. Leiner & Sons, America, Inc.
Perny, Inc.
Riches-Nelson, Inc.
Swift Edible Oil Co., Food Ingredients Products
V.G.F. Chemical Corp.
Vyse Gelatin Co.

UK

Arthur Branwell & Co., Ltd.
Brenntag (UK), Ltd.
Chemical Exchange (UK), Ltd.
Croda Food Ingredients, Ltd.
L.J. Rickards & Co., Ltd.
Leiner Gelatin, Ltd.
Oury, Miller & Co., Ltd.
Rousselot, Ltd.

8. Method of Manufacture

Type A Gelatin (acid process): Most type A gelatin produced in the United States is made from pork skins. The material is washed in cold water for a few hours to remove extraneous matter, and is then digested in dilute mineral acid (HCl, H_2SO_4, H_2SO_3, H_3PO_4 at pH 1-3) at 15-20°C until maximum swelling has occurred. This requires a period of approximately 24 hours. The swollen stock is washed with water to remove the excess acid and adjusted to pH of 3.5-4.0 for the conversion to gelatin by hot water extraction.

The hydrolytic extraction is carried out in batch-type operation with successive portions of hot water at progressively higher temperatures until the maximum yield is obtained. The gelatin solutions are chilled into jelled sheets and dried in temperature-controlled ovens. The dried gelatin is then ground to the desired particle size.

Type B Gelatin (alkaline process): The raw material, ossein or skin stocks is held in a calcium hydroxide (lime) slurry for a period of one to three months at 15-20°C. At the end of the liming, the stock is washed with cold water to remove as much lime as possible. It is then neutralized with acid (HCl, H_2SO_4, H_3PO_4). The ensuing process is the same as for the acid-treated pork skins.

9. Description

Appearance, color, odor, and taste: Gelatin is nearly tasteless and odorless. It is a vitreous, brittle solid, and is faintly yellow in color.

10. Pharmacopeial Specifications

Test	USP	BP
Identification	+	+
Microbial limits:		
Total bacterial count	≤1,000/g	—
Salmonella species	Negative	Negative
E. coli	Negative	Negative
Residue on ignition	≤2.0%	—
Odor & water-insoluble substances	+	—
Sulfur dioxide	≤0.15%	≤200 ppm
Arsenic	≤0.8 ppm	≤2 ppm
Heavy metals	≤0.005%	—
Copper	—	≤10 ppm
Lead	—	≤5ppm
Zinc	—	≤25 ppm
Jelly strength	—	≥150
Odor & taste of solution	—	+
Loss on drying	—	≤16.0%
Ash	—	≤3.25%

11. Typical Properties

Academy HPE Laboratory Project Data				
		Method	Lab #	Results (%)
Moisture	Content	MC-11	14	10.6[a]
"	"	MC-26	18	10.6[b]
"	"	MC-10	28	8.815[b]
"	"	MC-10	28	11.015[b]
"	"	MC-10	28	11.75 [a]
EMC Plot (Pharmagel A)		EMC-1	18	Fig. 18-EMC-3 K
SDI Plot		SDI-1	14	Fig. 14-SDI-3 L

Suppliers: Leiner[a]; Kind & Knox[b].

Amphoteric character: Gelatin, a typical protein, acts both as an acid and as a base. Thus, it is an amphoteric substance and can be titrated with acids and with alkalis.

Isoelectric point: In a strongly acidic solution, an ampholite such as gelatin is positively charged and migrates as a cation in an electric field. In a strongly alkaline solution, it is negatively charged and migrates as an anion. There is an intermediate point where the net charge is zero and no movement occurs. This point is known as the isoelectric point (IEP) and is designated in pH units.

Gelatin as a colloid: A very important, characteristic property of gelatin is its ability to form a gel or jelly in aqueous solution at temperatures below 35-40°C. At higher temperatures, the system exists as a sol. The gel-sol system is heat reversible, the melting temperature being slightly higher than the setting point.

Viscosity: In certain applications the viscosity of a solution of gelatin in water is as important as the ability of the solution to form a gel.

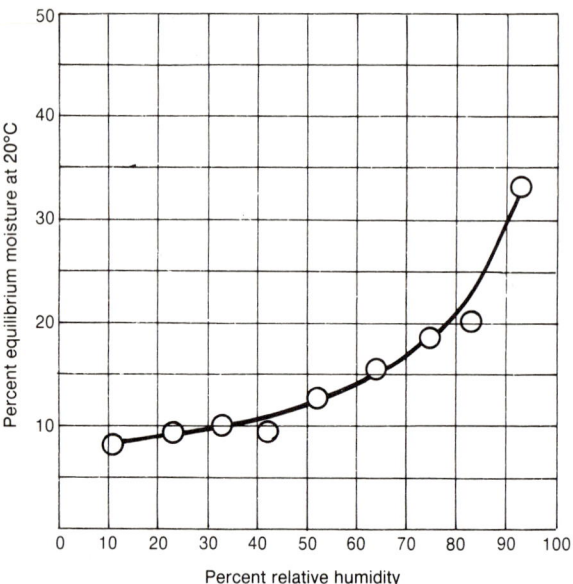

Gelatin USP, *Pharmagel A* (Kind & Knox)
Figure: 18-EMC-3

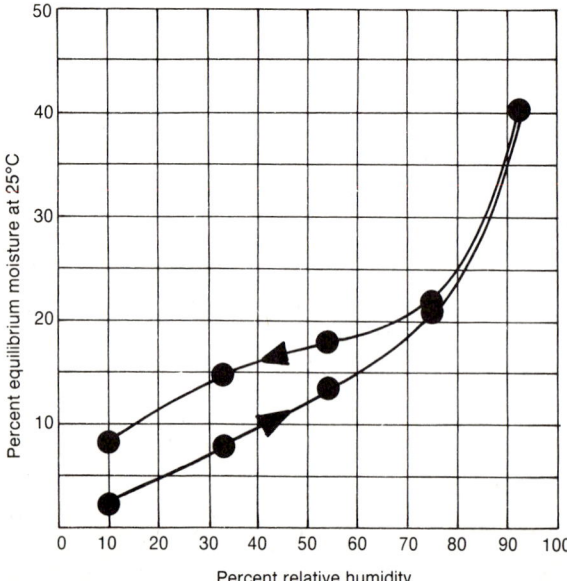

Gelatin (Leiner, Lot #627)
Figure: 14-SDI-3 **Method:** SDI-1

General Physical Properties:

Property	Type A	Type B
pH (1% solution at 25°C)	3.8-6.0	5.0-7.4
Isoelectric point		
USP method	9.0-9.2	4.8-5.0
BP method	8.9-9.2	4.8-5.2
Gel strength, Bloomgrams		
USP method	75-300	75-275
BP method	50-320	50-300
Viscosity, cP	2.0-7.5	2.0-7.5

Capsules: There are two types of gelatin capsules: elastic, or soft capsules, and two-piece hard capsules.

General Properties of Soft Capsules:

Property	Type A	Type B
Gel strength, Bloomgrams	170-180	150-175
Viscosity (mp)	30-35	35-40
pH	5.0-5.5	5.5-7.3
% ash	≤0.5 max.	≤2.0 max.
Total bacterial count	10,000 per gram max.	
Coliform count	Absent in 0.01 g. gelatin	

General Properties of Hard Capsules:

Property	Type A	Type B
Gel strength, Bloomgrams	250-280	220-250
Viscosity (mp)	45-50	45-60
pH	4.5-5.5	5.3-7.3
Total bacterial count	10,000 per gram max.	
Coliform count	Absent in 0.01 g. gelatin	

Density: Beckmann Air Pycnometer (mean of 3 samples): Acid processed = 1.325 g/cm³; Lime processed = 1.283 g/cm³

Solubility: (a) In water—At 25°C, absorbs up to 10 times its volume of water but does not dissolve; at 37°C, up to 20% readily dissolves; at 100°C, slowly breaks down in solution, with changes in viscosity and other physical properties. Up to 50% can be dispersed. (b) in other solvents: ethanol—insoluble; isopropanol—insoluble; 50% glycerol—up to 10%, depending on mol. wt. of gelatin; methanol—insoluble; acetone—insoluble; acids and alkalis—acetic acid will dissolve at least 5%. Strong acid and alkali tend to precipitate.

12. Stability and Storage Conditions

Pure, dry gelatin stored at room temperature in a tight container will retain its properties unchanged for years. Aqueous solutions of gelatin carefully stored under cool, sterile conditions are stable for long periods of time.

Possible slow depolymerization in aqueous solution at temperatures above 50°C and lowering of gel rigidity on resetting may occur. Depolymerization becomes more rapid at temperatures above 65°C, and gel strength may be reduced by 50% when heated at 80°C for 1 hour. The rate and extent of depolymerization depends on molecular weight, with lower molecular weight material decomposing more rapidly.

13. Incompatibilities

Prolonged heating above 40°C; presence of excess acid or alkali (below pH 2 and above pH 10); contact with proteolytic enzymes, bacteria, plasticizers, preservatives, electrolytes, surfactants, alcohols, metal ions, anionic and cationic polymers and aldehydes; precipitated by ether, alcohols, tannic acid, chloroform and mercury salts.

14. Safety

None found in the literature. However, parenteral solutions that contain gelatin have been associated with anaphylactic reactions.

15. Handling Precautions

—

16. Regulatory Acceptance

NF XVI; BP 1980

17. Applications in Pharmaceutical Formulation or Technological Use

Encapsulating agent; suspending agent; tablet binder and coating agent.

18. Related Substances

—

19. Comments

Store dry in an air-tight container. Stable for long periods at room temperature and low humidity. Sterilized by dry heat treatment. Simple coacervation occurs with dehydrating agents such as ethanol or 7% sodium sulfate solution at temperatures above 40°C. First adjust to isoelectric point, then add dehydrating agent slowly over a period of one hour. Might be necessary to construct triangular diagram to determine area of maximum coacervation. Complex coacervation between gelatin and acacia requires dilute solutions of the two colloids not greater than 2% each and of equal concentrations. Temperature should be 40°C and pH adjusted to between 3.8 and 4.6, depending on the system being encapsulated.

20. Specific References

1. "Gelatin", Gelatin Manufacturers Institute of America, Inc.; 515 Fifth Avenue, Suite 507, New York, NY 10036.
2. "The macromolecular chemistry of gelatin", A. Vies Ed., Academic Press 1964.
3. "The rheology of gelatin", F. R. Eirich Ed., Academic Press, Vol. 1, 1958.
4. N. A. Armstrong, K. C. James and W. K. L. Pugh, Drug migration in soft gelatin capsules, *J. Pharm. Pharmacol.*, 34 Suppl. 5P (1982).
5. J. C. Callahan, G. W. Cleary, M. Elefant, G. Kaplan, T. Kensler and R. A. Nash, Equilibrium moisture content of pharmaceutical excipients, *Drug Development and Industrial Pharmacy*, 8: (3), 355-369 (1982).
6. "The science and technology of gelatin", A. G. Ward and A. Courts Ed., Academic Press, 1977.

USA: M. Elefant*; J. C. Robinson**; R. E. Dempski**; Z. Chowhan**
UK: J. R. Nixon*

Liquid Glucose

1. Nonproprietary Name
NF: Liquid glucose

2. Functional Category
USP: Flavoring agent; tablet binder
Others: Coating agent

3. Synonyms
Corn syrup; starch syrup; glucose syrup

4. Chemical Names and CAS Registry Number
Liquid glucose is an aqueous solution of several compounds. These are principally dextrose, dextrins and maltose.

5. Empirical Formula
—

6. Structural Formula
—

7. Commercial Availability
USA
A. E. Staley Co.
American Maize Products Co.
Corn Products Co.
Corn Sweeteners

UK
CPC (UK) Ltd.
Gatton & Sons & Co., Ltd.
Tunnel Refineries Ltd.

8. Method of Manufacture
Liquid glucose is prepared by the incomplete acidic or enzymatic hydrolysis of starch.

9. Description
A nearly colorless, odorless, viscous liquid with a sweet taste.

10. Pharmacopeial Specifications

Test	NF
Identification	+
Acidity	+
Water (Karl Fischer)	≤21%
Residue on ignition (sulfates)	≤0.5%
Sulfite	+
Arsenic	≤1 ppm
Heavy metals	≤0.001%
Starch	+

11. Typical Properties
Density at 20°C: 1.43 g/cm^3
Viscosity at 37.8°C: 13-14.5 Ns/m^2 at 21°C
Dextrose equivalent: 39-43
Miscibility: Water—miscible in all proportions; ethanol (90%)—partially miscible

12. Stability and Storage Conditions
Store in an airtight container.

13. Incompatibilities
Incompatible with strong oxidizing agents.

14. Safety
Generally safe for non-diabetic consumption.

15. Handling Precautions
Avoid heat and strong oxidizing agents.

16. Regulatory Acceptance
NF XVI

17. Applications in Pharmaceutical Formulations

Use	Concentration (%)
Granulating agent	Usually 5-10
Tablet coating	Usually 10-20
Oral syrup vehicle	Usually 20-60

18. Related Substances
—

19. Comments
Corn syrup is classified according to its dextrose equivalent (DE) into four types:
Type I   : 20 to 38 DE
Type II   : 38 to 58 DE
Type III : 58 to 73 DE
Type IV : Above 73 DE

20. Specific References
1. R. X. Hoynak and G. N. Bolcenback, "This is Liquid Sugar," 2nd Ed., Refined Syrup and Sugars, Inc., Yonkers, N.Y., 1966, pp. 205 and 226.
2. W. R. Junk and H. M. Pancoast, "Handbook of Sugars," 1966, p. 103, 111, 319.
3. J. D. Commerford, Preparation of Liquid Glucose. In: Symposium, "Sweeteners," G. E. Inglett, Ed., Westport AVI, 1974, p. 78.
4. J. M. Newton and E. K. Wardrip, *ibid.*, p. 87.
5. G. A. Brooks *et al.*, *ibid.*, p. 97.
6. "Nutritive Sweeteners from Corn," Corn Refiners Association, Inc., Washington, D.C.

USA: A. Yu*; K. R. Heimlich**
UK: P.C. Record*

Glycerin

1. Nonproprietary Names

USP: Glycerin
BP/EP: Glycerol

2. Functional Category

USP: Humectant; solvent; plasticizer; tonicity agent
BP/EP: Lubricant
BPC: Demulcent, emollient, preservative

3. Synonyms

—

4. Chemical Names and CAS Registry Number

1, 2, 3-Propanetriol; propane-1,2,3-triol; Trihydroxypropane glycerol [56-81-5]

5. Empirical Formula   Molecular Weight

$C_3H_8O_3$ [C = 39.12%,
H = 8.75%, O = 52.12%]   92.09

6. Structural Formula

$CH_2OH \cdot CHOH \cdot CH_2OH$

7. Commercial Availability

USA

Colgate-Palmolive Company
Dow Chemical Company
Emery Industries
FMC Corporation
Lever Brothers Company
Mallinckrodt Chemicals—Washine Division
Procter & Gamble Distribution Company
Shell Chemical Co., Chemical Sales Division

UK

Croda Universal, Ltd.
Food Industries, Ltd.
Proctor & Gamble, Ltd.
Unichema Chemicals, Ltd.

8. Method of Manufacture

As a by-product from the hydrolysis of fats and oils in the manufacture of soaps and fatty acids. From natural sources (via fermentation) by the fermentation of sugar beet molasses in the presence of large quantities of sodium sulfite. By the synthetic chlorination and saponification of propylene.

9. Description

A clear, colorless, odorless, syrupy and hygroscopic liquid.

10. Pharmacopeial Specifications

Test	USP	BP/EP
Identification	+	+
Specific gravity	≥1.249	—
Relative density	—	1.258-1.263
Color	+	—
Clarity & color of solution	—	+
Acidity	—	+
Refractive index	—	1.470-1.475
Residue on ignition	≤0.01%	—
Sulfated ash	—	≤0.01%
Chloride	≤0.001%	≤10 ppm
Sulfate	≤0.002%	—
Arsenic	≤1.5 ppm	—
Heavy metals	≤5 ppm	≤5 ppm
Halogenated compounds	—	≤35 ppm
Chlorinated compounds (as chloride)	≤0.003%	≤5 ppm
Aldehydes and related compounds	—	+
Esters	—	+
Fatty acids and esters	+	—
Sugars	—	+
Assay	95.0%-101.0%	—

11. Typical Properties

Boiling point: 760 mm: 290°C (with decomposition)
Burning point: 204°C (98% purity)
Drop no.: 1 g = 23 drops
Flash point: 177°C (98% purity)
Freezing points: Freezing points of aqueous solutions (w/w) are: 10%: 1.6°C; 30%: 9.5°C; 50%: 23°C; 60%: 46.5°C; 80%: 20.3°C; 90%: 1.6°C.
Hygroscopicity: Medium-high.
Melting point: 17.9°C.
Solubility: Miscible with water, alcohol and methanol. One part of glycerin dissolves in 11 parts of ethyl acetate and in about 500 parts of ethyl ether. Insoluble in benzene, chloroform, ether, mineral oil, fixed and volatile oils, halogenated hydrocarbons and aromatic hydrocarbons.
Surface tension: 63.4 dyn/cm at 20°C for 98% purity.
Vapor density: 3.17.
Viscosity: 1490 cps at 20°C; 954 cps at 25°C.

Academy HPE Laboratory Project Data		
Method	Lab #	Results
VIS-1	27	515 ± 19 cps[a]
VIS-1	27	1,034 ± 19 cps[b]

Suppliers: Star[a]; Superol[b]

12. Stability and Storage Conditions

Pure glycerin decomposes on heating, with the evolution of toxic acrolein. Mixtures of glycerin with water, ethyl alcohol and propylene glycol are chemically stable. Preserve in a tight container to avoid moisture absorption.

13. Incompatibilities

An explosion may occur if glycerin is triturated with strong oxidizing agents, such as chromium trioxide, potassium chlorate and potassium permanganate. In dilute solution, the reaction proceeds at a slower rate, with several oxidation products forming. Black coloration occurs in contact with zinc oxide and basic bismuth nitrate in the presence of light. An iron contaminant in glycerin is responsible for the darkening of the color in mixtures containing phenols, salicylates, tannin. etc. Glycerin forms a complex with boric acid as glyceroboric acid, which is a stronger acid than boric acid.

14. Safety

Very large oral doses can exert systemic effects, such as headache, thirst and nausea. Injection of large doses may induce convulsions, paralysis and hemolysis. Oral LD_{50} (mice) = 31.5 g/kg; IV (mice) = 7.45 g/kg.

15. Handling Precautions

Avoid excessive exposure to air, since glycerin is hygroscopic. Dry heat sterilization should be avoided. Intimate contact with strong oxidizing agents, such as chromium trioxide, potassium permanganate, etc., causes explosion; therefore, avoid contact or exposure with such agents.

16. Regulatory Acceptance

USP XXI; BP/EP 1980

17. Applications in Pharmaceutical Formulation or Technology

Use	Concentration (%)
Emollient, humectant	Up to 30
Plasticizer in tablet film coating	Varying concentration
Preservative in liquid pharmaceuticals	Above 20
Solvent for parenteral formulations	Up to 50
Sweetener in high alcoholic elixirs	Up to 20

18. Related Substances

—

19. Comments

—

20. Specific References

—

USA: D. M. Patel*; P. Bernardo**; J. Cooper
UK: R. B. Forrester*

Glyceryl Monostearate

1. Nonproprietary Names
NF: Glyceryl monostearate
BP/EP: Glyceryl monostearate

2. Functional Category
NF: Emulsifying and/or solubilizing agent
BP/EP: Pharmaceutical aid
Other: Emollient; stabilizer

3. Synonyms
Monostearin; glycerol stearate; glycerol monostearate; α-monostearin; *Tegin; Zerol;* GMS; *Abracol* (various grades); *Cerasynt* (various grades); *Cithral* (various grades); *Empilan* (various grades); *Imwitor* (various grades); *Myverol*

4. Chemical Name and CAS Registry Number
Octadecanoic acid, monoester, with 1,2,3-propane-triol. [31566-31-1]

5. Empirical Formula and Molecular Weight
Glyceryl monostearate is a mixture of mono-, di- and triglycerides of stearic and palmitic acids. It contains not less than 90 percent of total fatty acid glycerides, of which at least 35 percent is monoglycerides, calculated as $C_{20}H_{40}O_4$. The molecular weight of pure glyceryl monostearate is 358.57.

6. Structural Formula

$$\begin{array}{l} CH_2\text{-}\underline{C}OOC_{17}H_{35} \\ | \\ CH\text{-}OH \\ | \\ CH_2\text{-}OH \end{array}$$

7. Commercial Availability
Glyceryl monostearate is commercially available in a variety of grades and types from various manufacturers. Following is a partial list of manufacturers:

USA
Ashland Chemical Company
Croda Chemicals
Cyclo Chemicals Corporation
Eastman Chemical (USA)
Glyco Chemicals, Inc.
A. Grass & Co., Div. of Millmaster Onyx Corp.
ICI Americas, Inc.
Inolex Corp., Personal Care Division
Witco Chemical Corporation

UK
Albright & Wilson
Alfa Chemicals
Bush Booke Allen
Croda (Goole), Ltd.
Croda (Leek), Ltd.
Dynamit Nobel (UK) Ltd.
Henkel (UK) Ltd.
Leek Chemicals Ltd.
Marchon
Van Dyke

8. Method of Manufacture
Glyceryl mono-fatty acids are manufactured by the esterification of glycerin with fatty acids, chiefly stearic acid. The commercial fatty acids used in the manufacturing process are not, in general, pure substances, but are associated with those substances which normally occur in a commercial acid of that type. For example, stearic acid will also contain palmitic and some oleic acids. Therefore, the final product would consist of mixed esters of stearates, palmitates and oleates. The products supplied by different manufacturers differ appreciably in properties.

9. Description
Glyceryl monostearate is a white to cream-colored, wax-like solid in the form of beads, flakes or powder. It is waxy to the touch and has a slight fatty odor and taste.

10. Pharmacopeial Specifications

Test	NF	BP/EP
Freezing point	—	54°-60°C
Melting range	≥55°C	—
Identification	—	+
Residue on ignition	≤0.5%	—
Acid value	≤6	≤3
Saponification value	155-165	162-173
Iodine value	≤3	≤3
Hydroxyl value	300-330	—
Arsenic	3 ppm	—
Heavy metals	≤0.001%	—
Sulfated ash	—	≤0.1%
Free glycerin	≤1.2%	≤6.0%
Monoglycerides of Fatty acids	≥90.0%	—
Water	—	≤2.0%
Assay (Monoglycerides) (as $C_{20}H_{40}O_4$)	—	≥35.0%

11. Typical Properties
A wide variety of glycol and glycerol esters are commercially available, as well as self-emulsifying grades which contain small amounts of soap or other surfactants. Most grades are tailored for specific applications or made to user specifications.
Flash point: 243°C
Solubility: Practically insoluble in water, but readily dispersible in hot water with the aid of an anionic or cationic agent. Soluble in hot alcohol, ether, chloroform, benzene, hot acetone, mineral oil and fixed oils.
HLB: Glyceryl monostearate   3.8
Glyceryl monostearate, self-emulsifying   5.5

12. Stability and Storage Conditions
Glyceryl monostearate should be stored in a light-resistant, tightly sealed container at cool temperatures. It will increase in acid value upon aging if stored at warm temperatures due to the saponification of the ester with trace amounts of water present. Effective anti-oxidants are butylated hydroxytoluene and propyl gallate.

13. Incompatibilities
The self-emulsifying grades of glyceryl monostearate are incompatible with acidic substances.

14. Safety

Glyceryl monostearate is non-toxic and edible. Patient-test subjects showed negative results toward it.

15. Handling Precautions

Protection from light and warm temperatures and storage in tightly sealed containers are recommended.

16. Regulatory Acceptance

NF XVI; BP/EP 1980.

17. Applications in Pharmaceutical Formulation and Technology

Glyceryl monostearate is an example of the non-dispersible type of non-ionic agents. It is used as a non-ionic emulsifier, stabilizer, emollient, plasticizer and anti-tack agent in a variety of food, pharmaceutical and cosmetic products. It acts as an effective stabilizer, i.e., as a mutual solvent for polar and non-polar compounds which may form water-in-oil or oil-in-water emulsions. These properties also make it useful as a dispersing agent of pigments in oils or of solids in fats, or as solvent for phospholipids, such as lecithin.

18. Related Substances

Self-emulsifying glyceryl monostearate; BP 1980, Addendum 1982.

Glyceryl monostearate is also supplied as a "self-emulsifying" grade in which manufacturers have added an emulsifying agent which may be a soluble soap, a salt of a sulfated alcohol, a non-ionic surface-active agent, a quaternary compound, etc. Mono-olein is listed in the Nordic Pharmacopeia and the Swiss Pharmacopeia. It is a mixture of oleic and other fatty acids, chiefly mono-olein ($C_{21}H_{40}O_4$). It contains $\geq 90\%$ of glycerides. It is typically a yellow, soft, granular mass which melts at 35-40°C. It has similar properties to glyceryl monostearate. Tegacid is a combination of glyceryl monostearate and a phosphoric acid derivative of an oleic acid derivative of an oleic acid amide of diethyl ethlenediamine. This combination is an effective emulsifying agent in acidic-type creams.

19. Comments

Glyceryl monostearate and other mono-fatty acids are not efficient emulsifiers as such. They are best regarded as useful emollients which are readily emulsified by the usual emulsifying agents and when other fatty materials are incorporated. The mono-esters in general endow the cream with smoothness and fine texture, and improve the stability.

In topical applications, glyceryl monostearate does not have as great a drying effect as straight stearate creams, and is not drying when used in protective applications.

20. Specific References

1. L. L. Ray and I. H. Blank, Results of patch tests with commonly used ointment bases, *Arch. Derm. Syph.*, 42: 285-289 (1940).
2. W. Wisniewski and Z. Golucki, *Acta Pol. Pharm.*, 22: 293 (1965).
3. E. Ehrenstein, *Am. Prof. Pharmacy*, 16: 874 (1950).
4. J. H. Beckerman et al., *Am. J. Hosp. Pharm.*, 24: 143 (1967).

USA: R. N. Acharya*; D. M. Wagenknecht*; C. W. Chong*
UK: G. M. Eccleston*

Glycofurol

1. Nonproprietary Name

None adopted. Glycofurol listed in Merck Index, 9th edition.

2. Functional Category

Solvent

3. Synonyms

Tetraglycol (also used for tetrahydrofurfuryl alcohol); tetrahydrofurfuryl alcohol polyethylene glycol ether; *Glycofurol 75*

4. Chemical Name and CAS Registry Number

α-(tetrahydrofuranyl)-ω-hydroxypoly(oxy-1,2-ethanediyl) [9004-76-6]

5. Empirical Formula   Molecular Weight

Average: $C_9H_{18}O_4$ Average: 190.24

6. Structural Formula

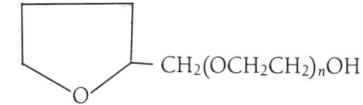

Glycofurol 75: $n = 1$-2

7. Commercial Availability

USA

Hoffmann-La Roche

UK

Becpharm, Ltd.

8. Method of Manufacture

Glycofurol is prepared by the reaction of tetrahydrofurfuryl alcohol with ethylene oxide (followed by a special purification process in the case of *Glycofurol 75*).

9. Description

Clear, colorless, almost odorless liquid, with a bitter taste and producing a warm sensation on the tongue.

10. Pharmacopeial Specifications

—

11. Typical Properties

Boiling point (Glycofurol 75): 80 - 100°C (at 40 N/m²)
Density: 1.070 - 1.090 g/cm³ (at 20°C)
Miscibility (Glycofurol 75):

Solvent	Miscibility (at 20°C)
Water	Miscible in all proportions*
Ethanol (96%)	Miscible in all proportions
Propylene glycol	Miscible in all proportions
Glycerol	Miscible in all proportions
Propan-2-ol	Miscible in all proportions
Castor oil	Miscible*
Arachis oil	Immiscible

*Cloudiness may occur

Solvent	Miscibility (at 20°C)
Polyethylene glycol 400	Miscible in all proportions
Isopropyl ether	Immiscible
Petroleum ether	Immiscible

Hydroxyl value: 300-400
Moisture content: Initial: ≤0.2%; at equilibrium with ambient humidity (about 30% RH), approximately 5%
Refractive index: 1.4545 (sodium D line, 589 nm) (at 40°C)
Viscosity (Glycofurol 75): 8 - 18 mN s/m² (at 20°C)

12. Stability and Storage Conditions

Stable if stored under nitrogen in a well-closed container protected from light.

13. Incompatibilities

Oxidizing substances.

14. Safety

When administered parenterally, quantities of glycofurol should not exceed 0.07 ml per kg of body weight per day (man).

15. Handling Precautions

—

16. Regulatory Acceptance

No known prohibitions by any regulatory bodies. Glycofurol is a component of a parenteral product marketed in several European countries.

17. Applications in Pharmaceutical Formulation or Technology

Glycofurol is used as a solvent in parenteral products for intravenous or intramuscular injection, in concentrations up to 50% v/v.

18. Related Substances

—

19. Comments

Grades other than *Glycofurol 75* may contain significant amounts of tetrahydrofurfuryl alcohol and other impurities. *Glycofurol 75* meets an analytical specification which includes a requirement that the fraction in which $n=1$-2 amounts to a minimum of 95%.

20. Specific References

1. H. P. Fiedler, "Lexikon der Hilfsstoffe für Pharmazie, Kosmetik und angrenzende Gebiete," 2nd Edition, Editio Cantor AG, 1971.
2. A. J. Spiegel and M. M. Noseworthy, *J. Pharm. Sci.*, 52 (10): 917 (1963).
3. H. Spiegelberg, R. Schlapfer, G. Zbinden and A. Studer, *Arzneim. Forsch.*, 6: 75 (1956).

USA: D. Walking*; E.L. Rowe**
UK: H.C. Worthington*

Guar Gum

1. Nonproprietary Name
NF: Guar gum

2. Functional Category
USP: Tablet binder; suspending and/or viscosity-increasing agent
Other: Table disintegrant

3. Synonyms
Guar flour; *Burtonite V-7-E; Supercol Guar Gums; Jaguar.*

4. Chemical Name and CAS Registry Number
—

Chemical Type
Galactomannan polysaccharide [9000-30-0]
Botanical Origin
Cyamopsis tetragonolobus (L.) Taub.

5. Empirical Formula   Molecular Weight
$(C_6H_{12}O_6)_n$ Approx. 220,000

6. Structural Formula
Linear chains of $(1\rightarrow4)$-β-D-mannopyranosyl units with α-D-galacto-pyranosyl units attached by $(1\rightarrow6)$ linkages. The ratio of D-galactose to D-mannose is 1:2.

7. Commercial Availability
USA

Burtonite Co.
Colony Import and Export Corp.
General Mills Chemical, Inc.
Hercules Company
Meer Corporation
S. B. Penick and Co.
Stein-Hall and Co., Inc.
Tragacanth Importing Corporation

UK

A.F. Suter
Arthur Branwell & Co.
Chemical Exchange, Ltd.
Speywood Laboratories
Steetley Chemicals

8. Method of Manufacture
The gum consists of the pulverized endosperm of the seed of *C. tetragonolobus.* The seed hull can be removed by grinding, after soaking in sulfuric acid or water, or by charring. The embryo (germ) is removed by differential grinding, since each component possesses a different hardness. The separated endosperm is ground to different particle sizes depending upon final application.

9. Description
Appearance and color: White to yellowish-white powder.
Odor: Odorless, or nearly so.
Taste: Bland

10. Pharmacopeial Specifications

Test	NF
Identification	+
Loss on drying	$\leq 15\%$
Ash	$\leq 1.5\%$
Acid-insoluble matter	$\leq 7\%$
Heavy metals	$\leq .002\%$
Arsenic	≤ 3 ppm.
Lead	$\leq .001\%$.
Protein	$\leq 10\%$
Starch	+
Galactomannans	$\geq 66\%$

11. Typical Properties
Chemical: Guar gum possesses the chemical properties typical of a polysaccharide.
Physical: Guar gum forms viscous colloidal dispersions (solutions) when hydrated in cold water. The optimum rate of hydration is between pH 7.5 and pH 9. The viscosity of a 1% solution ranges from 2,000 to 22,500 cps.; the sol is thixotropic. Finely-milled powders are more difficult to disperse. Two to four hours in water at room temperature are required to develop maximum viscosity.

12. Stability and Storage Conditions
Guar gum is stable in solution over a pH range of 1-10.5. Prolonged heating degrades the viscosity. Bacteriological stability can be improved by the addition of a mixture of 0.15% methyl and 0.02% propyl paraben, or by 0.1% benzoic acid or sodium pentachlorophenate. Store in a well-closed container.

13. Incompatibilities
Acetone, alcohol, tannins, strong acids and alkalis. Borate ions, if present in the dispersing water, will prevent hydration of guar. The addition of borate ions to hydrated solutions produces cohesive structural gels, which prevents further hydration. The gel can be liquefied by reducing the pH below 7.

14. Safety
Guar gum is recognized by the FDA as a substance added directly to human food and has been affirmed as generally recognized as safe. Specific limits in various foods are established; however, alkylated guar gums are not covered by appropriate FDA regulations.

15. Handling Precautions
—

16. Regulatory Acceptance
NF XVI

17. Applications in Pharmaceutical Formulation or Technology

Use	Concentration (%)
Thickener for lotions & creams	up to 2.5
Tablet binder	up to 10
Emulsion stabilizer	1

18. Related Substances

—

19. Comments

—

20. References

1. W. Feinstein and A. J. Bartilucci, Comparative study of selected disintegrating agents, *J. Pharm. Sci.*, 55 (3): 332-334 (1966).
2. A. M. Goldstein, E. N. Alter and J. K. Seaman, Guar Gum. In: "Industrial Gums," 2nd Ed., Chapter 14, R. L. Whistler and J. N. BeMiller, eds., Academic Press, New York, 1973.
3. A. M. Sakr and H. M. Elsabbagh, Evaluation of guar gum as a tablet additive: a preliminary report, *Pharm. Ind. 39* (4): 399-403 (1977).
4. Product literature from:
   Colony Import and Export Corp., New York City.
   General Mills Chemicals, Inc., Minneapolis, Minn.
   Meer Corporation, North Bergen, N.J.
   S. B. Penick and Co., Lyndhurst, N.J.
   Stein-Hall and Co., Inc., New York City.
   Swift Edible Oil Company, Chicago, Illinois.
   The Burtonite Company, Inc., Nutley, N.J.

USA: L.C. Schramm*; R.E. Dempski**

Hydrochloric Acid

1. Nonproprietary Names
NF: Hydrochloric acid
BP/EP: Hydrochloric acid

2. Functional Category
USP: Acidifying agent

3. Synonym
Concentrated hydrochloric acid

4. Chemical Name and CAS Registry Number
Hydrochloric Acid [7647-01-0]

5. Empirical Formula   Molecular Weight
HCl   36.46

6. Structural Formula
—

7. Commercial Availability
USA
Allied Chemical Corp.
Ashland Chemical Co.
Baker Chemical Co., J. T.
Conoco Chemicals Co.
Continental Water Systems Corps.
Dow Chemical Co.
E. I. du Pont de Nemours & Co.
FMC Corp./Industrial Chemicals Div.
Hooker Chemicals & Plastics Corp.
McKesson Chemical Co.
Monsanto Co.
Pfaltz & Bauer, Inc.
PPG Inudstries, Inc., Chemical Divs.
Ruger Chemical Co.
Shell Chemical Co.
Stauffer Chemical Co.
Thompson-Hayward Chemical Co.
Velsicol Chemical Corp.

UK
Berk Spencer Aids, Ltd.
Imperial Chemical Industries
Stavely Chemicals, Ltd.

8. Method of Manufacture
Hydrochloric acid is an aqueous solution of hydrogen chloride gas produced: (a) from the reaction of sodium chloride and sulfuric acid; (b) from the constituent elements; (c) as a by-product: (i) from the electrolysis of sodium hydroxide, or (ii) during the chlorination of hydrocarbons.

9. Description
Clear, colorless, fuming liquid with a pungent odor.

10. Pharmacopeial Specifications

Test	NF	BP
Identification	+	+
Clarity of solution (1 in 5)	—	+
Color	—	+
Residue on ignition	$\leq 0.008\%$	—
Arsenic	≤ 1 ppm	≤ 2 ppm
Heavy metals	≤ 5 ppm	≤ 2 ppm
Free chlorine	absence	≤ 4 ppm
Free bromine	absence	—
Bromide	absence	—
Iodide	absence	—
Sulfite	absence	—
Sulfate	absence	≤ 20 ppm
Assay limits w/w	36.5-38.0%	35.0-39.0%
Residue on evaporation	—	$\leq 0.01\%$

11. Typical Properties
Boiling point: 110°C (constant boiling mixture 20.24% w/w HCl)
Density at 20°C: Approximately 1.18 g/cm³
Freezing point: Approximately -24°C
pH: 0.1 (diluted 1 in 10, by volume, in water)
Refractive index at 20°C: 1.342 (diluted 1 in 10, by volume, in water)

12. Stability and Storage Conditions
Store in tight glass or other inert container at a temperature below 30°C. Avoid storage in close proximity to concentrated alkalis, metals and cyanides.

13. Incompatibilities
Hydrochloric acid reacts violently with alkalis, with the evolution of a large amount of heat. It attacks many metals, liberating hydrogen.

14. Safety
Very corrosive. Can cause severe damage on contact with eyes and skin, or if ingested. Fumes cause coughing and irritation to the eyes, nose and throat. Prolonged exposure may damage lungs.

15. Handling Precautions
Protect against burns, vapors and eye damage.

16. Regulatory Acceptance
NF XVI; BP/EP 1982 Add.

17. Applications in Pharmaceutical Formulation or Technology
Used for the preparation of the diluted form and as an acidifying agent.

18. Related Substances
NF XVI: Diluted hydrochloric acid: Contains 9.5–10.5% w/v; BP/EP 1980: Dilute hydrochloric acid: Contains 9.5–10.5% w/w.

19. Comments
—

20. Specific References
—

USA: F. A. Restaino*
UK: J. E. Jeffries*; W. Lund**

Hydroxyethyl Cellulose

1. Nonproprietary Name
NF: Hydroxyethyl cellulose

2. Functional Category
NF: Suspending and/or viscosity-increasing agent
Others: Binder; film-former; thickener

3. Synonyms
Natrosol; *Cellosize*

4. Chemical Names and CAS Registry Number
Cellulose, 2-hydroxyethylether
Cellulose hydroxyethylether [9004-62-01]

5. Empirical Formula
$(C_{12}H_{21.5}O_8)_n$

Molecular Weight
A wide variety of molecular weights are available. See the section on properties for typical grades available.

6. Structural Formula

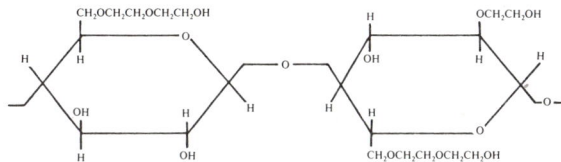

Idealized structure of hydroxyethyl cellulose (M.S. 2.5)

7. Commercial Availability

USA

Hercules, Inc.
Union Carbide Corporation

UK

B. P. Chemicals, Ltd.
Henkel Chemicals, Ltd.
Hercules, Ltd.

8. Method of Manufacture
A purified form of cellulose is reacted with sodium hydroxide to produce a swollen alkali cellulose. This alkali-treated cellulose is chemically more reactive than untreated cellulose. By reacting the alkali cellulose with ethylene oxide, a series of hydroxyethyl cellulose ethers is produced.

The manner in which ethylene oxide is added to cellulose can be described by two terms: Degree of Substitution (D.S.) and Molar Substitution (M.S.). The Degree of Substitution designates the average number of hydroxyl positions on the anhydroglucose unit that have been reacted with ethylene oxide. Since each anhydroglucose unit of the cellulose molecule has three hydroxyl groups, the maximum value for D.S. is 3. Molar Substitution is defined as the average numbr of ethylene oxide molecules that have reacted with each anhydroglucose unit. Once a hydroxyethyl group is attached to each unit, it can further react with additional groups in an end-to-end formation. This reaction can continue and, theoretically, there is no limit for Molar Substitution.

9. Description
Light tan or cream to white powder, odorless and tasteless. It may contain suitable anti-caking agents.

SEM-MF-20
Excipient: Hydroxyethyl cellulose (*Natrosol*)
Supplier: Hercules

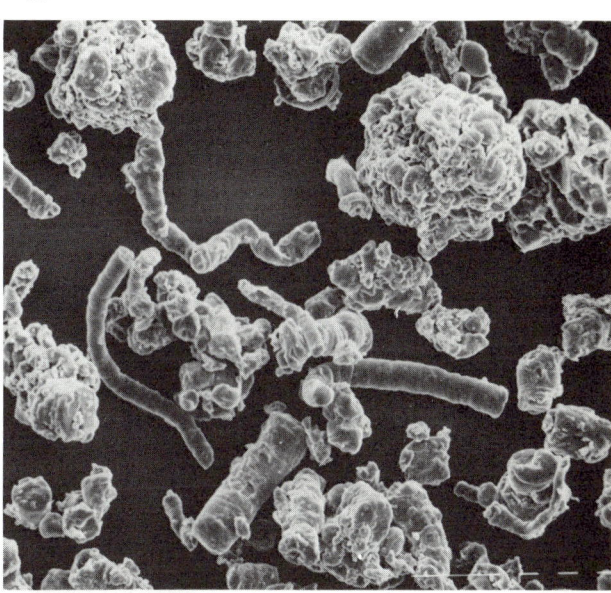

Magnification: 120×

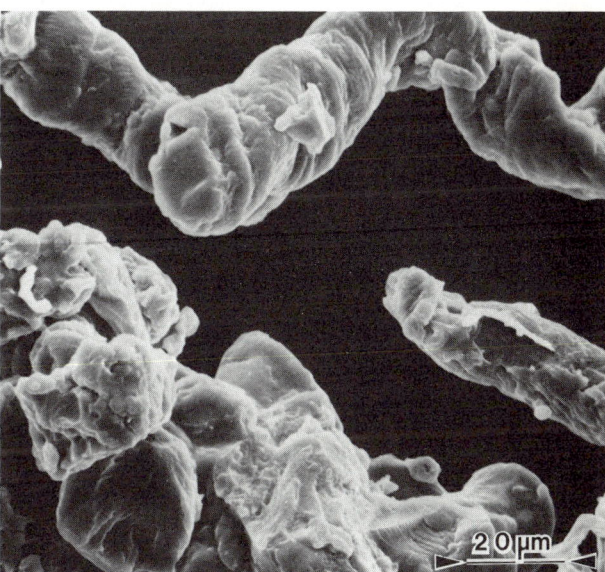

Magnification: 600×

10. Pharmacopeial Specifications

Test	NF
Identification	+
Viscosity	50–150% of label
pH (1 in 100)	6–8.5
Loss on drying	≤10.0%
Lead	≤3ppm
Residue on ignition	≤5.0%
Arsenic	≤3ppm
Heavy metals	≤0.004%

11. Typical Properties

Ash content: Natrosol—3.5% by weight (as Na_2SO_4); *Cellosize*—2.5% by weight (as Na_2CO_3).

Browning temperature: Natrosol—205-210°C; *Cellosize*—approximately 400°F.

Bulk density: Natrosol—39 lbs. per cu. ft. (0.6 g/ml); *Cellosize*—22 to 38 lbs. per cu. ft.

Microbiological properties: Hydroxyethyl cellulose is subject to enzymatic degradation, with consequent loss of viscosity of its solutions. Enzymes which catalyze this degradation are produced by many bacteria and fungi present in the environment. If prolonged storage of an aqueous solution is contemplated, a preservative is recommended.

Moisture content: The moisture level of all grades of hydroxyethyl cellulose as packaged does not exceed 5% by weight. Hydroxyethyl cellulose can absorb moisture from the atmosphere. The amount of moisture absorbed depends on the initial moisture content of hydroxyethyl cellulose and on the relative humidity of the surrounding air. Typical equilibrium moisture values are listed below.

Equilibrium moisture content of *Natrosol 250* at 73°F:

At 50% relative humidity . . . 6%

At 84% relative humidity . . .29%

Particle size: Natrosol—5% retained on U.S. 40 mesh; *Cellosize*—all through U.S. 80 mesh.

pH (in 1% solution): 6 to 7 (*Cellosize*); 6.5 to 8.5 (*Natrosol*)

Softening temperature: Natrosol—135-140°C; *Cellosize*—140.5°C.

Solubility: Hydroxyethyl cellulose dissolves in water, either cold or hot, to form clear, smooth, uniform solutions. As normally substituted, hydroxyethyl cellulose is insoluble in most organic solvents. In a few of the polar solvents, such as the glycols, it either swells or is partially soluble.

Solutions in water: Natrosol: specific gravity, 2% solution: 1.0033 g/ml; refractive index, 2% solution: 1.336; surface tension, 0.1% (250L): 66.8 dynes/cm; surface tension, 0.001% (250L): 67.3 dynes/cm; surface tension, 0.1% (180L): 66.7 dynes/cm; surface tension, 0.001% (180L): 69.8 dynes/cm; interfacial tension, 0.001% (250L) *vs.* fractol: 25.5 dynes/cm; interfacial tension, *0.001% (180G) vs.* fractol: 23.7 dynes/cm. *Cellosize:* specific gravity at 20°C, 2% sol.: 1.0033 g/ml; refractive index, 2% solution: 1.330.

Surface tension: Dynes/cm at 25°C:

Conc. (%)	WP-02	09	300	QP4400	52000	100M
0.01	65.8	65.7	66.4	66.3	65.9	66.1
0.1	65.3	65.4	65.8	65.3	65.4	65.4
1.0	64.4	65.1	65.5	65.8	66.1	66.3
2.0	64.2	65.0	66.3	67.3	—	—
5.0	64.1	64.7	—	—	—	—
10.0	64.4	65.9	—	—	—	—

Viscosity: A wide range of viscosity types is available. For example, *Cellosize* is manufactured in eleven regular viscosity grades. The grades differ principally in their aqueous solution viscosities, which range from 2 to almost 200,000 centipoises at a 2 percent concentration. Two types of *Cellosize* are produced: a WP-type, which is a normal-dissolving material, and a QP-type, which is a rapid-dispersing material. The lowest viscosity grade (02) is available only in the WP-type. Five viscosity grades (09, 3, 40, 300 and 4400) are produced in both WP- and QP-types. Five high-viscosity grades (10,000, 15,000, 30,000, 52,000, and 100M) are produced only in the QP-type. The table below shows the standard grades and types commercially available and their respective viscosity ranges in aqueous solution.

Type	Viscosity Grade	Concentration, Weight % on Dry Basis	Brookfield Viscosity (cps) at 25°C (Approximate)	
			L Range[a]	H Range[a]
WP	02	5	7-14	14-20
WP and QP	09	5	60-100	100-140
	3	5	220-285	285-350
	40	2	70-110	110-150
	300	2	250-325	325-400
	4400	2	4200-4700	4700-5200
QP	10,000	2	5700-	6500
	15,000	2	15000-18000	18000-21000
	30,000	1	950-1230	1230-1500
	52,000	1	1500-1800	1800-2100
	100M	1	2500-	3000

[a]*Cellosize* viscosity grades are available in narrower ranges, as noted by the L (low) and H (high) designation.

Natrosol is produced in four degrees of substitution, 1.5, 1.8, 2.5 and 3.0, designated, respectively, as *Natrosol 150*, *Natrosol 180*, *Natrosol 250* and *Natrosol 300*. *Natrosol 180* and *Natrosol 250* are produced in the ten viscosity types as listed in the following table.

Type	Brookfield Viscosity at 25°C, cps at Varying Concentrations of *Natrosol 250*		
	1%	2%	5%
HH	3400-5000	—	—
H4	2600-3300	—	—
H	1500-2500	—	—
MH	1000-1500	—	—
M	—	4500-6500	—
K	—	1500-2500	—
G	—	150-400	—
E	—	25-105	—
J	—	—	150-400
L	—	—	75-150

Natrosol 150 and *Natrosol 300* are made in several, but not all, viscosity types.

Academy HPE Laboratory Project Data

	Method	Lab #	% w/v	Visco-meter	Min/Max Range
Natrosol					
250L	VIS-4	6	5	RVT	150-225cps
250L	VIS-4	6	5	HBT	128-232cps
250MR	VIS-4	6	1	RVT	190-375cps
250MR	VIS-4	6	1	HBT	224-480cps
250MR	VIS-4	6	2	RVT	4250-7250cps
250MR	VIS-4	6	2	HBT	1776-4000cps
250HHR	VIS-4	6	1	RVT	3275-5875cps
250HHR	VIS-4	6	1	HBT	1296-3200cps

	Method	Lab #	% w/w	Factor	Spindle	cps
Natrosol						
250L	VIS-3*	28	2	1	1	13.6
250L	VIS-3	28	2	1	1	15.7
250MR	VIS-3	28	2	100	3	4120.0
250MR	VIS-3	28	2	100	3	4270.0
250HHR	VIS-3	28	2	1000	4	68200.0
250HHR	VIS-3	28	2	1000	4	61106.0

*Brookfield

Particle Friability	Method	Lab #	Results
Natrosol 250L	PF-1	36	0.050
Natrosol 250MR	PF-1	36	0.000
Natrosol 250HHR	PF-1	36	0.008

Supplier: Hercules

12. Stability and Storage Conditions

Variations in pH between about 2 and 12 have little effect on the viscosity of solutions of *Cellosize*. Solution viscosities tend to be lower beyond these limits. They may also be less stable if hydrolysis occurs at low pH or if oxidation occurs at high pH. Hydroxyethyl cellulose powder should be stored in a tightly closed container and in a dry atmosphere to prevent any increase in the moisture content.

13. Incompatibilities

As normally substituted, hydroxyethyl cellulose is insoluble in most organic solvents. It is partially compatible with the following water-soluble compounds: casein, starch, methyl cellulose, polyvinyl alcohol and gelatin. Hydroxyethyl cellulose is incompatible with zein. Hydroxyethyl cellulose can be used with a wide variety of water-soluble preservatives. However, it has been reported that *Dowicide G* (sodium pentachlorophenate) shows an immediate viscosity increase when added to *Natrosol* 250. Hydroxyethyl cellulose can be salted out of solution like other organic solutes. The following salt solutions will precipitate a 10% solution of *Cellosize WP-09* and a 2% solution of *Cellosize WP-4400*: sodium carbonate (50%) and saturated solutions of potassium ferrocyanide; disodium phosphate; aluminum sulfate; ammonium sulfate; chromic sulfate; magnesium sulfate; sodium sulfate; zinc sulfate; sodium sulfite; and sodium thiosulfate. Certain fluorescent dyes or optical brighteners and certain quaternary disinfectants will increase the viscosity of *Natrosol* 250 solutions. *Natrosol* can be dissolved in many salt solutions that will not dissolve other water-soluble polymers. Data indicate that *Natrosol* is soluble in most 10% salt solutions (except sodium carbonate and sodium sulfate) and many 50% salt solutions (except aluminum sulfate, ammonium sulfate, diammonium phosphate, disodium phosphate, ferric chloride, magnesium sulfate, potassium ferrocyanide, sodium metaborate, sodium nitrate, sodium sulfite, trisodium phosphate and zinc sulfate). *Natrosol* 150 is generally more tolerant of dissolved salts than *Natrosol* 250. Solubility is not affected by the viscosity type of *Natrosol* used.

14. Safety

Acute oral toxicology studies indicate that hydroxyethyl cellulose showed no toxic effects on rats. Subacute oral tests showed no gross signs of toxicity in rats. Inclusion in the rat diet at a level of 5% for 90 days caused no detectable harm. Gross and microscopic examinations of organs and tissues did not reveal any abnormalities that could be attributed to the feeding of hydroxyethyl cellulose. Hydroxyethyl cellulose is neither absorbed nor hydrolyzed in the rat gastrointestinal tract. Hydroxyethyl cellulose produces no more skin irritation in patch tests or in repeat-insult tests on humans than does commercial wheat starch, and showed no evidence of causing sensitization. Contact with the human eye may be expected to cause a reaction no more severe than a moderate degree of inflammation. Moderate eye irritation was observed on albino rabbits, but it cleared within 24 hours. It is not recommended for use in the preparation of parenteral preparations.

15. Handling Precautions

Dusts of hydroxyethyl cellulose are explosive if mixed with air in critical proportions and in the presence of an ignition source. These dusts represent a hazard quite similar to that of other cellulosic derivatives and to many widely used organic solids.

16. Regulatory Acceptance

NF XVI; neither *Natrosol* nor *Cellosize* has been cleared for direct use as a component of food products. Hydroxyethyl cellulose is presently approved by the U.S. Food and Drug Administration for use in indirect food applications, such as food packaging, adhesives and can and paper coatings. The reason for not being cleared for direct food use is probably that the residuals of ethylene glycol, which are formed during the manufacturing process, are too high.

17. Applications in Pharmaceutical Formulation or Technology

Hydroxyethyl cellulose is an effective film former, binder, thickener, stabilizer and dispersant in shampoos, hair sprays, neutralizers, creams and lotions. The concentration to be used is dependent on the solvent and molecular weight of the grade used.

18. Related Substances

—

19. Comments

The fact that hydroxyethyl cellulose is not approved for direct food use limits its scope of utility in pharmaceuticals.

20. Specific References

1. *Natrosol, Hydroxyethyl Cellulose, A Nonionic Water-Soluble Polymer, Physical and Chemical Properties*, Hercules, Inc., Wilmington, Delaware (1978).
2. *Cellulose Gum and Natrosol in Cosmetics*, Hercules, Inc., Wilmington, Delaware (1964).
3. *Cellosize, Hydroxyethyl Cellulose*, Union Carbide Corp., New York (1968).
4. M. G. Wirick, Study of the substitution pattern of hydroxyethyl cellulose and its relationship to enzymic degradation, *J. Polymer Science, Part A-1*, 6: 1705-1718 (1968).
5. E. D. Klug, Some properties of water-soluble hydroxyalkyl cellulose and their derivatives, *J. Polymer Science, Part C, Polymer Symposia No. 36*, 491-508 (1971).
6. A. J. Desmarais, Chapter 24, Hydroxyalkyl derivatives of cellulose. In: *Industrial Gums*, 2nd ed., Academic Press, New York, 1973, pp. 649-672.

USA: R. J. Harwood*; G. J. Papariello**; K. R. Heimlich**
UK: J. F. Pickard**

Hydroxypropyl Cellulose

1. Nonproprietary Name

NF: Hydroxypropyl cellulose

2. Functional Categories

USP: Suspending and/or viscosity-increasing agent; coating agent

Others: Emulsifier; film former; protective colloid; stabilizer; suspending agent; thickener; binder; and granulating agent

3. Synonym

Klucel

4. Chemical Names and CAS Registry Number

Cellulose, 2-hydroxypropyl ether

Cellulose, hydroxypropyl ether [9004-64-2]

5. Empirical Formula   Molecular Weight

$(C_{15}H_{28}O_8)_n$ Molecular weight range: 50,000–1,250,000

For M.S. = 3.0   (See section on properties for typical grades available.)

6. Structural Formula

Idealized structure of hydroxypropyl cellulose (M.S. 3.0)

7. Commercial Availability

USA

Biddle Sawyer Corp.
Hercules, Inc.
Shin-Etsu Chemical Co.

UK

Hercules, Ltd.
Shin-Etsu Chemical Co., Ltd.
Stancourt, Sons and Muir, Ltd.

8. Method of Manufacture

Hydroxypropyl cellulose is manufactured by reacting alkali cellulose with propylene oxide at elevated temperatures and pressures. The propylene oxide can be substituted on the cellulose through an ether linkage at the three reactive hydroxyls present on each anhydroglucose monomer unit of the cellulose chain. Published information suggests that etherification takes place in such a way that hydroxypropyl substituent groups contain almost entirely secondary hydroxyls. The secondary hydroxyl present in the side chain is available for further reaction with the oxide, and chaining-out may take place. This results in the formation of side chains containing more than one mole of combined propylene oxide.

9. Description

White to slightly yellowish powder, odorless and tasteless.

SEM-MF-21
Excipient: Hydroxypropyl cellulose (*Klucel*)
Supplier: Hercules

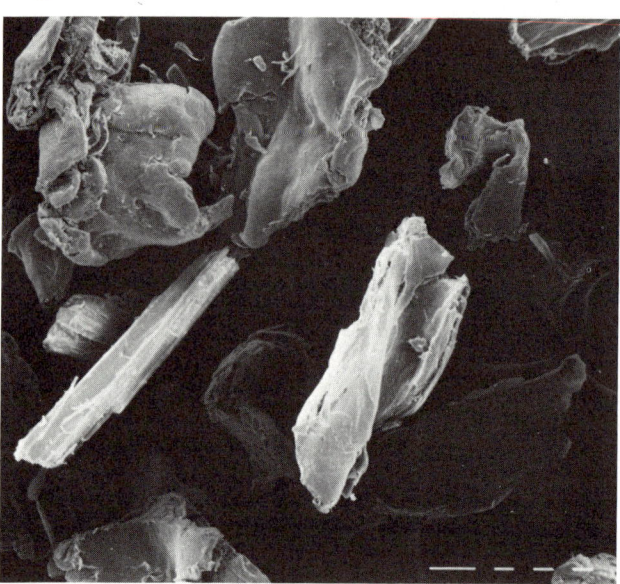

Magnification: 60×

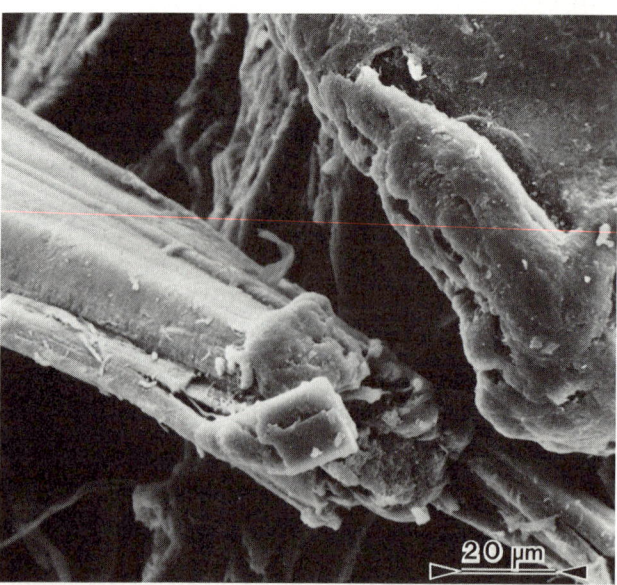

Magnification: 600×

10. Pharmacopeial Specifications

Test	NF
Identification	+
pH (1 in 100 solution)	5.0 - 8.0
Loss on drying	≤5.0%
Residue on ignition	≤0.2%
Arsenic	≤3 ppm
Heavy metals	≤0.004%
Lead	≤0.001%
Apparent viscosity	Conforming to label
Assay	≤80.5% of hydroxypropyl groups
Silica or other	≤0.6%
suitable anti-caking agents	

11. Typical Properties

Microbiological: The high level of substitution of hydroxypropyl cellulose improves the resistance of the polymer to degradation by molds and bacteria. However, aqueous solutions are susceptible to degradation under severe conditions, and a viscosity decrease may result. Certain enzymes, produced by microbial action, will degrade hydroxypropyl cellulose in solution. If prolonged storage is contemplated, a preservative is recommended. Solutions of hydroxypropyl cellulose in organic solvents do not generally require preservatives.

Moisture content: Maximum 5% from Hercules, Inc. (usually 2-3%). Maximum 10% from Shin-Etsu, Inc. Hydroxypropyl cellulose absorbs moisture from the atmosphere. The amount absorbed depends on the relative humidity and temperature of the environment. Typical equilibrium moisture content values are: at 50% R.H./73°F - 4%; at 84% R.H./73°F - 12%.

Ash content: Not more than 0.5% (if no silicone dioxide, an anti-caking agent, is added) for *Klucel.* ≤1% for L-HPC.

Bulk density: 0.5 g/ml (will vary with the type of hydroxypropyl cellulose).

Burnout temperature: Hydroxypropyl cellulose burns out completely at 450° to 500°C in nitrogen or oxygen.

Particle size:

Klucel	L-HPC
95% through 30 mesh	99.5% through 80 mesh
99% through 20 mesh	98% through 100 mesh

pH (1% solution): 5.0 to 8.5

Softening temperature: 130°C

Solubility: Soluble in water below 38°C. Soluble in many polar organic solvents, such as ethanol, propylene glycol, dioxane, methanol, isopropyl alcohol (95%), dimethyl sulfoxide and dimethyl formamide.

Insoluble in hot water, it is precipitated as a highly swollen floc at a temperature between 40 and 45°C. All types have excellent solubility in either hot or cold polar organic liquids. There is no tendency for precipitation in hot organic solvents. The grade of hydroxypropyl cellulose can have a marked effect upon solution quality in an organic liquid, that is, a borderline solvent (e.g., tertiary butanol, cyclohexanol, acetone, methylethyl ketone, methylacetate, isopropyl alcohol (99%), methylene chloride, butyl acetate, butyl cellosolve and lactic acid). The higher viscosity types may give slightly inferior solutions. The solution quality in borderline solvents can often be greatly improved through the use of small quantities of a co-solvent (5-15%). For example, methylene chloride is a borderline solvent for *Klucel HF*, and solutions are granular. The addition of 10% methanol results in a smooth solution. Hydroxypropyl cellulose is insoluble in aliphatic hydrocarbons, aromatic hydrocarbons, petroleum distillates, glycerin and oils. Hydroxypropyl cellulose is compatible with a number of high molecular weight, high-boiling waxes and oils, and can be used to modify certain properties of these materials. Examples of materials that are good solvents for hydroxypropyl cellulose at an elevated temperature are: acetylated monoglycerides, glycerides, polyethylene glycol, polypropylene glycol and pine oil.

Solutions in water:

Specific gravity, 2% solution at 30°C	1.010
Refractive index, 2% solution	1.337
Surface tension, 0.1% solution	43.6 dynes/cm
Interfacial tension, 0.1% solution	12.5 dynes/cm vs. refined mineral oil

Molecular weight range:

Klucel EF	60,000
Klucel LF	100,000
Klucel JF	125,000
Klucel GF	300,000
Klucel MF	600,000
Klucel HF	1,000,000

Viscosity: A wide range of viscosity types is available as indicated by the table below.

Viscosity of aqueous solutions at 25°C (centipoise) (Measured on Brookfield LVF Viscometer)

Concentration in Water by Weight

Type	1%	2%	5%	10%
Klucel HF	1,500-2,500			
Klucel MF		4,000-6,500		
Klucel GF		150-400		
Klucel JF			150-400	
Klucel LF			75-150	
Klucel EF				300-700

Brookfield Settings

RPM	Spindle No.	*Klucel* Type
60	2	EF
30	1	LF
60	2	JF
60	2	GF
60	4	MF
30	3	HF

Academy HPE Laboratory Project Data

	% w/v	Visco-meter*	Lab #	Viscosity Max/Min Range
Klucel EF	10	RVT	6	410-740 cps
Klucel EF	10	HBT	6	416-744 cps
Klucel GF	2	RVT	6	360-615 cps
Klucel GF	2	HBT	6	288-540 cps
Klucel GF	3	RVT	6	1350-1625 cps
Klucel GF	3	HBT	6	960-2320 cps
Klucel HF	1	RVT	6	180-325 cps
Klucel HF	1	HBT	6	240-300 cps
Klucel HF	2	RVT	6	2325-3300 cps
Klucel HF	2	HBT	6	1408-4320 cps

*Brookfield
Supplier: Hercules Inc.

Academy HPE Laboratory Project Data continued

	Method	Lab #	Results
EMC Plot (*Klucel*)[b]	EMC-1	15	Fig:15-EMC-3
SDI Plot (Type LH11)[a]	SDI-1	14	Fig:14-SDI-4
SDI Plot (*Klucel HF*)[b]	SDI-1	14	Fig:14-SDI-4
SDI Plot (*Klucel MF*)[b]	SDI-1	14	Fig:14-SDI-4
SDI Plot (*Klucel GF*)[b]	SDI-1	14	Fig:14-SDI-5
SDI Plot (*Klucel JF*)[b]	SDI-1	14	Fig:14-SDI-5
SDI Plot (*Klucel LF*)[b]	SDI-1	14	Fig:14-SDI-5
Type LH2[a]	MC-7	14	3.81
Klucel HF[b]	MC-7	14	4.27
Klucel MF[b]	MC-7	14	1.52
Klucel GF[b]	MC-7	14	1.67
Klucel JF[b]	MC-7	14	1.44
Klucel LF[b]	MC-7	14	2.21
Klucel EF[b]	MC-7	14	0.59
Solubility:[c]	SOL-7	32	
Water (25°C)			500.0 mg/ml
Water (37°C)			500.0 mg/ml
Alcohol (25°C)			0.14 mg/ml
Alcohol (37°C)			0.24 mg/ml
Prop. glycol (25°C)			1.00 mg/ml
Prop. glycol (37°C)			1.00 mg/ml
Hexane (25°C)			1.00 mg/ml
Hexane (37°C)			1.00 mg/ml
Particle friability[c]	PF-1	36	0.125

Suppliers: Biddle Sawyer Corp.[a]; Hercules, Inc.[b]; Shin-Etsu Chemical Co.[c]

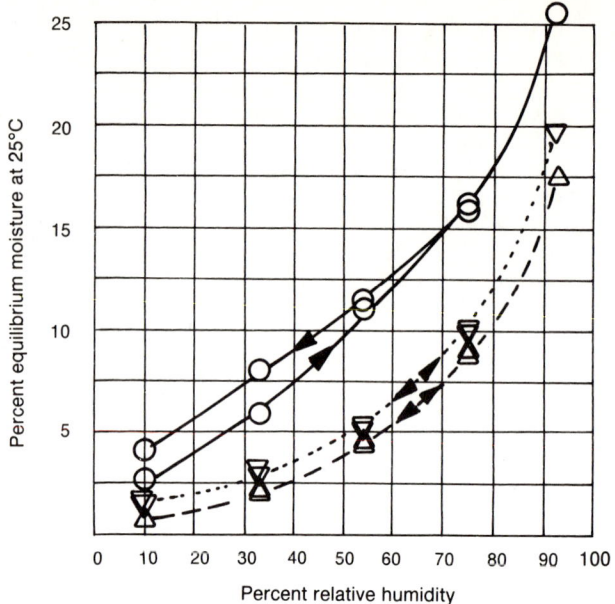

O: Hydroxypropyl cellulose, type LH 11 (Biddle Sawyer, lot #8069)
△: Hydroxypropyl cellulose, *Klucel HF* (Hercules, lot #1061)
▽: Hydroxypropyl cellulose, *Klucel MF* (Hercules, lot #1294)

Figure: 14-SDI-4   **Method:** SDI-1

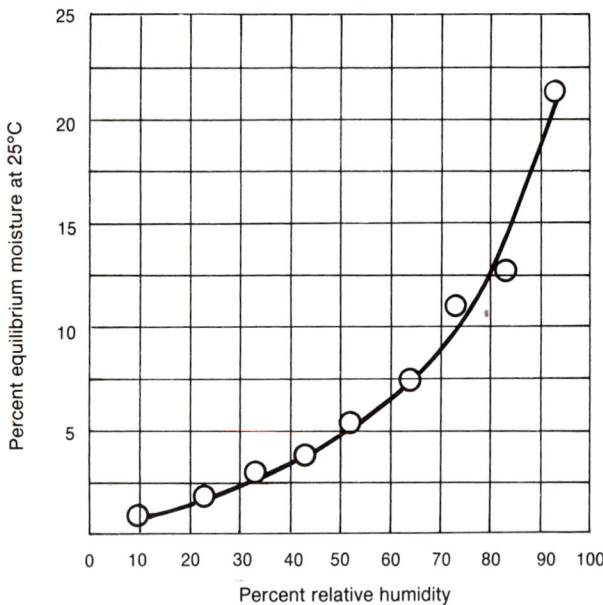

Hydroxypropyl cellulose, *Klucel* (Hercules, lot #6387)

Figure: 15-EMC-3   **Method:** EMC-1

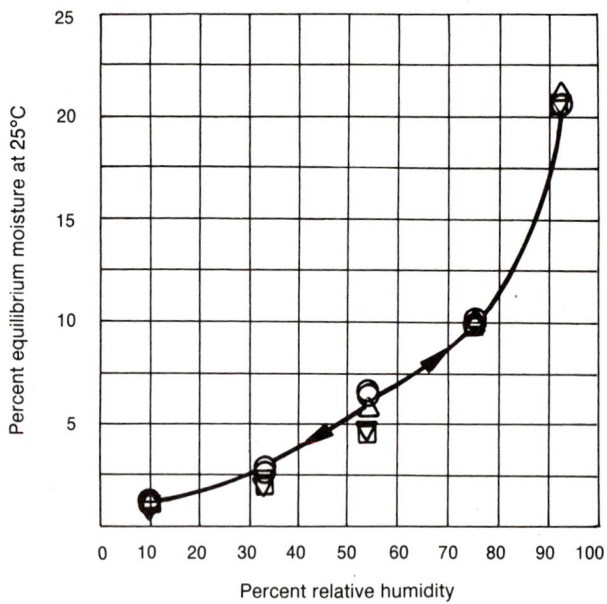

O: Hydroxypropyl cellulose, *Klucel GF* (Hercules, lot #4996)
△: Hydroxypropyl cellulose, *Klucel JF* (Hercules, lot #4753)
▽: Hydroxypropyl cellulose, *Klucel LF* (Hercules, lot #4965)
□: Hydroxypropyl cellulose, *Klucel EF* (Hercules, lot #1223)

Figure: 14-SDI-5   **Method:** SDI-1

12. Stability and Storage Conditions

Aqueous solutions of hydroxypropyl cellulose possess the best viscosity stability when the pH is maintained between 6.0 and 8.0 and the solutions are protected from light, heat and the action of micro-organisms. Hydroxypropyl cellulose in aqueous solution is susceptible to both chemical and biological degradation. Hydroxypropyl cellulose in solution is susceptible to acid hydrolysis, which causes chain scission and loss in solution viscosity. The rate of hydrolysis increases with increasing temperature and hydrogen ion concentration. Alkali-catalyzed oxidative degradation will also degrade the polymer and result in a decrease in viscosity of the solution. This degradation can result from the presence of dissolved oxygen or oxidizing agents in the solution. Light (U.V.) will degrade hydroxypropyl cellulose, and solutions will undergo some decrease in viscosity if exposed to light for several months. Hydroxypropyl cellulose powder should be stored in a tight container in a dry atmosphere to prevent any increase in moisture content.

13. Incompatibilities

Hydroxypropyl cellulose may not tolerate high concentrations of other dissolved materials. The balance of hydrophilic-lipophilic properties of the polymer, which are required for dual solubility, reduces its ability to hydrate with water. It tends to be "salted out" in the presence of a high concentration of other dissolved materials. It has been reported that when hydroxypropyl cellulose is combined with anionic polymers, higher viscosity values are obtained. The precipitation temperature is lower in the presence of relatively high concentrations of other dissolved materials that compete for the water in the system. The data in the table below illustrate this.

Ingredients and Concentrations	Precipitation Temperature, °C
1% *Klucel H*	41
1% *Klucel H* + 1.0% NaCl	38
1% *Klucel H* + 5.0% NaCl	30
0.5% *Klucel H* + 10% Sucrose	41
0.5% *Klucel H* + 30% Sucrose	32
0.5% *Klucel H* + 40% Sucrose	20
0.5% *Klucel H* + 50% Sucrose	7

Hydroxypropyl cellulose in solution demonstrates some incompatibility with substituted phenol derivatives, such as methyl and propyl parahydroxybenzoate

14. Safety

Toxicity testing indicates that hydroxypropyl cellulose is physiologically inert. The results of repeat insult patch tests on humans disclose no evidence that it is either a primary skin irritant or skin-sensitizing agent. Hydroxypropyl cellulose is considered nutritionally equivalent to purified cellulose, in that neither material is metabolized. Estimated acceptable daily intake: up to 25 mg/kg of body weight as the sum of total modified celluloses.

15. Handling Precautions

Store in a well-closed container.

16. Regulatory Acceptance

NF XVI; Hydroxypropyl cellulose is recognized in the *Federal Register* (Title 21, 121.1160).

17. Applications in Pharmaceutical Formulations or Technology

Granulating agent (binder)—*Klucel E* or *L*, 2 to 4% concentration. Film coating—*Klucel E* or *L*, 5% concentration in methylene chloride or isopropanol.
Thickener—Concentration is dependent on solvent. Micro-encapsulation—higher molecular weight grades used.

18. Related Substances

L-HPC is a low molecular weight, cross-linked hydroxypropyl cellulose. It is used as a tablet disintegrant.

19. Comments

Hydroxypropyl cellulose is a thermoplastic polymer that can be processed by virtually all fabrication methods used for plastics.

20. Specific References

1. *KLUCEL, Hydroxypropyl Cellulose, Physical and Chemical Properties*, by Hercules, Incorporated, 1976.
2. A.J. Desmarais, Chapter 24, Hydroxyalkyl derivatives of cellulose. In: *Industrial Gums*, 2nd Edition, Academic Press, N.Y., 1973, pp. 649-672.
3. M.G. Wirick, Study of the enzymic degradation of CMC and other cellulose ethers *J. Polymer Science: Part A-1: 6*, 1965-1974, July (1968).
4. E.D. Klug, Some properties of water soluble hydroxyalkyl celluloses and their derivatives, *J. Polymer Science, Part C*, No. 36: 491-508 (1971).
5. "L-HPC" Product Bulletin, by Shen-Etsu Chemical Company, Cellulose Division.
6. H. Delonca, J. Joachim and A. Mattha, Effect of temperature on disintegration and dissolution time of tablets with a cellulose component as a binder, *J. Pharm. Belg.*, 33: 171-8 (1978).
7. Y. Machida, Pharmaceutical interactions in dosage form and processing. 1. Directly compressed tablets containing hydroxypropyl cellulose in addition to starch and lactose, *Chem. Pharm. Bull.*, 22: 2346-51 (1974).
8. O. Nils Lindberg, Water vapour transmission through free films of hydroxypropyl cellulose, *Acta. Pharm. Svecica*, 8: 541-8 (1971).
9. J.W. Stafford, J.F. Pickard and R. Zink, Temperature dependence of the disintegration times of compressed tablets containing hydroxypropyl cellulose as binder, *J. Pharm. Pharmacol.*, 30: 1-5, (1978).
10. H. Delonca, J. Joachim and A.G. Mattha, Binding activity of hydroxypropyl cellulose (200,000 and 1,000,000 mol. wt.) and its effect on the physical characteristics of granules and tablets, *Farmaco Ed. Prat.*, 32: 157-71 (1977).
11. G. Banker, G. Peck, E. Williams, D. Taylor and P. Pirakitikulr, Microbiological considerations of polymer solutions used in aqueous film coating, *Drug Devel. and Ind. Pharm.*, 8(1): 41-51 (1982).
12. N. Kitamori and T. Makino, Improvement in pressure-dependent dissolution of tredibutone tablets by using intragranular disintegrants, *Drug Devel. & Ind. Pharm.*, 8(1): 125-139 (1982).

USA: R.L. Harwood*; A.A. Monaco**; Z. Chowhan**
UK: J. Wylth**

Hydroxypropyl Methylcellulose

1. Nonproprietary Names

USP: Hydroxypropyl methylcellulose 2208, 2906, 2910
BPC: Hypromellose

2. Functional Categories

USP: Suspending and/or viscosity-increasing agent; tablet binder; coating agent
BP: Viscosity-increasing agent; adhesive anhydrous ointment ingredient
Others: Film-former; emulsion stabilizer

3. Synonyms

Methyl hydroxypropylcellulose; propylene glycol ether of methylcellulose; methylcellulose propylene glycol ether

4. Chemical Names and CAS Registry Number

Cellulose, 2-Hydroxypropylmethylether
Cellulose Hydroxypropylmethylether [9004-65-3]

5. Empirical Formula   Molecular Weight

$C_8H_{15}O_6$ - $(C_{10}H_{18}O_6)n$ - $C_8H_{15}O_5$ Approx. 86,000

6. Structural Formula

7. Commercial Availability

USA

Aldrich Chemical Co.
Ashland Chemical Co.
Biddle Sawyer Corp.
Dow Chemical

UK

British Celanese, Ltd.
Colorcon, Ltd.
Henkel Chemicals, Ltd.
K & K Greeff Chemicals, Ltd.
Shin-Etsu Chemical Co., Ltd.
Stancourt, Sons & Muir, Ltd.

8. Method of Manufacture

Cellulose fibers, obtained from cotton linters or wood pulp, are treated with caustic (sodium hydroxide) solution. The alkali cellulose thus obtained is in turn treated with methyl chloride and propylene oxide to produce methylhydroxypropyl ethers of cellulose. The fibrous reaction product is then purified and ground to a fine, uniform powder or granules.

9. Description

An odorless, tasteless, white or creamy-white fibrous or granular powder.

SEM: KY-25
Excipient: Hydroxypropyl Methylcellulose
Manufacturer: Shin-Etsu Chemicals **Lot no:** 83214

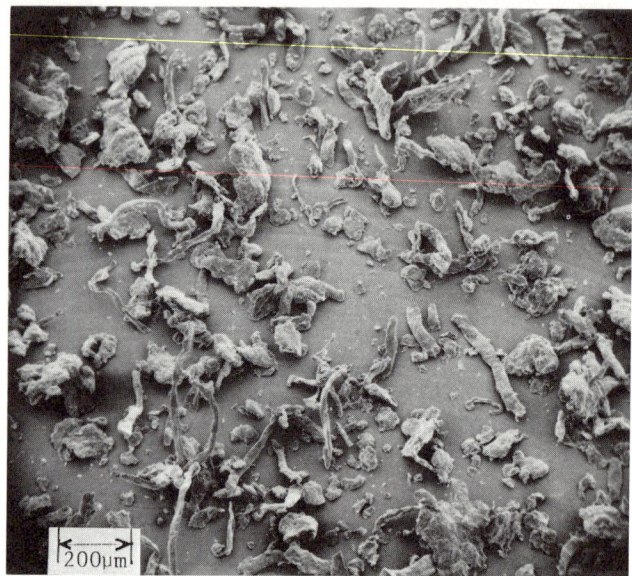

Magnification: 60× **Voltage:** 10kV

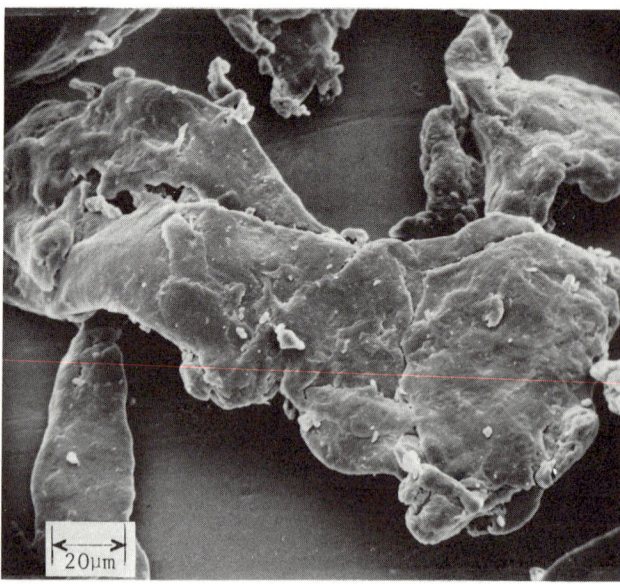

Magnification: 600× **Voltage:** 10kV

10. Pharmacopeial Specifications

Test	USP	BPC
Identification	+	+
pH	—	6.0-8.0

Apparent viscosity

Viscosity Grade	Viscosity at 20° C	Viscosity Grade	Viscosity at 20° C
100 cps or less	80.0-120.0%	20 cps 50	15-15 40-60
higher than 100 cps	75.0-140.0%	125	110-140
		450	350-550
		1500	1200-1800
		4500	3750-5250
		15,000	12,000-18,000

Test	USP	BPC
Loss on drying	≤5.0%	≤10.0%
Residue on ignition	≤1.5% for viscosity grade greater than 50 cps ≤3% for viscosity grade 50 cps or less	—
Arsenic	≤3 ppm	≤2 ppm
Heavy metals	0.001%	—
Lead	—	≤5 ppm
Sulfated ash	—	≤1.0%

Content of hydroxy-propoxy

Grade	Content	
2208	4.0-12.0%	
2906	4.0- 7.5%	4.0-7.5%
2910	7.0-12.0%	

Content of methoxy

Grade	Content	
2208	19.0-24.0%	
2906	27.0-30.0%	27.0-29.0%
2910	28.0-30.0%	

11. Typical Properties

Apparent density: 0.25-0.70 g/cm³
Browning temperature: 190-200° C (374-392° F)
Charring temperature: 225-230° C (437-446° F)
Enzyme resistance: Comparatively enzyme-resistant, providing excellent viscosity stability during long-term storage.
Gel formation: Undergoes a reversible transformation from sol to gel upon heating and cooling, respectively.
Gel-Point: 50° C - 90° C, depending upon the grade.
Ionic charge: No ionic charge (i.e., not a polyelectrolyte). Will not complex with metallic salts and ionic organics to form insoluble precipitates, thus presenting less compatibility problems.
Ash: 1.5%-3.0%, depending upon the grade.
Relative flammability in a furnace at 700° C (1292° F): 90+
Solubility: Soluble in cold water, forming a viscous colloidal solution; insoluble in alcohol, ether and chloroform, but soluble in mixtures of methyl alcohol and methylene chloride. Certain grades are soluble in aqueous acetone, mixtures of methylene chloride and isopropyl alcohol and other organic solvents.
Specific gravity: Approximately 1.3.
Surface activity: Provides some surfactancy in solutions. Surface tensions for such solutions range from 42 to 56 dynes per cm (a typical surfactant has a surface tension of 30 dynes per cm).
Equilibrium moisture: See Figure 15-EMC-4.

Academy HPE Laboratory Project Data			
	Method	Lab #	Results
Moisture content	MC-20	15	2.10[a]
Moisture content	MC-20	15	3.10[b]
EMC-Plot	EMC-1	15	Fig:15-EMC-4[a]

Supplier: Dow[a]; Hercules[b]

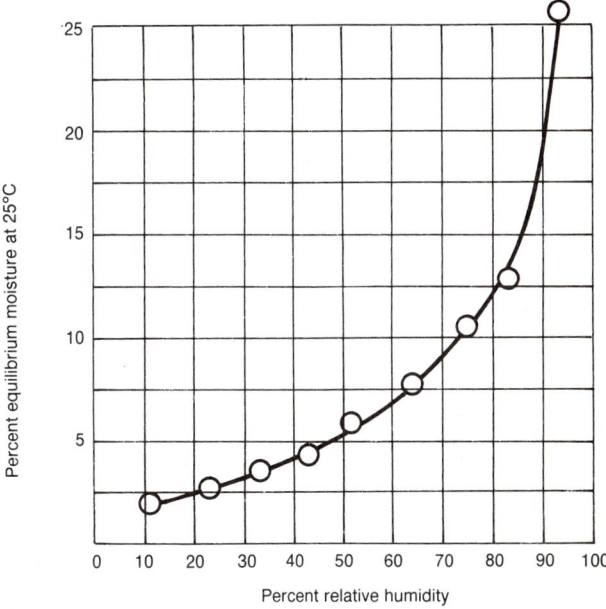

Hydroxypropyl methylcellulose, methocel E 15 (Dow, Lot # QP0502-801-E)

Figure: 15-EMC-4   **Method:** EMC-1

12. Stability and Storage Conditions

Very stable in dry conditions. Solutions are stable at pH 3.0-11.0. Aqueous solutions are liable to be affected by microorganisms. When used as a viscosity-increasing agent in ophthalmic solutions, an anti-microbial agent, such as benzalkonium chloride, should be incorporated. Store in a tight container, in a cool place.

13. Incompatibilities

Extreme pH conditions; oxidizing materials.

14. Safety

Human and animal feeding studies have shown hydroxypropyl methylcellulose to be safe.

15. Handling Precautions

—

16. Regulatory Acceptance

USP XXI; BPC

17. Applications in Pharmaceutical Formulation or Technology

Film-former in tablet film coating (perhaps the most commonly used film forming agent). Lower viscosity grades are used in aqueous film coating and higher viscosity grades are used in solvent film coating. The concentration varies from 2 to 10% depending upon the viscosity grade of the polymer. Binder in tablet granulations: 2-5%. High-viscosity grades are used to retard the release of water-soluble drugs. Thickening agent added to vehicles for eye drops and artificial tear solutions at 0.45-1.0% concentrations. Protective colloid which prevents droplets and particles from coalescing or agglomerating, thus inhibiting the formation of sediments. Emulsifier, suspending agent and stabilizer in gels and ointments. Adhesive in plastic bandages.

18. Related Substances

Hydroxypropyl methylcellulose, surface-treated powder or granular. These products are dispersible in cold water, and the dissolution rate can be controlled by a shift in pH. They are useful for slow-release or enteric coated formulations.

19. Comments

For USP grade hydroxypropyl methylcellulose, the name is followed by a four-digit number. The first two digits refer to the approximate content of the methoxy group ($-OCH_3$) in percent. The second two digits refer to the approximate content of the hydroxypropoxy group ($-OCH_2CHOHCH_3$) in percent, calculated on a dried basis. Maximum acceptable daily intake is 25 mg per kg of body weight. Hydroxypropyl methylcellulose is used as a food and drug additive without the addition of calories in the diet, because it is not metabolized. For BPC grade hypromellose, the name is followed by a number indicating the approximate viscosity of a 2% solution at 20° C. To prepare an aqueous solution, it is recommended to disperse and thoroughly hydrate Hydroxypropyl Methylcellulose in about 1/5 to 1/3 of the required amount of water at 80-90° C and add ice while stirring vigorously. Then add cold water to volume. When a water-miscible organic solvent such as alcohol, glycol, or mixtures of alcohol and methylene chloride is called for in the formulation, hydroxypropyl methylcellulose may be dispersed into the organic solvent first (at a ratio of 5-8 parts of solvent to 1 part of hydroxypropyl methylcellulose), followed by the addition of cold water. Aqueous solutions may be sterilized by autoclaving. The coagulated polymer must be redispersed by shaking on cooling.

20. Specific References

1. Seventeenth Report of FAO/WHO Expert Committee on Food Additives, Tech. Ref. Serv., Wld. Hlth. Org., No. 539, 1974.
2. R. C. Rowe, The adhesion of film coatings to tablet surfaces: the effect of some direct compression excipients and lubricants, *J. Pharm. Pharmacol.*, 29: 723 (1977).
3. Z. Chowhan, Role of binders in moisture-induced hardness increase in compressed tablets, and its effect on *in vitro* disintegration and dissolution, *J. Pharm. Sci.* 69: 1 (1980).
4. J. F. Pickard, An investigation of selected cellulose ethers as film coatings for pharmaceutical tablets, Ph.D. Dissertation, the Council for National Academic Awards, Feb. 1979.
5. Handbook on Methocel Cellulose Ether Products (Form No. 192-702), Dow Chemical Company.
6. Pharmacoat, Shin-Etsu Chemical Co., 1977.
7. G. K. Greminger and A. B. Savage. In: "Industrial Gums," R. L. Whistler, ed., London Academic Press, 1959, pp. 565-596.
8. R. C. Rowe, *J. Pharm. Pharmac.*, 32: 116-119 (1980).
9. A. O. Okhamafe and P. York, Moisture permeation mechanism of some aqueous-based film coats, *J. Pharm. Pharmacol.*, 34 Suppl: 52P (1982).
10. J. G. Hardy, J. W. Kenerley, M. J. Taylor, C. G. Wilson and S. S. Davis, Release rates from sustained-release buccal tablets in man, *J. Pharm. Pharmacol.*, 34 Suppl: 91P (1982).
11. G. Banker, G. Peck, E. Williams, D. Taylor, P. Pirakitikular, Microbiological considerations of polymer solutions used in aqueous film coating, *Drug Devel. and Ind. Pharm.*, 8(1):41-51 (1982).

USA: L. Y. Lin*; A. L. Monaco**; Z. Chowhan**
UK: R. C. Rowe*

Hydroxypropyl Methylcellulose Phthalate

1. Nonproprietary Name

NF: hydroxypropyl methylcellulose phthalate (200731 and 220824)

2. Functional Categories

NF: Coating agent; viscosity and/or suspending agent; film former
Others: Enteric coating agent

3. Synonyms

HPMCP; monophalic acid ester or hydroxypropyl methylcellulose 200731

4. Chemical Name and CAS Registry Number

Cellulose, hydroxypropyl methyl, 1,2-benzenedicarboxylate.

5. Empirical Formula   Molecular Weight

See structural formula

The molecular weights of all commercial grades are in the range 2,000-100,000 but average values are as follows:

Grade	Average Molecular Weight
HP-45	20,000
HP-50	20,000
HP-55	20,000
HP-55 F	20,000
HP-55 S	33,000

6. Structural Formula

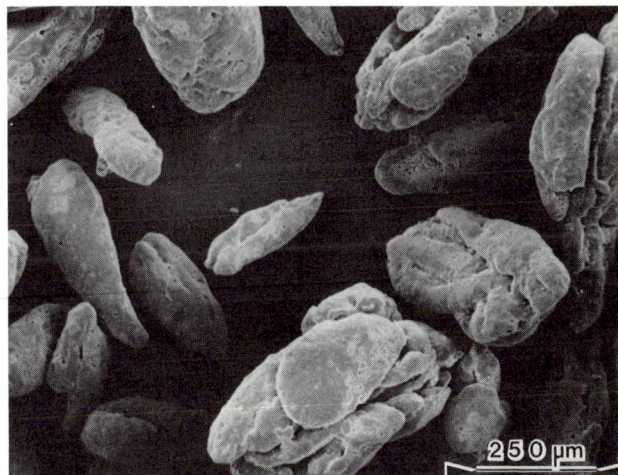

Degree of substitution	Content (%)		
	HP-45	HP-50	HP-55
Methoxy groups	19-24	20-25	18-22
Hydroxypropoxy groups	5.5-9.5	5-10	4-9
Carboxybenzoyl groups	18.5-21.0	20-24	27-35

7. Commercial Availability

USA
Biddle Sawyer Corp.

UK
Mitsui & Co. Europe, S.P.A.
Shin-Etsu Chemical Co., Ltd.
Stancourt, Muir & Sons, Ltd.

8. Method of Manufacture

Hydroxypropyl methylcellulose phthalate is prepared by esterification of hydroxypropyl methylcellulose with phthalic anhydride. The degree of alkyloxy and carboxybenzoyl substitution determines its polymer properties and in particular the pH at which it dissolves in aqueous media.

9. Description

White to off-white granular powder, odorless, with a barely detectable taste.

SEM-MF—19
Excipient: Hydroxypropyl cellulose phthalate-55

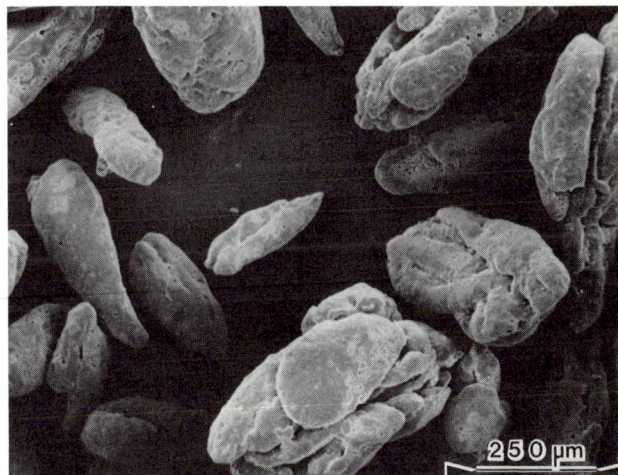

Magnification: 60×

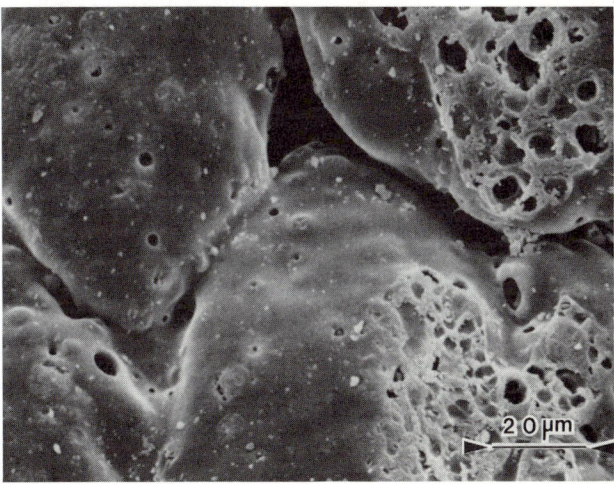

Magnification: 600×

10. Pharmacopeial Specifications

Test	NF
Identification	+
Clarity and color of solution	+
Viscosity	80–120% of label
Loss on drying (105°, 1 hour)	≤5% by wt.
Residue on ignition	≤0.20%
Chloride	≤0.07%
Arsenic	≤2 ppm
Heavy metals	≤0.001%
Free phthalic acid	≤1.0%
Assay	
Methoxy	
200731	18–22%
220824	20–24%
Hydroxy-propoxy	
200731	5–9%
220824	6–10%
Phthalyl	
200731	27–35%
220824	21–27%

11. Typical Properties

Contents of residue on ignition at 500 C:

SiO_2: 69-75 ppm
Na_2O: 8-12 ppm
Fe_2O_3: 8-13 ppm
CaO: 17 ppm
MgO: 3 ppm

Density:

Property	HPMCP grade:	
	HP-50	HP-55
True density, g/cm³	1.82	1.65
Poured bulk density, g/cm³	0.29	0.26
Tapped (consolidated) bulk density, g/cm³	0.34	0.32

Viscosity: 240 ± 48 mN s/m² (HP-50)
190 ± 38 mN s/m² (HP-55)
Determined in 15% solutions in methylene chloride: methanol (1:1) at 20°C using a Brookfield viscometer.

Methoxyl content: 20.0-25.0 (HP-50)
(wt.%) 18.0-22.0 (HP-55)

Hydroxypropoxyl content: 5.0-10.0 (HP-50)
(wt.%) 4.0- 9.0 (HP-55)

Carboxybenzoyl content: 20.0-24.0 (HP-50)
(wt.%) 27.0-35.0 (HP-55)

Loss on drying: ≤5%
Viscosity (2% aqueous solution): 192-288 cps (HP-50)
(15%, CH_2Cl_2/CH_3OH=1/1, w/w, 20°C): 152-228 cps (HP-55)

Moisture sorption: See Figure 1
Heavy metals: ≤10 ppm
Lead: ≤5ppm

Moisture content: a) Loss on drying: ≤5% (after 2 hours at 105°C). b) Hygroscopicity: HPMCP takes up between 2% and 5% moisture at ambient temperature and humidity conditions. The moisture sorption isotherm of HP-50 measured at 25°C (see Figure 1) indicates a sorption/desorption hysteresis.

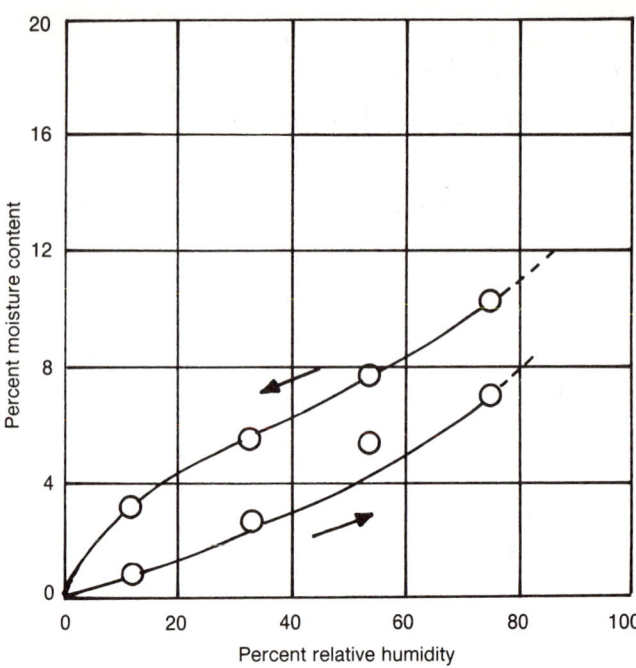

Figure 1: Moisture sorption isotherms

Phthalic acid (free): ≤1%
Softening point: 200°-210°C

Solubility: Readily soluble in a mixture of acetone and methyl or ethyl alcohol (1:1 by weight), in a mixture of methyl alcohol and methylene chloride (1:1 by weight) and in aqueous alkali. It is insoluble in hexane, water and aqueous acid. The solubility guide for a range of organic solvents is given in the following table:

Solvent	HP-55	HP-50
Acetone	+	/
Acetone/water (95:5)	+	+
Acetone/methanol (1:1)	+	+
Acetone/ethanol (1:1)	+	=
Acetone/propan-2-ol (1:1)	+	=
Acetone/methylene chloride (1:1)	+	/
Methylene chloride	/	/
Methylene chloride/methanol (1:1)	+	+
Methylene chloride/ethanol (1:1)	+	+
Methylene chloride/propan-2-ol (1:1)	+	=
Ethyl acetate	/	X
Ethyl acetate/methanol (1:1)	+	+
Ethyl acetate/ethanol (1:1)	+	=
Ethyl acetate/propan-2-ol (1:1)	+	/
Benzene/methanol (1:1)	+	+
Methyl ethyl ketone	+	/
Dioxane	+	+
Methanol	/	/
Ethanol	/	/
Propan-2-ol	/	X

Note: + ... Soluble, clear solution
= ... Slightly soluble, cloudy solution
/ ... Swells but insoluble
X ... Insoluble

12. Stability and Storage Conditions

HPMCP is chemically and physically stable at ambient conditions for at least 3 to 4 years, and at 40°C/75% RH for 2 to 3 months. After 10 days at 60°C/100% RH, 8% degradation occurred. It is stable after exposure to UV light for up to 3 months at 25°C/70% RH. The microbial content of HPMCP is ≤100 micro-organisms per g, with absence of any pathogens. At ambient storage conditions HPMCP is not susceptible to microbial attack.

13. Incompatibilities

Specific incompatibilities are unknown. Splitting of film coatings has been reported rarely, but notably with coated tablets containing microcrystalline cellulose and calcium carboxymethylcellulose. Film splitting can be avoided by a careful choice of the coating solvent and by the addition of a plasticizer. HPMCP is compatible with many commonly used tablet excipients and with plasticizers such as di- and tri-acetin, diethyl and dibutyl phthalate, castor oil, acetyl monoglyceride and polyethylene glycols.

14. Safety

Several published articles on these aspects of HPMCP may be summarized under the following headings.

Absorption, distribution, metabolism, excretion (ADME): In two Japanese studies (1,2), the ADME in rats of orally-administered HPMCP was investigated using the C^{14}-labeled compound. In both cases more than 90% of the product was excreted unchanged in the feces within 72 hours. Cumulative urinary excretion, usually as phthalic acid, was ≤1% for male rats and approximately 1.2% for female rats 72 hours after administration. There was no evidence of widespread radioactivity in the blood and body tissues, with the exception of the liver and kidney, in which very low levels of radioactivity were detected. The peak levels of radioactivity in these tissues were the same in both studies, but the time after administration depended on which part of the molecule had been labeled with C^{14}.

Acute and sub-acute toxicities: The acute and sub-acute toxicities of HPMCP in rats of both sexes were studied by Kitagawa and coworkers (3). The toxicity of HPMCP was so low that no fatalities were registered in the study group at dosages of up to 1.5 g per kg, and LD_{50} values were therefore not obtained. In the second part of the study, different groups of rats were administered HPMCP orally at levels of 1.3, 2.0, 3.0, 4.5 or 10 g per kg of body weight. The groups receiving 10 g per kg and the corresponding control group of animals receiving the solution vehicle used to administer HPMCP exhibited severe diarrhea and ataxia, and all animals died within 10 days and 16 days, respectively. This effect was attributed to the large volumes of vehicle (1.5% sodium bicarbonate solution) used to administer the HPMCP by stomach tube. Using the criteria survival, behavioral studies, body weight change, food consumption, tissue weight of major organs, urinary analysis, hematological analysis and pathological analysis of the major organs, there was no evidence of toxicity in the animals receiving dose levels of HPMCP up to 4.5 g per kg of body weight. Bacterial infection of the lungs found in test and control animals was not attributed to HPMCP.

Chronic toxicity: Chronic toxicity studies with HPMCP were carried out in rats by Kitagawa (4) and in dogs by Woodward (5). In the first of these studies, three groups of rats of both sexes were administered daily HPMCP doses of 1.5, 3 and 5 g per kg of body weight for six months. From the behavioral pattern, body weight gain, weight gain of the major organs, hematological studies, urinary analysis and patho-histological examination of the major organs, the authors concluded that there was no evidence of toxicity from HPMCP during this study. In the second study on chronic toxicity, HPMCP was administered in the diet to groups of three male and three female beagles for fifty-three weeks at daily dosage levels of 0.75, 1.5 and 3 g per kg of body weight. A control group of three male and three female beagles was treated similarly to the test animals. The animals were assessed using the criteria survival, body weight gain, food consumption, physical/pharmacological examination, hematological analysis, urine and serum analysis, physiological analysis of body function, weight change in the major organs and histopathological observations. It was concluded that there were no changes in the dogs which could be ascribed to the administration of HPMCP.

Teratogenicity: These studies were conducted by Ito (6) after the administration of HPMCP to female donryu rats and ddN mice during pregnancy. He examined the fetuses at the termination of pregnancy and the offspring not later than three weeks after birth. No change was observed in the percentage appearance of dead embryos, body weight of fetuses, external malformation, post-natal development, differentiation, behavior and growth rates. In the skeletons only a small percentage of spontaneous abnormalities was found in the sternum of both test and control animals. It was concluded that HPMCP produced no malformations.

15. Handling Precautions

No restrictions specified.

16. Regulatory Acceptance

NF XVI

17. Applications in Pharmaceutical Formulation or Technology

HPMCP can be used alone or in combination with other soluble or insoluble binders in the preparation of granules with sustained drug release properties. The release rate is pH-dependent.

Film former:

Water vapor transmission:
HP-50 : 246 g/m²/day
HP-55 : 213 g/m²/day
(Using Japanese Industrial Standard Z - 0208)

Mechanical properties:

	Tensile strength kg/mm²	Elongation %
HP-50	7.7	6.1
HP-55	7.9	5.6

(Using Japanese Industrial Standard K - 6301)

HPMCP is a useful enteric coating material which is completely insoluble in gastric fluid in film coatings which comprise approximately 5% to 10% of the tablet weight. Such coatings dissolve rapidly in the upper intestine. It can normally be applied to tablets and granules without the inclusion of a platicizer, using established coating techniques. Enteric coatings can also be applied using a dispersion of HPMCP in aqueous solutions of triacetin and a wetting agent.

18. Related Substances

Hydroxypropyl methylcellulose

19. Comments

HPMCP is approved in the USA, West Germany, Switzerland, Austria, Denmark, France, Australia, Spain, Poland and Japan. It is at present under review in the USSR. No specific prohibitions by regulatory bodies are known. The number following HP in each grade designation refers to the pH value (×10) at which the polymer dissolves in aqueous buffer solutions. The designation S in HP-55 S indicates a higher molecular weight grade, to give films with greater resistance to cracking. The designation F in HP-55 F indicates a product with smaller particle size, the mean size being approximately 20 microns. Aspirin tablets coated with HPMCP were chemically and physically stable after 4 weeks at 50°C in closed containers and at 40°C and 75% RH. Under the same storage conditions, coated erythromycin tablets were also physically stable. Coated pancreatin tablets were chemically and physically stable during 4 years in closed containers at room temperatures.

20. Specific References

1. Kitagawa H., Satoh T., Yokoshima T and Nanbo T., *Pharmacometrics*, 5: 1 - 4 (1971).
2. Kitagawa H., Yokoshima T., Nanbo T and Hasegawa M., *Pharmacometrics*, 8: 1123-1132 (1974).
3. Kitagawa H., Kawana H., Satoh T and Fukuda Y., *Pharmacometrics*, 4: 1017-1025 (1970).
4. Kitagawa H., Yano H and Fukuda Y., *Pharmacometrics* 7: 689-701 (1973).
5. Woodward, G. "HP-50 and HP-55, repeated oral administration of each test material to dogs for 53 weeks." Final report by Woodward Research Corporation.
6. Ito R and Toida S., *J. Med. Soc. Toho-Univ.*, 19: 453-461 (1972).
7. L Ehrhardt, V. Hartmann and L. Patt, *Deutsche Apotheker-Zeitung*, 112: 2005-2009 (1972).
8. L. Ehrhardt, L. Patt and E. Schindler, *Pharm. Ind.*, 35: 719-722 (1973).
9. L. Patt and V. Hartmann, *Pharm. Ind.*, 38: 902-906 (1976).
10. L. Ehrhardt, *Acta Pharm. Technol.*, Suppl. 1, 125-140 (1976).
11. J.P. Delporte and F. Jaminet, *J. Pharm. Belg.*, 31: 263-276 (1976).
12. Patents:
    Japan   - 43-65949, 43-65950, 44-18152
    France   - 69.31091
    UK   - 1 268 658
    US   - 3 629 237
    Germany - 19 46 170

USA: A. L. Monaco**; Z. Chowhan**
UK: J. F. Pickard*

Isobutane

1. Nonproprietary Name
NF: Isobutane

2. Functional Category
NF: Aerosol propellant

3. Synonym
A-31

4. Chemical Names and CAS Registry Number
Iso-butane; methyl propane

5. Empirical Formula
C_4H_{10}

Molecular Weight
58.12

6. Structural Formula

7. Commercial Availability
USA

Aeropres Corporation
Diversified Chemical and Propellant Company
Exxon Company
Industrial Hydrocarbons, Inc.
Phillips Chemical Company
Shell Chemical Company

UK
Air Products Ltd.

8. Method of Manufacture
See butane

9. Description
Isobutane is a liquefied gas, and exists as a liquid at room temperature when contained under its own vapor pressure, or as a gas when exposed to room temperature and atmospheric pressure. It is essentially a clear, colorless, odorless liquid, but may have a slight ethereal odor.

10. Pharmacopeial Specifications

Test	NF
Identification	+
Water	≤0.001%
High boiling residues	≤5ppm
Acidity of residue	+
Sulfur compounds	+
Assay	≥95% isobutane (C_4H_{10})

11. Typical Properties
Melting point °F: −255.3
Melting point °C: −159.4
Boiling point °F: 10.9
Boiling point °C: −11.7
Vapor pressure (psig at 70°F): 30.4
Vapor pressure (psig at 130°F): 96.0
Liquid density (g/cm³ at 70°F): 0.56
Vapor density (air = 1): 2.01
Kauri butanol value: 25
Solubility parameter: 7.1
Viscosity (Cps at 68°F): 0.156
Flammability in air: lower limit (vol %): 1.8; upper limit (vol %): 8.4
Flash point °F: −117

12. Stability and Storage Conditions
See butane. Isobutane is highly flammable and explosive. Preserve in tight cylinders and prevent exposure to excessive heat.

13. Incompatibilities
See butane

14. Safety
See butane

15. Handling Precautions
See butane

16. Regulatory Acceptance
NF XVI

17. Applications in Pharmaceutical Formulation or Technology
See butane

18. Related Substances
See butane

19. Comments
See butane

20. Specific References
See trichloromonofluoromethane.
"International Encyclopedia of Pressurized Packaging," A. Herzka, Ed., Pergamon Press, 1966.

USA: J. J. Sciarra*; A. C. Shah**

Isopropyl Alcohol

1. Nonproprietary Name
USP: Isopropyl alcohol
BP: Isopropyl alcohol

2. Functional Categories
USP: Solvent
Other: Local disinfectant

3. Synonyms
Isopropanol; alcohol isopropylicum; petrohol; dimethyl carbinol; 2-propanol; propan-2-ol; *sec*-propyl alcohol.

4. Chemical Name and CAS Registry Number
2-Propanol [67-63-0]

5. Empirical Formula   Molecular Weight
C_3H_8O 60.1

6. Structural Formula
$CH_3CH(OH)CH_3$

7. Commercial Availability
USA
Allied Chemical Corp.
ARCO Chemical Co. Div. Atlantic Richfield Co.
Ashland Chemical Co.
Baker Chemical Co., J. T.
Eastman Chemical Products, Inc.
Ingredient Technology Corp., Flavor & Fragrance Div.
Pfaltz & Bauer, Inc.
Publicker Industries, Inc.
Quad Chemical-Lonza Specialty Chemicals
Ruger Chemical Co.
Shell Chemical Co.
Stoney-Mueller, Inc.
Thompson-Hayward Chemical Co.
Union Carbide Corp.

UK
Alcohols, Ltd.
B. P. Chemicals, Ltd.
Carless Chemicals, Ltd.
Esso Chemicals, Ltd.
I.C.I., Plc.
Shell Chemicals, Ltd.
Unalco, Ltd.

8. Method of Manufacture
Isopropyl alcohol is prepared by absorption of propylene in sulfuric acid and hydrolysis to the alcohol; by catalytic reduction of acetone; and by certain fermentations of carbohydrates.

9. Description
Transparent, colorless, mobile, volatile, flammable liquid with a characteristic, spiritous odor resembling that of a mixture of ethanol and acetone, and a slightly bitter taste.

10. Pharmacopeial Specifications

Test	USP	BP
Identification	+	+
Specific gravity	0.783-0.787	—
Refractive index (20°C)	1.376-1.378	1.377–1.378
Acidity or alkalinity	+	+
Nonvolatile residue	≤0.005%	≤0.0016% (w/v)
Assay	≥99.0%	—
Weight per ml	—	0.784–0.786 g
Distilling range	—	81°–83°
Water-soluble matter	—	+
Water	—	≤0.5% (w/v)

11. Typical Properties
Auto-ignition temp: 425°C in air
Boiling point: bp_{760}=82.4°C; change in bp=0.0333°C/mm
Dielectric constant: D^{20}=18.62
Explosive limits: Lower limit=2.5% v/v in air, upper limit=12.0% v/v in air
Flammability: Flammable
Flash point: Closed cup, 11.7°C; water azeotrope, 16.0°C
Freezing point: −89.5°C
Melting point: −88.5°C
Microbiological: Isopropyl alcohol is bactericidal. Bactericidal effects increase steadily as its concentration approaches 100% (Reference 2). Isopropyl alcohol should not be relied upon to destroy such spore-bearing organisms as *Clostridium tetani, Clostridium welchii* or *bacillus anthracis*.
Refractive index: n_D^{20}=1.37723; n_D^{25}=1.3749.
Solubility: Miscible with water, ethanol, benzene, chloroform, ether, and glycerin. Insoluble in salt solutions. Soluble in acetone. Forms an azeotrope with water (bp_{760}=80.37°C, d_4^{20}=0.8158; composition isopropyl alcohol 87.7% w/w, 91.3% v/v).
Specific gravity: 25°C/25°C=0.783–0.787, 0.78505^{20}_4, 0.78084^{25}_4, 0.72883^{4}.
Vapor density: 2.07
Vapor pressure: −26.1°C=1.0 mm Hg; 20°C=32.4 mm Hg; 24°C=40 mm Hg; 39.5°C=100 mm Hg
Water content: Commercial grades: 0.1% to 13% w/w (13% corresponds to the water azeotrope).

12. Stability and Storage Conditions
Store in a tight container, remote from heat and protected from light.

13. Incompatibilities
Oxidizing agents like hydrogen peroxide and nitric acid decompose isopropyl alcohol. It may be salted out from aqueous mixtures by the addition of sodium chloride, sodium sulfate and other salts, or by sodium hydroxide.

14. Safety
Isopropyl alcohol acts as a local irritant and, in high concentrations, as a narcotic. It is about twice as toxic as ethyl alcohol, and the symptoms of intoxication appear to be similar, except that isopropyl alcohol has no initial euphoric action, and gastritis and vomiting are more prominent. Humans have been injected with up to 20 ml diluted with water and noticed only a sensation of heat and a slight lowering of the blood pressure. There are, however, reports of serious illness from as little as 10 ml given internally. 100 ml can be fatal. The LD_{50} orally in rats is 5.8 g/kg. Isopropyl alcohol can cause corneal burns and often eye damage. It causes a mild irritation of the eyes, nose and throat at concentration levels of 400 ppm. It may induce a mild

narcosis, the effects of which are usually transient, and it is somewhat less toxic than the normal isomer, but is twice as volatile. It is not considered an important toxic hazard. There is some evidence that personnel can acquire a slight tolerance to this material, and single or repeated applications of it on the skin of rats, rabbits, dogs or human beings induces no untoward effects. It acts very much like ethanol in regard to its absorption, metabolism and elimination, but with a stronger narcotic action. Chronic injuries due to it have been detected in animals. The maximum concentration of isopropyl alcohol vapor for an eight-hour exposure for workers has been estimated at 200 ppm, although the threshold limit value as recommended by the American Conference of Government and Industrial Hygienists is 400 ppm in air. The time-weighted average for the threshold limit value and the short term exposure limit TLV as recommended by the Health and Safety Executive (UK) are 400 ppm (980 mg/m^3) and 500 ppm (1225 mg/m^3) respectively. It is readily absorbed from the gastrointestinal tract and persists in the circulation somewhat longer than ethyl alcohol. It is slowly absorbed through the intact skin. Some isopropyl alcohol is converted in the body to acetone, which is slowly excreted in the breath and urine. Acetone may be further oxidized to acetate, formate and carbon dioxide. Unchanged isopropyl alcohol and its glucuronide may be excreted in the urine, especially following large doses.

15. Handling Precautions

Protect from heat.

16. Regulatory Acceptance

USP XXI; BP 1980. Isopropyl alcohol has not been sanctioned for food products, except as stated in Federal Regulation 173.240, nor is it recommended for use in products intended for internal consumption.

17. Applications in Pharmaceutical Formulation or Technology

Isopropyl alcohol can be used for pre-operative skin cleansing and as a disinfectant. Other uses: Ingredient in lotions, but its marked degreasing properties may limit its usefulness in preparations used repeatedly. Solvent for film coating, cosmetics and perfumes. Satisfactory non-aqueous moistening agent for tablet granulation if the alcohol is subsequently evaporated.

18. Related Substances

1-Propanol; isopropyl rubbing alcohol

19. Comments

—

20. Specific References

1. W. R. Brode, *J. Phys. Chem.*, 30:61 (1926).
2. *J. Am. Med. Assoc.*, 128:986 (1945).
3. E. Browning, "Toxicity and Metabolism of Industrial Solvents, Elsevier, New York, 1965, pp. 335-341.
4. H. F. Smyth, Jr. and C. P. Carpenter, *J. Ind. Hyg. Toxicol.*, 30:63-68 (1948).
5. K. W. Nelson, J. F. Ege, Jr., M. Ross, L. E. Woodman and L. Silverman, *J. Ind. Hyg. Toxicol.*, 25:282-5 (1943); C.A. 39. 5001[4] (1945).
6. Guidance Note EH 15/78 from Health and Safety Executive, U.K. Threshold Limit Values for 1978.

USA: D. G. Pope*; J. Byrne**; S. C. Valvani**
UK: R. B. Forrester*

Isopropyl Myristate

1. Nonproprietary Name
NF: Isopropyl myristate
BP: Isopropyl myristate

2. Functional Categories
USP: Oleaginous vehicle
Others: Solvent, emollient

3. Synonym
Isopropyl ester of myristic acid

4. Chemical Names and CAS Registry Number
Tetradecanoic acid, 1-methylethyl ester [110-27-0]

5. Empirical Formula   Molecular Weight
$C_{17}H_{34}O_2$ 270.45

6. Structural Formula
$CH_3(CH_2)_{12}COOCH(CH_3)_2$

7. Commercial Availability
USA
Chemical Dynamics Corp.
Costec, Inc.
Croda, Inc.
Emery Industries
Fanning Corp., The
Gallard-Schlesginer Chemical Mfg. Corp.
Givaudan Corp.
Henkel Corp.
ICN K & K Labs, Inc.
Ingredients International, Inc.
Inolex Chemical Co.
Lanaetex Products, Inc.
Lipo Chemicals, Inc.
Pfaltz & Bauer, Inc.
Polyesther Corp.
Ruger Chemical Co.
Stepan Chemical Co.

UK
Fluorochem, Ltd.
R.W. Unwin and Co. Ltd.

8. Method of Manufacture
Isopropyl myristate is prepared by esterification of myristic acid with isopropyl alcohol.

9. Description
Transparent, colorless, almost odorless, mobile liquid with a bland taste. Consists of esters of isopropyl alcohol and saturated high molecular weight fatty acids, principally myristic acid.

10. Pharmacopeial Specifications

Test	NF	BP
Identification	+	+
Specific gravity	0.8460-0.854	—
Refractive index (20°C)	1.432 to 1.436	1.434 to 1.437
Residue on ignition	≤0.1%	—
Acid value	≤1	≤0.5%

Test	NF	BP
Saponification value	202-212	—
Iodine value	≤1	≤1.0
Assay	≥90%	—
Relative density	—	0.850-0.855
Related substances	—	+
Ester value	—	+

11. Typical Properties
Chemical: Resistant to oxidation and hydrolysis, and does not become rancid.
Flash point (closed cup): 153.5°C
Solidification point: Approximately 3°C
Boiling point: 140.2°C
Solubility: Miscible with liquid hydrocarbons, fixed oils, waxes, fats and fatty alcohols. Soluble 1 in 3 in 90% alcohol at 20°C. Insoluble in water, glycerin and propylene glycol.
Viscosity: 7 cps at 25°C

12. Stability and Storage Conditions
Store in a closed container at room temperature.

13. Incompatibilities
In contact with rubber, there is a drop in viscosity with concomitant swelling and partial dissolution of the rubber. With plastics, e.g., nylon and polyethylene, swelling is experienced. Incompatible with hard paraffin.

14. Safety
Acute toxicity studies indicate a very low order of toxicity; e.g., attempts to establish an LD_{50} in mice failed when dosages equivalent to 100 ml/kg did not affect the test animals. Isopropyl myristate shows a very low degree of irritability and exhibits no sensitizing properties in rabbits and guines pigs following topical and parenteral administration. It is better tolerated than sesame or olive oil.

15. Handling Precautions
Observe all normal hygienic procedures.

16. Regulatory Acceptance
NF XVI; BP 1980; BP 1983 addendum

17. Applications in Pharmaceutical Formulation or Technology
Isopropyl myristate may be used in external preparations in place of vegetable oils and in emollient ointments and creams, yielding products which are relatively free from greasiness. It is a solvent for many substances applied externally, and is of value as a vehicle when direct contact and penetration of the medication is required[3]. It is absorbed fairly readily by the skin.

18. Related Substances
—

19. Comments
—

20. Specific References
1. *Drug and Cosmetic 1982 Catalog*, Harcourt Brace Jovanovich, 1982, p. 116.
2. E. L. Platcow and E. Voss, *J. Am. Pharm. Assoc., Sci. Ed.,* 43: 690 (1954).
3. F. Brunner, *Pharm. Rundschau,* 7: 248 (1965).

USA: D. G. Pope*; J. B. Byrne**
UK: J. E. Jeffries**

Isopropyl Palmitate

1. Nonproprietary Name
NF: Isopropyl palmitate

2. Functional Category
NF: Oleaginous vehicle

3. Synonym
Isopropyl ester of palmitic acid

4. Chemical Name and CAS Registry Number
Hexadecanoic acid, 1-methylethyl ester [142-91-6]

5. Empirical Formula   Molecular Weight
$C_{19}H_{38}O_2$ 298.51

6. Structural Formula
$CH_3(CH_2)_{14}COOCH(CH_3)_2$

7. Commercial Availability
USA
Bage, Inc.
Costec, Inc.
Croda Chemicals, Inc.
Emery Industries
Fanning Corp., The
Gallard-Schlesinger Chemical Mfg. Corp.
Gross & Co., A., Millmaster Onyx Group, Kewanee Inds., Inc.
Henkel Corp.
Ingredients International, Inc.
Inolex Chemical Co.
Lanaetex Products, Inc.
Lipo Chemicals, Inc.
Pfaltz & Bauer, Inc.
Polyesther Corp.
Ruger Chemical Co.
Stepan Chemical Co.-Specialty Chemicals Dept.
Union Camp Corp., Terpene & Aromatics Div.
Wickhen Products, Inc.

UK
Bush, Boake, Allen Ltd.
Croda Chemicals Ltd.
Fluorchem Ltd.
RW Unwin & Co.

8. Method of Manufacture
Isopropyl palmitate is prepared by the esterification of palmitic acid with isopropyl alcohol.

9. Description
Colorless to very pale yellow, oily, practically odorless liquid. Isopropyl palmitate has a slightly higher viscosity and a higher freezing point than isopropyl myristate. If the product is stored below 15°C, it will solidify.

10. Pharmacopeial Specifications

Test	NF
Identification	+
Specific gravity	0.850-0.855
Refractive index	1.435-1.438
Residue on ignition	≤0.1%
Acid value	≤1.0
Iodine value	≤1.0
Saponification value	183-193
Assay	≥90.0%

11. Typical Properties
Chemical: Resistant to oxidation and hydrolysis and does not become rancid.
Solidification point: Approximately 15°C
Solubility: Soluble in anhydrous ethanol and isopropyl alcohol, acetone, ethyl acetate, mineral oil, silicone oils, vegetable oils, aliphatic and aromatic hydrocarbons. Insoluble in water, glycerols and glycols.
Viscosity: 7 cps at 25°C

12. Stability and Storage Conditions
Store in a tight, light-resistant container above 16°C.

13. Incompatibilities
Similar to those for isopropyl myristate.

14. Safety
Dermatologically innocuous.

15. Handling Precautions
Observe all normal hygienic procedures.

16. Regulatory Acceptance
NF XVI

17. Applications in Pharmaceutical Formulation or Technology
Isopropyl palmitate is used either alone or in combination with isopropyl myristate in many cosmetic products. Isopropyl palmitate imparts improved spreading properties.

18. Related Substances
—

19. Comments
—

20. Specific References
—

USA: D. G. Pope*; J. Byrne**

Kaolin

1. Nonproprietary Names

USP: Kaolin
BP: Light kaolin, light kaolin (natural)
BP/EP: Heavy kaolin

2. Functional Categories

USP: Tablet and/or capsule diluent
Others: Suspending agent

3. Synonyms

Kaolinite; kaolinum leve; kaolinum ponderosum; china clay; bolus alba; porcelain clay; white bole

4. Chemical Name and CAS Registry Number

Hydrated aluminum silicate [1332-58-7]

5. Empirical Formula   Molecular Weight

$Al_2H_4O_9Si_2$ 258.16

6. Structural Formula

$Al_2O_3.2SiO_2.2H_2O$

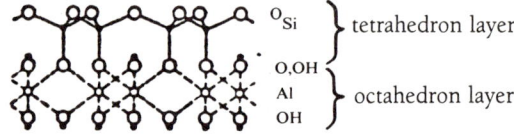

7. Commercial Availability

USA

Engelhard Minerals and Chemicals Corporation
Georgia Kaolin Company
J. T. Baker Chemical Company
Mallinckrodt, Incorporated
Thiele Kaolin Company

UK

Boots Ltd.
Chemical Exchange Ltd.
R. A. Watts Ltd.
Whitfield & Sons Ltd.

8. Method of Manufacture

Kaolin is a native hydrated aluminum silicate. Large deposits are mined in Georgia, U.S.A. and in Cornwall, England. It is powdered and freed of coarse, gritty particles by elutriation or by screening. Impurities such as ferric oxide, calcium carbonate and magnesium carbonate are removed with an electromagnet and by treatment with hydrochloric acid and/or sulfuric acid.

9. Description

White to greyish-white, unctuous powder free from gritty particles; characteristic earthy or clay-like taste and, when moistened with water, becomes darker and develops a clay-like odor.

SEM: KY-26
Excipient: Kaolin NF
Manufacturer: Georgia Kaolin Co. **Lot no.:** 1672

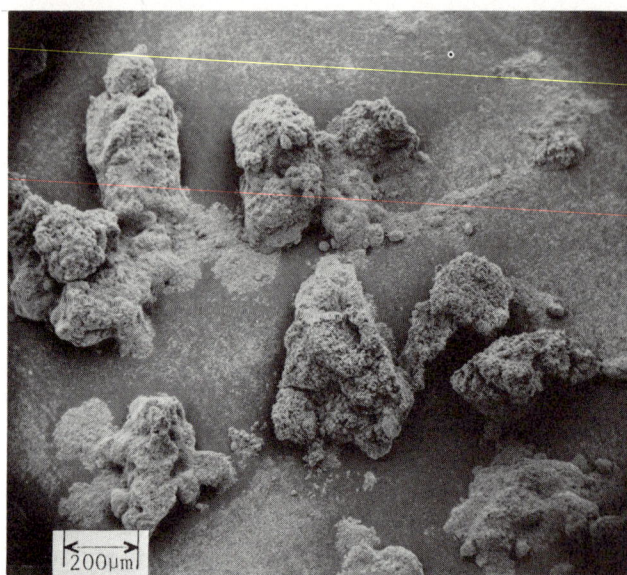

Magnification: 60×   **Voltage:** 10kV

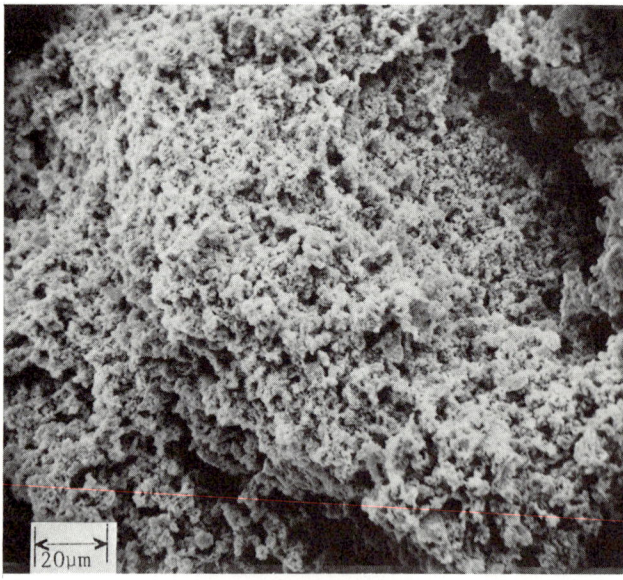

Magnification: 600×   **Voltage:** 10kV

10. Pharmacopeial Specifications

Test	USP	(Heavy Kaolin) BP/EP	(Light Kaolin) BP	(Light Kaolin) Natural BP
Identification	+	+	+	+
Acid-soluble substances	≤2.0%	≤1.0%	≤1.0%	≤1.0%
Loss on drying	—	—	≤1.5%	≤1.5%
Loss on ignition	≤15.0%	—	≤15.0%	≤15.0%
Lead	≤0.001%	—	—	—
Heavy metals	—	≤25 ppm	≤20 ppm	≤20 ppm

Pharmacopeial Specifications continued

Test	USP	(Heavy Kaolin) BP/EP	(Light Kaolin) BP	(Light Kaolin) Natural BP
Chloride	—	≤250 ppm	≤350 ppm	≤350 ppm
Arsenic	—	—	≤2 ppm	≤2 ppm
Iron	+	—	—	—
Calcium	—	≤250 ppm	—	—
Sulfate	—	≤0.1%	—	—
Carbonates	+	—	—	—
Coarse particles	—	—	≤0.5%	≤0.5%
Fine particles	—	—	+	+
Alkaline or acid impurities	—	+	—	—
Organic impurities	—	—	—	—
Adsorption power	—	+	—	—
Swelling power	—	1:1 triturate with water does not flow	—	—
Microbial limit test	Negative to *E. coli*	—	—	—
Readily carbonizable substances	—	+	—	—

11. Typical Properties

Abrasion index: Very low; 2 on Mohs' Hardness Scale.

Bacterial contamination: Unless sterilized, kaolin may be heavily contaminated with pathogenic micro-organisms, such as *Bacillus anthracis*, *Clostridium tetani* and *Clostridium welchii*.

Hygroscopicity: At relative humidities between about 15% and 65%, the equilibrium moisture content at 25°C is about 1%, but at relative humidities above about 75%, kaolin absorbs small amounts of moisture.

pH: 4.0-7.5 (20% aqueous slurry).

Particle size: Median: 0.6 to 0.8 μm.

Refractive index: 1.56

Solubility: Practically insoluble in water and organic solvents. Insoluble in mineral acids and solutions of alkali hydroxides.

Specific gravity: 2.6

Sterilization: Sterilized by maintaining the whole at a temperature not less than 160°C for not less than one hour.

Viscosity of suspension: 300 cps (70% solids, 10 rpm Brookfield viscometer).

Whiteness: 85% to 90% of the brightness of MgO.

12. Stability and Storage Conditions

Stable. Store in a well-closed container.

13. Incompatibilities

The absorbent properties of kaolin may influence the adsorption of other orally-administered drugs. Drugs reportedly affected by kaolin include cimetidine, lincomycin, tetracycline and digoxin. Warfarin adsorption by rat intestine *in vitro* was not affected by kaolin. With clindamycin, the rate (but not the amount) of absorption was affected by kaolin.

14. Safety

Disease of the lung due to chronic inhalation of kaolin dust (silicosis or kaolinosis) has been reported. Orally administered kaolin is harmless.

15. Handling Precautions

No restrictions specified.

16. Regulatory Acceptance

USP XXI; BP 1980

17. Applications in Pharmaceutical Formulation or Technology

Use	Concentration (%)
Adsorbent	7.5 to 55
Dusting powder	25
Poultice	53

18. Related Substances

Bentonite - A hydrated aluminum silicate used as a suspending agent. Talc - A hydrated magnesium silicate used as a dusting powder. Pumice - A complex aluminum potassium sodium silicate of volcanic origin used as a dental abrasive.

19. Comments

A distinction is made in *Chemical Abstracts* and in some other places between kaolin and kaolinite. Kaolin is the clay, presumably unprocessed, which historically was used in pharmaceuticals and in the manufacture of fine china dishes. Kaolin is in the general subject index of *Chemical Abstracts*, is given the empirical formula $AlHO_8Si_3K$ and has CAS registry number 1332-58-7.

Kaolinite is the processed mineral: it is the hydrated aluminum silicate. It is listed in the chemical subject index of *Chemical Abstracts*, is given the empirical formula $Al_2H_4O_9Si_2$ and has CAS registry number 1318-74-7.

Kaolin is listed as such in all the pharmacopeias. Kaolinite is what is available, and is used by the pharmaceutical industry. Kaolinite passes all the pharmacopeial specifications for kaolin. A typical chemical analysis follows:

Aluminum oxide	38.38%
Silicon dioxide (combined)	45.30%
Ignition loss at 950°C (combined water)	13.97%
Iron oxide	0.30%
Titanium dioxide	1.44%
Calcium oxide	0.05%
Magnesium oxide	0.25%

Sodium oxide	0.27%
Potassium oxide	0.04%

Authors in the scientific literature have not necessarily distinguished between kaolin and kaolinite.

20. Specific References

1. F. Ganjian, A.J. Cutie and T. Jachsberger, *In vitro* adsorption studies of cimetidine, *J. Pharm. Sci.*, 69: 352 (1980).
2. J.G. Wagner, Design and data analysis of biopharmaceutical studies in man, *Can. J. Pharm. Sci.*: 1: 55 (1966).
3. K.A. DeSante *et al*, The influence of kaopectate concentrate on tetracycline serum levels, *Academy of Pharmaceutical Sciences Abstracts*, 7: 116 (1977).
4. K.S. Albert *et al*, Influence of kaolin-pectin suspension on digoxin bioavailability, *J. Pharm. Sci.*, 67: 1582 (1978).
5. J.C. McElnay *et al*, The interaction of warfarin with antacid constituents in the gut, *Experientia*, 35: 1359 (1979).
6. K.S. Albert *et al*, Pharmacokinetic evaluation of a drug interaction between kaolin-pectin and clindamycin, *J. Pharm. Sci.*, 67: 1579, (1978).
7. M. Lesser *et al*, Silicosis in kaolin workers and firebrick makers," *South. Med. J.*, 71: 1242 (1978).
8. Technical Bulletin, "Hydrite Kaolinites," Georgia Kaolin Company.

USA: K. Wolter*; J. E. Carter*; A. L. Monaco**; J. Cooper**

Lactose

1. Nonproprietary Name
NF: Lactose
BP/EP: Lactose

2. Functional Category
USP: Tablet and/or capsule diluent

3. Synonyms
Milk sugar; *saccharum lactis*

4. Chemical Names and CAS Registry Number
4-O-β-D-galactopyranosyl-α-D-glucopyranose
4-(β-D-galactosido)-D-glucose
Anhydrous [63-42-3]
Monohydrate [64044-51-5]

5. Empirical Formula   Molecular Weight
$C_{12}H_{22}O_{11}$ (anhydrous)   342.30
$C_{12}H_{22}O_{11}H_2O$ (monohydrate) 360.31

6. Structural Formula

α - lactose   β - lactose

7. Commercial Availability
USA
Alba Chemical, Inc.
Bage, Inc.
Fallek Chemical Co.
Foremost Whey Products, Div. Wisconsin Dairies
Gallard-Schlesinger Chemical Mfg. Corp.
Ingredients International, Inc.
McKesson Chemical Co.
Pfaltz & Bauer, Inc.
Reisman Corp., H.
Robesco Chemicals, Inc.
Ruger Chemical Co.
Samrack Chemical
Sheffield Products
United States Biochemicals Corp.

UK
Becpharm, Ltd.
Dairy Crest
Hollandsche Melksuikerfabriek BV
Humko Products
K&K Greeff Chemicals, Ltd.
Meggle Milchindusrie veghel
Die Melkindustrie Veghel
National Co-operative Zinvelverkoopcentrale
Uromilk
Zimmermann Hobbs, Ltd.

8. Method of Manufacture
Obtained commercially from the whey of cows' milk. A number of distinct forms are produced by various crystalli-zation and drying processes. Forms can vary in their contents of crystalline and amorphous lactose, in the amounts of α and β lactose, and in their chemical state (hydrous or anhydrous). The most common form is α-lactose, but commercial grades of lactose do contain some β-lactose. β-lactose is obtained by crystallizing concentrated solutions of α-lactose at temperatures above 93.5°C.

9. Description
White to off-white or creamy-white crystalline particles or powder. Odorless; sweet-tasting. Lactose occurs in three forms: α-monohydrate (also known as ''α-lactose''); α-anhydrous; β-anhydrous (also known as ''β-lactose''). Lactose BP is described as the α-monohydrate. The NF refers to both the anhydrous and the monohydrate forms. Commercial lactose is mainly the α-monohydrate. Spray-dried lactose contains a proportion of amorphous material. β-lactose is more soluble and slightly sweeter than the α form, and is found only as the anhydrous form.

SEM:KY-27
Excipient: Lactose 80S
Supplier: Sheffield   **Lot no.:** 58A-12 (9 NK 18)

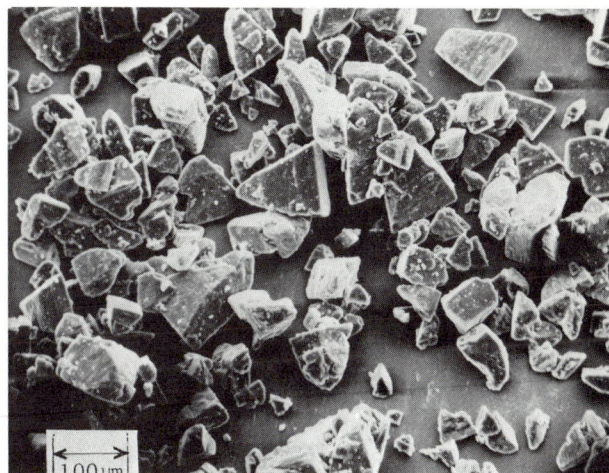

Magnification: 120× **Voltage:** 20kV

SEM:KY-28
Excipient: Lactose 60S
Supplier: Sheffield   **Lot no.:** 58A-13 (9 NJ 16)

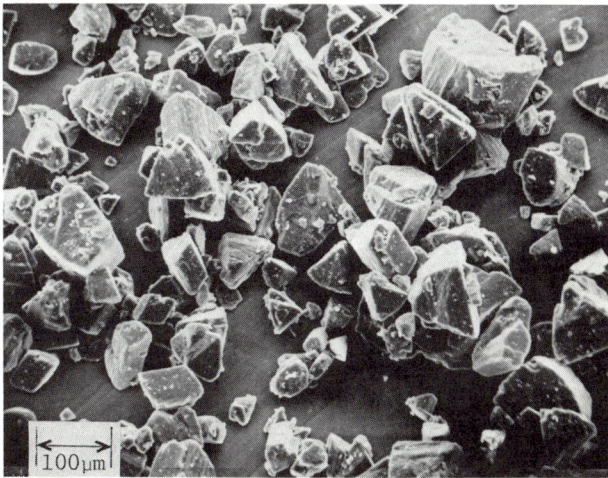

Magnification: 120× **Voltage:** 20kV

SEM:KY-29
Excipient: Lactose 80M
Supplier: Sheffield   **Lot no.:** 58A-11 (9 NL 18)

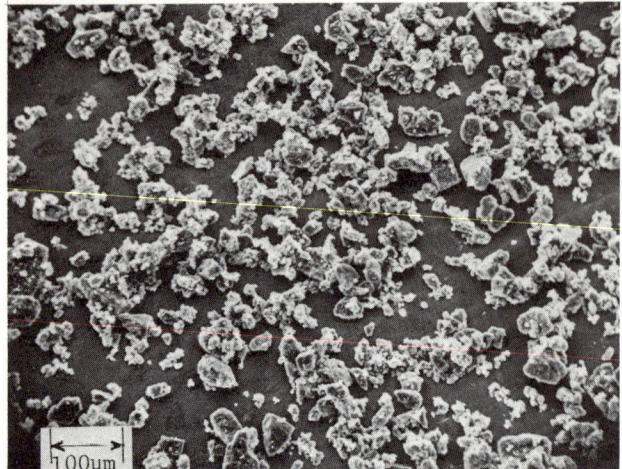

Magnification: 120× **Voltage:** 20kV

SEM:KY-30
Excipient: Lactose—capsule grade
Supplier: Sheffield   **Lot no.:** 58A-10 (9 NL 20)

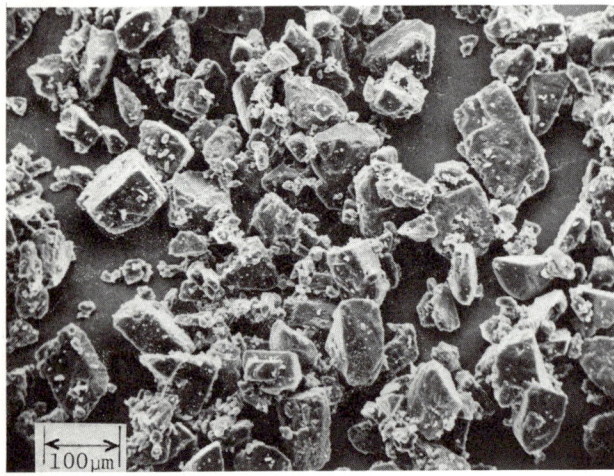

Magnification: 120× **Voltage:** 20kV

SEM:KY-31
Excipient: Lactose—anhydrous
Supplier: Sheffield   **Lot no.:** 58A-15 (0 NC 28)

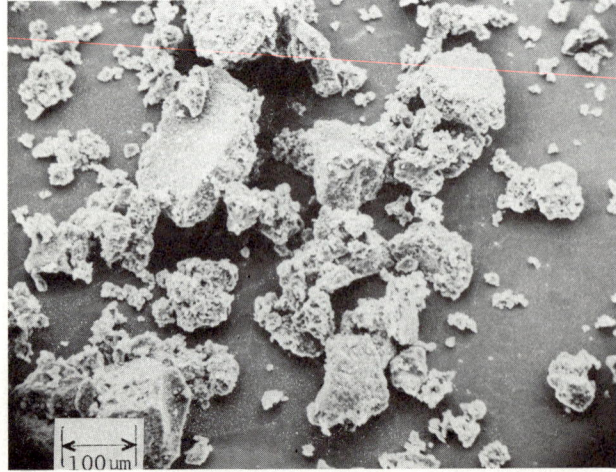

Magnification: 120× **Voltage:** 20kV

SEM:KY-32
Excipient: Lactose—impalpable
Supplier: Sheffield   **Lot no.:** 58A-14 (9 NH 22)

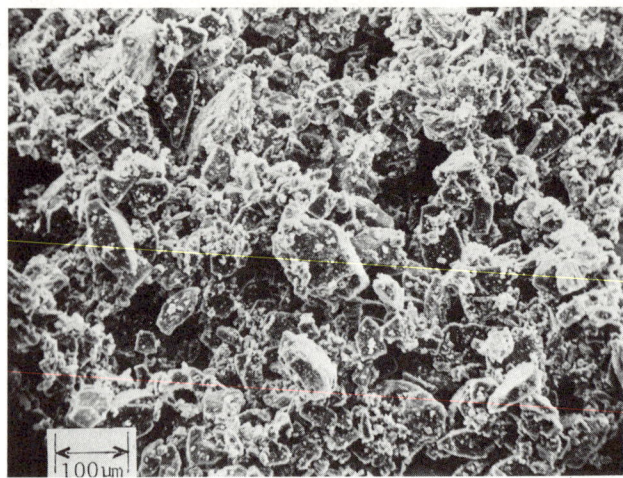

Magnification: 120× **Voltage:** 20kV

SEM-M-1
Excipient: Lactose D30
Supplier: Meggle

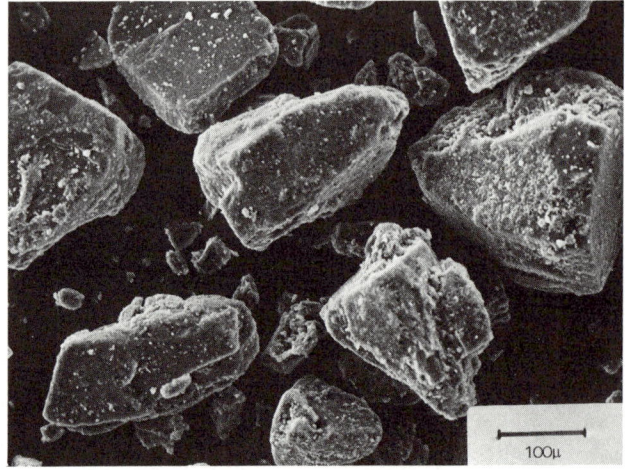

SEM-M-2
Excipient: Lactose G200
Supplier: Meggle

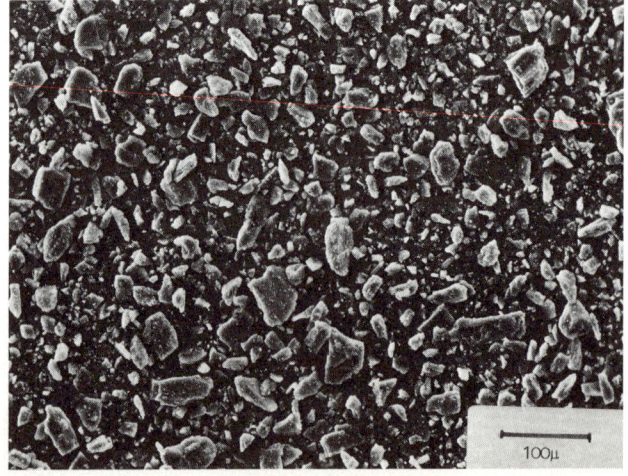

SEM-M-3
Excipient: Lactose—tabletto grade
Supplier: Meggle

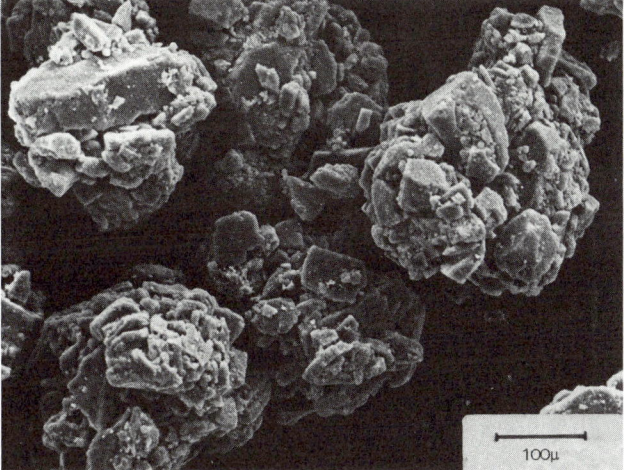

100μ

10. Pharmacopeial Specifications

Test	NF	BP/EP
Identification	+	+
Specific rotation	between +54.8° and +55.0° (calculated on anhydrous)	+52.2° to +°52.8° (monohydrate)
Microbial limits total bacterial count	≤100 per g	
Salmonella sp.	test negative	
Escherichia coli	test negative	
pH	4.0 - 6.5 (10% solution)	—
Water		
anhydrous	≤1.0%	—
monohydrate	≤5.5%	—
Residue on ignition	≤0.1%	—
Alcohol - soluble residue	≤20 mg/10 g	≤24 mg/5 g
Heavy metals	≤5 ppm	
Clarity and color solution	Solution of 3 g in 10 ml of boiling water is clear, colorless or nearly colorless, and odorless	Solution of 15 g in 50 ml of boiling water is clear, odorless, and colorless
Acidity or alkalinity	—	+
Arsenic	—	≤1 ppm
Lead	—	≤0.5 ppm
Sulphated ash	—	≤0.1%

11. Typical Properties

Density:
a) Particle   1.52 g/cm^3 (α-lactose monohydrate)
b) Bulk   1.77 g/cm^3 (anhydrous, Humko Sheffield)
               1.42 g/cm^3 (spray-dried, Die Melkindustrie Veghel)
c) Tapped   1.36 g/cm^3 (anhydrous, Humko Sheffield)
               1.12 g/cm^3 (spray-dried, Die Melkindustrie Veghel)

Hygroscopicity: Lactose monohydrate is only slightly influenced by atmospheric humidity at room temperature. Anhydrous lactose, however, becomes monohydrate at 70% relative humidity.

Melting point:
202°C α-monohydrate
223°C α-anhydrous
252°C β-anhydrous

Microbiological Contamination:
(Manufacturers' specifications)

	Dairy Crest	Foremost	Die Melkindustrie Veghel	Humko Sheffield
		(NF)	(NF)	(NF hydrous & anhydrous)
Standard plate count	≤500/g	≤100/g	≤50/g	20 typical
Coliform count	—	≤10g	—	Neg.
Molds /10 mg	≤50/g	—	≤5/g	Neg.
Yeasts/10 mg				
Escherichia coli	Neg. (in 0.1 g)	Neg.	Neg. (in 10 g)	—
Salmonella	—	Neg.	Neg. (in 100 g)	—

Moisture content: Anhydrous lactose normally contains ≤1% water, of which approximately 0.1 to 0.2% is adsorbed moisture. Lactose monohydrate contains approximately 5% water of crystallization, and approximately 0.1% of adsorbed water. Lactose monohydrate loses 75% of its water of crystallization at 103-105°C, and 100% at 120°C. Drying at 80°C removes the adsorbed water only.

Particle size analysis: Size distributions of commercially available grades of lactose are shown in *Table 1*.

Solubility:

Water	Cold	Boiling
(α-lactose monohydrate)	20g in 100ml	38.4g in 100ml
(β-lactose)	45g in 100ml	91g in 100ml

Soluble in ammonia and acetic acid. Slightly soluble in dilute alcohols. Insoluble in chloroform, ether and absolute alcohol.

Sweetness: α-lactose has about 15% the sweetness of sucrose; β-lactose is sweeter than the α form.

Table 1—Size distributions of commercial grades of lactose

Grade	Particle size (µm)	Fraction (%)
a. Die Melkindustrie Veghel		
Lactose NF:		
35/40 mesh	>400	> 90
	>600	< 10
45/50 mesh	>200	> 90
	>500	< 10
80 mesh	> 63	> 93
	>100	82 - 96
	>160	52 - 80
	>250	10 - 30
	>315	1.5 - 7
	>400	0
100 mesh	> 63	> 88
	>100	60 - 80
	>160	10 - 30
	>250	0 - 1
125 mesh	> 32	92 - 95
	> 45	75
	> 63	< 50
	>100	0.5
	>160	0 - 0.5
150 mesh	> 45	60 - 70
	> 63	35 - 40
	>100	12 - 18
	>160	2 - 4
	>250	0.2 - 0.5
	>315	0
200 mesh	> 45	40 - 50
	> 63	17 - 22
	>100	1 - 7
	>160	0 - 1
	>250	0
350 mesh	> 45	< 30
	> 63	< 15
	>100	< 4
	>160	< 0.5
b. Humko Sheffield Chemical		
Lactose NF monohydrate		
Grade 30 S	< 74	20 - 35
	74 - 177	5 - 20
	177 - 250	30 - 60
	>250	10 - 30
Grade 60S	< 74	15 - 35
	74 - 105	5 - 15
	105 - 149	22 - 45
	149 - 177	10 - 20
	177 - 250	10 - 25
	>250	0 - 3
Grade 80S	< 74	20 - 35
	74 - 105	10 - 20
	105 - 149	25 - 50
	149 - 177	10 - 25
	177 - 250	1 - 7
	>250	0 - 0.7
Grade 80M	< 74	65 - 90
	74 - 105	10 - 30
	105 - 149	2 - 5
	149 - 177	0.5 - 5
	>177	0 - 2

Grade		Particle size (µm)	Fraction (%)
Capsulating grade		< 74	55 - 70
		74 - 149	25 - 45
		149 - 177	1 - 8
		>177	0 - 1
Impalpable		< 74	> 90
		74 - 105	5 - 10
		105 - 149	1 - 3
		>149	0 - 1.5
Lactose NF anhydrous			
Direct tabletting		< 74	15 - 30
		74 - 105	6 - 20
		105 - 149	10 - 25
		149 - 177	7 - 15
		177 - 250	15 - 30
		>250	10 - 20
c. Meggle Milchindustrie GmbH			
Lactose NF monohydrate			
Tablettose (αlactose)		<630	100
d. Foremost Whey Products			
Lactose NF (αlactose monohydrate, 100% crystalline)			
Coarse granular	311	< 74	20 - 35
		>177	3 - 10
Regular	310	> 74	40 - 70
		>177	> 2
Impalpable	312	> 74	< 5
		>105	< 1
Impalpable	313	< 44	< 10
		> 74	< 1
Lactose NF (αlactose monohydrate and amorphous lactose)			
Spray process	315	< 74	< 60
		>105	0
		>595	0
"Fast-Flo" spray-dried	316	< 74	15 - 45
		>105	25 - 65
		>420	0
e. Dairy Crest			
Lactose BP: Crystalline 30 grade		< 75	10 - 20
		75 - 150	25 - 35
		150 - 250	30 - 50
		>250	5 - 15
50 grade		< 75	20 - 30
		75 - 150	40 - 55
		150 - 250	20 - 40
		>250	0 - 4
Powder regular grade		< 53	20 - 35
		53 - 90	25 - 35
		90 - 125	15 - 25
		125 - 212	15 - 30
		>212	0 - 5
120 grade		< 53	70 - 80
		53 - 90	15 - 30
		90 - 125	2 - 6
		125 - 212	1 - 2
		>212	0

Grade	Particle size (µm)	Fraction (%)
170 grade	< 53	93 - 96
	53 - 90	3 - 7
	90 - 125	1 - 2
	>125	0
350 grade	< 45	97 - 99
	45 - 90	1 - 3
	> 90	0
Spray-dried	< 53	20
	53 - 90	31
	90 - 125	26
	125 - 150	13
	150 - 212	9
	>212	1

f. B V Hollandsche Melksuikerfabriek

Pharmaceutically pure
Lactose

Crystalline coarse	<297	< 1
	297 - 475	5 - 15
	475 - 690	60 - 80
	>690	10
Fine	<177	< 5
	177 - 250	20 - 30
	250 - 420	55 - 75
	>420	5 - 10
Extra fine	< 74	20 - 30
	74 - 105	15 - 25
	105 - 149	25 - 35
	149 - 250	20 - 30
	>250	< 1
Powder coarse	< 74	25
	74 - 105	15
	105 - 177	30
	177 - 420	30
Fine	< 74	70
	74 - 149	25
	149 - 190	5
Impalpable	< 74	92
	> 74	8

Meggle Pharma-Lactose-Types
Quality covers all pharmaceutical Pharmacopeia

No.	Type	Mesh-size	Bulk density g/l	Tap density g/l
1	*Microtose*	400 mesh micronized	360	420
2	G 200	200 mesh impalpable special	500	590
3	D 80	200 mesh impalpable	500	590
4	G 100	100 mesh special fine	700	820
5	D 30	80 mesh fine	720	850
6	GK	80 mesh regular special	700	870
7	D 20	60 mesh coarse	600	720
8	D 10	40 mesh very coarse	540	600
9	*Tablettose*	special granulation for direct compression	550	630

Academy HPE Laboratory Project Data

	Method	Lab #	Results
Anhydrous[a]	BTD-5	6	B:0.570 g/cm³
			T:0.756 g/cm³
Impalpable[a]	BTD-5	6	B:0.485 g/cm³
			T:0.788 g/cm³
Impalpable 312[a]	BTD-8	36	B:0.476 g/cm³
Capsule grade	BTD-5	6	B:0.629 g/cm³
			T:0.876 g/cm³
Anhydrous[a]	BTD-6	8	Volume: 20.5%
Anhydrous[a]	BTD-6	8	Weight: 18.0%
Hydrous[a]	BTD-6	8	Volume: 20.0%
Hydrous[a]	BTD-6	8	Weight: 15.0%
Anhydrous[b]	BTD-8	36	B:0.493 g/cm³
			T:0.663 g/cm³
Coarse 311[c]	BTD-8	36	B:0.712 g/cm³
			T:0.841 g/cm³
Fast Flo 316[c]	BTD-8	36	B:0.691 g/cm³
			T:0.743 g/cm³
Impalpable 313[c]	BTD-8	36	B:0.438 g/cm³
			T:0.642 g/cm³
Regular 310[c]	BTD-8	36	B:0.677 g/cm³
			T:0.839 g/cm³
Spray process 315[c]	BTD-8	36	B:0.726 g/cm³
			T:0.782 g/cm³
60S	BTD-5	6	B:0.701 g/cm³
			T:0.904 g/cm³
80S	BTD-5	6	B:0.705 g/cm³
			T:0.896 g/cm³
80M	BTD-5	6	B:0.563 g/cm³
			T:0.922 g/cm³
Anhydrous[a]	DE-S4	36	1.4217
Anhydrous[a]	FLO-3	24	NO FLOW
Anhydrous[a]	FLO-1	14	NO FLOW
Fast Flo 316[c]	FLO-1	14	39g/sec.
Impalpable 312[c]	FLO-1	14	NO FLOW
Impalpable 313[c]	FLO-1	14	NO FLOW
Regular 310[c]	FLO-1	14	NO FLOW
Spray process 315[c]	FLO-1	14	41g/sec.
Anhydrous[a]	SI-1	13	Fig:13-SI-8
Capsule grade[a]	SI-1	13	Fig:13-SI-8
Anhydrous[b]	SI-1	13	Fig:13-SI-8
Coarse[c]	SDI-1	14	Fig:14-SDI-6
Fast Flo[c]	EMC-1	2	Fig:2-EMC-2,3,4,5
Hydrous[c]	SI-1	13	Fig:13-SI-8
Hydrous, fast-flow[c]	SDI-1	14	Fig:14-SDI-6
Hydrous, spray process[c]	SDI-1	14	Fig:14-SDI-6
Impalpable C[c]	SDI-1	14	Fig:14-SDI-6
Impalpable[c]	SDI-1	14	Fig:14-SDI-6
Regular[c]	SDI-1	14	Fig:14-SDI-6
Spray dried[c]	EMC-1	2	Fig:2-EMC-2,3,4,5
Anhydrous[d]	EMC-1	2	Fig:2-EMC-2,3,4,5
Anhydrous[d]	SDI-1	14	Fig:14-SDI-6
Monohydrate[e]	EMC-1	2	Fig:2-EMC-2,3,4,5
Anhydrous[a]	COM-7	12	Fig:12-COM-34
Anhydrous[a]	COM-3	20	Fig:20-COM-1
Anhydrous[b]	PSD-2	21	Fig:21-PSD-2
Fast Flo[c]	COM-4,5,6	29	Fig:29-COM-23
Hydrous[c]	COM-3	20	Fig:20-COM-2
Impalpable C[c]	COM-4,5,6	29	Fig:29-COM-22
Impalpable 312[c]	COM-4,5,6	29	Fig:29-COM-20
Spray process[c]	COM-3	20	Fig:20-COM-8
Spray process[c]	COM-4,5,6	29	Fig:29-COM-21
Anhydrous[e]	COM-2	21	Fig:21-COM-29

Academy HPE Laboratory Project Data

	Method	Lab #	Results
Spray dried[f]	COM-1	21	Fig:21-COM-30
Crystalline	COM-1	21	Fig:21-COM-28
Anhydrous[a]	PSD-2	5	152.0 μm
Anhydrous[b]	PSD-2	5	132.0 μm
Anhydrous[b]	PSD-5A	21	44 μm:64%
Anhydrous[b]	PSD-5A	21	44-74 μm:30%
Anhydrous[b]	PSD-5A	21	74-149 μm:6%
Hydrous[c]	PSD-2	5	76.0 μm
Regular[c]	PSD-7	24	38.5 μm
Spray process 315[a]	PF-1	36	0.018
Coarse 311[c]	PF-1	36	0.022
Fast Flo 316[c]	PF-1	36	0.000
Regular 310[c]	PF-1	36	0.026
Anhydrous[a]	MC-16	14	0.69%
Anhydrous[a]	MC-3	14	0.64%
Anhydrous[c]	MC-3	2	0.20%
Anhydrous, spray dried[c]	MC-20	2	0.20%
Coarse 311[c]	MC-3	25	5.18%
Coarse 311[c]	MC-16	14	5.09%
Coarse 311[c]	MC-3	14	5.10%
Fast Flo 316[c]	MC-16	14	5.10%
Fast Flo[c]	MC-20	2	0.20%
Hydrous, spray dried[c]	MC-16	14	5.30%
Hydrous, spray dried[c]	MC-3	14	5.01%
Impalpable 313[c]	MC-16	14	5.04%
Impalpable 313[c]	MC-3	14	5.12%
Regular[c]	MC-3	25	5.06%
Regular 310[c]	MC-16	14	5.13%
Regular 310[c]	MC-3	14	5.27%
Anhydrous[d]	MC-3	25	1.06%
Monohydrate[e]	MC-20	2	0.20%

Suppliers: Sheffield Products[a]; May and Baker[b]; Foremost McKesson[c]; Humko[d]; Mallinckrodt[e]; Tennants[f]

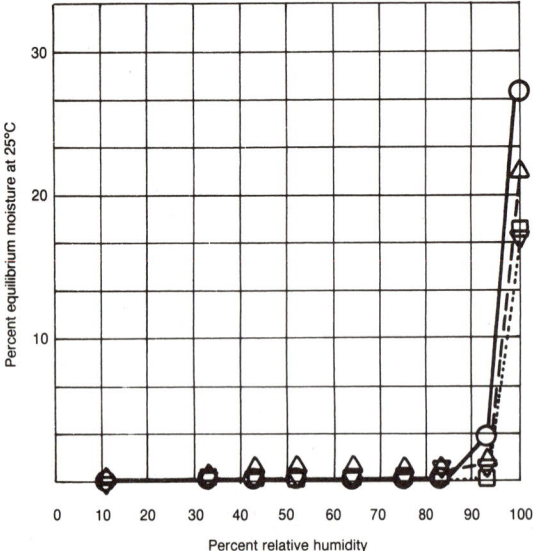

○: Lactose USP, anhydrous (Kraft-Humko, Lot #8NH22-211)
△: Lactose USP, spray dried (Foremost, Lot #56165)
▽: Lactose USP, beadlets (Fast-Flo), (Foremost, Lot #RB806)
□: Lactose USP, monohydrate (Mallinckrodt, Lot #B1523)
Figure: 2-EMC-2,3,4,5   **Method:** EMC-1

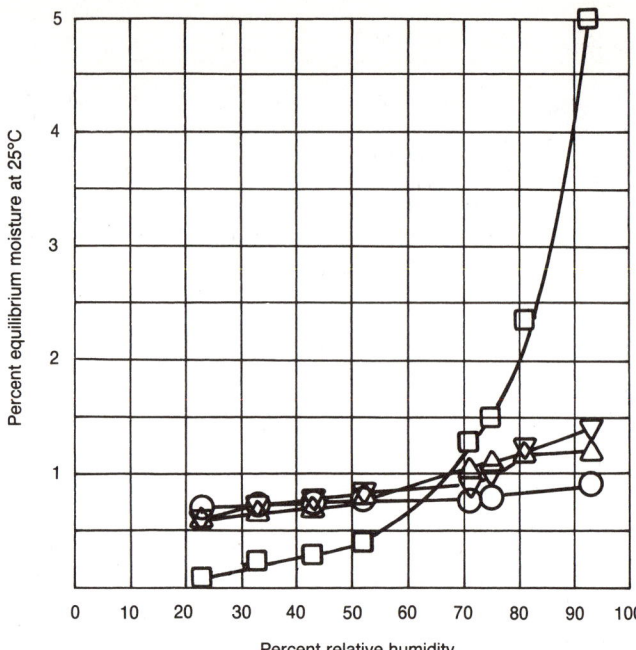

○: Lactose, hydrous (Foremost, Lot #SE812)
△: Lactose, capsule grade (Sheffield, Lot #9W18)
□: Lactose, anhydrous (Sheffield, Lot #7W 48-68)
▽: Lactose, anhydrous (May & Baker, Lot #0120)
Figure: 13-SI-8   **Method:** SI-1

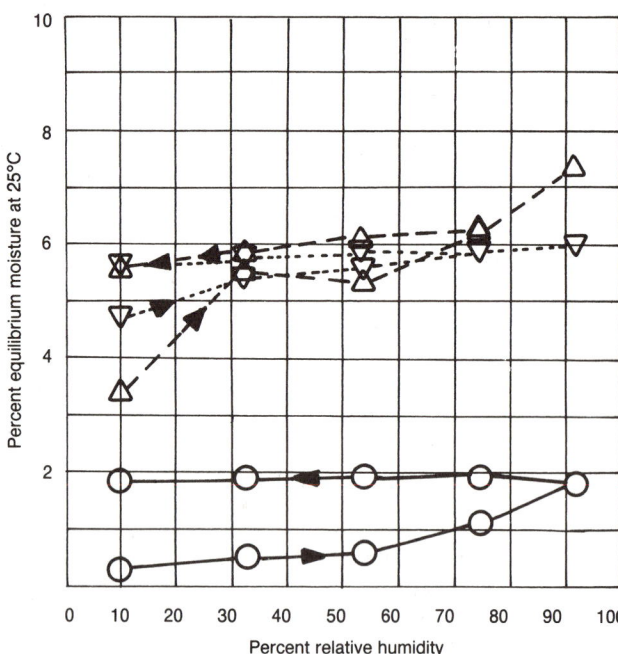

○: Lactose USP, anhydrous (Humco Sheffield, Lot #7N4868)
△: Lactose, spray process, hydrous (Foremost, Lot #RH914)
▽: Lactose USP, regular (Foremost, Lot #SF927)
The results of the following were similar to ▽:
   Lactose USP, Fast-Flo, hydrous (Foremost, Lot #RE917); Lactose USP, impalpable C (Foremost, Lot #SK819); Lactose USP, coarse (Foremost, Lot #SM828); Lactose USP, impalpable (Foremost, Lot #SM827).
Figure: 14-SDI-6   **Method:** SDI-1

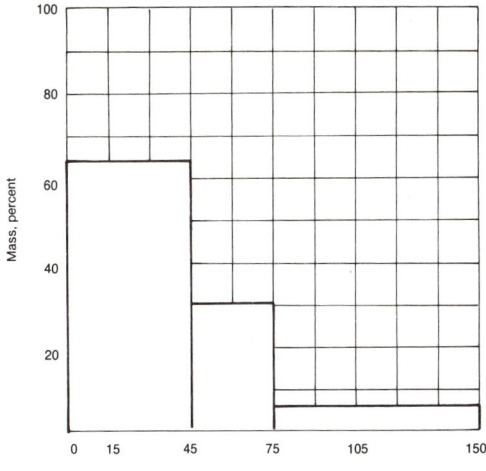

Lactose, USP, anhydrous (May & Baker, Canada, Lot #0120)
Figure: 21-PSD-2   **Method:** PSD-2

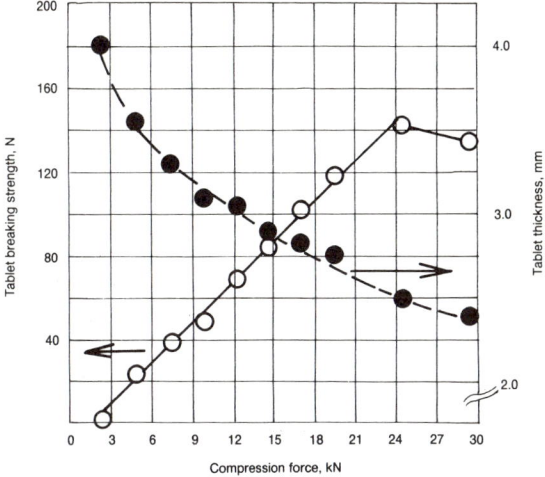

Lactose, powder, hydrous USP (Foremost, Lot #SE812)
Mean tablet weight: 488 mg
Minimum compressional force for compaction: 1.15 kN
Compressional force resulting in capping: 29.4 kN
Figure: 20-COM-2   **Method:** COM-3

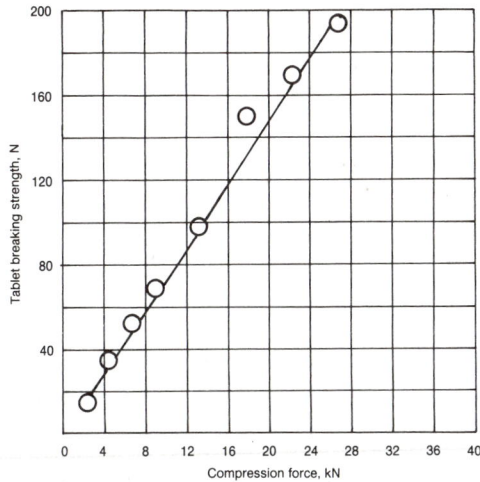

Lactose, anhydrous (Sheffield, Lot #ONC-28)
Tablet weight: 500 mg
Figure: 12-COM-34   **Method:** COM-7

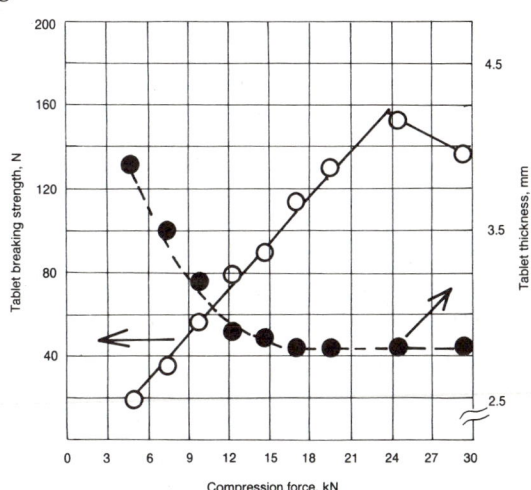

Lactose, spray process (Foremost, Lot #RL921)
Mean tablet weight: 511 mg
Minimum compressional force for compaction: 4.9 kN
Compressional force resulting in capping: 29.4 kN
Figure: 20-COM-8   **Method:** COM-3

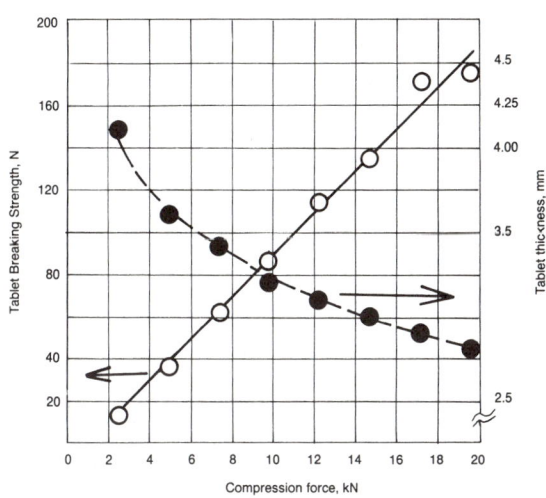

Lactose, anhydrous, USP (Sheffield, Lot #17N4868)
Mean tablet weight: 500 mg
Minimum compressional force for compaction: 0.77 kN
Compressional force resulting in capping: 29.4 kN
Figure: 20-COM-1   **Method:** COM-3

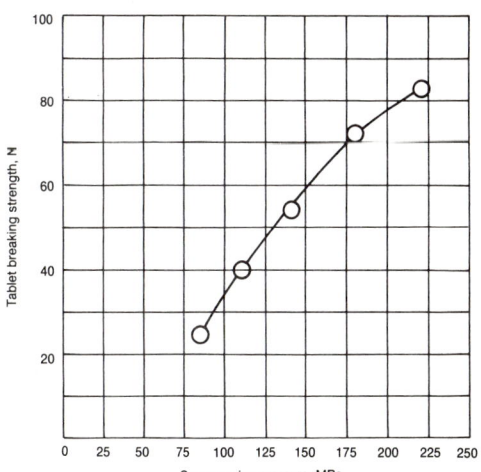

Lactose, crystalline (Condensfabrief, Holland, Lot #2498)
Weight range of tablets: 675–720 mg
Figure: 21-COM-28   **Method:** COM-1

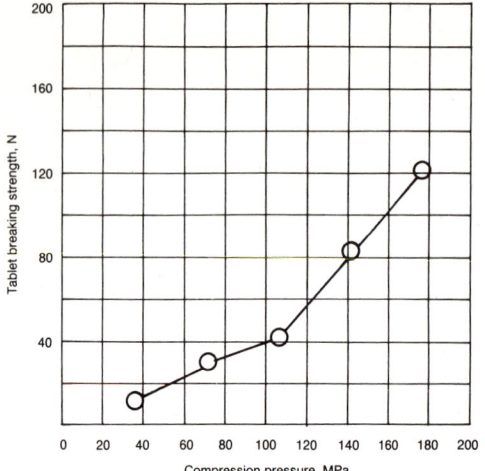

Lactose, anhydrous (Mallinckrodt, Canada, Lot #TFH204)
Tablet weight: 700 mg
Figure: 21-COM-29   **Method**: COM-2

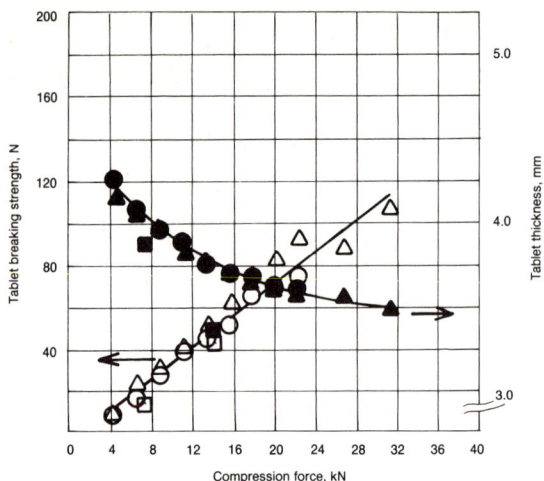

Lactose #312 impalpable USP (Foremost, Lot #SG-923)
○ ●: Unlubricated, Carver Laboratory Press (COM-5)
△ ▲: Lubricated, Carver Laboratory Press (COM-6)
□ ■: Lubricated, Instrumented Stokes Model F–single punch
   press (COM-4)
Figure: 29-COM-20   **Methods**: COM-4,5,6

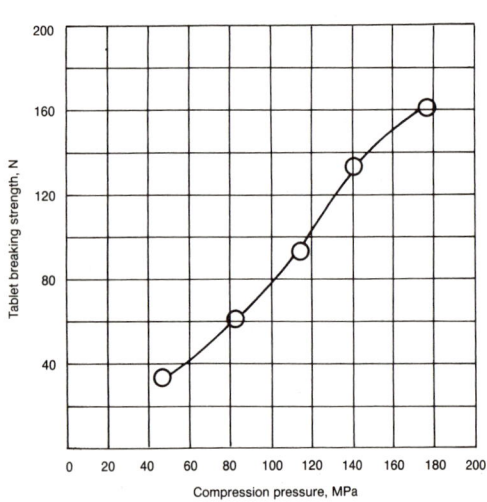

Spray dried lactose (Charles Tennant, Canada, Lot #RK720)
Weight range of tablets: 660–700 mg
Figure: 21-COM-30   **Method**: COM-1

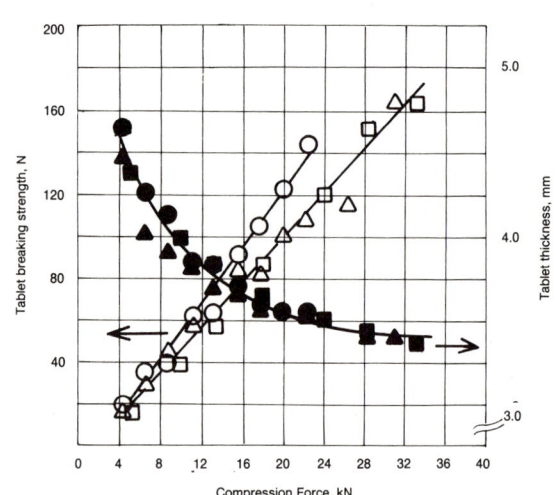

Lactose #315, spray process USP (Foremost, Lot #RH-914)
○ ●: Unlubricated, Carver Laboratory Press (COM-5)
△ ▲: Lubricated, Carver Laboratory Press (COM-6)
□ ■: Lubricated, Instrumented Stokes Model F–single punch
   press (COM-4)
Figure: 29-COM-21   **Methods**: COM-4,5,6

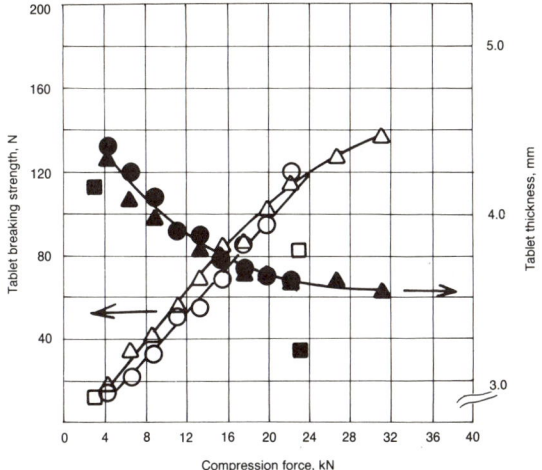

Lactose #313 impalpable C USP (Foremost, Lot #SL-924)
○ ●: Unlubricated, Carver Laboratory Press (COM-5)
△ ▲: Lubricated, Carver Laboratory Press (COM-6)
□ ■: Lubricated, Instrumented Stokes Model F–single punch press (COM-4)
Figure: 29-COM-22   Methods: COM-4,5,6

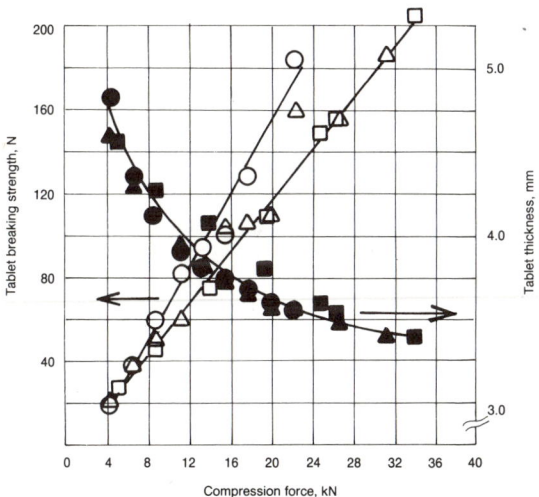

Lactose #316 Fast-Flo USP (Foremost, Lot #RK-923)
○ ●: Unlubricated, Carver Laboratory Press (COM-5)
△ ▲: Lubricated, Carver Laboratory Press (COM-6)
□ ■: Lubricated, Instrumented Stokes Model F–single punch press (COM-4)
Figure: 29-COM-23   Methods: COM-4,5,6

12. Stability and Storage Conditions

Store in a well-closed container to prevent absorption of moisture and of odors. Under humid conditions (80% RH and above), mold growth may occur.

Lactose may develop a brown coloration on storage (see also section 13). This reaction is accelerated by warm, damp conditions. Saturated solutions of β-lactose may precipitate crystals of α-lactose on standing. Shows mutarotation. Equilibrium mixture (containing 62% β-isomer and 38% α-isomer) obtained instantly on the addition of a trace of ammonia.

13. Incompatibilities

A Maillard-type condensation is likely to occur between lactose and compounds with a primary amino group (e.g., amphetamines and amino acids) to form brown-colored products. This reaction occurs more readily with amorphous than crystalline lactose, and the spray-dried material (which contains about 10% amorphous lactose) is more prone to discoloration. The "browning reaction" is base-catalyzed and may, therefore, be accelerated if alkaline lubricants are used. Lactose may also develop a yellow-brown color in the absence of amines (again, browning occurs most rapidly in spray-dried material, possibly due to the formation of 5-hydroxymethyl-2-furfural. Colored products are formed with arsenic-containing compounds and with glyceryl trinitrate.

14. Safety

Intolerance to lactose occurs in persons with a deficiency of intestinal lactase and may lead to abdominal cramps, diarrhea, distension and flatulence. In lactose-tolerant individuals, the enzyme lactase hydrolyzes lactose in the small intestine to glucose and galactose, which are then absorbed. It is not uncommon for humans to lose the ability to hydrolyze lactose as they mature. The incidence of adult lactase deficiency (hypolactasia) varies considerably among different populations. Northern and Central Europeans and the white populations of North America and Australia commonly show persistent lactase activity. Persistent lactase activity is rare or absent in Mongolian populations (including American Indians and Eskimos), in tropical Africa, in Melanesian peoples and in the Middle East. Between these 2 extremes, 30-70% of individuals of Southern European origin show persistent lactase activity.

In addition to variations in frequency of lactose intolerance among populations, variations in degree occur among individuals. Approximately 10-20% of lactose-intolerant individuals in two studies (8, 9) became symptomatic upon receiving only 3 to 5 g. of lactose. In one of these studies (8), 75% of the patients had symptoms with 12 gm. of lactose (equivalent to 8 ounces of milk). In the other study (9), 8 of 13 individuals developed diarrhea after the administration of 20 g. of lactose, and 9 out of 13 after the administration of 25 g. "Drug-induced diarrhea" due to lactose intolerance has been reported as a result of the lactose in pharmaceutical formulations.

15. Handling Precautions

No restrictions specified.

16. Regulatory Acceptance

NF XVI; BP/EP 1980

17. Applications in Pharmaceutical Formulation or Technology

Solid dosage forms. Diluent, bulking agent, filler and excipient for compressed and molded tablets and capsules (both oral and inhalation); an ingredient of infant foods, animal feed products and powders presented in sachets. Direct-compression grades of lactose (particularly certain spray-dried lactoses and anhydrous lactose) are also commonly used in tablets. These grades are more fluid and more compressible than crystalline or powdered lactose. Compressibility depends on the method of crystallization and ratio of amorphous/crystalline forms. They may be combined with microcrystalline cellulose or starch, and usually require a tablet lubricant. Concentrations of lactose generally used in these formulations are from 65 to 85%.

A range of mesh sizes is available for special application in encapsulating mixtures or as a tablet diluent. The particle size range selected for capsules is often dependent upon the type of encapsulating machine used. Usually, finer sizes are used in the preparation of tablets by the wet granulation method or when milling during processing is carried out. *Film-coating.* Can be used to modify the properties of non-disintegrating polymers in film coatings. *Lyophilized products.* Added to freeze-dried solutions to increase plug size and aid caking. *Sugar coating.* Lactose is used in combination with sucrose (approx. 1:3) for sugar-coating solutions.

18. Related Substances

None

19. Comments

Some manufacturers include limits for fat and protein content of their products. Lactose is described in the Pharmacopeias of the following countries: Argentina, Austria, Belgium, Brazil, Chile, China, Czechoslovakia, France, West Germany, Hungary, India, Italy, Japan, Yugoslavia, Mexico, the Netherlands, Nordic countries, Poland, Portugal, Rumania, Spain, Switzerland and USSR.

20. Specific References

1. N. H. Batuyios, Anhydrous lactose for direct compression, *J. Pharm. Sci.*, 55: 727 (1966).
2. J. T. Fell and J. M. Newton, The characterization of the form of lactose in spray dried lactose, *Pharm. Acta Helv.*, 45: 520 (1970).
3. J. T. Fell and J. M. Newton, The production and properties of spray dried lactose, *Pharm. Acta Helv.*, 46: 226 and 425 (1971).
4. O. Alpar, J. A. Hersey, and E. Shotton, The compression properties of lactose, *J. Pharm. Pharmacol.*, 22: 15 (1970).
5. S. M. Blaug and W. Huang, Interaction of dextroamphetamine sulphate with spray dried lactose, *J. Pharm. Sci.*, 61: 1770 (1972).
6. G. K. Bolhuis and C. I. Lerk, Comparative evaluation of excipients for direct compression, *Pharm. Weekbld.*, 108: 469 (1973).
7. C. F. Lerk, G. K. Bolhuis and A. M. DeBoer, Comparative evaluation of excipients for direct compression, *Pharm. Weekbld.*, 109: 945 (1974).
8. M. S. Bedine and T. M. Bayless, Intolerance of small amounts of lactose by individuals with low lactase levels, *Gastroenterology*, 65: 735 (1973).
9. E. Gudmand-Hyer and K. Simong, Individual sensitivity to lactose in lactose malabsorption, *Am. J. Dig. Dis.*, 22: 177 (1977).
10. Technical Report: Lactose (Saccharum Lactis) hydrous, pharmaceutically pure, B.V. Hollandsche Melsuikerfabriek, Uitgeest, Holland (1975).
11. Booklet: Lactose, physical and chemical properties, Foremost Foods Company.
12. Brochure: Lactose USP Fast-Flo®, Foremost Foods Company.
13. Technical Data: Lactose USP Hydrous, Humko Sheffield Chemical.
14. Technical Data: Lactose USP Anhydrous—Direct Tableting, Humko Sheffield Chemical.
15. R. W. Chilankurti, C. T. Rhodes and J. B. Schwartz, Some studies on compression properties of tablet matrices using a computerized instrumented press, *Drug Devel. & Ind. Pharm.*, 8:(1), 63-86 (1982).
16. A. M. Molokhia, M. A. Moustafa and M. W. Gouda, Effect of storage conditions on the hardness, disintegration and drug release from some tablet bases, *Drug Devel. & Ind. Pharm.*, 8:(1), 63-86 (1982).
17. N. Kitamori and T. Makino, Improvement in pressure-dependent dissolution of trepibutone tablets by using intragranular disintegrants, *Drug Devel. & Ind. Pharm.*, 8:(1), 125-139 (1982).
18. Z. T. Chowan, A. A. Amaro and Y. P. Chow, Tablet-to-tablet dissolution variability and its relationship to the homogeneity of a water-soluble drug, *Drug Devel. and Ind. Pharm.*, 8:(2), 145-168 (1982).

USA: F. Goodhart*; K. R. Middleton**; Z. Chowhan**
UK: T. M. Jones*

Lanolin

1. Nonproprietary Names
USP: Lanolin
BP/EP: Hydrous wool fat

2. Functional Category
USP: Ointment base

3. Synonym
Hydrous lanolin

4. Chemical Name and CAS Registry Number
Lanolin [8020–84–6]

5. Empirical Formula   Molecular Weight
—   —

6. Structural Formula
—

7. Commercial Availability
USA
Amerchol Corp.
Emery Industries, Inc.
R. W. Greeff & Co., Inc.
Lanaetex Products, Inc.
Maybrook, Inc.
Rita Corp.
Robinson Wagner Co., Inc.
Arthur C. Trask Corp.

UK
Croda Chemicals, Ltd.
Charles Page & Co., Ltd.
Westbrook Lanolin Co.

8. Method of Manufacture
Anhydrous lanolin is melted, and sufficient purified water is added gradually with constant stirring.

9. Description
A yellowish-white, sticky, unctuous substance with a faint characteristic odor.

10. Pharmacopeial Specifications

Test	USP	BP
Identification	—	+
Acidity	+	—
Acid value	—	≤0.8
Alkalinity	+	—
Melting point	—	38°–44° C
Water content	25–30%	—
Peroxide value	—	≤15
Ammonia	+	—
Saponification value	—	67–79
Petrolatum	+	—
Water absorption capacity (in 10 g)	—	≥20 ml
Iodine value	18–36	—
Paraffins (in 3.0 g)	—	≤30 mg
Chloride	≤0.035%	≤115 ppm
Water-soluble oxidizable substances	—	+
Water-soluble acids and alkalis	+	+
Butylated hydroxytoluene	—	≤150 ppm
Non-volatile matter	—	72.5–77.5%
Sulfated ash	—	≤0.15%

11. Typical Properties
Solubility: Insoluble in water, chloroform and ether; only fat content dissolves. About equal weight of water may be incorporated in hydrous wool fat without affecting its consistency.

12. Stability and Storage Conditions
USP: Store in a tightly-sealed, preferably rustproof, container at controlled room temperature. BP: Store in a well-closed container at 25° C or below.

13. Incompatibilities
See lanolin anhydrous.

14. Safety
See lanolin anhydrous.

15. Handling Precautions
No restrictions specified.

16. Regulatory Acceptance
USP XXI; BP/EP 1980, Addendum 1983

17. Applications in Pharmaceutical Formulation or Technology
See lanolin anhydrous

18. Related Substances
Lanolin anhydrous, USP; wool alcohols, BP; wool fat, BP.

19. Comments
See lanolin anhydrous

20. References
See lanolin anhydrous

USA: N. L. Henderson*, J. Cooper**
UK: S. S. Davis*

Lanolin Alcohols

1. Nonproprietary Names
NF: Lanolin alcohols
BP: Wool alcohols

2. Functional Category
NF: Emulsifying and/or solubilizing agent

3. Synonym
Wool wax alcohols

4. Chemical Name and CAS Registry Number
Lanolin alcohol is a crude mixture of steroids and triterpene alcohols, including 28-34% cholesterol and 10-13% iso-cholesterol. Lanolin alcohol also contains 500-1,000 ppm of antioxidant, either butylated hydroxyanisole or butylated hydroxytoluene.

5. Empirical Formula
—

6. Structural Formula
—

7. Commercial Availability
USA
Amerchol Corp.
Croda, Inc.
Emery Industries
UK
Croda Chemicals, Ltd.
P. F. Anstead
Westbrook Lanolin Co.

8. Method of Manufacture
Lanolin alcohols are prepared by the saponification of the wool grease of sheep and subsequent separation of the fraction containing cholesterol and other alcohols.

9. Description
Golden-brown solid, plastic when warm, but brittle when cold; faint characteristic odor.

10. Pharmacopeial Specifications

Test	NF	BP
Identification	+	+
Melting range	$\geq 56°C$	$\geq 58°C$
Acidity and alkalinity	+	—
Loss on drying	$\leq 0.5\%$	$\leq 0.5\%$
Residue on ignition	$\leq 0.15\%$	$\leq 0.5\%$
Copper	≤ 5 ppm	≤ 10 ppm
Acid value	≤ 2.0	≤ 2.0
Saponification value	+	≤ 12
Soap: mineral acid	—	+
Sulfated ash	—	≤ 0.15

Test	NF	BP
Assay: cholesterol	$\geq 30.0\%$	≥ 30.0
Assay: suitable anti-oxidant	$\leq 0.1\%$	—
Assay: butylated hydroxyanisole or butylated hydroxytoluene	—	500-1,000 ppm

11. Typical Properties
Solubility: Practically insoluble in water; very slightly soluble in alcohol; completely soluble in 25 parts of boiling dehydrated alcohol; soluble in ether, chloroform and light petroleum.

12. Stability and Storage Conditions
Store in a well-closed, light-resistant container at controlled room temperature (approximately 20-25°C). There is a risk of gradual autoxidation during storage.

13. Incompatibilities
Incompatible with 1% phenol, 5% ichthamol and 1% coal tar. Separation occurred in 2 weeks with 1% ichthammol and 5-10% resorcinol.

14. Safety
Sensitization may occur in some individuals. Patients suspected to be allergic to lanolin should be patch tested against lanolin alcohols.

15. Handling Precautions
Lanolin alcohols sometimes have a slight irritant action, and in rare instances may give rise to a bullous eruption. Occasional cases of skin sensitivity have occurred.

16. Regulatory Acceptance
NF XVI; BP 1980

17. Applications in Pharmaceutical Formulation or Technology
Used as a hydrophobic vehicle and in the preparation of water-in-oil creams. The proportion of water that can be incorporated in soft paraffin is increased three-fold by the addition of 5% lanolin alcohols. Such emulsions do not crack upon the addition of citric, lactic or tartaric acid.

18. Related Substances
Cetyl alcohol, stearyl alcohol and hexadecyl alcohol

19. Comments
Water-in-oil emulsions prepared with lanolin alcohols, unlike those made with anhydrous lanolin, do not show surface darkening, nor do they develop an objectionable odor in hot weather.

20. Specific References
—

USA: J. Cooper*; Z. Chowhan**
UK: S. S. Davis*

Lecithin

1. Nonproprietary Name
NF: Lecithin

2. Functional Categories
USP: Emulsifying and/or solubilizing agent.
Others: wetting and dispersing agent; emollient; digestible surfactant; moisturizer

3. Synonyms
Soybean phospholipids; mixed soybean phosphatides; soybean lecithin; vegetable lecithin; egg lecithin; ovolecithin.

4. Chemical Name and CAS Registry Number
Phosphatidylcholine—commercially, a mixture of phosphatidylcholine, phosphatidylethanolamine, phosphatidylinositol, phytoglycolipids, other phosphatides, carbohydrates, triglycerides and other components. [8002-43-S]

5. Empirical Formula   Molecular Weight
—   —

6. Structural Formula

$$CH_2OCOR$$
$$CHOCOR \quad O^-$$
$$CH_2O—P—OCH_2CH_2\overset{+}{N}(CH_3)_3$$
$$O$$

α—phosphatidylcholine β—phosphatidylcholine

7. Commercial Availability
USA

American Lecithin
Central Soya Co.
Spencer-Kellogg

UK

Alembic (Lovelock) Products
Steetley Chemicals, Ltd.

8. Method of Manufacture
Crude soybean lipids are obtained by the solvent extraction of soybeans. Lecithin is obtained as a water extract of these crude soybean lipids. This crude lecithin is then upgraded by various techniques. Lecithin can also be made from corn, peanut, cottonseed, castor seed and coffee beans. It has been made from egg, known as egg lecithin. Synthetic lecithins are also made.

9. Description
Lecithin is brown to light yellow, depending on whether it is unbleached or bleached. It has practically no odor and a bland to nut-like taste, similar to soybean oil. In consistency, it may vary from plastic to fluid depending on the free fatty acid content.

10. Pharmacopeial Specifications

Test	NF
Water (method I)	≤1.5%
Arsenic	≤3 ppm
Lead	≤0.001%
Heavy metals (method II)	≤0.004%
Acid value	≤36
Hexane-insoluble matter	≤0.3%
Acetane-insoluble matter	≤50.0%

11. Typical Properties
Isoelectric point: Approximately 3.5
Miscibility: When mixed with water, lecithin hydrates to form an emulsion. It readily forms imbibitions (taking up liquid without a measurable increase in volume) with almost any solvent.
pH: Approx. 6.6 (soybean phosphatides)
Solubility: Soluble in aliphatic and aromatic hydrocarbons, halogenated hydrocarbons, mineral oil and fatty acid. Insoluble in polar solvents and water. Practically insoluble in cold vegetable and animal oils.
Physical form: Liquid or granule (oil-free lecithin)
Density: Liquid lecithin, 0.97 g/cm^3; granule lecithin, 0.5 g/cm^3
Iodine value: Liquid lecithin, 95-100; granule lecithin, 82-88
Saponification value: 196

12. Stability and Storage Conditions
Fluid lecithin grades should be stored at room temperature or above (22°-49°C) in well-closed containers. Temperatures of 160-180°C will cause degradation within 24 hours. Temperatures below 10°C may cause separation. Lecithins are hygroscopic; keep containers closed to prevent moisture pickup. Lecithin is subject to microbial degradation. Exposure to light should be avoided. A shelf life of several years can be expected when stored at ambient temperatures.

13. Incompatibilities
Lecithin decomposes at extreme pH. When heated, it oxidizes, darkens and decomposes. It is hydrolyzed by esterases.

14. Safety
Lecithin is recognized as a multiple purpose food substance by the FDA.

15. Handling Precautions
—

16. Regulatory Status
NF XVI

17. Applications in Pharmaceutical Formulation or Technology
Lecithins are used as dispersing and emulsifying agents for intramuscular injections. They are used in creams and ointments as dispersing, wetting, emulsifying and emollient agents.

18. Related Substances
—

19. Comments
Since lecithin contains a variety of unspecified materials, care should be exercised in the use of unpurified lecithin in injectable or topical dosage forms, as interaction with the active ingredient or formulation excipients may occur.

20. Specific References
1. P. Sartoretto, Lecithin. In "Encyclopedia of Chemical Technology," 2nd Ed., Kirk & Othmer eds., Vol. 12, John Wiley and Sons, Inc., 1967, New York, p. 343.
2. G. B. Ansell and J. N. Hawthorne, "Phospholipids," Elsevier, New York, 1964.

USA: W. Han*; A. Palmieri**; A. L. Monaco**

Magnesium Aluminum Silicate

1. Nonproprietary Name

NF: Magnesium aluminum silicate
BP: Aluminum magnesium silicate

2. Functional Categories

NF: Suspending and/or viscosity-increasing agent
BP: Pharmaceutical aid
Others: Thickening agent; binder; disintegrant; emulsion stabilizer; adsorbent; thixotropic agent

3. Synonyms

Magnesium aluminum silicate, colloidal; Magnesium aluminum silicate, complex colloidal; *Veegum*

4. Chemical Names and CAS Registry Number

Magnesium aluminum silicate [1327-43-1]
Aluminum magnesium silicate [12511-31-8]

5. Empirical Formula

A polymeric complex of Mg, Al, Si and O (OH).
The average chemical analysis is conventionally expressed as oxides:

Silicon dioxide	61.1%
Magnesium oxide	13.7%
Aluminum oxide	9.3%
Titanium dioxide	0.1%
Ferric oxide	0.9%
Calcium oxide	2.7%
Sodium oxide	2.9%
Potassium oxide	0.3%
Carbon dioxide	1.8%
Water of combination	7.2%

6. Structural Formula

The complex is composed of a three-lattice layer of octahedral alumina and two tetrahedral silica sheets. The aluminum is substituted to varying degrees by Mg (with Na or K for balance of electrical charge).
Additional elements present in small amounts include Fe, Li, Ti, Ca and C.

7. Commercial Availability

USA
Engelhard Minerals & Chemicals Corp.
Georgia Kaolin Company
R. T. Vanderbilt Co., Inc.

UK
K&K Greeff Chemicals, Ltd.

8. Method of Manufacture

Magnesium aluminum silicate is obtained from silicate ores of the montmorillonite group which show high magnesium content. The ore is blended with water to form a slurry to remove impurities and separate out the colloidal fraction. The refined colloidal dispersion is drum-dried to form a small flake. The flake is then micro-atomized to form various powder grades.

9. Description

Off-white to creamy white, odorless, tasteless, soft, slippery small flakes or fine (micronized) powder. Flakes vary in shape and size from about 0.3 by 0.4 mm to 1.0 by 2.0 mm and from about 25 to 240 μm thick. Many flakes are perforated by scattered circular holes ranging from 20 to 120 μm in diameter. Under dark field polarized light, innumerable bright specks are observed scattered over the flakes. Powder varies from 50 to 325 mesh.

SEM:KY-33
Excipient: Magnesium aluminum silicate (*Veegum*)
Manufacturer: R. T. Vanderbilt   **Lot number:** 61A-1

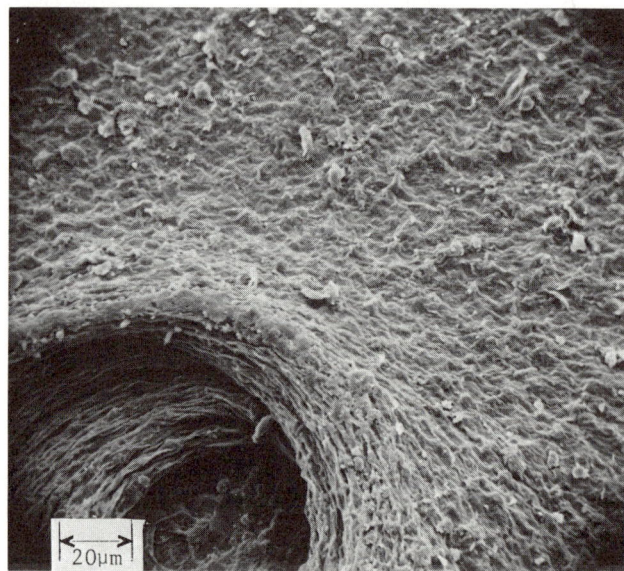

Magnification: 600×   **Voltage:** 10 kV

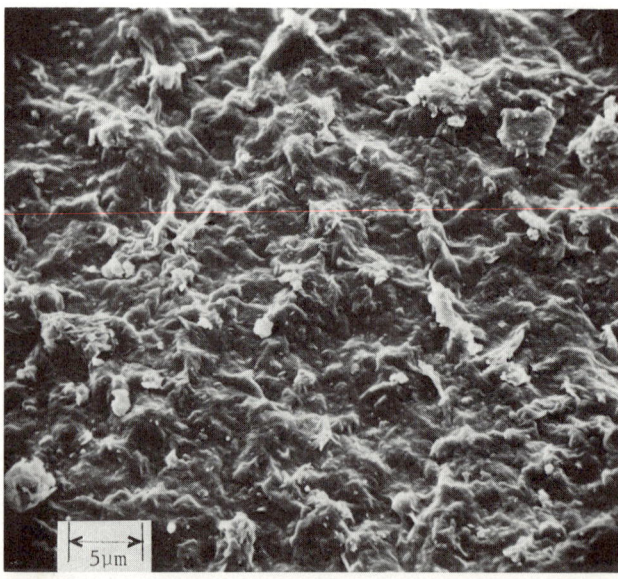

Magnification: 2400×   **Voltage:** 10 kV

SEM:KY-34
Excipient: Magnesium aluminum silicate (*Veegum F*)
Manufacturer: R. T. Vanderbilt **Lot number:** 61A-2

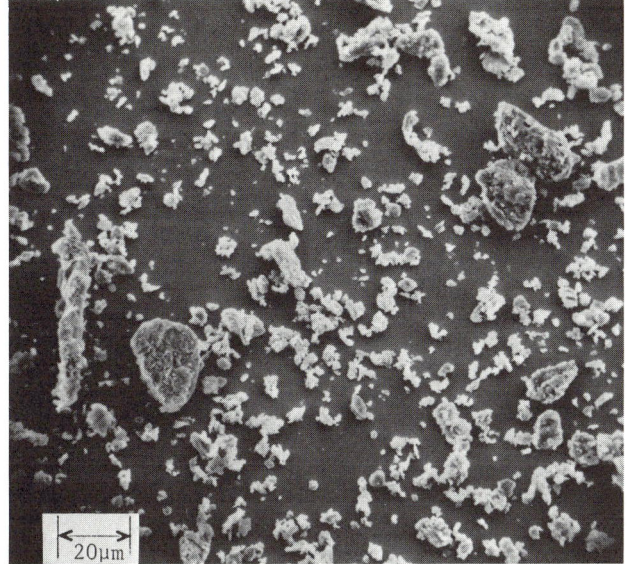

| 20μm |

Magnification: 600× **Voltage:** 10 kV

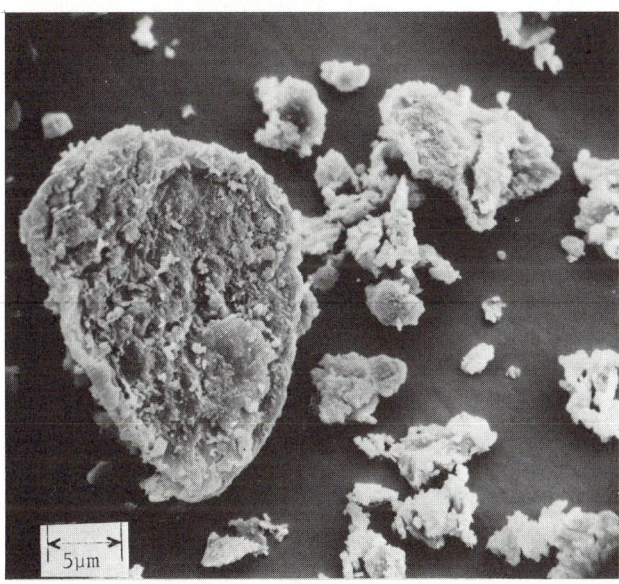

| 5μm |

Magnification: 2400× **Voltage:** 10 kV

10. Pharmacopeial Specifications

	NF	BP	
Identification	—	+	
Alkalinity	—	+	
Arsenic	≤ 3 ppm	—	
Loss on drying	≤ 8.0%	≤ 10.0%	
Loss on ignition	—	≤ 17.0%	
Viscosity	+	—	
Microbial limits			
Total aerobic count	≤ 1000 per g	—	
E. coli	Absent	—	
pH (5 in 100			
suspension)	9.0–10.0	—	
Acid demand	+	—	
Lead	≤ 0.0015%	—	
Al/Mg content	+	—	

Type	Viscosity (cps) Min.	Viscosity (cps) Max.	Al content/ Mg content Min.	Al content/ Mg content Max.
IA	225	600	0.5	1.2
IB	150	450	0.5	1.2
IC	800	2200	0.5	1.2
IIA	100	300	1.4	2.8
IIIA	250	500	3.5	5.5
IIIB	40	200	3.5	5.5

11. Typical Properties

Solubility: Insoluble in water or alcohols; swells to many times its original volume to form colloidal dispersions; practically insoluble in organic solvents.
Acid demand: 6 to 8 ml of 0.1 N HCl is required to reduce the pH of 1 g to pH 4.
Swellability: Swells to many times its original volume.
Rheology: Dispersions in water at the 1%-2% level are thin colloidal suspensions. At 3% and above, dispersions are opaque. As the concentration is increased above 3%, the viscosity of such aqueous dispersions increases rapidly. At 4-5%, dispersions are thick, white colloidal sols, and at 10% firm gels are formed. Dispersions are thixotropic at levels above 3%. Viscosity of the suspension increases with heating, addition of electrolytes and at higher concentrations with aging.

Viscosity of Various Grades of Colloidal					
Grade	Viscosity (cps)* Min.	Viscosity (cps)* Max.	Al content/Mg content Min.	Al content/Mg content Max.	Acid Demand
Veegum	225	600	0.5	1.2	6-8
Veegum F	150	450	0.5	1.2	6-8
Veegum HV	800	2200	0.5	1.2	6-8
Veegum K	100	300	1.4	2.8	<3.5
Veegum S728	250	500	3.5	5.5	6.9
Veegum HS	40	200	3.5	5.5	<2.5

*Centipoise at a concentration of 25 g in 475 ml of water.

Academy HPE Laboratory Project Data			
	Method	Lab #	Results
Moisture content[b]	MC-22	2	6.00%
Moisture content[b]	MC-13	18	6.85%
Moisture content[b]	MC-13	18	9.98%
Particle size dist.[b]	PSD-2	5	260 μm
Particle size dist.[b]	PSD-2	5	636 μm
EMC Plot (*Veegum HV*)[b]	EMC-1	2	Fig:2-EMC-6
SDI Plot (*Pharmasorb*)[a]	SDI-2	26	Fig:26-SDI-2
SDI Plot[c]	SDI-2	26	Fig:26-SDI-3
SDI Plot (*Colloidal*)[a]	SDI-2	26	Fig:26-SDI-4

Suppliers: Englehard Minerals & Chemicals Corp.[a]; R. T. Vanderbilt Co., Inc.[b]; ICD[c]

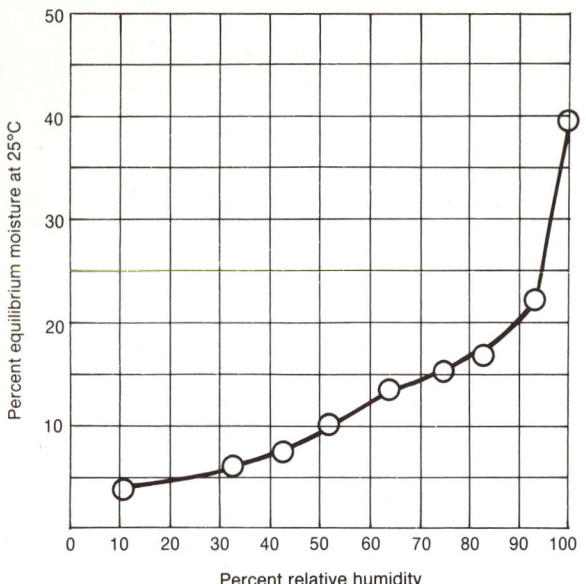

Magnesium aluminum silicate, NF, Veegum HV (Vanderbilt, Lot No. NV1640)

Figure: 2-EMC-6   **Method:** EMC-1

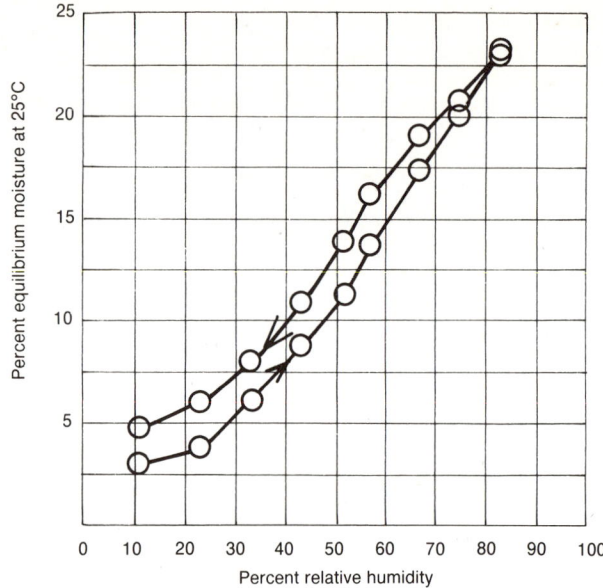

Magnesium aluminum silicate (ICD, Lot No. MAK-378)

Figure: 26-SDI-3   **Method:** SDI-2

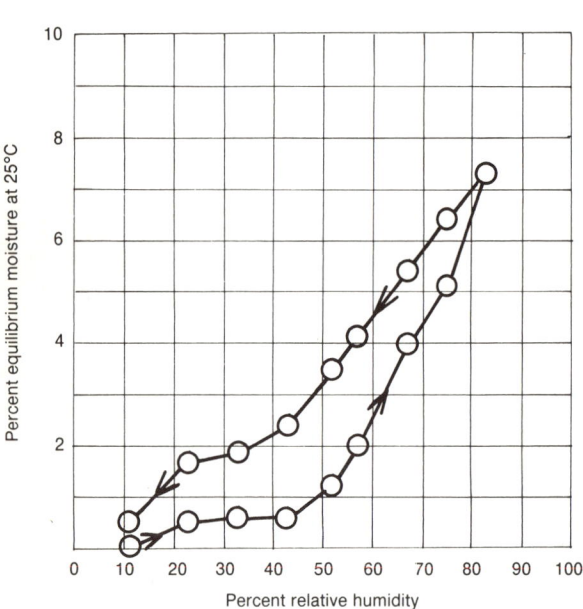

Magnesium aluminum silicate (Englehard, Pharmasorb, Lot No. 160-9-5)

Figure: 26-SDI-2   **Method:** SDI-2

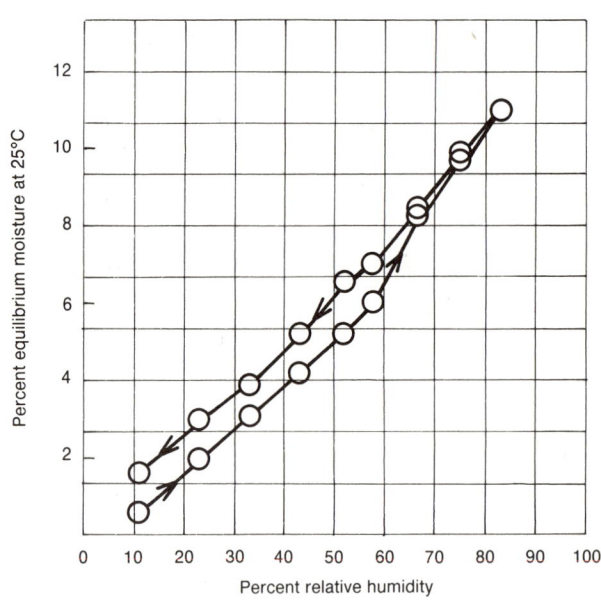

Magnesium aluminum silicate (Englehard, *Pharmasorb*, Collodial, Lot No. 349-9-3)

Figure: 26-SDI-4   **Method:** SDI-2

12. Stability and Storage Conditions

Magnesium aluminum silicate is stable indefinitely when stored under dry conditions. Store in a well-closed container.

13. Incompatibilities

Due to its inert nature, magnesium aluminum silicate has few incompatibilities. It is generally unsuitable for acidic drugs below pH 3.5. Magnesium aluminum silicate, as with other clays, may absorb active drugs. This may result in low bioavailability if the drug is tightly bound or slowly desorbed.

14. Safety

Nontoxic. Non-irritating. Magnesium aluminum silicate presents few if any toxicological problems. Sub-acute testing in rats and dogs at 10% of ration for 90 days was negative, including autopsy and histo-pathological examinations.

15. Handling Precautions

—

16. Regulatory Acceptance

NF XVI; BP 1980

17. Applications in Pharmaceutical Formulation or Technology

Use	Concentration (%)
Suspending agent (topical)	1-10
Suspending agent (oral)	0.5-2.5
Adsorbent	10-50
Stabilizing agent	0.5-2.5
Binding agent	2-10
Disintegrating agent	2-10
Emulsion stabilizer (topical)	2-5
Emulsion stabilizer (oral)	1-5
Viscosity modifier	2-10

18. Related Substances

Pharmasorb, Colloidal, Engelhard Minerals and Chemical Corp.; #2472 *Calcined Clay*, Wittaker, Clark & Daniels, Inc.; *Magnesium Alumino Silicate*, Tomita Pharmaceutical Co., Ltd.

19. Comments

This excipient can alter the bioavailability of some drugs. Additional characteristics: stable over a wide pH range; has base-exchange capacity; absorbs some organic substances; is compatible with organic solvents; is a valuable modifier for organic gums.

20. Specific References

1. *Veegum, The Versatile Ingredient*, Section II, Bibliography, R. T. Vanderbilt Co., Inc.
2. *Pharmaceutical Applications of Veegum*, R. T. Vanderbilt Co., Inc.
3. J. W. McGinity and J. L. Lach, *In vitro* adsorption of various pharmaceuticals to *Veegum*, J. Pharm. Sci., 65: 896 (1976).
4. H. Yokoi, S. Enomoto and H. Takahashi, Effect of magnesium aluminosilicate on fluidity of pharmaceutical powder, Yakugaku Zasshi, 98: 48 (1978).
5. J. Pawlaczyk and M. Goszozynska, Rheological studies on some dispersing agents used in the pharmaceutical industry, Ann. Pharm., 12: 45 (1977).
6. K. Sakai, K. Moriguchi, Effect of magnesium alumino silicate administered to pregnant mice on pre- and postnatal development of offsprings, Oyo Yakri 9: 703 (1975).
7. J. W. McGinity and J. L. Lach, Sustained-release applications of montmorillonite interaction with amphetamine sulfate, J. Pharm. Sci., 66: 63 (1977).
8. J. W. McGinity and M. R. Harris, Optimization of slow-release tablet formulations containing montmorillonite I. Properties of tablets, Drug Dev. Ind. Pharm., 6: 399 (1980).
9. J. W. McGinity and M. R. Harris, Increasing dissolution rates of poorly-soluble drugs by adsorption to montmorillonite, Drug Dev. Ind. Pharm., 6: 35 (1980).
10. B. C. Carlson, Stabilizers in creams and lotions, Cosmetic Technology, p. 27, November, 1980.
11. J. Polon, The mechanisms of thickening by inorganic agents, J. Soc. Cosmetic Chem., 5: 347 (1970).

USA: F. L. Grab*; J. H. Johnson**; A. L. Monaco**
UK: A. J. Winfield*

Magnesium Carbonate

1. Nonproprietary Name
USP: Magnesium carbonate
BP/EP: Heavy magnesium carbonate
Light magnesium carbonate

2. Functional Category
Filtering aid for alkaline solutions; direct compression tableting excipient; adsorbent in tablet of drug extracts which contain oily component.

3. Synonyms
Carbonic acid, magnesium salt (1:1), mixture with magnesium hydroxide, hydrate; magnesia alba; magnesium carbonate hydroxide; magnesium carbonate basic; heavy magnesium carbonate; light magnesium carbonate; carbonic acid, magnesium salt (1:1), hydrate; magnesium carbonate hydrate; magnesium carbonate dihydrate; normal magnesium carbonate; carbonic acid, magnesium salt (1:1); magnesium carbonate; magnesium carbonate anhydrous.

4. Chemical Name and CAS Registry Number
Carbonic acid, magnesium salt (1:1), mixture with magnesium hydroxide, and magnesium hydrate [39409-82-0]
Carbonic acid, magnesium salt (1:1), hydrate [23389-33-5]
Carbonic acid, magnesium salt anhydrous (1:1) [546-93-0]

5. Empirical Formula   Molecular Weight

Magnesium carbonate hydroxide $(MgCO_3)_4 \cdot Mg(OH)_2 \cdot 5H_2O$	485.65
Heavy magnesium carbonate $(MgCO_3)_3 \cdot Mg(OH)_2 \cdot 4H_2O$	383.32
Light magnesium carbonate $(MgCO_3 \cdot Mg(OH)_2 \cdot 3H_2O$	365.30
Normal magnesium carbonate $MgCO_3 \cdot xH_2O$	various
Magnesium carbonate anhydrous $MgCO_3$	84.31

6. Structural Formula
—

7. Commercial Availability
USA
American International Chemical, Inc.
Austin Chemical Co.
Baker Chemical Co., J.T.
Delamar, Inc.
Gallard–Schlesinger Chemical Mfg. Corp.
Generichem Corp.
Glyco, Inc.
Mallinckrodt, Inc.

McKesson Chemical Co.
Merck & Co., Merck Chemical Div.
Pfaltz and Bauer, Inc.
Ruger Chemical Co.
Sitco (Shah International Trading Corp.)
Tamms Industries Co.
Thompson-Hayward Chemical Co.
Uhe Co., George
Whittaker, Clark & Daniels, Inc.

UK
Croxton & Garry Ltd.
Dunn Bros. Manchester Ltd.
John & E. Sturge Ltd.

8. Method of Manufacture
Note: Depending on the variables of the manufacturing process, the composition of the product obtained varies between that of a basic hydrated magnesium carbonate, to which the formula $(MgCO_3)_4 \cdot Mg(OH)_2 \cdot 5 H_2O$ has been assigned, and that of normal hydrated magnesium carbonate $(MgCO_3 \cdot xH_2O)$.

Method A
An aqueous suspension of dolomite $(MgCO_3 \cdot CaCO_3)$ is saturated with CO_2 under pressure. On increasing the temperature, $CaCO_3$ precipitates almost entirely. The filtered solution is heated to boiling, the magnesium bicarbonate loses CO_2 and H_2O, and magnesium carbonate precipitates.

Method B
Precipitation of a solution of a soluble magnesium salt, such as magnesium chloride or magnesium sulfate, with a soluble carbonate, such as sodium carbonate.

Light magnesium carbonate is usually produced by Method A, and heavy magnesium carbonate is usually produced by Method B, using concentrated solutions of magnesium salts. Use of more dilute magnesium salts in Method B will produce less dense material.

9. Description
Light, white friable masses or bulky white powder; odorless, but having a highly absorptive ability; will absorb odor; slight earthy taste. The material usually referred to as magnesium carbonate is not one homogenous compound. The USP recognizes three types of magnesium carbonate: anhydrous magnesium carbonate, which is rarely seen; basic magnesium carbonate, probably the most common form, a product which can vary between light magnesium carbonate, $(MgCO_3)_3 \cdot Mg(OH)_2 \cdot 3H_2O$ and magnesium carbonate hydroxide, $(MgCO_3)_4 \cdot Mg (OH_2) 5H_2O$; and normal magnesium carbonate, which is an hydrous magnesium carbonate with a varying amount of water, $MgCO_3 \cdot Mg(OH)_2 \cdot H_2O$. The BP and EP are more specific, and list magnesium carbonate as one of two basic forms: light magnesium carbonate, which has a varying composition corresponding approximately to the formula $(MgCO_3)_3 \cdot Mg(OH)_2 \cdot 3H_2O$; and heavy magnesium carbonate, which has a varying composition corresponding approximately to the formula $(MgCO_3)_3 \cdot Mg(OH)_2 \cdot 4H_2O$.

SEM: KY-35
Excipient: Magnesium carbonate USP
Supplier: Mallinckrodt **Lot No.:** KJGJ

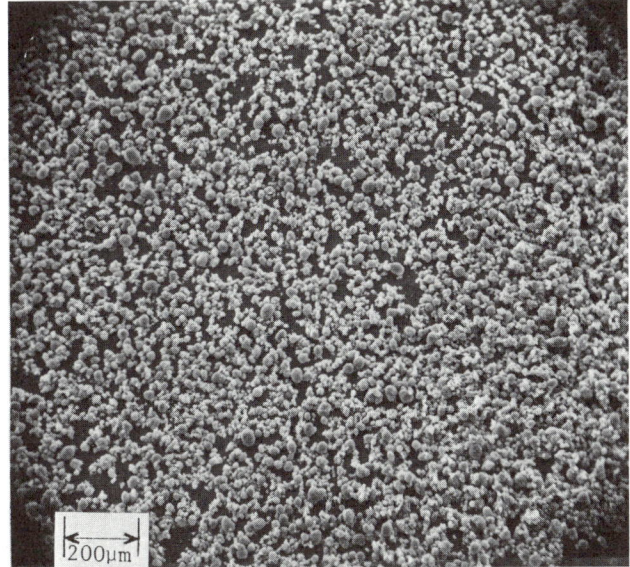

Magnification: 60× **Voltage:** 20 kV

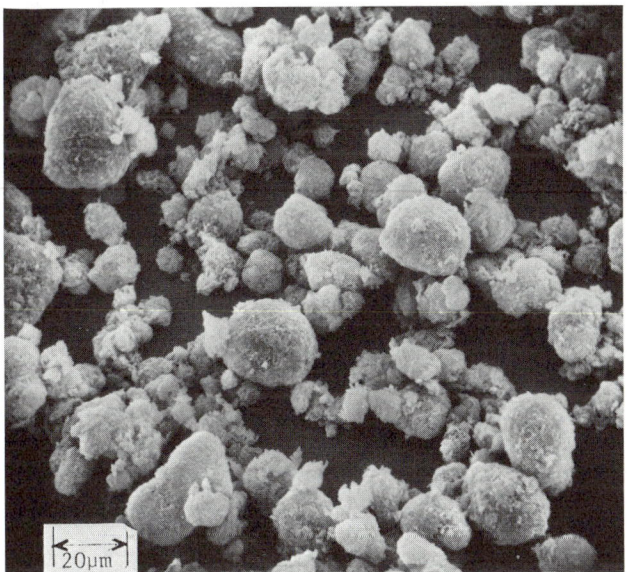

Magnification: 600× **Voltage:** 20 kV

10. Pharmacopeial Specifications

Test	USP	BP/EP Heavy	Light
Identification	+	+	+
Solubility	—	+	+
Soluble salts	≤1.0%	—	—
Soluble substances	—	≤1.0%	≤1.0%
Acid-insoluble substances	≤0.05%	—	—

Test	USP	BP/EP Heavy	Light
Heavy metals	≤0.003%	≤20 ppm	≤20 ppm
Arsenic	≤4 ppm	≤2 ppm	≤2 ppm
Iron	≤0.02%	≤400 ppm	≤400 ppm
Calcium	≤0.45%	≤0.75%	≤0.75%
Chloride	—	≤0.07%	≤0.07%
Sulfate	—	≤0.6%	≤0.3%
Color of solution	—	+	+
Assay (as MgO)	40.0-43.5%	40.0-45.0%	40.0-45.0%
Microbial limit, *E. coli*	Absent	—	—

11. Typical Properties

Solubility: Magnesium carbonate is practically insoluble in water and other solvents. Dilute acids dissolve it with effervescence. It is soluble in water containing CO_2 and insoluble in alcohol.

Academy HPE Laboratory Project Data

	Method	Lab #	Results
Compression Plot[a]	COM-5,6	29	Fig:29-COM-25[a]
Compression Plot[b]	COM-1	21	Fig:21-COM-31[b]
Compression Plot[a]	COM-7	12	Fig:12-COM-35[a]

Suppliers: [a]Mallinckrodt, Inc.; [b]Merck & Co.

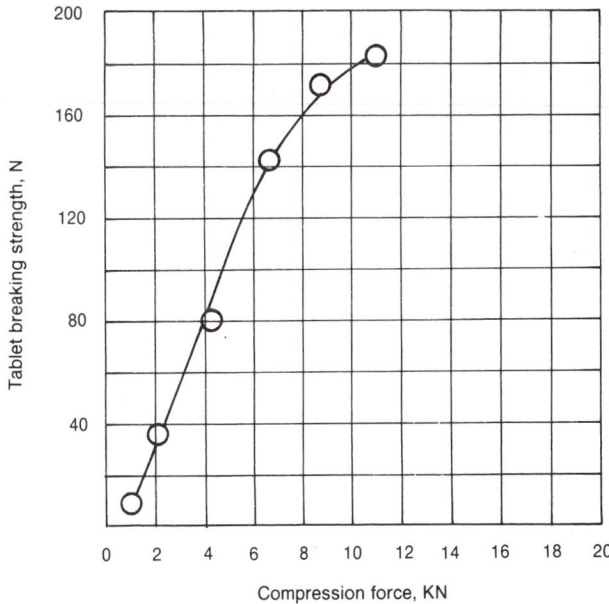

Magnesium carbonate (Mallinckrodt, Lot #KJGJ)
Tablet weight: 300 mg

Figure: 12-COM-35   **Method:** COM-7

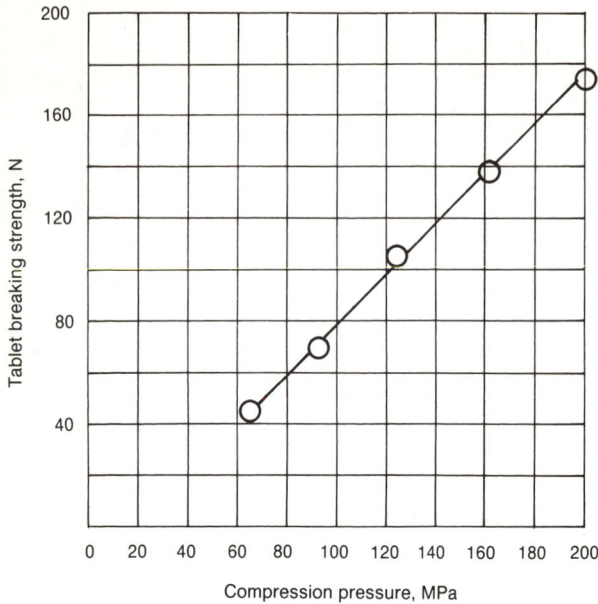

Magnesium carbonate, heavy powder, BP (Merck, Lot #351386)
Weight range of tablets: 625-650 mg

Figure: 21-COM-31   **Method:** COM-1

12. Stability and Storage Conditions

Magnesium carbonate is stable in dry air and light, and should be stored in a tightly closed container.

13. Incompatibilities

Acids will dissolve magnesium carbonate, with the liberation of CO_2. Slight alkalinity is imparted to water, and suspensions of it will cause precipitation of insoluble free alkaloids from solutions of alkaloidal salts.

14. Safety

Magnesium carbonate is fairly safe as a drug. It is contraindicated as an antacid for those individuals whose stomachs cannot tolerate the evolution of CO_2. The usual dose as an antacid is 250 to 600 mg and as a laxative, 2 to 8 g. A maximum safe dose has not been determined, but laxation usually limits the total daily dose to 8 to 15 g. Safe under ordinary occupational exposure.

15. Handling Precautions

Avoid dilute acids and moisture.

16. Regulatory Acceptance

USP XXI; BP 1980

17. Applications in Pharmaceutical Formulations or Technology

Use	Concentration %
Tablet excipient (direct compression)	≤45%
Adsorbent of liquid, such as flavors, in tabletting	0.5-1.0%

18. Related Substance

—

19. Comments

—

20. Specific References

1. R. F. Haines-Nutt, *J. Pharm. Pharmacol.* 28: 469 (1976).

USA: L. Wilken*; C. B. Peot**

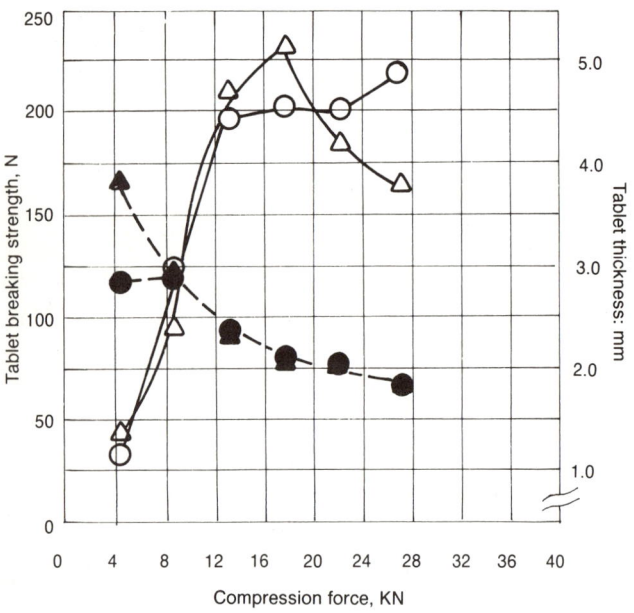

Magnesium carbonate, heavy powder, NF (Mallinckrodt, Lot #KJGJ)
○ ● : Unlubricated, Carver Laboratory Press (COM-5)
△ ▲ : Lubricated, Carver Laboratory Press (COM-6)

Figure: 29-COM-25   **Methods:** COM-4, 5, 6

Magnesium Stearate

1. Nonproprietary Name
NF: Magnesium stearate
BP/EP: Magnesium stearate

2. Functional Category
USP: Tablet and/or capsule lubricant
BP/EP: Lubricant; pharmaceutical aid
Others: Glidant; anti-adherent

3. Synonyms
Metallic stearate; magnesium salt

4. Chemical Names and CAS Registry Number
Octadecanoic acid; magnesium salt; magnesium stearate
[557-04-0]

5. Empirical Formula
$C_{36}H_{70}MgO_4$

Molecular Weight
591.3

6. Structural Formula
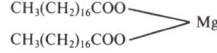

7. Commercial Availability

USA
Alba Chemical, Inc.
Austin Chemical Co.
Browning Chemical Corp.
ICN K & K Labs, Inc.
Mallinckrodt, Inc.
McKesson Chemical Co.
Pfaltz and Bauer, Inc.
Ruger Chemical Co.
SITCO (Shah International Trading Corp.)
Tenneco Chemicals, Inc.
VGF Chemical Corp.
Whittaker, Clark & Daniels, Inc.
Witco Chemical Corp., Organics Div.

UK
Frederick Allen and Sons, Ltd.
Durham Raw Materials, Ltd.
Megret, Ltd.
Witco Chemical, Ltd.
Wilfred Smith (Fine Chemicals), Ltd.

8. Method of Manufacture
Interaction of aqueous solutions of magnesium chloride and sodium stearate.
Interaction of magnesium oxide, hydroxide or carbonate with stearic acid at elevated temperatures.

9. Description
Fine, white, precipitated or milled, impalpable powder of low bulk density. Odor and taste are slight but characteristic. The powder is unctuous, and readily adheres to the skin.

SEM: KY-36
Excipient: Magnesium stearate USP

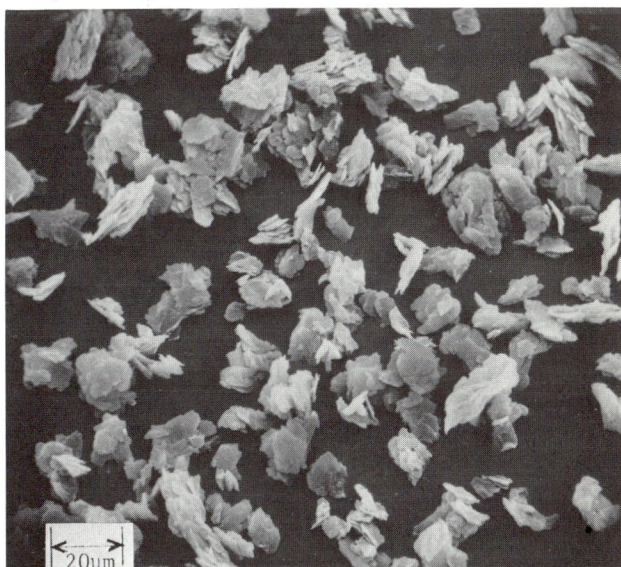

Magnification: 600×

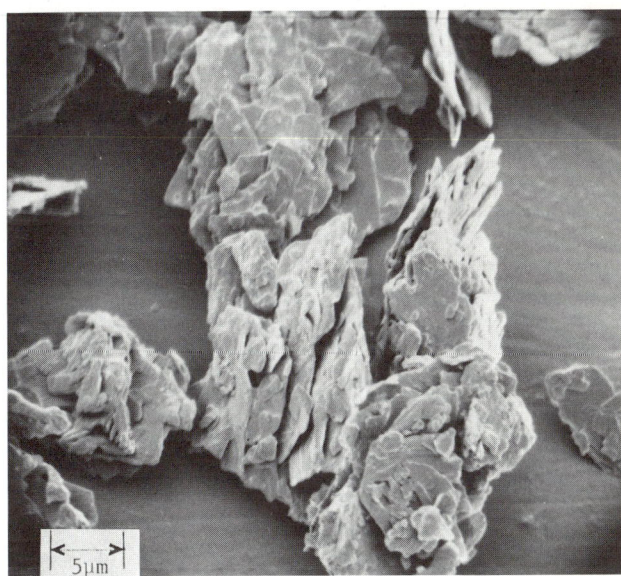

Magnification: 2,400×

SEM: UK-2
Excipient: Magnesium stearate BP
Supplier: Dart Chemicals, Ltd.; Otto Breyer, Holland
Lot no: 0734J

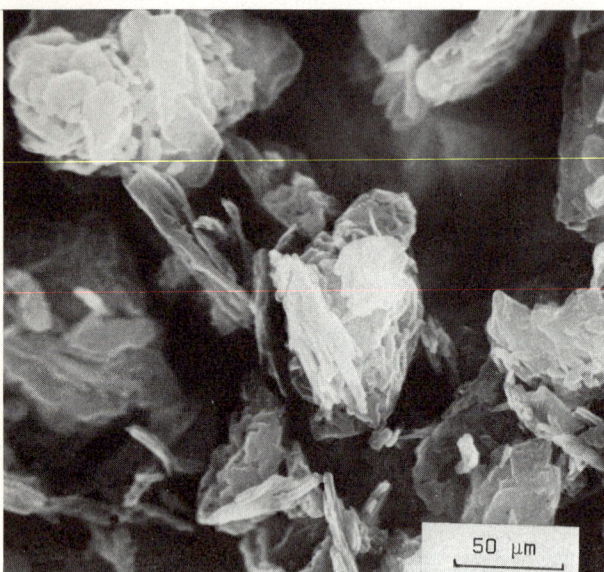

Magnification: 360×

Academy HPE Laboratory Data

	Method	Lab #	Results
Moisture content	MC-12	5	3.00%[b]
Moisture content	MC-12	1	3.85%[a]
Bulk/tap density	BTD-2	1	B: 0.143 g/cm³[a]
			T: 0.224 g/cm³[a]
Bulk/tap density	BTD-7	14	B: 0.160g/cm³[a]
			T: 0.180 g/ml[a]
Bulk/tap density	BTD-6	8	Volume: 7.0%[a]
			Weight: 8.0%[a]
Density	DE-1	7	1.08 ± 0.02[a]
Solubility (Water 25°C)	SOL-1	1	0.040 mg/ml[a]
(Alcohol 25°C)			0.160 mg/ml[a]
(n-Hexane 25°C)			0.018 mg/ml[a]
Compression			
(at 63.5-235 MN/m²)	COM-1	21	No compacts[c]
(at 500 lbs.)	COM-7	12	Lamination[a]
EMC Plot	EMC-1	5	Fig:5-EMC-3[b]

Suppliers: Mallinckrodt, Inc.[a]; Penick[b]; Witco Chemical Corp.[c]

10. Pharmacopeial Specifications

Test	NF XVI	BP/EP
Identification	+	+
Acidity or alkalinity	—	pH: 6.2-7.4
Loss on drying	≤4%	≤6%
Acid value of fatty acids	—	195-210
Chloride	—	≤250 ppm
Lead	≤0.001%	—
Heavy metals	—	≤20 ppm
Sulfate	—	≤0.25%
Zinc stearate	—	≤0.5%
Assay	6.8-8.3% MgO	3.8-5.0% Mg
Color of solution	—	+
Clarity and color of solution of fatty acids	—	+
Microbial limits: total bacteria count	≤1000/g	—
Microbial limits: *E. coli*	Negative	—

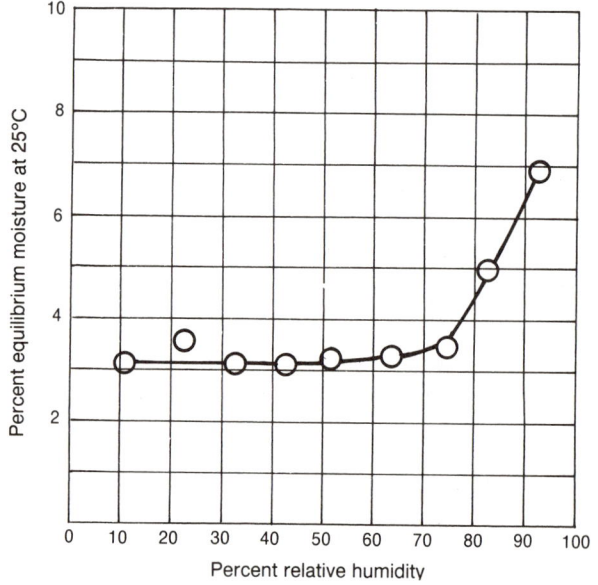

Magnesium stearate NF (Manufacturer: Penick, Lot No. 338-NB5-003)

Figure: 5-EMC-3   **Method:** FMC-1

11. Typical Properties

Density (He): 1.03 - 1.08 g/cm³
Bulk volume: 3.0 - 8.4 ml/g
Tapped volume: 2.5 - 6.2 ml/g
Melting point: 88.5°C
Solubility: Insoluble in water, alcohol and ether. Slightly soluble in hot alcohol and benzene.
Moisture sorption: Negligible
Ignition: Yields carbon monoxide, carbon dioxide and magnesium oxide.
Specific surface area: 2.45 - 7.93 m²/g
     2.45 - 16.0 m²/g (UK)
Polymorphic forms: A trihydrate, acicular form and a dihydrate, lamellar form have been isolated, with the latter possessing the better lubricating power (Reference #6).
Flowability: Poorly flowing, cohesive powder.

12. Stability and Storage Conditions

Stable, non-self-polymerizable. Store in a cool, dry place in a well-closed container.

13. Incompatibilities

Acidic substances; alkaline substances; iron salts. Avoid mixing with strong oxidizing materials. Use with caution with drugs which are incompatible with alkali.

14. Safety

Magnesium stearate is described as an inert or nuisance dust. Classified as non-hazardous by the Department of Transportation Regulations. Generally considered not to be a health hazard under normal conditions of use. OSHA has adopted limits of 15 mg/m^3 for the total dust and 5 mg/m^3 for the respirable fraction. Dust clouds of magnesium stearate may be explosive.

15. Handling Precautions

—

16. Regulatory Acceptance

NF XVI; BP/EP 1980

17. Applications in Pharmaceutical Formulation or Technology

Use	Concentration
Tablet and capsule lubricant, glidant or anti-adherent	0.25 - 2.0%

18. Related Substances

Other metallic stearates (see monograph on calcium stearate)

19. Comments

Due to its hydrophobic nature, magnesium stearate may retard the dissolution of a drug from a solid dosage form, and it is therefore advisable to use as low a concentration as possible. There is often considerable variation between batches of magnesium stearate, but it has not been possible to conclusively correlate these findings with the observed lubricity. There is evidence that the hydrophobic nature of the magnesium stearate can vary from batch to batch due to the presence of water-soluble, surface-active impurities. Batches containing only very low concentrations of these impurities (mainly sodium stearate) have been shown to retard the dissolution of a drug to a greater extent than when using batches containing more of these impurities.

An increase in the coefficient of variation of mixing and a decrease in the dissolution rate was observed when magnesium stearate was blended with the tablet granulation. A large decrease in dissolution rate occurred during the first minutes of mixing. The tablet crushing strength also decreased continuously during the first 10 minutes of mixing with magnesium stearate. Magnesium stearate may also increase tablet friability. Blending times with magnesium stearate should be carefully controlled.

20. Specific References

1. Material Safety Data Sheet, Diamond Shamrock Chemical Company.
2. Butcher, A.G. and Jones, T.J., Some physical characteristics of magnesium stearate, *J. Pharm. Pharmac.*, 24, Suppl. 1P (1972).
3. Caldwell, Henry C., Dissolution of lithium and magnesium from lithium carbonate capsules containing magnesium stearate, *J. Pharm. Sci.*, 63: 770 (1974).
4. Levy, G. and Gumtow, R.H., The effect of certain formulation factors on dissolution rate of the active ingredient, III: Tablet lubricants, *J. Pharm. Sci.*, 52: 1139 (1963).
5. Ganderton, David, The effect of distribution of magnesium stearate on the penetration of a tablet by water, *J. Pharm. Pharmac.*, 21: Suppl. 95P (1969).
6. Jones, T.M., The effect of glidant addition on the flowability of bulk particulate solids, *J. Soc. Cosmet. Chem.*, 21: 483 (1970).
7. Hanssen, D. *et al.*, Evaluation of magnesium stearate as a tablet lubricating agent by electronic pressure measurements, *Pharm. Ind.*, 32: 97 (1970).
8. Pilpel, N., Metal stearates in pharmaceutical and cosmetics, *Manuf. Chem. and Aerosol News*, 37: Oct. (1971).
9. Muller, B.W., Tribological conformity with natural law and tabletting technology, Part 2, *Pharm. Ind.*, 38: 394 (1976).
10. Billany, M.R., Hydrophobicity of magnesium stearate and its effect on the dissolution rate of a model drug from solid dosage forms, *Proc. 2nd Inter. Conf. on Pharm. Tech.*, Paris (1980).
11. Carr, R.L., Compressibility Index, British Chemical Engineering, 1970, Vol. 15, p. 1541.
12. T.A. Miller, P. York and T.M. Jones, Manufacture and characterization of magnesium stearate and palmitate powders of high purity, *J. Pharm. Pharmacol*, 34: Suppl. 8P (1982).
13. A.F. Asker, M.M. Abdel-Khalek and I. Machloof, Effect of scaling-up and formulation factors on the qualities of prednisone tablets, *Drug Develop. & Indust. Pharm.*, 7(1): 79-111 (1981).
14. M. Sheikh-Salem and J.T. Fell, The influence of magnesium stearate on time-dependent strength changes in tablets, *Drug Develop. & Indust. Pharm.*, 7(6): 669-674 (1981).
15. K. Tong, T. Mitrevej and L.L. Augsberger, Adhesion of tablets in a rotary tablet press II. Effect of blending time, running time and lubricant concentration, *Drug Develop. & Indust. Pharm.*, 8(2): 237-282 (1982).
16. Z.T. Chowhan, A.A. Amaro and Y.P. Chow, Tablet-to-tablet dissolution variability and its relationship to the homogeneity of a water soluble drug, *Drug Develop. & Indust. Pharm.*, 8(2): 145-168 (1982).
17. G.K. Bolhuis, A.J. Smallenbroek and C.F. Lerk, Interaction of tablet disintegrants and magnesium stearate during mixing I: Effect on tablet disintegration, *J. Pharm. Sci.*, 70(12): 1328-1338 (1981).
18. J. Bossert and A. Stamm, Effect of mixing on the lubrication of crystalline lactose by magnesium stearate, *Drug Develop. & Indust. Pharm.*, 6 (6): 573-589 (1980).
19. N.R. Bohidar, F.A. Restaino and J.B. Schwartz, Selecting key pharmaceutical formulation factors by regression analyses, *Drug Develop. & Indust. Pharm.*, 5(2): 175-216 (1979).
20. J.L. Ford and M.H. Rubinstein, An investigation into some pharmaceutical interactions by differential scanning colorimetry, *Drug Develop. & Indust. Pharm.*, 7(6): 675-682 (1981).
21. P.J. Stewart, Effect on magnesium stearate on the homogeneity of a prednisone granule, *Drug Develop. & Indust. Pharm.*, 7 (5): 485-495 (1981).
22. G.K. Bolhuis, C.F. Lerk and P. Broersma, Mixing action and evaluation of tablet lubricants in direct compression, *Drug Develop. & Indust. Pharm.*, 6(1): 15-33 (1980).
23. R.F. Shangraw, J.W. Wallace and F.M. Bowers, Morphology and functionality in tablet excipients for direct compression: Part II, *Powder Technology*, 5(10): 44-60 (1981).
24. P.J. Jarosz and E.L. Parrott, Effect of tablet lubricants on axial and radial work of failure, *Drug Develop. & Indust. Pharm.*, 8(3): 445-453 (1982).

USA: W. Han*; D. Liebe*; J. Cooper*; A. Bruno**; D. Hovermale**; J. Mollica**

UK: M. Billany*; T.M. Jones*; W. Lund**

Malic Acid

1. Nonproprietary Name
NF: Malic acid

2. Functional Category
NF: Acidifying agent
Others: Antioxidant; flavoring agent; synergist

3. Synonym
Apple acid, DL-malic acid

4. Chemical Names and CAS Registry Number
Hydroxybutanedioic acid
Hydroxysuccinic acid
Malic acid [6915-15-7]

5. Empirical Formula   Molecular Weight
$C_4H_6O_5$ 134.09

6. Structural Formula

HOCHCOOH
|
CH_2COOH

7. Commercial Availability
USA

American International Chemical, Inc.
Atomergic Chemetals Corp.
Chemical Dynamics Corp.
Fallek Chemical Corp.
Gallard-Schlesinger Chemical Mfg. Corp.
ICN/K & K Labs, Inc.
Pfaltz and Bauer, Inc.
United States Biochemicals Corp.

UK

BDH Chemicals, Ltd.
Croda Food Ingredients, Ltd.
Fisons, Ltd.

8. Method of Manufacture
Malic acid is manufactured by hydrating maleic and fumaric acids in the presence of suitable catalysts and separating the malic acid from the equilibrium product mixture.

9. Description
White or nearly white, crystalline powder or granules having a slight odor and a strongly acidic taste. Synthetic material is a racemic mixture. Naturally occurring material is levorotatory.

10. Pharmacopeial Specifications

Test	NF
Identification	+
Specific rotation	$-0.1°$ and $+0.1°$
Residue on ignition	$\geq 0.1\%$
Water insoluble substances	$\leq 0.1\%$
Heavy metals	0.002%
Fumaric acid	$\leq 1.0\%$
Malic acid	$\leq 0.05\%$
Assay	99.0-100.5%

11. Typical Properties
Buffering index: 3.26
Dissociation constants: $pk_{a1}=3.40$ (25° C)
$pk_{a2}=5.05$ (25° C)
pH of 1% aqueous solution at 25° C: 2.4-2.5
Solubility: Freely soluble in water. A saturated solution contains about 56% malic acid at 20°C. Readily soluble in ethanol (28% at 25° C).

Solvent	Solubility (mg/ml)
Water	500-664
Ethanol (95%)	390
Propylene glycol	534
Methanol	830

Specific gravity: d_4^{20}: 1.601 g/cm³
Specific gravity (saturated solution at 25° C): 1.250
Viscosity (50% aqueous solution at 25° C): 6.5 cps
Melting range: 130°-132° C
Bulk density: 0.81 g/cm³
Tapped density: 0.92 g/cm³

12. Stability and Storage Conditions
Malic acid is stable when heated to 150° C. At temperatures above 150° C, it begins to lose water very slowly to yield fumaric acid. Since malic acid is deliquescent, it should be stored in a well-closed container. It is readily degraded by many aerobic and anaerobic micro-organisms.

13. Incompatibilities
No information found.

14. Safety
Malic acid is in no sense a dangerous material, but it can be an irritant, especially in concentrated solutions. It is one of the miscellaneous and/or general-purpose food additives recognized as GRAS by the FDA.

15. Handling Precautions
Dust and aqueous solutions may irritate skin, eyes, and mucous membranes. Avoid contact with eyes.

16. Regulatory Acceptance
NF XVI. FDA-approved excipient (levorotatory form) for drug use and as a synthetic flavoring agent. In the UK, malic acid has been approved for use as a general acidulant by *Miscellaneous Additives in Food Regulations* (1974).

17. Applications in Pharmaceutical Formulation or Technology
General purpose acidulant. Flavor enhancer, in masking bitter taste. Used as an alternative to citric acid in effervescent powders, mouthwashes and tooth-cleaning tablets. Has chelating and antioxidant properties. Used as a synergist with butylated hydroxytoluene to retard oxidation in vegetable oils.

18. Related Substances
Fumaric acid; D-malic acid; L-malic acid

19. Comments
None

20. References
1. "Malic Acid," Alberta Gas Chemicals Technical Bulletin.
2. "Malic and Fumaric Acids," *Manufacturing Chemist and Aerosol News*, 35: 57-59, December (1964).

USA: D. M. Patel*; G. T. Popp**
UK: S. Williamson*; W. Lund**

Mannitol

1. Nonproprietary Name
USP: Mannitol
BP: Mannitol

2. Functional Category
USP: Tonicity agent, tablet and/or capsule diluent, sweetening agent
Others: Filler for tablets, especially chewable tablets; vehicle (bulking agent) for lyophilized preparations

3. Synonyms
Mannite; manna sugar; manita

4. Chemical Names and CAS Registry Number
1,2,3,4,5,6-Hexanehexol
D-Mannitol [69-65-8]

5. Empirical Formula | Molecular Weight
$C_6H_{14}O_6$ 182.17

6. Structural Formula

```
        CH₂OH
         |
   HO—C—H
         |
   HO—C—H
         |
    H—C—OH
         |
    H—C—OH
         |
        CH₂OH
```

7. Commercial Availability
USA
Aceto Chemical Co.
American Roland Corp.
Aroma Resources, Div. of Biddle Sawyer Corp.
Austin Chemical Co.
Bage, Inc.
Delamar, Inc.
Gallard-Schlesinger Chemical Mfg. Corp.
Greeff & Co., R. W.
ICC Industries, Inc.
ICI Americas, Inc.
ICN K & K Labs, Inc.
Ingredients International, Inc.
McKesson Chemical Co.
Pfaltz and Bauer, Inc.
Reisman Corp., H.
Robeco Chemicals, Inc.

Ruger Chemical Co.
SITCO (Shah International Trading Corp.)
S.S.T. Corp.
Tri-K Industries, Inc.
United States Biochemicals Corp.

UK
Atlas Chemical Industries (UK), Ltd.
BDH Chemicals Ltd.
Chemical Exchange (UK) Ltd.
Steetley Chemicals Ltd.

8. Method of Manufacture
Mannitol may be extracted from the dried sap of manna and other natural sources by means of hot alcohol or other selective solvents. It is commercially produced by the catalytic or electrolytic reduction of monosaccharides such as mannose and glucose.

9. Description
A hexanydril alcohol related to mannose. It is isomeric with sorbitol. A white, odorless, crystalline powder, or free-flowing granules. Appears microscopically as orthorhombic needles when crystallized from alcohol. One-half as sweet as sucrose and about as sweet as glucose.
Color—Hunter Colorlab tester. L = +82.2
                                     a = +0.9
                                     b = +0.3

SEM-MF-14
Excipient: Mannitol
Supplier: Triangle Import & Export Co.

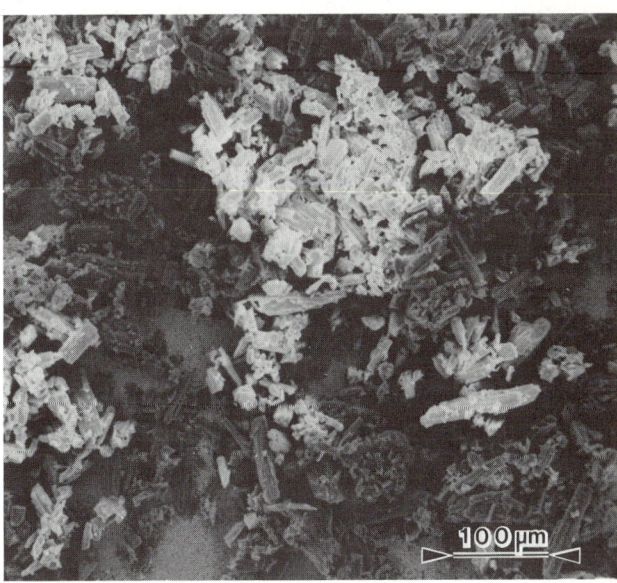

Magnification: 120×

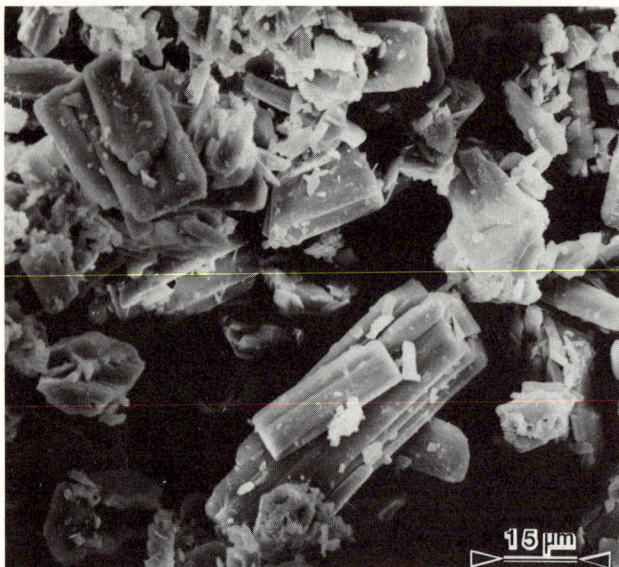

Magnification: 600×

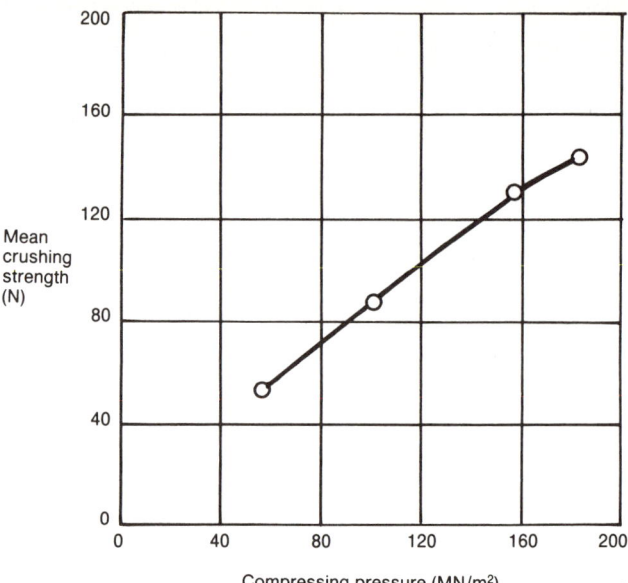

Figure 1: Compression characteristics

10. Pharmacopeial Specifications

Test	NF	BP
Identification	+	+
Melting range	165° to 169°C	+165° to 168°C
Specific optical rotation	+137° to +145°	+23° to +24°
Acidity	+	
Loss on drying	≤0.3%	≤0.5%
Chloride	≤0.007%	70 ppm
Sulfate	≤0.01%	120 ppm
Arsenic	≤1 ppm	≤2 ppm
Absence of reducing sugars	+	+
Assay	98.0-102.0%	98.0-102.0%
Sulphated ash	—	≤0.1%

11. Typical Properties

Compression characteristics: See Figure 1
Compression machine: Manesty E2
Speed of compression: 50 strokes per minute
(Note: Punches and die were lubricated after each compression cycle; hence, machine was not running continuously. However, the speed of the top punch when it entered the die was equal to that of a continuously running machine.)

Diameter of compacts: 12.5 mm
Weight of compacts: 610 ± 10 mg
Tablet strength instrument: Schleuniger
Lamination was not noted over the pressure range studied.
Density: Particle: 1.48 g/cm³ (helium pycnometer); bulk: 0.401 g/cm³; tapped: 0.58 g/cm³ (1250 taps)
Flowability: Cohesive (powder), free flowing (granules).
Melting point: 166°C
Moisture content: (a) Karl Fischer 0.1%; (b) Moisture sorption isotherm. See Figure 2 (sample dried at 60°C for 24 hours over silica gel.)
Particle size distribution: See Figure 3.

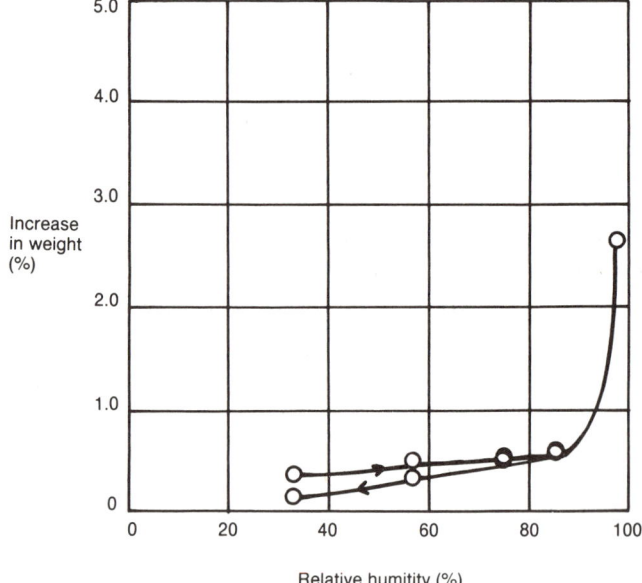

Figure 2: Moisture sorption desorption isotherm

Solubility:

Solvent	g in 100/ml (at 25°C)	(at 60°C)
Purified water	16.7	—
Aqueous buffers-over pH range 2 to 9; Teore 11 and Stenhagen phosphate—citrate—borate	16.7	40
Ethanol	1.3	
Propan-2-ol	1.0	
Glycerol	5.6	

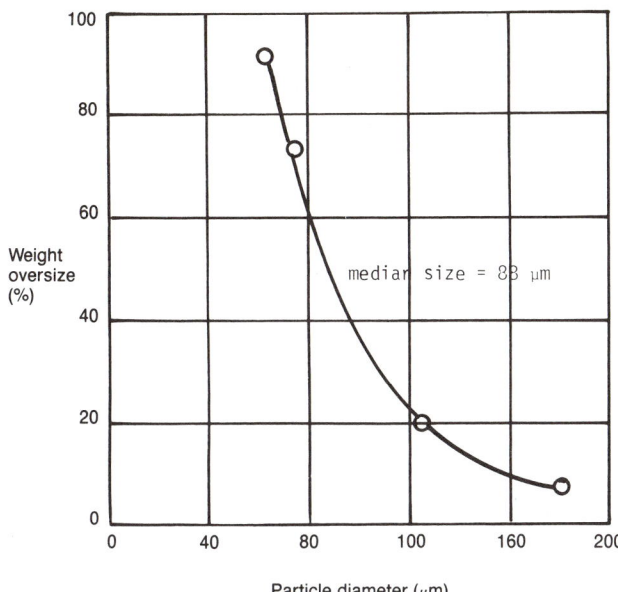

Figure 3: Particle size distribution

Specific surface area: 0.60m²/g (Micromeritics model 2205)
Flash point: Above 150°C.
Fire point: Above 150°C.
Heat of combustion: 3960 ± 5 calories/g.
Heat of solution: 28.9 calories/g at 25°C.
K_a: 3.4 × 10⁻¹⁴ at 19°C.

Academy HPE Laboratory Project Data

	Method	Lab #	Results
Moisture Content[b]	MC-29	23	0.277%
Bulk/Tap density[a]			
Granular USP	BTD-5	6	B:0.573 cm³
Powder USP[e]	BTD-5	6	B:0.381 cm³
			T:0.599 cm³
Powder USP[a]	BTD-5	6	B:0.429 cm³
			T:0.679 cm³
Powder USP[b]	BTD-5	6	B:0.420 cm³
			T:0.633 cm³
USP[c]	BTD-6	6	Volume:17.5%
USP	BTD-6		Weight: 18.0%
Particle size dist.[b]	PSD-7	24	12.5µm
Solubility[b]	SOL-6	23	
Water (25°C)			0.1798 g/ml
Water (37°C)			0.2234 g/ml
Alcohol (25°C)			0.0133 g/ml
Alcohol (37°C)			0.0139 g/ml
Prop. Glycol (25°C)			0.100-0.200 g/ml
Prop. Glycol (37°C)			0.100-0.200 g/ml
Hexane (25°C)			<0.001
Hexane (37°C)			<0.001
Average flow rate[b]	FLO-3	24	NO FLOW
Compression plot[a] (Gran.)	COM-3	20	Fig:20-COM-10
Compression plot[d] (Gran.)	COM-2	21	Fig:21-COM-32

Suppliers: Atlas Chemical Industries (UK)[a], Ltd.; Pfizer[b]; ICI Americas, Inc.[c]; Triangle[d]; George Lihe[e]

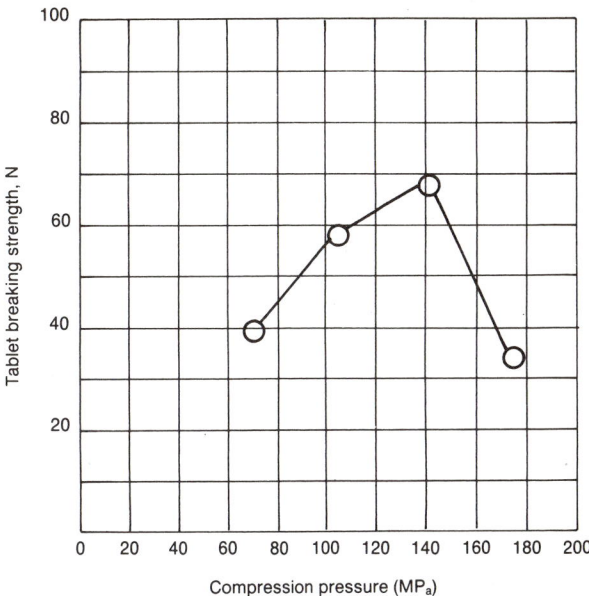

Mannitol (Triangle Import & Export, Lot #1233R8060791)
Tablet weight: 500 mg

Figure: 21-COM-32   **Method:** COM-2

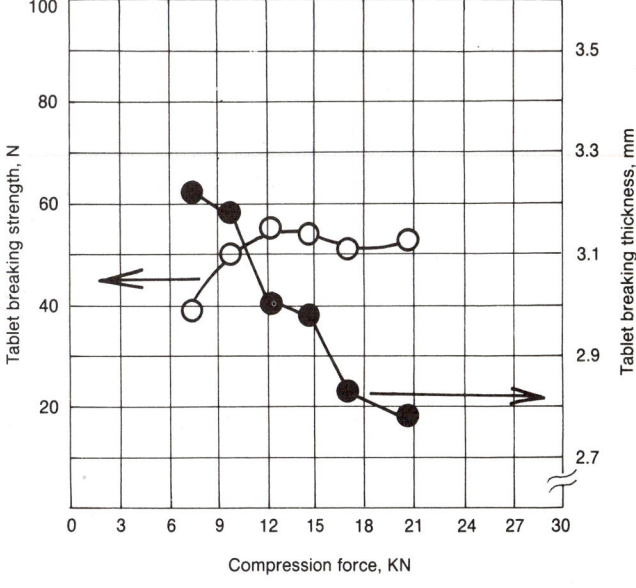

Mannitol, granular, USP (Atlas, Lot #2022BO)
Mean tablet weight: 500 mg
Minimum compressional force for compaction: 7.35 KN
Compressional force resulting in capping: 24.5 KN

Figure 2: 20-COM-10   **Method:** COM-3

12. Stability and Storage Conditions

Mannitol is stable in the dry state and in aqueous sterile solutions. In solution it is not attacked by cold, dilute acids or alkalis, nor by atmospheric oxygen in the absence of catalysts. No special storage conditions are required. Store in a well-closed container.

13. Incompatibilities

None reported in the dry state. Sodium cephapirin at 2 mg and 30 mg/ml is not compatible with 20% mannitol in water. Mannitol has also been reported to be incompatible with a xylitol infusion. It is reported to form complexes with some metals (Fe, Al, Cu).

14. Safety

Mannitol is a naturally occuring sugar alcohol found in animals and plants and present in small quantities in almost all vegetables. Mannitol is not absorbed from the gastrointestinal tract. After IV injection, mannitol is not metabolized to any appreciable extent, and is minimally reabsorbed by the renal tubule. About 80% of a dose is excreted in the urine in three hours. When used in foods as a bodying agent, if daily ingestion of over 20 grams is foreseeable, the label must bear the statement "Excess consumption may have a laxative effect." GRAS listed (up to 5%—special dietary foods).

15. Handling Precautions

None

16. Regulatory Acceptance

USP XXI; BP 1980

17. Applications in Pharmaceutical Formulation or Technology

Mannitol is used as a filler (10-90%) for conventional tablets. It is of special value when moisture-sensitive drugs are being tabletted because of its non-hygroscopicity; the granular form is easily dried. Mannitol has an even wider application in the manufacture of chewable tablets because of its negative heat of solution, its sweetness and its "mouth feel." The granular form was developed especially as a directly compressible vehicle for tablets. Mannitol is specified as the basis for glyceryl trinitrate tablets of the BP 1980. In lyophilized injectable preparations, mannitol has been included as a carrier (20-90%). Mannitol (up to 7%) has been used to prevent the thickening of aqueous suspensions of aluminum hydroxide intended as an antacid. It has also been suggested as a plasticizer in soft gelatin capsules. Granular mannitol flows well and imparts improved flow to materials which do not. Usually, however, it cannot be used with concentrations of other materials exceeding 25% by weight. Recommended levels of lubricant are 1% Calcium stearate or 2% magnesium stearate. Suitable binders for preparing granulations of powdered mannitol are gelatin, methylcellulose 400, starch paste, povidone and sorbitol. Usually 3-6 times as much magnesium stearate or 1.5-3 times as much calcium stearate is needed for lubrication of mannitol granulations than is needed for other excipients.

18. Related Substances

Mannitol is an isomer of sorbitol. The difference between the two polyols occurs in the planar orientation of the OH group on the second carbon atom. Each isomer is characterized by its own individual set of properties. The most important difference is the response to moisture. Sorbitol is much more mygroscopic. Mannitol resists moisture sorption, even at high relative humidities.

19. Comments

Mannitol is described in monographs of the pharmacopeias of the following countries: Brazil, Italy, Nordic countries, Portugal, Spain and Switzerland.

20. Specific References

1. Anon. "Atlas Mannitol, USP—Tablet Excipient," ICI America, Inc. (LM-28 7M 8/73).
2. R. W. Mendes, S. Goll and C. Q. An, *Drug and Cosmetic Ind.,* 122: 36 (1978).
3. K. N. Wai, H. G. DeKay and G. S. Banker, Stability of vitamins A, B, and C in selected vehicle matrices, *J. Pharm. Sci.,* 51: 1076 (1962).
4. R. G. Daoust and M. J. Lynch, *Drug Cosmet. Ind.,* 93: 26 (1963).
5. J. L. Kanig, Properties of fused mannitol in compressed tablets, *J. Pharm. Sci.,* 53: 188 (1964).
6. E. J. Mendell, *Manufacturing Chemist,* 43, 43 (1972).
7. J. F. Weidenheimer and F. M. Callahan, U.S. patent 2,770,553, Nov. 13, 1956.
8. A. M. Molokhia, M. A. Moustafa and M. W. Gouda, Effect of storage conditions on the hardness, disintegration and drug release from tablet bases, *Drug Develop. & Indust. Pharm.,* 8:(2), 283-293 (1982).
9. H. H. El-Shattawy, D. O. Kildsig and G. E. Peck, Differential scanning colorimetry of aspartame-mannitol mixtures, *Drug Develop. and Indust. Pharm.,* 8:(3), 429-443 (1982).
10. M. J. Miralles, J. W. McGinity and A. Martin, Combined water soluble carriers for coprecipitates of Tolbutamide, *J. Pharm. Sci.,* 71:(3), 302-304 (1982).

USA: G. E. Reier*; A. B. Rednick**; Z. Chowhan**

UK: N. A. Armstrong*

Methylcellulose

1. Nonproprietary Name
USP: Methylcellulose
BP: Methylcellulose

2. Functional Category
USP: Suspending agent and/or viscosity-increasing agent; tablet binder; coating agent

3. Synonym
Cellulose methyl ether; *Celacol*; *Methocel A*; *Metholose*

4. Chemical Name and CAS Registry Number
Cellulose methyl ether [9004-67-5]

5. Empirical Formula
Long-chain-substituted cellulose, ether of 50-1,500 anhydroglucose units containing 26-32% methoxyl groups (CH_3O)

6. Structural Formula

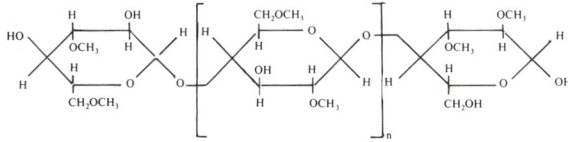

The degree of substitution (DS) is the average number of methoxyl groups attached to each anhydroglucose unit along the chain. The DS is characteristic of material from a particular source and affects the solubility of the material.
For Celacol, the DS ranges from 1.6 to 1.9.
For Methocel, the DS ranges from 1.1 to 2.0.

7. Commercial Availability
USA
Aceto Chemical Co.
Biddle Sawyer Corp.
Chemcentral Corp.
Dow Chemical Co.
Hampden Color & Chemical Co.
UK
British Celanese Ltd.
Colorcon, Ltd.
Shin-Etsu Chemical Co. Ltd.

8. Method of Manufacture
Methylcellulose is prepared from wood pulp or chemical cotton by treatment with alkali and methylation of the alkali cellulose with methyl chloride.

9. Description
White to slightly off-white, essentially odorless and tasteless powder or granules.

SEM:KY-37
Excipient: Methylcellulose
Manufacturer: Dow Chemical Co.; **Lot No.:** MM-090271-A

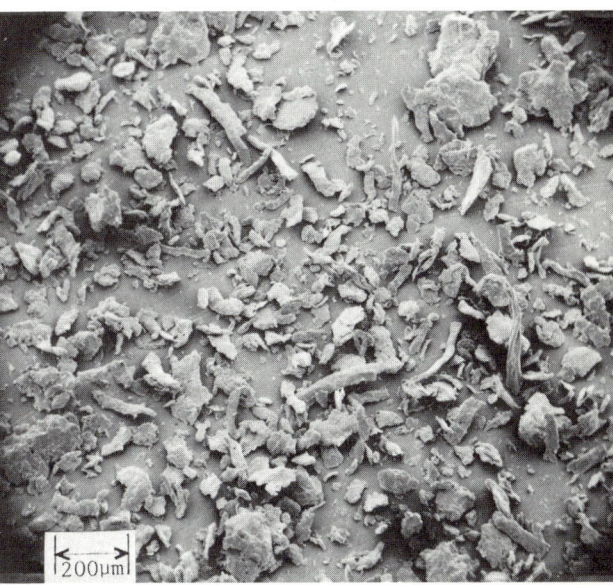

Magnification: 60× **Voltage:** 10 kV

SEM:KY-37
Excipient: Methylcellulose
Manufacturer: Dow Chemical Co.; **Lot No.:** MM-090271-A

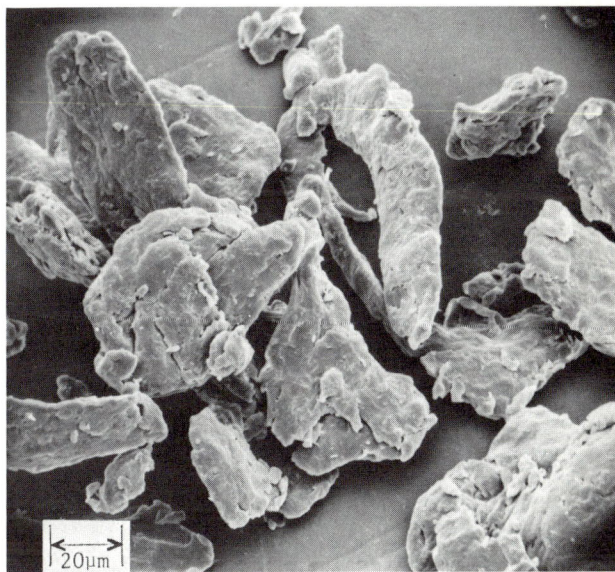

Magnification: 600× **Voltage:** 10 kV

10. Pharmacopeial Specifications

Test	USP	BP
Identification	+	+
Clarity and color of solution	—	+
Loss on drying	≤5%	≤10%
Chloride	—	≤0.5%
Residue on ignition	≤1.5%	—
Sulfated ash	—	≤1.0%
Heavy metals	≤0.001%	≤20 ppm
Arsenic	≤3 ppm	—
Acidity or alkalinity (pH) (1% solution)	—	5.5 - 8.0
Apparent viscosity	75-140% of stated value	75-140% of stated value
Viscosity types of 100 cps or less	80-120% of label	—
Viscosity types higher than 100 cps	75-140% of label	—
Assay range (methoxyl-calculated on dry basis)	27.5 to 31.5% of methoxy (OCH₃) groups	Varies with grade

11. Typical Properties

Viscosity: Methylcellulose swells in cold water and produces a clear to opalescent, viscous, colloidal suspension. Insoluble in hot water, saturated salt solutions, alcohol, ether and chloroform. Soluble in glacial acetic acid and in a mixture of equal volumes of alcohol and chloroform. Salts of mineral acids and particularly of polybasic acids, phenols and tannins coagulate solutions of methylcellulose, but this can be prevented by the addition of alcohol or glycol diacetate.
Viscosity grades available:
Approximate viscosity of 2%:

Solution at 20°C/cps	Material	Solvent
20	Celacol M20 GP	Water
450	Celacol M450 GP	Water
1000	Celacol M1000 GP	Water
2500	Celacol M2500 GP	Water
5000	Celacol M5000 GP	Water
10000	Celacol M10000 GP	Water
10	Celacol MM10 GP	Water
100	Celacol MM100 GP	Water
20*	Celacol M20B PC	
450*	Celacol M450 BPC	
15*	Methocel A15 Premium	Water
400*	Methocel A4C Premium	Water
1500*	Methocel A15C Premium	Water
4000*	Methocel A4M Premium	Water

*Calculated with reference to dried material.

Solution properties:
Specific gravity, 20°/4°C: 1% 1.0012; 5% 1.0117; 10%–1.0245. Refractive index (2%): 1.336. Gelatin temperature (2%): 48°C. Surface tension, 25°C: 47-53 dynes/cm. Interfacial tension (paraffin oil), 25°C: 19-23 dynes/cm. Freezing point (2%): 0.0°C. pH (1% @ 25°C): 6-8.
Unplasticized film properties (Methocel):
Specific gravity: 1.39. Area factor, in²/lb/mil: 24,000. Moisture-vapor transmission rate, 100°F, 90-100%. RH: 67.5 g/100 in²/24 hr/mil. Oxygen transmission rate, 75°F: 25 cc/100 in²/24 hr/mil. Tensile strength, 75°F, 50% RH: 8,500-11,400 lb/in². Elongation, 75°F, 50% RH: 10-15%. Stability to ultraviolet light (500 hrs., Fade Ometer exposure): Excellent. Resistance to oils and most solvents: Excellent. Ultraviolet transmission: 400: 55%; (2 mil film) 290: 49%; 210: 26%. Refractive index, n_D²⁰°C: 1.49. Melting point: 290-305°C. Charring temperature: 290-305°C.
Equilibrium moisture:
See Figure 13-SI-9.

Academy HPE Laboratory Project Data			
	Method	Lab #	Results
Moisture content	MC-14	28	3.87%[a]
Particle friability			
Metolose SM-15	PF-1	36	0.261[b]
Metolose SM-400	PF-1	36	0.323[b]
Metolose SM-4000	PF-1	36	0.204[b]

Method	% w/w	Meter	Spindle	Factor	Results
VIS-3	2.0	LVT*	2	5	20 cps[c]
Sorption plot	SOR-1	13			Fig:13-SI-9[a]

*Brookfield
Suppliers; Dow[a]; Shin-Etsu[b]; Hercules[c]

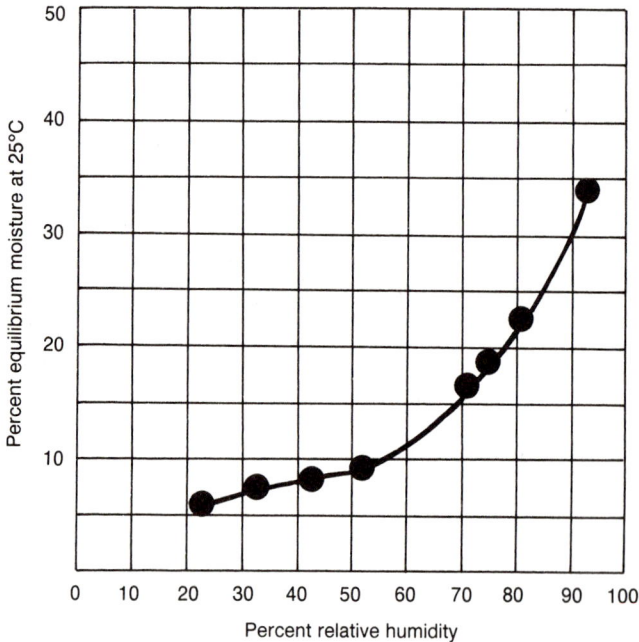

Methylcellulose (DOW, Lot # MM032364-A)
Figure: 13-SI-9   **Method:** SI-1

12. Stability and Storage Conditions

Methylcellulose powder is slightly hygroscopic and should be stored in a well-closed container. Solution is stable to alkalis and dilute acids over a pH range of 2-12 at room temperature. Irreversible decreases in viscosity are caused by heating and cooling. Solutions gel around 55°C. Stored solutions should contain suitable antimicrobial preservatives.

13. Incompatibilities

Incompatibilities have been reported with aminacrine hydrochloride, chlorocresol, mecuric chloride, phenol, resorcinol, tannic acid, silver nitrate, cetylpyridinium chloride, *p*-hydrox benzoic acid, *p*-aminobenzoic acid, methyl *p*-hydroxybenzoate, propyl *p*-hydroxybenzoate and butyl *p*-hydroxybenzoate. Complexation of methylcellulose has also been found with highly surface-active compounds, such as tetracaine and dibutoline sulfate. Large amounts of electrolytes increase the viscosity of methylcellulose mucilages owing to the salting out of methylcellulose. In very high concentrations of electrolytes, the methylcellulose may be completely precipitated in the form of a discrete or continuous gel.

14. Safety

Methylcellulose has a toxicity ranking of 1 (practically nontoxic). The probable oral lethal dose in humans is greater than 15 mg/kg. The FAO/WHO 17th Report on food additives allows up to 25 mg/kg of body weight daily, as sum of total modified celluloses. Methylcellulose is biologically inert aside from mechanical actions. It is not absorbed from the bowel. Given parenterally, methylcellulose produces glomerulonephritis and hypertension in rats.

15. Handling Precautions

Methylcelluloses are organic polymers that will burn under the right conditions of air and oxygen. Good housekeeping is required to prevent dust in the air from reaching possibly explosive levels.

16. Regulatory Acceptance

USP XXI; BP 1980

17. Applications in Pharmaceutical Formulation or Technology

Binder: Low or medium viscosity grades preferred. May be used in solution or as part of a powder mix. May be used to modify disintegration/dissolution patterns. Usual concentration: 1 to 20%.

Gelling agent: High viscosity grades preferred for thickening gels and creams.

Suspending and thickening agent: Used to delay the settling of suspensions and increase contact time of drugs such as antacids in the stomach. Solutions used as replacements for sugar syrups and extemporaneous suspension bases. Low viscosity grades preferred at low concentration, up to 5% for thickening.

Tablet coating: Highly substituted, low viscosity grades are preferred for film coating. Also used for sealing tablet cores prior to sugarcoating.

Disintegrant: High viscosity grades may act as disintegrants by swelling on contact with the disintegration medium. Usual concentration: 2-10% by weight.

Emulsifying agent: Low viscosity grades preferred, as the surface tension of the solution is lower. Usual concentrations: 1-5%.

Ophthalmic solutions: 0.5-1% high viscosity grades are preferred for eye-drop vehicles. Also used for contact lens wetting and soaking solutions.

18. Related Substance

Hydroxypropyl methylcellulose

19. Comments

The material is usually supplied in grades corresponding to a narrow viscosity range for a 2% solution.

20. Specific References

1. Technical Manual CC 1000, British Celanese Ltd., Derby, UK.
2. Handbook on Methocel Cellulose Ether Products (Form No. 192-702-78), The Dow Chemical Co.

USA: S. P. Ericksen*; A. L. Monaco**
UK: F. E. J. Sendall*

Methylparaben

1. Nonproprietary Names
NF: Methylparaben
BP: Methyl hydroxybenzoate
EP: Methylis parahydroxybenzoas

2. Functional Category
NF: Antimicrobial preservative
BP: Antimicrobial preservative

3. Synonyms
Methyl chemosept, Methyl parasept

4. Chemical Names and CAS Registry Number
4-Hydroxybenzoic acid methyl ester
Methyl *p*-hydroxybenzoate [99-76-3]
Methyl 4-hydroxybenzoate

5. Empirical Formula   Molecular Weight
$C_8H_8O_3$ 152.15

6. Structural Formula

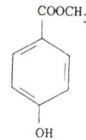

7. Commercial Availability

USA
Bayer
Beta Chemical Corporation
R. W. Greeff & Company, Inc.
Inolex Chemical Co.
Mallinckrodt, Inc.
Naarden
Napp Chemicals
Nipa Labs Inc.
Protameen Chemicals, Inc.
Tenneco Chemical, Inc.
Zimmerli

UK
BDH Chemicals
Nipa Laboratories
Sigma (London) Chemical Co.

8. Method of Manufacture
Methylparaben is prepared by the esterification of *p*-hydroxybenzoic acid with methanol.

9. Description
White, almost odorless powder with a slight burning taste.

SEM: MF-9
Excipient: Methylparaben
Supplier: Bate Chemical Co. Ltd.; Lot No.: N.A.

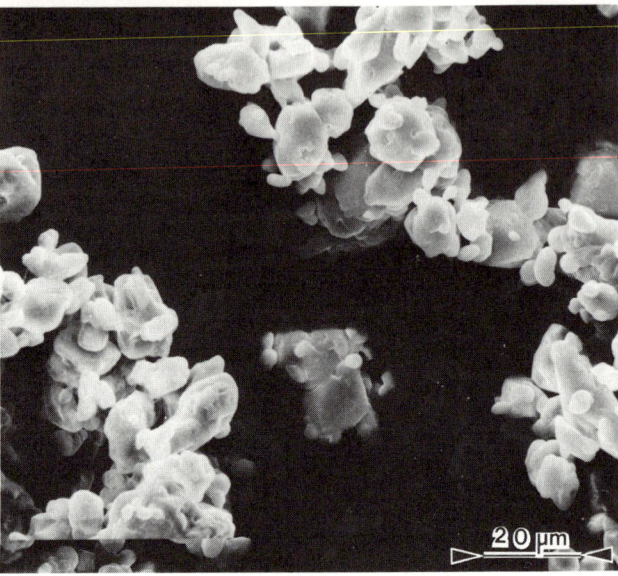

Magnification: 600×

10. Pharmacopeial Specifications

Test	NF	BP/EP
Identification	+	+
Melting range	125–128°C	125–128°C
Acidity	+	+
Loss on drying	≤0.5%	—
Residue on ignition	≤0.05%	—
Assay	99.0–100.5%	99.0–101.0%
Sulfated ash	—	≤0.1%
Clarity & color of solution	—	+

USP Reference standard available

11. Typical Properties
Solubility:

Solvent (at 25°C)	Solubility (g/100 g solvent)
Water	0.25
Methanol	59.0
Propylene Glycol	22.0
Glycerin	1.7
Peanut Oil	0.5
Ether	23.0

pKa Value: 8.4 (22°C)
Oil/Water Partition Coefficients:

Solvent	Oil/Water Partition Coefficient
Liquid Paraffin	0.03
Almond Oil	7.5
Castor Oil	6.0
Lanolin	7.0
Isopropyl Myristate	18.0
Diethyl Adipate	200

Note: Values for vegetable oils vary considerably and are affected by the purity of the oil.

Academy HPE Laboratory Project Data

	Method	Lab #	Results
Solubility (water)	SOL-8	30	0.24%

12. Stability and Storage Conditions

Methylparaben should be stored in a well-closed container. Aqueous solutions at pH 3-6 can be sterilized at 120°C for 20 minutes without decomposition. Aqueous solutions at pH 3-6 are stable (less than 10% decomposition) for up to about four years at room temperature. Aqueous solutions at pH 8 or higher are subject to rapid hydrolysis (10% or more after about 60 days at room temperature).

Predicted rate constant and half-life of hydrolysis at 25°C:

Concentration of HCl (N)	Rate Constant $k \pm \sigma^*$ (HR^{-1})	Half-Life, $t^{1/2} \pm \sigma^*$ (Day)
0.1	$(1.086 \pm 0.0005) \times 10^{-4}$	266 ± 13
0.01	$(1.16 \pm 0.12) \times 10^{-5}$	2490 ± 260
0.001	$(6.1 \pm 1.5) \times 10^{-7}$	47000 ± 12000
0.0001	$(3.27 \pm 0.64) \times 10^{-7}$	88000 ± 17000

* indicates the standard error

Some pharmaceutical preparations containing parabens require autoclave sterilization under pressure at 121.5°C for 20 minutes. Predicted results are shown below:

Concentration of HCl	Rate Constant $k \pm \sigma^*$ (HR^{-1})	Predicted Residual % after Sterilization
0.1	$(4.96 \pm 0.16) \times 10^{-1}$	84.77 ± 0.46
0.01	$(4.49 \pm 0.37) \times 10^{-2}$	98.51 ± 0.12
0.001	$(2.79 \pm 0.57) \times 10^{-3}$	99.91 ± 0.02
0.0001	$(1.49 \pm 0.57) \times 10^{-3}$	99.95 ± 0.01

* indicates the standard error

13. Incompatibilities

The antimicrobial properties of methylparaben are reduced in the presence of nonionic surfactants, a reduction which can be of considerable magnitude. For example, approximately 80% of the total methylparaben present in the aqueous phase is bound, and, thus, inactivated in the presence of 5% Tween 80. Adsorption of methylparaben by plastics has been reported, with the amount adsorbed dependent upon the type of plastic and the vehicle. In general, low and high density polyethylene bottles did not adsorb methylparaben. Propylene glycol (30%) reduced adsorption. Methylparaben is discolored in the presence of iron and subject to hydrolysis by weak alkalis and strong acids.

14. Safety

In rare instances methylparaben can elicit skin sensitization and induce cutaneous allergic responses. Allergy from ingestion or parenteral administration has not been reported. Methylparaben (5% in propylene glycol) causes no primary irritation. The acute and chronic oral toxicity of methylparaben is low.

15. Handling Precautions

—

16. Regulatory Acceptance

NF XVI; BP 1980

17. Applications in Pharmaceutical Formulations or Technology

Methylparaben (0.05 to 0.25%), alone or in combination with other esters of *p*-hydroxybenzoic acid or with other antimicrobial agents, is used as a preservative in cosmetic and pharmaceutical preparations and in foods. Methylparaben [0.18% together with propylparaben (0.02%)] has been used for the preservation of various parenteral drugs. As a rule, the preservative effect is increased in combination with other *p*-hydroxybenzoate esters or by the addition of 2-5% propylene glycol.

18. Related Substances

Butylparaben; ethylparaben; propylparaben.
Sodium methyl hydroxybenzoate (BP), the sodium salt of methylparaben, may be used instead of methylparaben because of its better water solubility, provided the pH of the preserved preparation does not rise.

Molecular Weight: 174.1
Solubility:

Solvent	g/100 g solvent
Water	50
Ethanol (96%)	2

19. Comments

The following tabulation lists the minimal concentration (% in water) of methylparaben required to inhibit growth.

Aerobacter aerogenes ATCC 8308	0.2
Aspergillus aryzae	0.06
Aspergillus niger ATCC 10254	0.1
Bacillus subtilis ATCC 6633	0.2
Bacillus cereus var. *mycoides* ATCC 6462	0.2
Candida albicans ATCC 10231	0.2
Escherichia coli ATCC 9637	0.2
Penicillium digitatum ATCC 10030	0.05
Proteus vulgaris ATCC 8427	0.2
Pseudomonas aeruginosa	0.1
Rhizopus nigricans ATCC 6227A	0.05
Saccharomyces cerevisiae ATCC 9763	0.1
Sarcina lutea	0.4
Staphylococcus aureus ATCC 6538P	0.08
Trichoderma lignorum ATCC 8678	0.025

The antimicrobial effectiveness decreases with increasing pH, due to the formation of phenolate anion.

20. Specific References

1. J. Schimmel and M. N. Slotsky, "Preservation of Cosmetics," 2nd Ed., M. S. Balsam and E. Sagarin, eds., Wiley-Interscience, New York, 1974, Vol. III, pp. 391-470.
2. H. Sokol, Recent developments in the preservation of pharmaceuticals, *Drug Standards*, 20: 89 (1952).
3. C. Matthews *et al.*, *p*-Hydroxybenzoic acid esters as preservatives II, *J. Am. Pharm., Assoc.*, 45: 260 (1956).
4. P. S. Jones *et al.*, *p*-Hydroxybenzoic acid esters as preservatives III, *J. Am. Pharm. Assoc.*, 45: 268 (1956).
5. S. R. Marouchoc, Cosmetic preservation, *Cosmetic Technology*, 2(10): 38-44 (1980).
6. A. Kamada, N. Yata, K. Kubo and M. Arakawa, Stability of *p*-Hydroxybenzoic acid esters in acidic medium, *Chem. Pharm. Bull.*, 21(9): 2073-2076 (1973).
7. E. L. Richardson, Preservatives: Frequency of use in cosmetic formulas as disclosed to FDA, *Cosmetic and Toiletries*, 92: 85-88 (1977).
8. H. B. Kostenbauder, Physical chemical aspects of preservative selection for pharmaceutical and cosmetic emulsions, *Development and Industrial Microbiology*, 1: 286-296 (1962).
9. K. Kakemi, H. Sezaki, E. Arakawa, K. Kimura and K. Ikeda, Interactions of Parabens and other pharmaceutical adjuvants with plastic containers, *Chem. Pharm. Bull.*, 19: 2523-2529 (1971).
10. H. W. Hibbot and J. Monks, Preservatives of emulsions, *J. Soc. Cosm. Chem.*, 12: 2 (1960).
11. T. R. Aalto, M. C. Firman and N. E. Rigler, *p*-Hydroxybenzoic Acid esters as preservatives, *J. Am. Pharm. Assoc.*, 42: 449 (1953). .
12. M. S. Allwood, The adsorption of esters of P-Hydroxybenzoil Acid by magnesium trisilicate, *Inter. J. Pharm.* 11: 101 (1982).

USA:M. Rieger*; P. Kotwal**; Z. Chowhan**
UK: M. C. Allwood*

Mineral Oil

1. Nonproprietary Names

USP: Mineral oil
BP: Liquid paraffin

2. Functional Category

USP: Solvent, oleaginous vehicle
Others: Lubricant for tablets, and mold-release agent for suppositories and capsule shells.

3. Synonyms

Heavy liquid petrolatum; liquid paraffin; liquid petrolatum; white mineral oil.

4. Chemical Name and CAS Registry Number

—

5. Empirical Formula   Molecular Weight

—   —

6. Structural Formula

A mixture of refined liquid hydrocarbons, essentially paraffins and naphthenic in nature, obtained from petroleum. It may contain a suitable stabilizer.

7. Commercial Availability

USA

Ashland Chemical Co.
Bage, Inc.
Camilli, Albert & Laloue
Ingredients International, Inc.
Marathon Morco Co.
McKesson Chemical Co.
Penreco
Ruger Chemical Co.
Strahl & Pitsch, Inc.

UK

Astor Chemicals
Burmah-Castrol Industries, Ltd.
Daltons Ltd.
Fina Chemicals Ltd.

8. Method of Manufacture

The lighter hydrocarbons are removed from petroleum by distillation. The residue is redistilled between 330° and 390°C. The distillate is then chilled and the solid fractions removed by filtration. The filtrate is then further purified and decolorized by high pressure hydrogenation (or sulfuric acid treatment) and filtered through adsorbents. The liquid portion is again distilled, rejecting that portion boiling below 360°C. A suitable stabilizer may be added.

9. Description

Transparent, colorless, viscous liquid. Practically tasteless and odorless when cold. Essentially free from fluorescence in daylight.

10. Pharmacopeial Specifications

Test	USP	BP
Specific gravity	0.845 to 0.905	—
Weight per ml	—	0.830 to 0.890
Viscosity	$\geq$34.5 cSt at 40.0°C	—
Kinematic viscosity	—	$\geq$64* cSt at 37.8°C
Neutrality	+	—
Acidity or alkalinity	—	+
Readily carbonizable substance	+	+
Limit of polynuclear compounds	+	—
Solid paraffin	+	+
Light absorption	—	$\leq$0.10%
Stabilizer addition	Label to indicate	$\leq$10 ppm†

*Kinematic viscosity of tocopherol or butylated hydroxytoluene
†Amount

11. Typical Properties

Solubility: Insoluble in water, glycerin and alcohol; soluble in benzene, chloroform, ether, carbon disulfide and petroleum ether. Miscible with most volatile oils and fixed oils, with the exception of castor oil. The addition of a small amount of a suitable surfactant may promote miscibility/solubilization.
Surface tension: Slightly less than 35 dynes/cm at 25°C
Refractive index: n_D^{20} = 1.4756 to 1.480
Pour point: between −12.2° and −9.4°C
Flash point: beween 210° and 224°C

Academy HPE Laboratory Project Data			
	Method	Lab No.	Results
Ervol[a]	VIS-1	27	47 ± 0.5 cps
Gloria[a]	VIS-1	27	86 ± 1.0 cps
Kaydol[a]	VIS-1	27	163 ± 2.0 cps
Protol[a]	VIS-1	27	75 ± 1.0 cps
Marcol 52[b]	VIS-1	27	10 ± 0.2 cps
Primol 355[b]	VIS-1	27	158 ± 2.0 cps

Suppliers: Witco[a]; Exxon[b]

12. Stability and Storage Conditions

When exposed to light and heat, mineral oil undergoes various reactions, the most common being oxidation. Oxidation begins with the formation of peroxides, and the process exhibits what is commonly known as an induction period. Under ordinary conditions, the induction period may take months or years. Once a trace of peroxide is formed, further oxidation is autocatalytic and proceeds very rapidly. Oxidation results in the formation of aldehydes and organic acids, which impart taste and odor. Stabilizers may be added to retard oxidation. α=Tocopherol, butylated hydroxyanisole (BHA) and butylated hydroxytoluene (BHT) are the most commonly used anti-oxidants. Any substance added as a stabilizer must be named on the label (USP).
Store in an airtight container. Protect from light (BP). Preserve in a tight container (USP).

13. Incompatibilities

Strong oxidizers

14. Safety

Mineral oil is considered safe by the FDA for direct use in food. Chronic use may impair appetite and interfere with the absorption of fat-soluble vitamins. It is absorbed to some extent when emulsified, leading to granulomatous reactions. The latter reactions are also caused upon injection of oil. The use of mineral oil or mineral oil-containing products is not recommended for oral and intranasal use by infants or children because of the possible hazard of causing lipid pneumonia.

15. Handling Precautions

Do not mix or store with strong oxidants. Do not handle or store near heat, sparks or flame. If spilled, recover the free liquid if possible. Add an absorbent to the spill area. Keep out of sewers and watercourses.

16. Regulatory Acceptance

USP XXI; BP 1980. The mineral hydrocarbons in Food Regulations, 1966, and The Mineral Hydrocarbons in Food (Scotland) Regulations, 1966, prohibit, subject to certain exemptions, the use in Great Britain of any mineral hydrocarbon in the composition or preparation of food.

17. Applications in Pharmaceutical Formulation or Technology

Use	Concentration (%)
Ingredient in ointments, creams and emulsions	As required
Solvent for medicinals in soft gelatin capsule	Up to 100

18. Related Substances

Light mineral oil. A variety of mineral oil which has a lower viscosity and a lower specific gravity than mineral oil (USP) or liquid paraffin (BP). Used as a tablet and/or capsule lubricant.

Related Substances Pharmacopeial Specifications

Test	NF
Specific gravity	0.818 to 0.880
Viscosity	$\leq$33.5 centistokes at 40°C
Neutrality	+
Readily carbonizable substances	+
Limit of polynuclear compounds	+
Solid paraffin	+
Stabilizer addition	Label to indicate

Typical Properties of Related Substance

Flash point: 152° to 199°C
Pour point: −9.4° to −1.1°C
Refractive index: n_D^{20}: 1.4577 to 1.4774
Viscosity (at 40°C): 6.5 to 30.2 centistokes

19. Comments

Effect of gamma irradiation: Liquid paraffin, in completely filled soft plastic tubes, showed bubbles of gas after irradiation, the bubbles being larger at the higher level of irradiation (25 Mrad). The iodine value was increased after irradiation at both high and low (2.5-Mrad) levels of irradiation.

20. Specific References:

1. "Oil-Based Effervescent Dentifrice", *French Demande* 2:327,762, May 13, 1977.
2. Antiperspirant composition and its preparation, *Jpn. Kokai Tokyo Koho*, 79(73): 114 (June 12, 1979).
3. E. Regdon, M. Kapas and G. Regdon, Effect of subsidiary materials on the physical properties and drug release of suppositories containing salicylic acid derivatives, *Acta. Pharm. Technol.*, 25: 101 (1979).
4. A.S. Nikolaev, V.A. Chlenov and A.I. Tentsova, Study of the properties of acetylsalicylic acid microcapsules, *Khim-Farm Z.H.*, 12: 121 (1978).
5. "Report of the MRC Carcinogenic Action of Mineral Oils Committee", Special Report Series No. 206, HM Stationery Office, London, 1968.

USA: D.A. Wadke*; G.E. Reier*; N.H. Batuyios**; F.A. Fus**
UK: A.J. Grace*

Mineral Oil and Lanolin Alcohols

1. Nonproprietary Names
Mineral oil and lanolin alcohols

2. Functional Category
W/o primary emulsifier; o/w auxiliary emulsifier or stabilizer; emollient; moisturizer; plasticizer

3. Synonyms
Mineral oil (and) lanolin alcohol (CTFA); *Amerchol L-101*

4. Chemical Name and CAS Registry Number
—

5. Empirical Formula   Molecular Weight
—   —

6. Structural Formula
—

7. Commercial Availability
USA
Amerchol Corporation
UK
D. F. Anstead, Ltd.

8. Method of Manufacture
Lanolin is saponified. The total alcohols are then fractionated, and a fraction containing surface-active alcohols (comprising cholesterol, agnosterol, lanosterol, 7-dehydrocholesterol and cerebrosterol) is extracted. This fraction is dissolved in mineral oil.

9. Description
A pale yellow, oily liquid with a faint characteristic sterol odor. It has an HLB value of about 8.

10. Pharmacopeial Specifications
—

11. Typical Properties
Solubility: Soluble in chloroform to the extent of 50%; soluble in corn oil and castor oil to the extent of 25%. A 1% solution can be made in mineral oil. It is insoluble in water and 95% ethanol and will precipitate in hexane. It is soluble in isopropyl palmitate in concentrations in excess of 10%.
Acid value: ≤ 1
Saponification value: ≤ 2
Hydroxyl value: ≥ 10
Iodine value: ≤ 12
Moisture: $\leq 0.2\%$
Ash: $\leq 0.2\%$
Water-soluble acids and alkalis: The aqueous layer remaining after treatment of the sample is neutral to litmus.
Specific gravity: ≥ 0.840 and ≤ 0.860 at 25°C
Heavy metals: ≤ 20 ppm
Arsenic content: ≤ 2 ppm
Microbiological count: The total bacterial count when packaged is $<10/g$ of sample.

12. Stability and Storage Conditions
Stable; store in a tight container in a cool place.

13. Incompatibilities
—

14. Safety
Acute oral toxicity: Not lethal when administered into the stomach of albino rats at doses ranging from 2.5 to 40 ml/kg of body weight. It has an acute oral LD_{50} in excess of 40.0 ml/kg.
Eye irritation: When instilled into the eyes of albino rats, it was found to be a mild, transient irritant to the rabbit eye when not followed by a washout after instillation. These conjunctival effects cleared within 48-72 hours.
Skin irritation: Found to be a mild irritant to both intact and abraded skin of albino rabbits. When applied to intact human skin in concentrations of from 20% to 100%, the results indicated that it was non-irritating and non-sensitizing.

15. Handling Precautions
—

16. Regulatory Acceptance
CTFA

17. Applications in Pharmaceutical Formulation or Technology

Use	Concentration (%)
Primary emulsifier in w/o creams and lotions	5.0-15.0
Auxiliary emulsifier/stabilizer in o/w creams and lotions	0.5-6.0
Emollient, moisturizer	3.0-6.0

18. Related Substances
Amerchol CAB, Amerchol H-9 and *Amerchol C* are mixtures of lanolin alcohols with petrolatum. They are semi-solids or soft solids and have similar applications to *Amerchol L-101.*

19. Comments
Also used in cosmetic products

20. Specific References
1. Amerchol Laboratory Handbook.
2. Amerchol Lanolin Derivatives.
3. Topicals.
All published and distributed by the manufacturer, Amerchol Corporation.

USA: S. Scheindlin*; J. Cooper**

Monoethanolamine

1. Nonproprietary Names
NF: Monoethanolamine
BP: Ethanolamine

2. Functional Category
Alkalizing agent; emulsifying agent (adjunct)

3. Synonyms
Ethanolamine; β-aminoethyl alcohol; 2-aminoethanol; β-hydroxyethylamine; 2-hydroxyethylamine

4. Chemical Names and CAS Registry Number
2-Aminoethanol [141-43-5]

5. Empirical Formula   Molecular Weight
C_2H_7NO 61.08

6. Structural Formula
$HO\text{-}CH_2\text{-}CH_2\text{-}NH_2$

7. Commercial Availability
USA
BASF
Dow Chemicals Co.
Olin Chemicals
Wyandotte Corp.
UK
Shell Chemical (UK) Ltd.
Unalco, Ltd.

8. Method of Manufacture
Production of the ethanolamines is accomplished by reacting ethylene oxide with ammonia to yield a mixture of the three compounds. By a series of separation procedures, monoethanolamine, diethanolamine and triethanolamine are obtained.

9. Description
Clear, colorless or pale yellow, moderately viscous liquid with mild, ammoniacal odor

10. Pharmacopeial Specifications

Test	NF	BP
Identification	—	+
Specific gravity	1.013-1.016	—
Distilling range	≥95% (167-173°C)	—
Residue on ignition	≤0.1%	—
Refractive index	—	1.453-1.459
Assay range	98.0-100.5%	≥98.0%
Weight per ml	—	1.014-1.023 g
Related substances	—	≤2.0%

11. Typical Properties
Physical properties:
Melting point, °C: 10.5
Boiling point, 760 mm, °C: 170.8
Flash point (open cup), °C: 93.0
Vapor pressure, 20°C, mm Hg: 0.4
Viscosity (absolute), 20°C, cps: 24.1
Surface tension, 20°C, dyn/cm: 48.8
pKa, 25°C: 9.47
pH (0.1N solution):   12.1
Solubility: Miscible with water and with ethanol (96%); slightly soluble in ether.
Hygroscopicity: Very hygroscopic.
Chemical properties: The ethanolamines are characterized by the presence of a basic nitrogen atom and hydroxy group(s). Thus, they are capable of undergoing reactions typical for both amines and alcohols. The amine group usually exhibits the greater activity whenever it is possible for a reaction to take place at either the amine or the hydroxy group. Monoethanolamine is a primary amine and displays the usual properties of this class of nitrogen bases.

12. Stability and Storage Conditions
The ethanolamines present no unusual problems in handling under ordinary conditions. In general, it is advisable to store them in a tight container protected from light, and storage temperatures should not exceed 50°C. Storage in milled steel is satisfactory for a limited time. However, stainless steel should be used if prolonged storage is anticipated. This will prevent discoloration. The color may develop due to the absorption of atmospheric oxygen. Thus, storage tanks should also be gas padded, if color is important. Ethanolamines are hygroscopic. If water content is to be minimized, a dry, inert gas pad under pressure should also be used when ethanolamines are to be stored in tanks.

13. Incompatibilities
Ethanolamines will react with acids to form salts and esters. Monoethanolamine will react with acids, acid anhydrides, acid chlorides and esters to form amide derivatives and with propylene carbonate or other cyclic carbonates to give the corresponding carbonates. As a primary amine, monoethanolamine reacts with aldehydes and ketones to yield aldimines and ketimines. Monoethanolamine reacts with copper to form complex salts. Discoloration and precipitation will take place in the presence of heavy metal salts.

14. Safety
All of the ethanolamines are capable of producing severe eye injuries. They may be health hazards primarily because of their instant action on the skin and in the eyes. The mono- and diethanolamines are also considered to be slightly hazardous from the standpoint of oral administration. Insofar as absorption through the skin is concerned, only pure monoethanolamine has a definite toxicity. In this respect, di- and triethanolamine are much less toxic. The table below summarizes the acute toxicity of monoethanolamine.

Acute oral LD_{50}, g/kg	2.7
Acute dermal LD_{50}, g/kg	2.0

15. Handling Precautions
Personal protective equipment should be used by personnel handling concentrated solutions of ethanolamines. Monoethanolamine has especially corrosive effects on the skin and mucous membranes.

16. Regulatory Acceptance
NF XVI; BP 1980

17. Applications in Pharmaceutical Formulation or Technology
As a pharmaceutical necessity, monoethanolamine is used for various buffering purposes, including the preparation of

emulsions. It can be used as a solvent for fats and oils. It is also being used to form salts with various acids. Monoethanolamine is used to prepare injections of ethanolamine oleate (BP), which is used as a sclerosing agent. A salt of monoethanolamine with vitamin C is used for intramuscular injection. The salicylate and undecenoate monoethanolamine salts are utilized in rheumatism and as a fungistat, respectively. Theophylline forms an additional compound with ethanolamine which is more soluble than theophylline alone. Monoethanolamine (1-8%) stabilized an injectable solution of sodium diphenylhydantoin containing dextrose. (H. C. Schneller, H. J. Levin and S. Sklar, *C. A.* 79, 129089w, 1973).

18. Related Substances

Diethanolamine; triethanolamine

19. Comments

—

20. Specific References

1. "Ethanolamines, Technical Brochure," Jefferson Chemical Co., Inc., 1972.
2. "Ethanolamines, Product Data," Olin Chemicals. "Monoethanolamine, Material Safety Date," Olin Chemicals, 1977.
3. "Ethanolamine Pure, Technical Leaflet," BASF AG, 1969. "Alkanolamines," BASF AG, 1972.

USA: E. Shek*; G. S. Brenner**

Paraffin

1. Nonproprietary Names
NF: Paraffin
BP: Hard paraffin

2. Functional Categories
NF: Stiffening agent
Others: Raises melting point of ointment.

3. Synonyms
Paraffin wax; paraffum durum; paraffum solidum; hard wax.
Note: The title "Paraffum Solidum," in certain pharmacopeias, such as the Swiss, refers to specially refined waxes, such as ceresin.

4. Chemical Name and CAS Registry Number
—

5. Empirical Formula and Molecular Weight
A mixture of hydrocarbons having the general formula C_nH_{2n+2}, obtained from petroleum or shale oil.

6. Structural Formula
See above

7. Commercial Availability
USA
Conoco Chemicals Co., Div. Conoco, Inc.
International Wax Refining Co.
Frank B. Ross Co.
Ruger Chemical Co.
Shell Chemical Co.
William H. Scheel, Inc.

UK
Burmah-Castrol Industries
British Wax Refining Co.
Daltons, Ltd.
Hopkin & Williams
Kerax Ltd.
Shell Chemicals UK Ltd.

8. Method of Manufacture
Manufactured by the distillation of crude petroleum or shale oil, followed by purification by acid treatment and filtration. Paraffins of different properties may be produced by controlling the distillation and subsequent congealing conditions.

9. Description
An odorless, tasteless, translucent, colorless to white solid. It feels slightly greasy and may show a brittle fracture. Microscopically, a mixture of bundles of microcrystals. When melted, it is essentially free of fluorescence, although a slight odor may be apparent. Hard paraffin burns with a luminous, sooty flame.

10. Pharmacopeial Specifications

Test	NF	BP
Identification	+	—
Congealing range	47-65° C	—
Solidifying point	—	50-57° C
Acidity or alkalinity (litmus)	—	+
Readily carbonizable substances	+	—
Sulfated ash	—	≤0.1%

11. Typical Properties
Density at 20°C: Approximately 0.84-0.89 g/cm^3
Solubility/Miscibility: Water: insoluble; ethanol: insoluble; acetone: insoluble; waxes: will mix with most waxes if melted together and cooled; chloroform, ether, oils and fats: soluble, particularly on warming near melting points; stays in solution on cooling.
Melting point: Various melting points (hardnesses) are available to suit users' needs. Pharmacopeial quality is more restricted.

12. Stability and Storage Conditions
Very stable. Store in well-closed containers and avoid exposure to excessive heat.

13. Incompatibilities
None known. Repeated melting/congealing may alter physical properties.

14. Safety
Paraffin presents few, if any, safety or toxicologic problems. It appears to be as inert biologically as it is inert chemically. Topically, paraffin is generally well accepted. If injected, it may cause a granulomatous reaction.

15. Handling Precautions
No restrictions specified.

16. Regulatory Acceptance
NF XVI; BP 1980

17. Applications in Pharmaceutical Formulation or Technology
As a component of creams and ointments. In the latter, it adds "body," that is, stiffens the ointment.

18. Related Substances
Petrolatum; purified waxes

19. Comments
Many of the uses of hard paraffin are being usurped by more highly purified waxes with specifically controlled properties of hardness, malleability, melting range, etc.

20. Specific References
—

USA: Z. Chowhan*
UK: A. J Grace**

Peanut Oil

1. Nonproprietary Names
NF: Peanut oil
BP: Arachis oil

2. Functional Category
NF: Solvent and oleaginous vehicle

3. Synonyms
Ground-nut oil; nut oil; earth-nut oil

4. Chemical Name and CAS Registry Number
Peanut oil — —

5. Empirical Formula and Molecular Weight
—

6. Structural Formula
A typical analysis of refined peanut oil indicates the composition of the acids, present as glycerol esters, to be: palmitic acid, 8.3%; stearic acid, 3.1%; arachidic acid, 2.4%; oleic acid, 56.0%; linoleic acid, 26.0%; behenic acid, 3.1%; and lignoceric acid, 1.1%.

7. Commercial Availability
USA

Camilli, Albert and Laloue
Canada Packers, Inc., Chemical Div.
Dormar Chemicals, Inc.
Ingredients International, Inc.
Ruger Chemical Co.
Tri-K Industries, Inc.
Welch, Holme & Clark Co.

UK

J. Bibby & Sons, Ltd.
M. Hamburger & Sons, Ltd.
E.J.R. Lovelock, Ltd.

8. Method of Manufacture
The refined peanut oil is obtained from the seeds of *Arachis hypogaea* (leguminosae). The seeds are separated from the peanut shells and are exposed to powerful expression in hydraulic presses. The crude oil thus obtained has a light yellow to light brown color. It requires purification before it is suitable for food or medicinal purposes.

9. Description
The colorless or pale yellow liquid has a faint nutty odor and a bland, nutty taste. At about 3°C it becomes cloudy, and partially solidifies at lower temperatures.

10. Pharmacopeial Specifications

Test	NF	BP
Acid value	—	≤0.5
Identification	+	+
Iodine value	84–100	86–106
Heavy metals	0.001%	—
Refractive index	1.462–1.464 at 40°C	1.468–1.472 at 19.5°C–20.5°C
Cottonseed oil	+	+
Sesame oil	—	+
Rancidity	+	—
Free fatty acids	+	—
Saponification value	185–195	188–196
Solidification range of fatty acids	26°–33°	—
Unsaponifiable matter	≤1.5%	—
Specific gravity at 20°C	0.912–0.920	—
Weight per ml		0.909–0.916

11. Typical Properties
Solubility: Almost insoluble in alcohol (95%); miscible with solvent ether, petroleum ether, chloroform, and light petroleum; soluble in benzene, carbon tetrachloride and oils.

Academy HPE Laboratory Project Data		
Method	Lab No.	Results
Viscosity		
VIS-2	30	39.44 cps[a]
VIS-2	30	42.96 cps[b]
Specific gravity		
DE-5	30	0.914[a]
DE-5	30	0.915[b]

Suppliers: Capital[a]; Welch[b]

12. Stability and Storage Conditions
Peanut oil is stable. It should be kept in an air-tight, light-resistant container, and exposure to excessive heat should be avoided. On exposure to air, peanut oil thickens very slowly and may become rancid. If it has solidified, it should be completely melted and mixed before use.

13. Incompatibilities
No citations in the literature.

14. Safety
Acute skeletal muscle necrosis and renal failure occurred in a 22-year-old man with a recent history of multiple drug abuse following intravenous administration of nearly 4 g of arachis oil.

15. Handling Precautions
Slight fire hazard.

16. Regulatory Acceptance
NF XVI; BP 1980

17. Applications in Pharmaceutical Formulation or Technology

Use	Concentration
Solvent for intramuscular injection	as required
Vehicle for liniments, ointments and soaps	as required

18. Related Substances
Cottonseed oil; corn oil; sesame oil

19. Comments
Peanut oil is sterilized by maintaining it at 150°C for one hour or by aseptic filtration.

20. Specific References:
None

USA: A. Rahman*; D. Sanvordeker**; F. A. Chrzanowski**

Petrolatum

1. Nonproprietary Names

USP: White petrolatum, petrolatum
BP/EP: White soft paraffin, yellow soft paraffin

2. Functional Category

USP: Ointment base
Other: Topical protective, emollient, sun-screen

3. Synonyms

Petroleum jelly; white petroleum jelly, yellow petrolatum, yellow petroleum jelly. Some pharmacopeias use the titles vaselinum album or vaselinum flavum. In the United States, the United Kingdom and many other countries, *Vaseline* is a trademark.

4. Chemical Name and CAS Registry Number

—

5. Empirical Formula and Molecular Weight

Primarily, C_nH_{2n+2}, in which chain branching is common. Petrolatum may also contain some cyclic alkanes and aromatics with paraffin side chains. The average molecular weight is dependent on the source. Petrolatum has been separated into n-, iso- and cyclic-paraffin fractions (2).

6. Structural Formula

See above

7. Commercial Availability

USA

Exxon Co., U.S.A.
McKesson Chemical Co.
Penreco, Division of Penzoil Oil Company
Quad Chemical-Lonsa Specialty Chemicals
Ruger Chemical Co.
Technical Petroleum Co.
Witco Chemical Corp., Sonneborn Div.

UK

Astor Chemicals, Ltd.
British Wax Refining Company, Ltd.
Burmah-Castrol Industries Ltd.
Fina Chemicals, Ltd.

8. Method of Manufacture

Petrolatum is manufactured from the semi-solid material that is left from the steam or vacuum distillation of petroleum. This residue is de-waxed and/or blended with stock from other sources and lighter fractions to give the appropriate consistency. Final purification is done by a combination of high-pressure hydrogenation (or sulfuric acid treatment) and filtration through adsorbents. White petrolatum is more highly refined than the yellow.

9. Description

Petrolatum is an unctuous, soft mass. White petrolatum is white to faintly yellow in color, while yellow petrolatum is pale yellow to yellow. Both types are odorless and almost tasteless, transparent in thin layers and not more than slightly fluorescent in daylight, even when melted.

10. Pharmacopeial Specifications

Test	USP	BP
Petrolatum-Yellow:		
Acidity or alkalinity	—	+
Light absorption (.05% soln)	—	≤0.75
Melting range	38°-60°C	38°-56°C
Foreign organic matter	—	+
Sulfated ash	—	≤0.1%
Specific gravity (at 60°C)	0.815-0.880	—
Alkalinity	+	—
Acidity	+	—
Residue on ignition	≤0.1%	—
Organic acids	+	—
Fixed oils, fats & rosin	+	—
Color	+	—
Consistency	100-300	—
Petrolatum-White:		
Acidity or alkalinity	—	+
Light absorption (.05% soln)	—	≤0.5
Melting range	38°-60°C	38°-56°
Foreign organic matter	—	+
Organic acids	+	—
Consistency	100-300	—
Residue on ignition	≤0.05%	—
Specific gravity	0.815-0.880	—
Alkalinity	+	—
Acidity	+	—
Fixed oil, fats & rosin	+	—
Sulfated ash	—	≤0.1%
Color	+	—

11. Typical Properties

Congealing point: between 48° and 51°C
Consistency: between 100 and 300 (Penetration Test: 10-30 mm)
Viscosity @ 98.9°C.:
White petrolatum: between 60 and 75 S.U.S.*
Yellow petrolatum: between 57 and 82 S.U.S.*
*Saybolt Universal Seconds
Color (Maximum, Lovibond Color–2″ Cell):
White petrolatum: 0.5 to 18 Y, 0.5 R
Yellow petrolatum: 35 Y, 7 R
Solubility: Almost insoluble in water, hot or cold alcohol, dehydrated alcohol, acetone and glycerol. Soluble in benzene, chloroform, ether, hexane, carbon disulfide, petroleum ether, turpentine oil and most fixed and volatile oils. The solution sometimes shows slight opalescence. An alcoholic extract is neutral to litmus.

The rheological properties of petrolatum are determined by the ratio of the three paraffin fractions, namely n-, iso- and cyclic-paraffins, to each other. Petrolatum, having a relatively lower content of n-paraffins and a higher content of iso-paraffins, is considered most suitable for use as a base in pharmaceutical ointments.

A rheological study of white petrolatum, USP, and white ointment, USP, has been reported to indicate that the spreading characteristics of these materials are related to their structural composition.

Academy HPE Laboratory Project Data Petrolatum, White			
	Method	Lab #	Results
18 Batches	PEN-1	4	180-286
19 Batches	PEN-1	4	150-280
Supplier: Penn Refining			

12. Stability and Storage Conditions

Preserve in a well-closed container. Petrolatums are inherently very stable because of the unreactive nature of their hydrocarbon components. Most stability problems are related to the presence of small quantities of impurities. These impurities may be oxidized by light to give a slight discoloration of the petrolatum and an undesirable odor. Recognizing this, the USP/NF allows a suitable stabilizer, such as α-tocopherol or butylated hydroxytoluene (BHT), to be added. The magnitude of the oxidation problem depends on the source and degree of refinement. It is inadvisable to heat petrolatum above 70°C or above the temperature of complete fluidity for extended periods.

Some attempts have been made to sterilize petrolatums using radiation. Although this can be done, the stability of the petrolatum to the radiation is not good. The radiation produces swelling, discoloration, odor and changes in the rheological properties of the petrolatum.

13. Incompatibilities

Because of its inert nature, petrolatum has few incompatibilites.

14. Safety

Petrolatum presents few, if any, safety or toxicologic problems. It appears to be as biologically inert as it is chemically inert. Its irritancy rating on skin is low. It has been implicated in a few rare allergic reactions, and may cause acne in susceptible individuals if used repeatedly on facial skin. No carcinogenic or any other toxic response resulted in mice undergoing single subcutaneous administration of 100 mg. of petrolatum blends. Similarly, no toxic effects were observed in a two-year rat study from the chronic feeding of diets containing 5% of petrolatum blends. Petrolatum has been tentatively implicated in the formation of spherulosis of the upper respiratory tract when a petrolatum-based ointment was used in packing after surgery. Injection into soft tissues causes granulomas. Taken orally it acts as a mild laxative, and may inhibit the absorption of lipids and lipid-soluble nutrients. In general, however, toxic effects are rare when petrolatum is used in the usual way as a topical ointment base or protective.

15. Handling Precautions

No restrictions specified.

16. Regulatory Acceptance

USP XXI; BP 1980

17. Applications in Pharmaceutical Formulation or Technology

Petrolatum is used primarily as an ointment base. Although it is usually combined with other ingredients to achieve the desired properties, it serves as the primary base for some of the official ointments. The BP lists a total of 14 or more monographs which include either white or yellow, or both, petrolatums. Although some of these ointments serve strictly for their emollient properties, in a majority of them petrolatum serves as a vehicle for the active drug substance. It has also been used as a base for ophthalmic ointments, and two such preparations are official in the BP. There are at least five official preparations in the USP containing petrolatum. These are white ointment, yellow ointment, hydrophilic ointment, hydrophilic petrolatum and petrolatum gauze.

Petrolatum is also used as an emollient in cream formulations. There are at least six such cream formulations official in the BP.

Guideline for use in ointments and creams:

Applications	Concentrations
Ointment base	up to 100%
Creams, etc. (as an emollient)	10% to 30%

18. Related Substances

Hard Paraffin, BP, is a mixture of solid hydrocarbons obtained from petroleum.

Liquid Paraffin, BP, is a mixture of liquid hydrocarbons obtained from petroleum.

19. Comments

Petrolatum USP refers to yellow petrolatum, while petrolatum is official in the USP as petrolatum, white. Petrolatum is a mixture of hydrocarbons characterized primarily by its semi-solid nature and inertness. It may exhibit a range of properties, depending on the composition of the mixture, which in turn depends on the starting material and the method of preparation. This means that a tabulation of properties can only give approximate values. Exact values can only be specified for a particular sample of petrolatum. Manufacturers can control the properties of their various grades of petrolatum within narrower limits, and their specifications should be consulted for the properties of a specific grade. USP allows petrolatum to contain a suitable stabilizer. Care is required in heating petrolatum because of its large coefficient of thermal expansion. It has been shown by both rheological and spectrophotometric methods that soft paraffins undergo phase transition at temperatures between 30° and 40°C. Additives, such as microcrystalline waxes, may be used to add body to the petrolatum.

20. Specific References

1. B. W. Barry and A. J. Grace, Grade variation in the rheology of white soft paraffin, BP, *J. Pharm. Pharmacol.*, 22: Supp., 147S (1970).
2. K. E. Schulte and M. A. Kassem, *Pharm. Acta. Helv.*, 38: 358 (1963).
3. J. C. Boylan, Rheological estimation of the spreading characteristics of pharmaceutical semi-solids, *J. Pharm. Sci.*: 56, 1164 (1967).
4. A. R. Longworth and J. D. French, Quality control of white soft paraffin, *J. Pharm. Pharmacol.*, 21: Supp. 1 (1969).
5. S. S. Davis, M. S. Khander, I. Adams, I. R. Colley, J. Cammack and P. Sanford, Effect of gamma radiation on rheological properties of pharmaceutical semi-solids, *J. Texture Studies*, 8: (1), 61 (1977).
6. B. P. Jacob and K. Leupin, Sterilization of eye-nose ointments by gamma radiation, *Pharm. Acta. Helv.*, 49: 12 (1974).
7. P. J. Frosch and A. M. Kligman, *Cutaneous Toxicity*, V. A. Drill and P. Lazar, Eds., Academic Press, New York, 1977, p. 127.
8. A. R. Verhagen, Pomade acne in black skin, *Arch. Dermatol.*, 110: (3), 465 (1974).
9. B. L. Oser, M. Oser and S. Carson, Toxicologic studies of petrolatum in mice and rats, *Toxicol. Appl. Pharmacol.*, 7: (13), 382 (1965).
10. J. Rosai, The nature of myospherulosis of the upper respiratory tract, *J. Am. Clin. Pathology*, 69, 475 (1978).
11. G. Barker, New trends in formulating with mineral oil and petrolatum, *Cosmetic and Toiletries*, 92: 43 (1977).
12. B. W. Barry and A. J. Grace, Structural, rheological and textural properties of soft paraffins, *J. Texture Studies*, 2: 259 (1971).

USA: H. L. Wells*; D. M. Baaske**; A. Y. Gore**
UK: A.J. Grace*

Petrolatum and Lanolin Alcohols

1. Nonproprietary Name
Petrolatum and lanolin alcohols

2. Functional Categories
Absorption base component; emollient; moisturizer; plasticizer

3. Synonyms
Petrolatum (and) lanolin alcohol (CTFA)

4. Chemical Name and CAS Registry Number
—

5. Empirical Formula   Molecular Weight
—   —

6. Structural Formula
—

7. Commercial Availability
USA
Amerchol Corporation

UK
D. F. Anstead, Ltd.

8. Method of Manufacture
Lanolin is saponified. The total alcohols are then fractionated, and a fraction containing surface-active alcohols (comprising cholesterol, agnosterol, lanosterol, 7-dehydrocholesterol, and cerebrosterol) is extracted. This fraction is then blended with petrolatum.

9. Description
A pale ivory, soft solid with a faint, characteristic sterol odor.

10. Pharmacopeial Specifications
Not official

11. Typical Properties
Solubility: Soluble to the extent of about 5% in chloroform and about 1% in mineral oil. It will precipitate at higher concentrations. It precipitates in water, 95% ethanol and hexane, and will form a gel in corn oil and castor oil. It can be dispersed in isopropyl palmitate.
Acid value: ≤ 1
Saponification value: ≤ 2
Hydroxyl value: ≥ 11 and ≤ 15
Moisture: $\leq 0.2\%$
Ash: $\leq 0.2\%$
Water-soluble acids and alkalis: The aqueous layer remaining after treatment of the sample is neutral to litmus. It has an HLB value of about 9.
Melting range: 40–46°C

Heavy metals: ≤ 20 ppm
Arsenic content: ≤ 2 ppm
Microbiological count: The total bacterial count when packaged is ≤ 10 per gram of sample.

Academy NHPE Laboratory Project Data Amerchol CAB		
Method	Lab #	Results
PEN-1	4	131.4

Supplier: Amerchol Co.

12. Stability and Storage Conditions
Stable; store in a tight container in a cool place.

13. Incompatibilities
No citations in the literature.

14. Safety
Acute oral toxicity: Not lethal when administered into the stomach of albino rats at doses ranging from 2.5 to 40 ml/kg of body weight. It has an acute oral LD_{50} in excess of 40 ml/kg.
Eye irritation: When instilled into the eyes of albino rabbits it was found to be a mild, transient irritant when not followed by a washout. This irritation disappeared within 48-72 hours.
Skin irritation: Found to be mildly irritating to both abraded and nonabraded skins of albino rabbits. When applied to intact human skin in concentrations ranging from 20 - 100%, the results indicated that it was nonirritating and nonsensitizing.

15. Handling Precautions
No restrictions specified.

16. Regulatory Acceptance
—

17. Applications in Pharmaceutical Formulation or Technology

Use	Concentration (%)
Absorption base component	10.0-50.0
Emollient, moisturizer, plasticizer in ointments	5.0-50.0

18. Related Substances
Amerchol L-101; Amerchol H-9; Amerchol C

19. Comments
A soft solid which is used in hypoallergenic preparations. It is suitable for use in medium-to-heavy creams and lotions. It is also used to aid the release of active ingredients. It will improve contact with tissue surfaces and maintain the natural condition of skin. It can also absorb serous exudates.

20. Specific References
1. Amerchol Laboratory Handbook.
2. Amerchol Lanolin Derivatives.
3. Topicals.
(All published and distributed by the manufacturer, Amerchol Corporation.)

USA: S. Scheindlin*; J. Cooper**

Phenylethyl Alcohol

1. Nonproprietary Name
USP: Phenylethyl alcohol

2. Functional Category
USP: Antimicrobial preservative

3. Synonyms
Phenethyl alcohol; benzyl carbinol; β-phenylethyl alcohol; β-hydroxyethyl benzene; benzene ethanol

4. Chemical Names and CAS Registry Number
Benzene ethanol
Phenylethyl alcohol [60-12-8]

5. Empirical Formula   Molecular Weight
$C_8H_{10}O$ 122.17

6. Structural Formula

7. Commercial Availability
USA

Aroma Resources, Div. of Biddle Sawyer Corp.
Chemical Dynamics Corp.
Floressence Perfumes Oils, Inc.
GAF Corp.
Givaudan Corp.
ICN K & K Labs, Inc.
International Flavors & Fragrances, Inc. (IFF)
Norda, Inc.
Orbis Products Corp.
Pfaltz and Bauer, Inc.
Polarome Mfg. Co.
Ungerer & Co.

UK

BASF (UK), Ltd.
Bush Boake Allen Ltd.
Givaudan and Co. Ltd.
Koch-Light Laboratories, Ltd.
Kodak, Ltd.

8. Method of Manufacture
Reduction of ethyl phenylacetate with sodium in absolute alcohol; hydrogenation of phenylacetaldehyde in the presence of a nickel catalyst; addition of ethylene oxide or ethylene chlorohydrin to phenylmagnesium bromide, followed by hydrolysis; phenylethyl alcohol occurs naturally in etheric oils (especially attar of roses).

9. Description
Clear, colorless liquid with an odor of rose oil. It has a burning taste which irritates and then anesthetizes mucous membranes.

10. Pharmacopeial Specifications

Test	USP
Identification	+
Specific gravity	1.017-1.020
Refractive index	1.531-1.534(20°C)
Residue on ignition	≤0.005% w/v
Chlorinated compounds	+
Aldehyde	+

11. Typical Properties
Antimicrobial activity: Moderate activity and relatively slow acting; not sufficiently active to be used alone.
Bacteria: Fair activity against gram positive bacteria; for *Staphylococcus aureus*, the MIC may be more than 5 mg/ml. Greater activity is shown against gram negative organisms. Typical MIC values are: *Salmonella typhi* 1.25 mg/ml; *Pseudomonas aeruginosa* 2.5 mg/ml; *Escherichia coli* 5.0 mg/ml. *Spores:* Inactive, e.g., at 0.6%, reported to be ineffective against spores of *Bacillus stearothermophilus* at 100°C for 30 minutes. *Molds and fungi:* Poor activity.
Effect of pH: Greatest activity at pH values below 5; inactive above pH 8.
Boiling point: 219-221°C
Freezing point: −27°C
Partition coefficients: Chloroform–water: 15.2; octanol–water: 21.5; heptane–water: 0.58.
Solubility/miscibility:

Solvent	Solubility (at 25°C)
Water	1 part in 60 parts
Ethanol (50%)	1 part in 1 part
Propylene glycol	Very soluble
Fixed oils	Miscible
Ether	Miscible
Liquid paraffin	Slightly soluble
Glycerin	Very soluble

Flash point: 102°C

12. Stability and Storage Conditions
Phenylethyl alcohol is stable in bulk, but is volatile and sensitive to light and oxidizing agents. It is reasonably stable in both acidic and alkaline solutions. Aqueous solutions may be sterilized by autoclaving. Store in a well-closed container, protected from light and in a cool place. If stored in low density polyethylene containers, phenylethyl alcohol may be taken up by the containers. Losses to polypropylene containers have been reported to be insignificant over 12 weeks at 30°C. Sorption to rubber closures is generally small.

13. Incompatibilities
Oxidizing agents; protein (e.g., serum); partially inactivated by polysorbates, but to a lesser extent than hydroxybenzoate esters.

14. Safety
LD_{50} (oral) in rats is 1,790 mg/kg. At concentrations used to preserve eye drops (about 0.5% w/v) or above, eye irritation may be experienced.

15. Handling Precautions
Slight fire hazard; avoid heat and oxidizing materials.

16. Regulatory Acceptance
USP XXI

17. Applications in Pharmaceutical Formulation or Technology

Preservative for parenteral and ophthalmic preparations, frequently at concentrations of 0.25 to 0.5% w/v in combination with other preservatives. Synergistic response has been claimed for combinations with benzalkonium chloride, chlorhexidine gluconate or diacetate, polymixin B sulfate and phenylmercuric nitrate. With either benzalkonium chloride or chlorhexidine, synergistic effects were observed against *Pseudomonas aeruginosa* and apparently additive effects against gram positive organisms. With phenylmercuric nitrate, the effect was additive against *Pseudomonas aeruginosa*. Phenylethyl alcohol has been used alone at concentrations up to 1% w/v in topical preparations (as an antimicrobial agent). Perfumery component (especially in rose perfumes).

18. Related Substances

None

19. Comments

Was also described in a monograph in the Nordic Pharmacopeia.

20. Specific References

1. C. K. Bahal and H. B. Kostenbauder, *J. Pharm. Sci.*, 53: 1027 (1964).
2. S.W. Goldstein, *J. Amer. Pharm. Ass., Pract. Ed.*, 14: 498 (1953).
3. W. H. Heller, N. E. Foss, D. E. Shay and C. T. Ichniowski, *J. Amer. Pharm. Ass., Pract. Ed.*, 16: 29 (1955).
4. S. R. Kohn, L. Gershenfeld and M. Barr, *J. Pharm. Sci.*, 52: 967 (1963).
5. B. D. Lilley and J. H. Brewer, *J. Amer. Pharm. Ass., Sci. Ed.*, 42: 6 (1953).
6. Murphy, *et al*, *Arch. Ophth.*, 53: 63 (1955).
7. R. M. E. Richards and R. J. McBride, *J. Pharm. Sci.*, 61: 1075 (1972).
8. R. M. E. Richards and R. J. McBride, *J. Pharm. Sci.*, 62: 585 (1973).
9. R. M. E. Richards and R. J. McBride, *J. Pharm. Sci.*, 62: 2035 (1973).
10. R. M. E. Richards and R. J. McBride, *J. Pharm. Sci.*, 63: 54 (1974).
11. S. Silver and L. Wendt, *J. Bact.*, 93: 560 (1967).

USA: S. Scheindlin*; J. Mennonna*; D. Hovermale**; J. Mollica**
UK: M. C. Allwood*; R. M. E. Richards*; J. Emerson**

Phenylmercuric Acetate

1. Nonproprietary Name
NF: Phenylmercuric acetate
BPC: Phenylmercuric acetate

2. Functional Category
USP: Antimicrobial preservative
BPC: Antibacterial and antifungal agent

3. Synonym
Acetoxyphenylmercury

4. Chemical Names and CAS Registry Number
Mercury, (acetato)phenyl
(Acetato)phenylmercury
, [62-38-4]

5. Empirical Formula   Molecular Weight
$C_8H_8HgO_2$ 336.74

6. Structural Formula

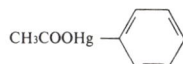

7. Commercial Availability

USA

Atomergic Chemetals Corp.
Burlington Bio-Medical Corp.
Conray Chemicals, Inc.
ICN K & K Labs, Inc.
Pfaltz and Bauer, Inc.
Ruger Chemical Co.
Uhe Co., George

UK

BDH Chemicals, Ltd.
Fisons Scientific Apparatus Ltd.
Koch-Light Laboratories, Ltd.
Steetley Chemicals Ltd.

8. Method of Manufacture
Phenylmercuric acetate is readily formed by heating benzene with mercuric acetate.

9. Description
Phenylmercuric acetate occurs as a white to creamy white, odorless or almost odorless, crystalline powder, or as small white prisms or leaflets.

SEM-MF-16
Excipient: Phenylmercuric acetate
Supplier: Eastman Chemicals

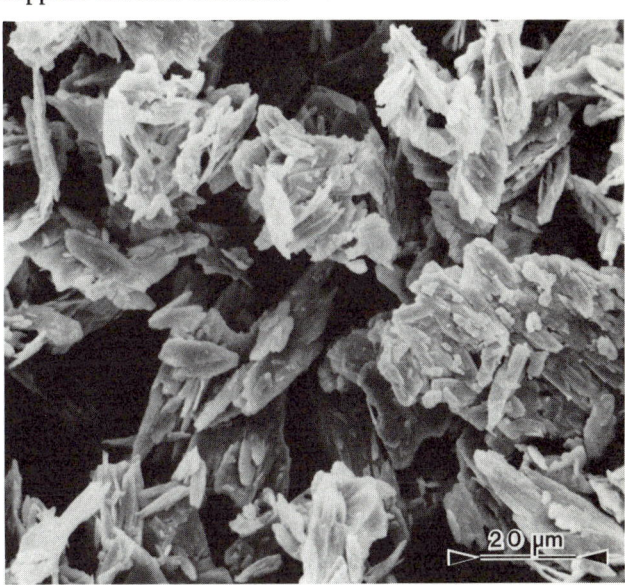

Magnification: 600×

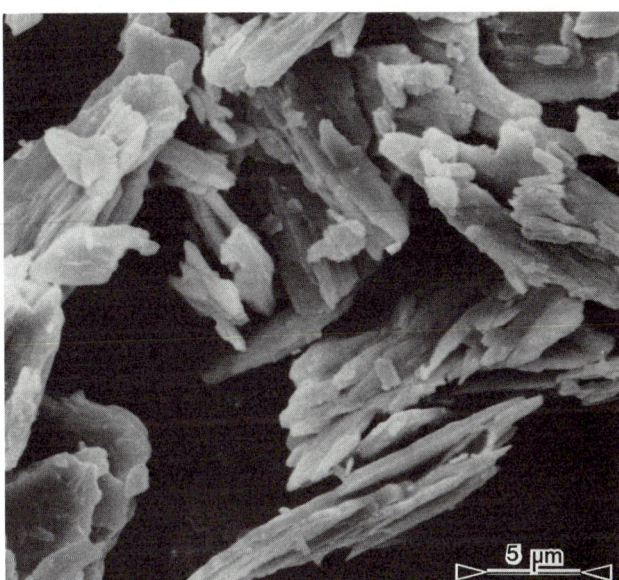

Magnification: 1,800×

10. Pharmacopeial Specifications

Test	NF	BPC
Identification	+	+
Assay	98.0–100.5%	≥98.0%
Mercury salts and heavy metals	+	+
Polymercurated benzene compounds	≤1.5%	≤1.5%
Melting range	149–153°C	149–153°C
Residue on ignition	≤0.2%	—
Sulfated ash	—	≤0.2%

11. Typical Properties

Acidity/alkalinity: (saturated aqueous solution) pH about 4
Antimicrobial activity: See phenylmercuric nitrate
Partition coefficient: Liquid paraffin: water = 0.1
Solubility:

Solvent		Solubility* (at 25°C unless otherwise stated)
Water	(20°C)	1 in 600
		1 in 200 (slightly soluble)
Ethanol	(20°C)	1 in 24
		1 in 225 (sparingly soluble)
Acetone	(20°C)	1 in 19
Chloroform		1 in 30
		1 in 6.8 (slightly soluble)
Ether		1 in 220

*Compendial values for solubility vary considerably and in most instances do not show close agreement with laboratory-determined values, which also vary. Descriptive terms (in parentheses) are appropriate to the solubility ranges determined experimentally.

12. Stability and Storage Conditions

All phenylmercuric compound solutions form a black residue of metallic mercury when exposed to light or after prolonged storage. Solutions may be sterilized by autoclaving. Phenylmercuric acetate should be stored in a tight, light-resistant container.

13. Incompatibilities

Phenylmercuric acetate may precipitate from acidic solutions. Phenylmercuric ion is incompatible with halide ions, particularly bromides and iodides, with which it forms less-soluble halogen compounds. At concentrations of 0.002%, precipitation may not occur in the presence of chlorides. It is also incompatible with aluminum and other metals, ammonia and ammonium salts and some sulfur-containing compounds (e.g., in rubber). Its antimicrobial activity may be reduced in the presence of anionic emulsifying agents and suspending agents. Organic mercurials are sorbed or otherwise removed from dilute aqueous solutions by rubber and plastic packaging components. Uptake is usually greatest to natural rubbers and polyethylene, and least to polypropylene.

14. Safety

LD_{50} (orally in rats): 30 mg/kg.
LD_{50} (orally in mice): 50 mg/kg.
Human toxicity—Local application in concentrated form may cause irritation and give rise to erythema and blistering 6 to 12 hours later.

15. Handling Precautions

Protect from ingestion, inhalation and contact with skin and eyes.

16. Regulatory Acceptance

NF XVI; BPC 1973

17. Applications in Pharmaceutical Formulation or Technology

Use	Concentration (%)
Bactericide in parenterals and eye drops	0.001–0.002
Spermicide in vaginal suppositories and jellies	0.02

18. Related Substances

Phenylmercuric nitrate; phenylmercuric benzoate; phenylmercuric borate; phenylmercuric chloride

19. Comments

—

20. Specific References

See phenylmercuric nitrate

USA: R. El-Rashidy*, J. Cooper*, D. Hovermale**
UK: M. C. Allwood*, S. Malcolm*, J. Emerson**, W. Lund**

Phenylmercuric Borate

1. Nonproprietary Name
BP/EP: Phenylmercuric borate

2. Functional Category
BP/EP: Antimicrobial preservative; antiseptic

3. Synonyms
Phenylmercuriborate; phenomerborum

4. Chemical Names and CAS Registry Number
Orthoborato(1-)-0-phenylmercury
(Dihydrogen borato)phenylmercury   [102-98-7]

5. Empirical Formula

		Molecular Weight
The BP 1980 material is an equi-molecular compound of phenyl-mercury hydroxide with either of the following borates, or a mixture of both:		
Phenylmercury orthoborate	$C_{12}H_{13}Hg_2B_4O$	633.2
Phenylmercury metaborate	$C_{12}H_{11}Hg_2B_3O$	615.2

6. Structural Formula

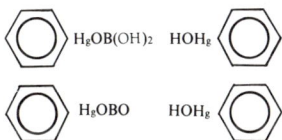

7. Commercial Availability
USA
Atomergic Chemetals Corp.
Burlington Bio-Medical Corp.
Pfaltz & Bauer, Inc.
Ruger Chemical Co.
Uhe Co., George

UK
Sigma London Chemical Co. Ltd.
Ward Blenkinsop Trading, Ltd.

8. Method of Manufacture
Heating benzene with mercuric borate. Evaporating to dry-ness under vaccum an alcoholic solution containing equimo-lar proportions of phenylmercuic hydroxide and boric acid.

9. Description
Colorless, shiny flakes or white or slightly yellow crystalline powder. Odorless.

10. Pharmacopeial Specifications

Test	BP
Identification	+
Clarity and color of solution	+
Ionized Mercury (as heavy metals)	≤50 ppm
Loss on drying (at 45°C)	≤3.5%
Assay: Mercury (Hg)	64.5-66.0%
Borates (H_3BO_3)	9.8-10.3%

11. Typical Properties
Acidity/alkalinity: (0.6% solution) pH 5.0-7.0
Antimicrobial activity: See phenylmercuric nitrate.
Melting point: 112-113°C
Solubility:

Solvent		Solubility* at 25°C unless otherwise stated
Water	(20°C)	1 in 125
		1 in 500
	(25°C)	1 in 500
	(100°C)	1 in 100
Ethanol	(20°C)	1 in 150
Propylene glycol		Soluble
Glycerol		Soluble

*Compendial values for solubility vary considerably.

12. Stability and Storage Conditions
All phenylmercuric compound solutions form a black resi-due of metallic mercury when exposed to light or after prolonged storage. Solutions may be sterilized by autoclav-ing. Phenylmercuric borate should be stored in a tight, light-resistant container.

13. Incompatibilities
Phenylmercuric borate may precipitate from acidic solu-tions. Phenylmercuric ion is incompatible with halide ions, particularly bromides and iodides, with which it forms less-soluble halogen compounds. At concentrations of 0.002%, precipitation may not occur in the presence of chlorides. It is also incompatible with aluminum and other metals, am-monia and ammonium salts and with some sulfur-contain-ing compounds (e.g., in rubber). Its antimicrobial activity may be reduced in the presence of anionic emulsifying agents and suspending agents. Organic murcurials are sorbed or otherwise removed from dilute aqueous solutions by rubber and plastic packaging components. Uptake is usually greatest to natural rubbers and polyethylene, and least to polypropylene.

14. Safety
Human toxicity—local application in concentrated form may cause irritation and give rise to erythema and blistering 6 to 12 hours later.

15. Handling Precautions
Protect from ingestion, inhalation and contact with the skin and eyes.

16. Regulatory Acceptance
BP/EP 1982 Addendum

17. Application in Pharmaceutical Formulations or Technology

Use	Concentration (%)
Antimicrobial agent in parenterals	0.002–0.125
Antimicrobial agent in ophthalmics	0.002–0.004

18. Related Substances
Phenylmercuric acetate, phenylmercuric benzoate, phenylmercuric nitrate, phenylmercuric chloride

19. Comments
—

20. Specific References
See phenylmercuric nitrate.

USA: R. El-Rashidy*; J. Cooper**
UK: M. C. Allwood*; S. Malcolm*; J. Emerson**; W. Lund**

Phenylmercuric Nitrate

1. Nonproprietary Name
NF: Phenylmercuric nitrate
BP: Phenylmercuric nitrate

2. Functional Category
USP: Antimicrobial preservative
BP: Antiseptic; antimicrobial preservative

3. Synonym
Merphenyl nitrate

4. Chemical Names and CAS Registry Number
Mercury, (nitrato-O)phenyl-
Nitratophenylmercury [55-68-5]

5. Empirical Formula   Molecular Weight
$C_{12}H_{11}Hg_2NO_4$ 634.45

6. Structural Formula

HgNO₃HO—Hg

7. Commercial Availability
USA

Atomergic Chemetals Corp.
Burlington Bio-Medical Corp.
Conray Chemicals, Inc.
ICN K&K Laboratories, Inc.
Pfaltz & Bauer, Inc.
Ruger Chemical Co.
Uhe Co., George

UK

BDH Chemicals, Ltd.
Fisons Scientific Apparatus
Koch-Light Labs, Ltd.
Kodak, Ltd.
Sigma Chemicals Ltd.

8. Method of Manufacture
Phenylmercuric nitrate is readily formed by heating benzene with mercuric acetate, then treating the resulting acetate with an alkali nitrate.

9. Description
Phenylmercuric nitrate is an equi-molecular compound of phenylmercuric hydroxide with phenylmercuric nitrate and occurs as a white, crystalline powder with a slight aromatic odor.

SEM-MF-17
Excipient: Phenylmercuric nitrate
Supplier: Eastman Chemicals

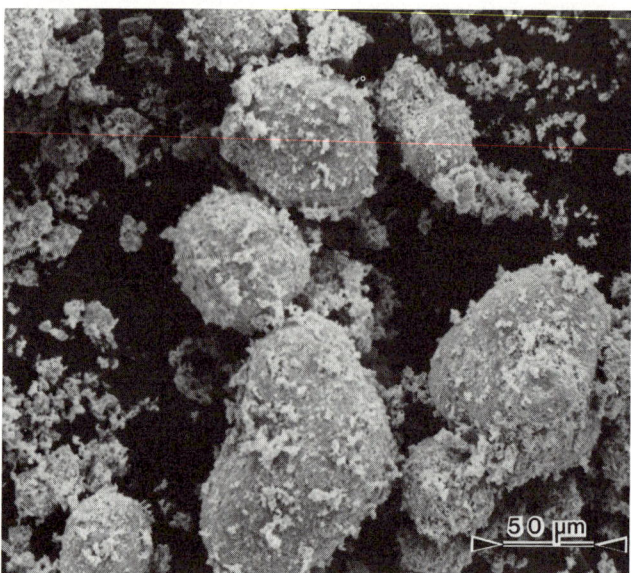

Magnification: 180×

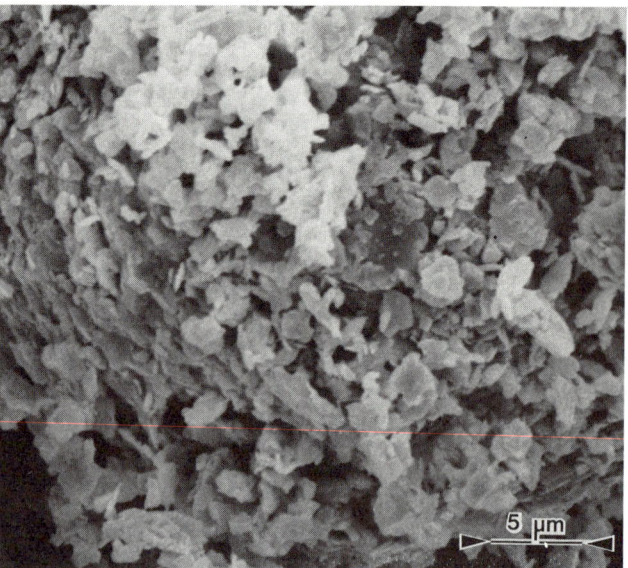

Magnification: 1,800×

10. Pharmacopeial Specifications

Test	NF	BP
Identification	+	+
Acidity (0.02% w/v soln)	—	+
Loss on drying	—	≤1.0%
Residue on ignition	≤0.1%	—
Mercuric salts & heavy metals	—	+
Mercury ions	+	—
Melting range	175°-185°C	—
Assay—		
Mercury	62.75-63.50%	—
Phenylmercuric ions	87.0-87.9%	—
Phenylmercuric nitrate (dried basis)	—	98.0-102.0% (as $C_{12}H_{11}Hg_2NO_4$)

11. Typical Properties

Solubility: Very slightly soluble in water; slightly soluble in alcohol and in glycerin. It is more soluble in the presence of either nitric acid or alkali hydroxides. Its saturated solution in water is acidic to litmus.

Antimicrobial activity: Broad spectrum growth-inhibiting agents at the concentrations normally used for preservation of pharmaceuticals. Slow bactericidal and fungicidal activity. *Bacteria:* Gram positive: good inhibition, more moderate cidal activity. MIC against *Staphylococcus aureus* 0.5 μg ml^{-1}. Gram negative: inhibitory activity for most gram negative bacteria is similar to that for gram positive bacteria. MIC approximately 0.3-0.5 μg ml^{-1}. Less active against some *Pseudomonas* species, and particularly *Pseudomonas aeruginosa*. Against *Pseudomonas aeruginosa* MIC approximately 12 μg ml^{-1}. *Spores:* May be active in conjunction with heat. The BP 1980 lists heating at 100°C for 30 minutes in the presence of 0.002% w/v PMA or PMN as a "sterilisation" method. However, in practice this may not be sufficient to kill spores. *Fungi:* Most fungi are inhibited by 0.3 -1 μg ml^{-1}; phenylmercuric salts exhibit both inhibitory and fungicidal activity. e.g., PMA against *Candida albicans* MIC 0.8 μg ml^{-1}. PMA against *Aspergillus niger* MIC approximately 10 μg ml^{-1}.

Effect on pH: Antimicrobial activity tends to increase with increasing pH; however, in solutions of pH 6 and below activity against *Pseudomonas aeruginosa* has been demonstrated and phenylmercuric salts are included in several compendial eye drops of acid pH.

Partition coefficients: PMA: liquid paraffin: water, 0.1; PMN: liquid paraffin: water, 0.58; Arachis oil: water, 0.4.

12. Stability and Storage Conditions

All phenylmercuric compound solutions form a black residue of metallic mercury when exposed to light or after prolonged storage. Phenylmercuric nitrate should be stored in a tight, light-resistant non-aluminum container. Phenylmercuric nitrate is absorbed by some types of plastic containers as well as by rubber stoppers.

13. Incompatibilities

Phenylmercuric ion is incompatible with halide ions, particularly bromides and iodides, with which it forms less-soluble halogen compounds. At concentrations of 0.002% phenylmercuric salt, precipitation may not occur in the presence of chlorides. It is also incompatible with aluminum and other metals, ammonia and ammonium salts and with some sulfur compounds (e.g., in rubber). Its antimicrobial activity may be reduced in the presence of anionic emulsifying agents and suspending agents.

14. Safety

LD_{50}—(SC in rat): 63 mg/kg; (IV in mice): 27 mg/kg; (oral in mice): 50mg/kg.

Human toxicity: local application of a more concentrated solution may cause irritation and may give rise to erythema and blistering 6 to 12 hours later. In a modified repeated insult patch test, a 2% solution was found to produce extreme sensitization of the skin. Eye drops containing phenylmercuric nitrate as a preservative should not be used continuously for prolonged periods.

15. Handling Precautions

Protect from ingestion, inhalation and contact with skin and eyes.

16. Regulatory Acceptance

NF XVI; BP 1980

17. Applications in Pharmaceutical Formulation or Technology

Use	Concentration (%)
Bactericide in parenterals	0.001
Preservative in eye drops	0.002
Bactericide in vaginal suppositories and jellies	0.02

18. Related Substances

Phenylmercuric acetate, phenylmercuric benzoate, phenylmercuric borate, phenylmercuric chloride

19. Comments

For compatibilities of organic phenyl mercurial agents, see Remington's "Pharmaceutical Sciences," 14th edition, p. 1573. For the spectrum of bacterial activities in ophthalmic preparations, see Remington's "Pharmaceutical Sciences," 15th edition, p. 1503.

Organic mercurials are sorbed or otherwise removed from dilute aqueous solutions by rubber and plastic packaging components; uptake is usually greatest to natural rubbers and polyethylene and least to polypropylene.

20. Specific References

1. J. Buckles, M. W. Brown and G. S. Porter, The inactivation of phenylmercuric nitrate by sodium metabisulphite," *J. Pharm. Pharmac.*, 23: (Supplement), 237S (1971).
2. R. M. E. Richards and J. M. E. Reary, Changes in antibacterial activity of thiomersal and PMN on autoclaving with certain adjuvants, *J. Pharm. Pharmac.*, 24: (Supplement), 84P (1972).
3. R. M. E. Richards, A. F. Fell and J. M. E. Butchart, Interaction between sodium metabisulphite and PMN, *J. Pharm. Pharmac.*, 24: 999 (1972).
4. A. Hart, Antibacterial activity of phenylmercuric nitrate in zinc sulphate and adrenaline eye drops BPC 1968, *J. Pharm. Pharmac.*, 25: 507 (1973).
5. N. T. Naido, C. H. Price and T. J. McCarthy, Preservative loss from ophthalmic solutions during filtration sterilization, *Austral. J. Pharm. Sci.*, NS1: (No. 1), 16 (1972).
6. J. Ingversen and V. S. Andersen, Transfer of phenylmercuric compounds from dilute aqueous solutions to vials and rubber closures, *Dansk Tidsskr. Farm.*, 42: 264 (1968).

7. K. Eriksson, Loss of organomercurial preservatives from medicaments in different kinds of containers, *Acta Pharm. Suecica*, 4: 261 (1967).

8. K. Christensen and E. Dauv, Absorption of preservatives by drip attachments in eye drop packages, *J. Mond. Pharm.*, 12: (1), 5 (1969).

9. J. A. Aspinall, T. D. Duffy, M. B. Saunders and C. G. Taylor, The effect of low density polyethylene containers on some hospital-manufactured eye drop formulations, I. Sorption of phenylmercuric acetate, *J. Clin. Hosp. Pharm.*, 5: 21 (1980).

10. E. O. Miezitis, A. E. Polack and M. S. Roberts, Concentration changes during autoclaving of aqueous solutions in polyethylene containers: An examination of some methods for reduction of solute loss, *Austral. J. Pharm. Sci.*, 8: (3), 72 (1979).

11. D. O. Jordan and A. E. Polack, The permeation of organic solutes in aqueous solution through polyethylene membranes, II. Effect of concentration, temperature and other variables, *Austral. J Pharm. Sci.*, NS1: 82 (1972).

12. T. J. McCarthy, Interaction between aqueous preservative solutions and their plastic containers, III, *Pharm. Weekblad*, 107: 1 (1972).

13. N. Grier, Mercurials—inorganic and organic. In: "Disinfection, Sterilization and Preservation," S. S. Block, Ed., Lea & Febiger, Philadelphia, 1977.

14. R. Dolder and F. S. Skinner, Eds., "Ophthalmica," Band II, Wissenschaftliche Verlagsgesellschaft mbH, Stuttgart, 1978, p. 464.

15. R. Barkman, M. Germanis, G. Karpe and A. S. Malmborg, Preservatives in eye drops, *Acta Ophthal.*, 47: 461 (1969).

16. N. R. Horn, T. J. McCarthy and E. Ramsted, Interactions between powder suspensions and selected quaternary ammonium and organomercurial preservatives, *Cosmet. & Toilet.*, 95, 69 (1980).

17. J. E. Aspinall, T. D. Duffy and C. G. Taylor, The effect of low density polyethylene containers on some hospital-manufactured eye drop formulations, II. Inhibition of the sorption of phenylmercuric acetate, *J. Clin. Hosp. Pharm.*, 8: 223 (1983).

USA: R. El-Rashidy*, J. Cooper*, J. Mollica**
UK: M. C. Allwood*, S. Malcolm*, J. Emerson**, W. Lund**

Polacrilin Potassium

1. Nonproprietary Names

NF: Polacrilin potassium

Polacrilin and polacrilin potassium are USAN names for *Amberlite IRP-64* and *Amberlite IRP-88*, respectively.

2. Functional Category

NF: Tablet disintegrant

Others: Drug carriers; taste modifiers; drug stabilizers; ion-exchange resins

3. Synonyms

Pharmaceutical grade resins	Parent resin
Amberlite IRP-69 and IRP-69M	*Amberlite* IR-120
Amberlite IRP-64 and IRP-64M	*Amberlite* IRC-50
Amberlite IRP-88	*Amberlite* IRC-50
Amberlite IRP-58 and IRP-58M	*Amberlite* IR-4B
Amberlite IRP-67 and IRP-67M	*Amberlite* IRA-400

4. Chemical Names and CAS Registry Number

2-propenoic acid; 2-methyl-; polymer with divinylbenzene; potassium salt.

Methacrylic acid polymer with divinylbenzene; potassium salt [39394-76-5]

5. Empirical Formula and Molecular Weight

—

6. Structural Formula

7. Commercial Availability

USA

Rohm & Haas Company

UK

Rohm & Haas (UK) Ltd.

8. Method of Manufacture

These resins are produced by copolymerization between styrene and divinylbenzene (*Amberlites* IRP-69, IRP-67, IR-120, and IRA-400), methacrylic acid and divinylbenzene (*Amberlites* IRP-64, IRP-88, and IRC-50) and phenolic-based polyamine condensates (*Amberlites* IRP-58 and IR-4B). The homogeneity of resin structures depends on the purity, nature and properties of copolymers used as well as the controls and conditions employed during the polymerization reactions. The nature and degree of cross-linking have significant influence on the physico-chemical properties of the resin matrix. The functional groups introduced on the matrix confer the property of ion-exchange. Depending upon the acidity or basicity of the functional groups, strongly acidic to strongly basic types of ion exchangers are produced.

9. Description

Pharmaceutical grade resins are supplied in two particle size ranges: 1) 100 to 500 mesh; and 2) finer than 325 mesh (which is denoted by the letter M). All pharmaceutical grade resins are free-flowing powders of a tan or off-white color. IRP-58 and IRP-58M have a mild amine odor; other pharmaceutical grade resins are odorless. The corresponding parent resins are free-flowing beads of a tan or off-white color.

10. Pharmacopeial Specifications

Test	NF
Identification	+
Loss on drying	$\leq$10.0%
Arsenic	$\leq$3ppm
Iron	$\leq$0.01%
Sodium	$\leq$0.20%
Heavy metals	$\leq$0.002%
Powder fineness	$\leq$1.0% on #100 sieve
	$\leq$30.0% on #200 sieve
Assay (for potassium)	20.6%-25.1%

11. Typical Properties

Physico-chemical properties of pharmaceutical grade resins and their parent resins are summarized in Tables I and II, respectively.

Table I — Summary of Physico-Chemical Properties of Pharmaceutical Grade *Amberlite* Resins

	Grade	Copolymer	Type	Functional Structure	Ionic Form	Particle Size (Mesh)	Parent Resin	% Moisture (Max)	pH Range	Max. Operation Temp. (F°)	Application
CATION	IRP-69	Styrene-DVB	Strongly acidic	-SO$_3$Na$^+$	Na$^+$	100-500	IR-120	10	0-14	250	Carrier for cationic drugs which are bases or salts.
	IRP-69M	Styrene-DVB	Strongly acidic	-SO$_3$Na$^+$	Na$^+$	<325	IR-120	10	0-14	250	
	IRP-64	Methacrylic acid DVB	Weakly acidic	-COO-H$^+$	H$^+$	100-500	IRC-50	10	5-14	250	Carrier for cationic drugs which are bases
	IRP-64M	Methacrylic acid DVB	Weakly acidic	-COO-H$^+$	H$^+$	<325	IRC-50	10	5-14	250	
	IRP-88	Methacrylic acid DVB	Weakly acidic	-COO-K$^+$	K$^+$	100-500	IRC-50	10	5-14	250	Tablet disintegrant.
ANION	IRP-58	Phenolic polyamine	Weakly basic	NH NH$_2$	free base	100-500	IR-4B	10	0-7	140	Carrier for anionic drugs, which are acids.
	IRP-58M	Phenolic polyamine	Weakly basic	<NH NH$_2$		<325	IR-4B	10	0-7	140	
	IRP-67	Styrene-DVB	Strongly basic Type I	-N(CH$_3$)$_3$$^+Cl^-$	Cl$^-$	100-500	IRA-400	10	0-12	140	Carrier for anionic drugs, which are acids or salts.
	IRP-67M	Styrene-DVB	Strongly basic Type I	-N(CH$_3$)$_3$$^+Cl^-$	Cl$^-$	<325	IRA-400	10	0-12	140	

Table II — Summary of Physico-Chemical Properties of Parent *Amberlite* Resins Used in the Manufacture of Pharmaceutical Grade Resins

Grade Matrix Structure	Ionic Forms Available	Densities Apparent g/cm³	(Wet) True g/cm³	Effective Size (mm)	Moisture Content (%)	pH Range	Maximum Operating Temp (°F)	Total Exchange Capacity* (a)g CaCO₃/ft³ (b)meq/ml (wet)	Swelling (%)* Typical values based on complete conversion
Amberlite IR-120 Styrene-DVB	Sodium or Hydrogen	0.85	1.26	0.47-0.62	44-48	0-14	250	(a) 41.4 (b) 1.9	$Na^+ \longrightarrow H^+$ 5-7
Amberlite IRC-50 Methacrylic acid-DVB	Hydrogen	0.69	1.25	0.33-0.50	43-53	5-14	250	(a) 76.3 (b) 3.5	$N^+ \longrightarrow Na^+$ 75-100 $H^+ \longrightarrow Ca^{++}$ 30-40
Amberlite IR-4B Phenolic	Free Base	0.58	—	0.35-0.45	42-47	0-7	140	(a) 69.8 (b) 3.2	$FB \longrightarrow Cl^-$ 75-100
Amberlite IRA-400 Styrene-DVB	Chloride	0.71	1.11	0.38-0.45	42-48	0-14 0-14	140(OH) 170(Cl)	(a) 30.5 (b) 1.4	$Cl^- \longrightarrow OH^-$ 18-22

*Minimum values

Solubility: Negligible in water

Specific gravity: Except for *Amberlite* IR-4B, resins are heavier than water. The specific gravity of IR-4B is 0.6.

Microbial level: Not available in a sterile and pyrogen-free form. They can be sterilized by conventional methods.

12. Stability and Storage Conditions

Resins are stable up to the maximum operation temperature (listed in Tables I & II). Under excessive heat, thermal decomposition of the resins may yield one or more oxides of carbon, nitrogen, sulfur and/or amines. Pharmaceutical grade resins must be stored in well-closed containers. Avoid repeated freeze-thaw storage conditions for the parent resins.

13. Incompatibilities

Avoid contact with concentrated nitric acid or any other strong oxidizing agent at all times.

14. Safety

Can disturb electrolyte balance.

15. Handling Precautions

No hazard up to the maximum operation temperature. Resin dust or particles may be as irritating to the eyes as any other foreign bodies. Dry resins expand when wetted, which may cause glass containers (columns) to shatter.

16. Regulatory Acceptance

NF XVI

17. Applications in Pharmaceutical Formulation or Technology

Resins are used as processing aids in the manufacture of pharmaceutical and food products for the purposes of isolation, purification and enrichment.

Amberlite IRP-88 is used as a tablet disintegrant at a level of about 2%.

Other pharmaceutical grade resins are used as excipients to stabilize drugs, to mask or modify the taste of drugs, to obtain sustained-release dosage forms and to perform as drug carriers.

18. Related Substances

None

19. Comments

When resins are used in the processing of any material which is to be consumed by human beings or animals, precautions must be taken to avoid contamination which may result from extractables, bacterial action or introduction of extraneous poisonous materials. Also, low molecular copolymers might be present in fresh, unconditioned resins. In order to comply with FDA Regulation #121.1148, dated July 13, 1964, such resins must be preconditioned.

20. Specific References:

1. K. Dorfner, *Ion Exchangers, Properties and Applications*, 3rd Ed., Ann Arbour Science Publishers, Michigan, 1972.
2. Technical data sheets and brochures from Rohm and Haas Company, Philadelphia.
3. F.C. Nachod and J. Schubert, *Ion Exchange Technology*, Academy Press, Inc., New York, 1956.
4. E.M. Rudnic, C.T. Rhodes, S. Welch and P. Bernardo, Evaluation of the mechanism of disintegrant action, *Drug Devel. & Indust. Pharm.*, 8(1):87-109 (1982).

USA: R. Acharga*; C. Bergstrom*: J. Cohen**; D. Hovermale**; J. Mollica**

Poloxamer

1. Nonproprietary Name
NF: Poloxamer

2. Functional Category
USP: Wetting and/or solubilizing agent; emulsifying and/or solubilizing agent
Others: Nonionic emulsifying, solubilizing, wetting, foaming and gel-forming agent

3. Synonyms
Pluronic F-68, Poloxalkol, Monolan, Supronic

4. Chemical Names and CAS Registry Number
Oxirane, methyl-, polymer with oxirane
Polyethylene-propylene glycol
α-Hydro-ω-hydroxypoly(oxyethylene)$_a$ poly(oxypropylene)$_b$ (27-31 moles) poly(oxyethylene)$_a$ block copolymer (a=2−130; b=15−67) CAS registry number [9003-11-6]

5. Empirical Formula and Molecular Weight
Poloxamer 188 is one of a series of poly (oxyethylene), poly (oxypropylene) block polymers with the general empirical formula

$$HO\ (CH_2CH_2O)_a \bullet (\underset{\underset{CH_3}{|}}{CH}-CH_2O)_b \bullet (CH_2CH_2O)_aH$$

For poloxamer 188: a=75 and b=30
Average molecular weight=8350

6. Structural Formula
See above

7. Commercial Availability
USA

BASF Wyandotte Corporation

UK

A.B.M. Chemicals, Ltd.
BASF (UK) Ltd.
Diamond Shamrock U.K., Ltd.
Pechiney Ugine Kuhlmann Ltd.

8. Method of Manufacture
Propylene oxide is condensed onto a propylene glycol nucleus, followed by condensation of ethylene oxide onto both ends of the poly (oxypropylene) base.

9. Description
White, waxy, free-flowing prilled granules or cast solid; practically tasteless and odorless.

10. Pharmacopeial Specifications

Test	NF
pH (1 in 40 solution)	5.0-7.5
Arsenic	$\leq$ 3 ppm
Heavy metals	$\leq$ 0.002%
Average molecular weight	90.0-110.0% of label (1,000-7,000)
	80.0-120.0% of label (above 7,000)
Polyoxypropylene number	85.0-115.0% of label
Polyoxyethylene number	Within 1 of label

11. Typical Properties
Antimicrobial action: nil; supports mold growth in aqueous solution
Aqueous gelation concentration: between 60 and 90% at room temperature
Cloud point (Aqueous, 1% and 10%): more than 100°C
Flash point: 260°C
HLB value: ~29
Interfacial tension: 25°C, 0.1%-19.8 dynes/cm; 0.01%-24.0 dynes/cm; 0.001%-26.0 dynes/cm
Loss on drying: ~0.5%
Melting point: 52°C
pH: between 6.0 and 7.4 (2.5% w/v)
Solubility: soluble in water, dilute acids and ethyl alcohol; slightly soluble in toluene and xylene; insoluble in propylene glycol, perchloroethylene, glycerin, mineral oil and liquid paraffin
Specific gravity: ~1.06 g/cm³ at 25°C
Surface tension: 25°C, 0.1%-50.3 dynes/cm; 25°C, 0.01%-51.2 dynes/cm; 25°C, 0.001%-53.6 dynes/cm
Viscosity: 1000 cps at 77°C as a melt (Brookfield)
Hygroscopicity: very slight
Flowability: free flowing

Academy HPE Laboratory Project Data Poloxamer 188 (Pluronic F-68)			
Test	Method	Lab #	Results (mg/cm³)
Solubility			
(Water 25°C)	SOL-7	32	500
(Water 37°C)			500
(Alcohol 25°C)			398
(Alcohol 37°C)			396
(Prop. Glycol 25°C)			1.0
(Prop. Glycol 37°C)			1.0
(Hexane 25°C)			0.05
(Hexane 37°C)			0.09
Moisture content	MC-3	32	0.33%
EMC Plot	EMC-1	15	Fig:15-EMC-5

Supplier: BASF Wyandotte Corp.

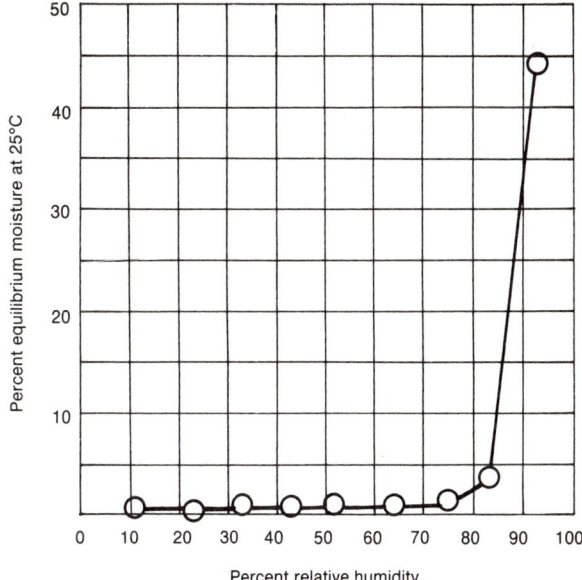

Poloxamer 188, Pluronic F-68 (BASF, Lot #WPEA535B)

Figure: 15-EMC-5   **Method:** EMC-1

12. Stability and Storage Conditions

Stable to aqueous acids, alkalis and metal ions

13. Incompatibilities

Depending on the relative concentration, poloxamer 188 is incompatible with phenols and parabens.

14. Safety

The oral LD_{50} for five species of animals is >15 g/kg of body weight. Directly applied to the eyes of rabbits in 5% and 10% concentrations, there was no irritation. No incidents have been reported concerning skin irritation or sensitization.

At concentrations of 5%, 10% and as a paste, there was no irritation or hyperemia in the gums of rabbits and dogs. No symptoms of toxicity were observed when injected IV into dogs at a dosage of 0.1 g/kg or into rabbits at a dosage of 1.0 g/kg. The IV LD_{50} is reported to be 5.5 g/kg for mice and 3.95 g/kg for rats when injected as a 5% solution.

In a 14-day study of IV administration to rabbits at concentrations up to 0.5 g/kg/day, there were no overt effects. A similar study with dogs showed no effects at dosage levels up to 0.5 g/kg/day.

The LD_{50} for mice when injected intraperitoneally is 5-10 g/kg.

Over a range of 0.001% to 10%, no hemolysis of human blood cells was observed over 18 hours at 25°C. Poloxamer 188 has been used as an emulsifier and as a stabilizer for emulsions which have been safely injected intravenously. It is not metabolized in the body.

Rats fed 3% or 5% in their food for up to two years did not exhibit significant symptoms of toxicity. Rats receiving 7.5% showed a decrease in growth rate.

15. Handling Precautions

No restrictions specified

16. Regulatory Acceptance

NF XVI

17. Applications in Pharmaceutical Formulation or Technology

Use	Concentration
Flavor solubilizer	0.3%
Antibiotic solubilizer	25-400% of antibiotic
Wetting agent	0.01-5%
Gelling agent	15-50%
Spreading agent	1%
Fat emulsifier	0.3%
Stabilizing agent	1-5%
Suppository base	4-6%, 90%
Tablet coating	10%
Tablet excipient	5-10%
Acetanilide solubilizer	—
Absorption promoter	—
Fluorocarbon emulsifier	2.5%

18. Related Substances

The poloxamer polyols are a series of closely related block copolymers whose molecular weights range from 1,100 to over 14,000. All are chemically similar in composition, differing only in the relative amounts of propylene and ethylene oxides added during manufacture. Their physical and surface active properties vary over a wide range.

19. Comments

Poloxamer 188 is used as a component of orally administered fecal stool softeners, injectable fat emulsions, injectable anesthetic emulsions, artificial blood, injectable radio-diagnostics, dentifrices and oral rinses.

20. Specific References

1. C. Carr, Acute toxicity studies with Pluronic F-68, BASF-Wyandotte report, June 29, 1951.
2. C. Carr, Chronic toxicity studies with Pluronic F-68, BASF-Wyandotte report, May 19, 1952.
3. Pluronic polyols—toxicity and irritation data, BASF-Wyandotte Corp., 05-3012, p. 765.
4. Improvements in or relative to pharmaceutical compositions containing Polyglycol, British Patent No. 897, 743, May 30, 1962.
5. N. Goldstein, A new method of tablet coating, B.S. thesis, Columbia University, 1954.
6. Method of granulating materials for subsequent forming into tablets, U.S. Patent No. 3, 308, 217, March 7, 1967.
7. J. H. Collett and E. A. Tobin, Relationships between poloxamer structure and the solubilization of some *p*-substituted acetanilides, *J. Pharm. Pharmacol.*, 31: 174-177 (1979).
8. J. H. Collett, J. A. Rees and D. L. Buckly, The influence of some structurally related Pluronics on the hydrolysis of aspirin, *J. Pharm. Pharmacol.*, 31: 80 (1979).
9. R. K. Reddy, S. A. Khalil and M. W. Gouda, Effect of dioctyl sodium sulfisoxazole and poloxamer 188 on dissolution and intestinal absorption of sulfadiazine and sulfasoxazole in rats, *J. Pharm. Sci.*, 65: 115 (1976).
10. J. Hadgraft and J. R. Howard, "Drug release from pluronic gels," *J. Pharm. Pharmacol.*, 34: Suppl., 3P (1982).
11. R. P. Geyer, "Bloodless rats through the use of artificial blood substitutes," *Fed. Proc.*, 34: 1499 (1975).

USA: D. Monkhouse*; G. E. Reier*; I. S. Gibbs**
UK: J. H. Collett*

Polyethylene Glycol

1. Nonproprietary Name

NF: Polyethylene glycol
BP: Macrogol 300; macrogol 1540; macrogol 4000

2. Functional Category

USP: Suppository base; solvent; tablet and/or capsule lubricant; ointment base
BP: Pharmaceutical aid

3. Synonyms

PEG; Macrogol; polyoxyethylene glycol

4. Chemical Name and CAS Registry Number

α-Hydro-ω-hydroxypoly-(oxy-1,2-ethanediyl)
Polyethylene glycol [25322-68-3]

5. Empirical Formula   Molecular Weight

Table 1
Structural Formula and Molecular Weight

$HOCH_2(CH_2OCH_2)n\ CH_2OH$

where n represents the average number of oxyethylene groups. The number which follows the name indicates the average molecular weight of the compound.

Grade	n	Average Molecular Weight
PEG 200	3	190 - 210
PEG 300	5 - 6	285 - 315
PEG 400	8 - 10	380 - 420
PEG 600	11 - 13	570 - 613
PEG 1000	20 - 24	950 - 1050
PEG 1500 ("pure")	30 - 36	1400 - 1600
*PEG 1500 (blend)		500 - 600
PEG 1540	28 - 36	1300 - 1600
PEG 2000	40 - 50	1800 - 2200
PEG 3000	60 - 75	2700 - 3300
PEG 4000	69 - 84	3000 - 4800
PEG 6000		5400 - 6600
PEG 8000	158 - 204	7000 - 9000
PEG 20000		15000 - 20000

* Macrogol 1500 of the Japanese Pharmacopeia is a blend of equal parts of the 300 and 1540 grades.
  Lanogen 1500 (Hoechst) is a blend of equal parts PEG 300 and PEG 1500.
  In this profile, the general term "liquid PEGs" is used for grades 200, 300, 400 and 600; grades of 1000 and upwards are referred to as "solid PEGs."

6. Structural Formula

See Table 1

7. Commercial Availability

USA

Ashland Chemical Co.
BASF Wyandotte Corp.
Diamond Shamrock Corp.
Durkee Industrial Foods/SCM Corp.
Gallard-Schlesinger Chemical Mfg. Corp.
Glyco, Inc.
Hodag Chemical Corp.
ICN K & K Labs, Inc.
Mazer Chemicals, Inc.
Olin Corporation
Pfaltz and Bauer, Inc.
Quad Chemical - Lonza Specialty Chemicals
Ruger Chemical Co.
Stoney-Mueller, Inc.
Thompson-Hayward Chemical Co.
Union Carbide Corp., Chemicals & Plastics Div.

UK

BASF AG
Hoeschst AG
Chemische Werke Huls AG
Pechiney Ugine Kuhlmann, Ltd.
Shell Chemicals UK, Ltd.

8. Method of Manufacture

Condensation polymers of ethylene oxide and water are progressively formed, under pressure, in the presence of a catalyst.

9. Description

Liquid PEGs (Grades 200 - 600)
Clear, colorless or slightly yellowish, viscous liquids. The odor is slight but characteristic, and the taste is bitter and slightly burning. PEG 600 can be solid at ambient temperatures.
Solid PEGs (Grades 1000 - 2000)
The solid grades are white or off-white in color, and range in consistency between pastes and waxy flakes. Their odor is faint and sweet. Grades of 6000 and above are available as free-flowing milled powders.

10. Pharmacopeial Specifications

	NF	BP 1980		
Test	Polyethylene Glycol	Macrogol 300	Macrogol 1540	Macrogol 4000
Completeness and/or color of solution	+	+	+	+
Viscosity	See Table 2	59-73 mm^2s^{-1} (at 25°C)	25-32 $mm^{2-1}s$ (at 100°C)	76-110 mm^2s^{-1} (at 100°C)
pH (5% solution)	4.5 - 7.5	—	—	—
Acidity or alkalinity	—	pH 4.0-7.0	pH 4.0-7.0	pH 4.5-7.5
Residue on ignition	≤0.1%	—	—	—
Arsenic	≤3ppm	—	—	—
Heavy metals	≤5ppm	—	—	—
Limit of ethylene glycol and diethylene glycol	≤0.25% (combined)	—	—	—
Ethylene oxide	≤0.02%	+	—	—

Test	NF Polyethylene Glycol	BP 1980 Macrogol 300	Macrogol 1540	Macrogol 4000
Average molecular weight (MW)	95.0-105.0% of nominal value (when MW < 1000) 90.0-110.0% of nominal value (when MW = 1000-7000) 87.5-112.5% of nominal value (when MW > 7000)	—	—	—
Hydroxyl value	—	356 - 394	70 - 86	30 - 36
Refractive index	—	1.462-1.466	—	—
Weight per ml	—	1.120-1.130 g	—	—
Sulphated ash	—	≤0.1%	≤0.1%	≤0.1%
Water	—	≤1.0%	—	—
Freezing point	—	—	42°-46°C	53°-56°C
Color of solution	—	+	+	+

10. Pharmacopeial Specifications

Table 2
NF Specification for Viscosity (at 98.9 ± 0.3°C)

Nominal Average Molecular Weight	Viscosity Range (cSt)
300	5.4 to 6.4
400	6.8 to 8.0
500	8.3 to 9.6
600	9.9 to 11.3
700	11.5 to 13.0
800	12.5 to 14.5
900	15.0 to 17.0
1000	16.0 to 19.0
1100	18.0 to 22.0
1200	20.0 to 24.5
1300	22.0 to 27.5
1400	24 to 30
1450	25 to 32
1500	26 to 33
1600	28 to 36
1700	31 to 39
1800	33 to 42
1900	35 to 45
2000	38 to 49
2100	40 to 53
2200	43 to 56
2300	46 to 60
2400	49 to 65
2500	51 to 70
2600	54 to 74
2700	57 to 78
2800	60 to 83
2900	64 to 88
3000	67 to 93
3250	73 to 105
3350	76 to 110
3500	87 to 123
3750	99 to 140
4000	110 to 158
4250	123 to 177
4500	140 to 200
4750	155 to 228
5000	170 to 250
5500	206 to 315
6000	250 to 390
6500	295 to 480
7000	350 to 590
7500	405 to 735
8000	470 to 900

11. Typical Properties

Density: Liquid PEGs: 1.11-1.14 g/cm^3 (25°C); Solid PEGs: 1.15-1.21 g/cm^3

Flash point: PEG 200: 182°C; PEG 300: 213°C; PEG 400: 238°C; PEG 600: 250°C.

Melting point:
PEG 1000: 37 - 40°C;
PEG 1500: 44 - 48°C;
PEG 1500 (blend 300/1500): 38 - 41°C;
PEG 1540: 40 - 48°C;
PEG 2000: 45 - 50°C;
PEG 3000: 48 - 54°C;
PEG 4000: 50 - 58°C;
PEG 6000: 55 - 63°C;
PEG 8000: 60 - 63°C;
PEG 20000: 60 - 63°C.

Moisture content: ≤1.0% (Karl Fischer)

Hygroscopicity: Liquid PEGs are very hygroscopic, but hygroscopicity decreases with increasing molecular weight. Solid grades of 4000 and above have low hygroscopicity.

Refractive index: n_D^{25} PEG 200: 1.459; PEG 300: 1.463; PEG 400: 1.465; PEG 600: 1.467.

Solidification point: PEG 200: Sets to glass below −65°C; PEG 300: −15 to −8°C; PEG 400: 4 to 8°C; PEG 600: 15 to 25°C.

Solubility/miscibility: All grades are soluble in water and miscible in all proportions with other PEGs (after melting, if necessary). Aqueous solutions of higher molecular weight grades may form gels.

Liquid PEGs are soluble in alcohols, glycols, acetone, glycerol and benzene.

Solid PEGs are soluble in methanol, ethanol, acetone and methylene chloride. They are slightly soluble in ether and aliphatic hydrocarbons, but insoluble in liquid paraffin, fats and fixed oils.

Surface tension: Liquid PEGs: approx 44 mN/m; Solid PEGs: approximately 55 mN/m (10% aqueous solution).

Viscosity:
a) Measured by capillary viscometer (mm^2/s)

	25°C	99°C
PEG 200	39.9	4.4
PEG 300	68.8	5.9
PEG 400	90.0	7.4
PEG 600	131	11.0
PEG 1000	solid	19.5
PEG 1500 (blend)	solid	15.0
PEG 2000	solid	47
PEG 4000	solid	180
PEG 6000	solid	580
PEG 20000	solid	6900

b) Measured by Höppler Falling Ball at 25°C (mN s/m^2)

PEG 200	46 - 53
PEG 300	66 - 74
PEG 400	85 - 95
PEG 600	13 - 15)
PEG 1000	19 - 23)
PEG 1500 ('pure')	29 - 34)
PEG 1500 (blend) 300/1500	15 - 20) 50% w/w
PEG 2000	40 - 48)aqueous solution
PEG 4000	90 - 120)
PEG 6000	170 - 220)
PEG 20000	2200 - 2800)

Volatility: Practically non-volatile.

Academy HPE Laboratory Project Data

	Method	Lab #	Results
Moisture content:			
PEG 1540[c]	MC-3	28	0.585%
PEG 4000 (Flakes)[c]	MC-19	1	0.290%
PEG 4000 (Powder)[c]	MC-19	1	0.290%
PEG 4000 (Powder)[b]	MC-20	2	0.300%
PEG 6000 (Flakes)[c]	MC-19	1	0.120%
PEG 6000 (Powder)[c]	MC-19	1	0.150%
PEG 4000 (Flakes)[c]	BTD-3	1	B:0.485cm^2
			T:0.575 cm^2
PEG 4000 (Powder)[c]	BTD-1	1	B:0.581 cm^2
			T:0.704 cm^2
PEG 6000 (Flakes)[c]	BTD-3	1	B:0.476 cm^2
			T:0.562 cm^2
PEG 6000 (Powder)[c]	BTD-1	1	B:0.481 cm^2
			T:0.581 cm^2
PEG 4000 (Powder)[c]	BTD-7	14	B:0.610 cm^2
			T:0.750 cm^2
PEG 6000 (Powder)[c]	BTD-7	14	B:0.510 cm^2
			T:0.570 cm^2
PEG E4000 (Prilled)[a]	BTD-6	8	VOLUME: 7.5%
			WEIGHT: 7.0%
PEG 4000 (Powder)[c]	BTD-6	8	VOLUME: 17.0%
			WEIGHT: 13.0%
PEG 4000 (Flakes)[c]	BTD-6	8	VOLUME: 13.0%
			WEIGHT: 12.0%
PEG 6000 (Polyol)[a]	BTD-6	8	VOLUME: 13.0%
			WEIGHT: 12.0%
PEG 6000 (Powder)[a]	BTD-6	8	VOLUME: 19.5%
			WEIGHT: 17.0%
PEG 6000 (Flakes)[c]	BTD-6	8	VOLUME: 15.0%
			WEIGHT: 14.0%
EG 4000 (Powder)[c]	PSD-1S	1	<44µm: 2.7%
			44- 62µm: 7.7%
			62- 90µm: 17.3%
			90-105µm: 15.0%
			105-125µm: 17.1%
			126-149µm: 9.2%
			149 & over: 31.0%
PEG 4000 (Flakes)	PSD-1	1	<149µm: 0.5%
			149-177µm: 0.2%
			177-250µm: 1.0%
			250-420µm: 5.9%
			420-595µm: 11.6%
			595-840µm: 29.5%
			840 & over: 51.3%

Academy HPE Laboratory Project Data

	Method	Lab #	Results
PEG 6000 (Powder)[c]	PSD-1S	1	<44µm: 2.2%
			44- 62µm: 4.9%
			62- 90µm: 10.9%
			90-105µm: 13.9%
			105-125µm: 15.0%
			125-149µm: 10.3%
			149 & over: 42.8%
PEG 6000 (Flakes)[c]	PSD-1	1	<149µm: 0.6%
			149-177µm: 0.9%
			177-250µm: 4.1%
			250-420µm: 19.6%
			420-595µm: 23.6%
			595-840µm: 26.9%
			840 & over: 24.3%

Solubility (at 25°C):			*mg/ml*
PEG 4000	(Water)	SOL-2 1	2.1×10^3
POWDER[c]	(Alcohol)	SOL-2 1	0.575
	(n-Hexane)	SOL-1 1	0.013
PEG 4000	(Water)	SOL-2 1	2.1×10^3
FLAKES[c]	(Alcohol)	SOL-2 1	0.575
	(n-Hexane)	SOL-1 1	0.006
PEG 6000	(Water)	SOL-2 1	1.9×10^3
FLAKES[c]	(Alcohol)	SOL-2 1	0.500
	(n-Hexane)	SOL-1 1	0.011
PEG 6000	(Water)	SOL-2 1	1.9×10^3
POWDER[c]	(Alcohol)	SOL-2 1	0.420
	(n-Hexane)	SOL-1 1	0.055

Viscosity:			
PEG 4000 Flakes[a] (Pluracol)	VIS-1	27	1.26±0.1 cps
PEG 4000 Flakes[b]	VIS-1	27	1.26±0.1 cps
PEG 4000 Powder[b]	VIS-1	27	1.26±0.1 cps

Density:			
PEG 4000[a] (Polyol Prilled)	DE-1	31	1.043
PEG 4000 (Sentry)[c]	DE-1	31	1.205
PEG E4000[a]	DE-1	31	1.094
PEG 6000 Powder (Sentry)[c]	DE-1	31	1.122
EMC Plot (PEG 4000 NF)[b]	EMC-1	2	Fig:2-EMC-7
SDI Plot (PEG 4000 Powd)[c]	SDI-2	26	Fig:26-SDI-6
SDI Plot (PEG E-4000)[a]	SDI-2	26	Fig:26-SDI-6
SDI Plot (PEG 6000 Powd)[c]	SDI-2	26	Fig:26-SDI-7
SDI Plot (PEG E-6000)[a]	SDI-2	26	Fig:26-SDI-7

Suppliers: [a]BASF Wyandotte Corp.; [b]McKesson; [c]Union Carbide Corp., Chemicals & Plastics Div.

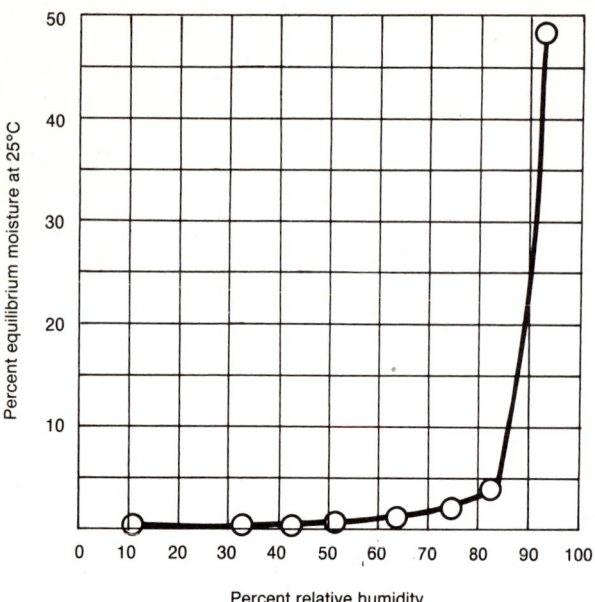

○ : Polyethylene glycol 4000 NF (McKesson, Lot #B192-8209)

Figure: 2-EMC-7 **Method:** EMC-1

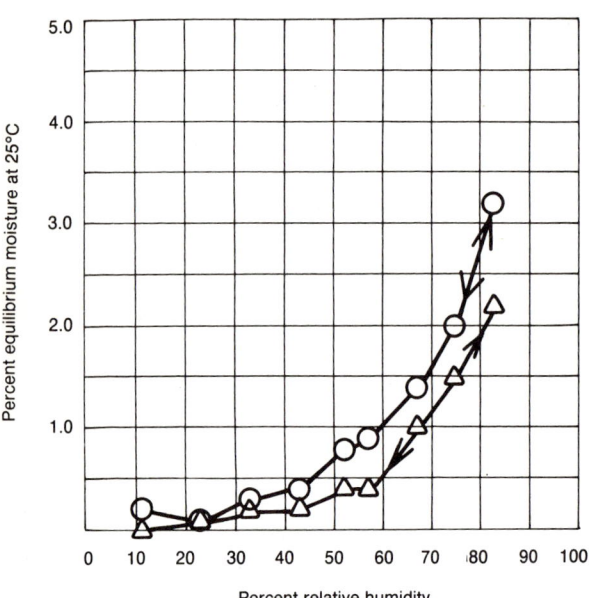

○ : Polyethylene glycol 4000 powder, Sentry (Union Carbide, Lot #B-251)

△ : Polyethylene glycol E-4000 (BASF, Lot #WPYA-575B)

Figure: 26-SDI-6 **Method:** SDI-2

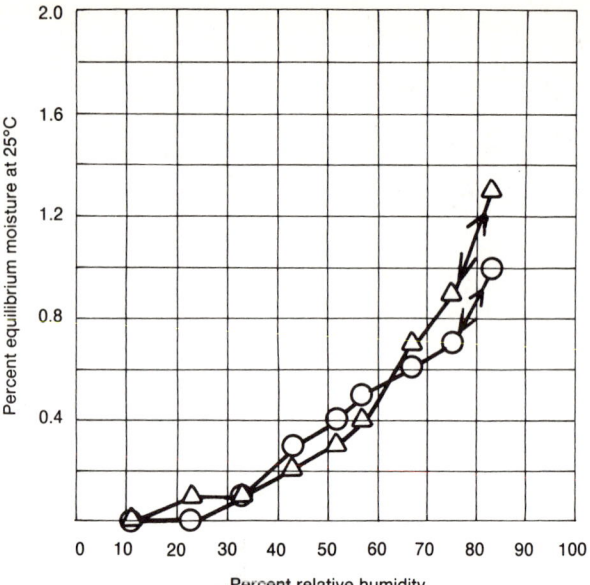

○ : Polyethylene glycol 6000 powder, Sentry (Union Carbide, Lot #B-507)

△ : Polyethylene glycol E-6000 (BASF, Lot #WPNY-124B)

Figure: 26-SDI-7 **Method:** SDI-2

12. Stability and Storage Conditions

Chemically stable in air and in solution. PEGs do not support microbial growth, nor become rancid. Stainless steel, aluminum, glass or lined steel are preferred for storage of liquid and low molecular weight products. Moisture may be absorbed, especially the grades of molecular weight less than 2000. These must be stored in well-closed containers. Aqueous solutions of PEGs can be sterilized by autoclaving or filtration. Sterilization of solid grades by dry heat at 150°C

for 1 hour may induce oxidation, darkening and the formation of acidic degradation products. Ideally, sterilization should be carried out in an inert atmosphere, or oxidation may be inhibited by the inclusion of a suitable anti-oxidant. If heated tanks are used to maintain solid PEGs in a molten state, care must be taken to avoid contamination with iron, which can lead to discoloration. Temperature must be kept to the minimum necessary to ensure fluidity. Oxidation may occur if PEGs are exposed for long periods to temperatures exceeding 50°C. Storage under nitrogen will reduce the possibility of oxidation.

13. Incompatibilities

The chemical reactivity of PEGs is mainly confined to the two terminal hydroxyl groups, which can be either esterified or etherified. However, all grades can exhibit an oxidizing activity due to the presence of peroxide impurities and secondary products formed by auto-oxidation.

Chemical incompatibilities occur with aspirin, carbonic acid, bismuth, mercury and silver salts, iodine, potassium iodide and theophylline derivatives.

With solid grades, phenobarbital forms a water-insoluble complex (by hydrogen bonding).

Liquid and solid grades are incompatible with FD & C Red No. 3 and Yellow No. 5. Additionally, the solid grades interact with FD & C Blue No. 1 and Red Nos. 1, 2 and 4. No reaction occurs with lakes of the above dyes.

The anti-bacterial activity of certain antibiotics, particularly penicillin and bacitracin, is reduced in PEG bases. Preservative effectiveness of hydroxybenzoate esters may also be impaired due to binding with PEGs.

Physical effects caused by PEG bases include softening and liquefaction in mixtures with phenol, tannic acid and salicylic acid, and discoloration of sulfonamides and dithranol. Sorbitol may be precipitated from mixtures. Plastics such as polyethylene, phenolformaldehyde, polyvinyl chloride and cellulose-ester membranes (in filters) may be softened or dissolved by PEGs. Migration of PEG can occur from tablet film coatings, leading to interaction with core components.

14. Safety

Toxicity is low; PEG is permitted as an additive to animal feeds and drinking water.

LD$_{50}$: PEG 200:28.9 ml/kg (rat, oral)
PEG 400:43.6 g/kg (rat, oral)
PEG 4000:59 g/kg, divided doses (rat, oral)
PEG 8000: > 50 g/kg (rat, oral)

The maximum recommended concentration of PEG 300 in parenteral solutions is approximately 30% (Katalog pharmazeutischer Hilfsstoffe). Hemolytic effects have been observed at concentrations greater than 40%.

Skin irritation is low, but PEGs can cause a local stinging effect when used as suppository bases due to their hypertonicity.

The activity of drugs dissolved in PEGs may be potentiated. For additional information on toxicity, see Reference 3.

15. Handling Precautions

Slight fire hazard, avoid heat and oxidizing substances.

16. Regulatory Acceptance

NF XVI; BP 1980

17. Applications in Pharmaceutical Formulation and Technology

Gelling agent: Solid PEGs are useful as water-soluble ointment bases. Consistency can be adjusted by mixture with lower molecular weight PEGs (e.g., macrogol ointment BP). As suppository bases, admixtures of PEGs offer the following advantages over fats:

a) The melting point is higher, so they can withstand exposure to warmer climates.
b) Release of the drug is not dependent upon melting point.
c) Physical stability on storage is better.
d) They are readily miscible with rectal fluids.

The disadvantage is that PEGs are more reactive chemically than are fats. Greater care is needed in processing to avoid inelegant contraction holes in suppositories. The rate of release of water-soluble medications decreases with the increasing molecular weight of the PEG. PEGs also tend to be more irritating than fats to mucous membranes.

Suspending agent: In aqueous vehicles, PEGs can be used to adjust viscosity and consistency. When used in conjunction with other emulsifiers, PEGs can act as emulsion stabilizers.

Solvent: Liquid PEGs are used as water-miscible vehicles for the contents of soft gelatin capsules. However, they may cause hardening of the shell by preferential absorption of moisture from the gelatin shells.

In concentrations up to 30%, PEGs 300 and 400 have been used as vehicles in parenteral dosage forms.

Solubilizer: The aqueous solubility or dissolution characteristics of poorly soluble compounds can be enhanced by making solid dispersions with an appropriate PEG. Studies have also been made in animals of the use of PEGs as solvents for steroids in osmotic pumps.

Binder: Higher molecular weight PEGs can enhance the effectiveness of tablet binders and impart plasticity to granules. However, they have only limited binding action when used alone, and can prolong disintegration if present in concentrations greater than 5%.

When used for thermoplastic granulations, a mixture of the powdered constituents with 10 to 15% PEG 6000 is heated

to 70 - 75°C. The mass becomes paste-like and forms granules if stirred while cooling. The technique is useful for dosage forms such as lozenges when prolonged disintegration is required.

Plasticizers in film coating: Solid grades can be used alone for film coating tablets, and can be useful as hydrophilic polishing materials. They are widely used as plasticizers in conjunction with film-forming polymers. The presence of PEGs, especially the liquid grades, in films tends to increase their water permeability, and may reduce protection against low pH in enteric coating films.

PEGs are useful as plasticizers in micro-encapsulated products to avoid rupture of the coating film when microcapsules are compressed into tablets.

Lubricant: Grades of 6000 and above can be used as lubricants, particularly in soluble tablets. The lubricant action is not as good as that of magnesium stearate, and stickiness may develop if the material becomes too warm during compression. An anti-adherent effect is also exerted, again subject to avoidance of over-heating.

18. Related Substances

Polyoxyethylene esters; polyoxyethylene alkyl ethers; polyoxyethylene sorbitan fatty acid esters (see separate profiles).

19. Comments

Polyethylene glycols of various molecular weights are described in the pharmacopeias of the following countries: Argentina, Austria, Belgium, Brazil, Czechoslovakia, France, West Germany, Hungary, Italy, Japan, Yugoslavia, Netherlands, Nordic countries, Poland, Portugal, Romania and Switzerland.

20. Specific References:

1. W. L. Chiou and S. Riegelman, Correlations between physical and drug release characteristics of polyethylene glycol suppositories, *J. Pharm. Sci.*, 60, 1281 (1971).
2. I. W. Kellaway and C. J. Marriott, Pharmaceutical applications of solid dispersion systems, *J. Pharm. Sci.*, 64, 1162 (1975).
3. H. F. Smyth, C. P. Carpenter, and C. S. Weil, The toxicity of the Polyethylene Glycols, *J. Am. Pharm. Assoc., Sci. Ed.*, 39, 349 (1950).
4. J. I. Wells, D. A. Bhatt and K. A. Khan, Improved wet massed tabletting using plasticized binder, *J. Pharm. Pharmacol.*, 34 Suppl., 46P (1982).
5. A. O. Okhamafe and P. York, Moisture permeation mechanism of some aqueous based film coats, *J. Pharm Pharmacol.*, 34 Suppl., 53P (1982).
6. J. L. Ford and M. H. Rubinstein, Formulation and aging of tablets prepared from indomethacin-polyethylene glycol 6000 solid dispersions, *Pharm. Acta Helv.*, 55 (1), 1-7 (1980).
7. H. F. Smith, Jr., C. P. Carpenter and C. S. Weil, The chronic oral toxicity of the Polyethylene Glycols, *J. Am. Pharm. Assoc., Sci. Ed.*, 44, 27 (1955).
8. T. W. Tusing, J. R. Elsea and A. B. Sauveur, The chronic dermal toxicity of a series of polyethylene glycols, *J. Am. Pharm. Assoc., Sci. Ed.*, 43, 489 (1954).
9. M. J. Miralles, J. W. McGinity and A. Martin, Combined water soluble carriers for coprecipitates of tolbutamide, *J. Pharm. Sci.*, 71 (3), 302-304 (1982).

USA: J. C. Price*; A. Y. Gore**; Z. Chowhan**
UK: R. L. Horder*

Polymethacrylates

1. Nonproprietary Names

NF: Methacrylic acid copolymer; polymeric methacrylates

2. Functional Category

Film former, tablet binder

3. Synonyms

Methacrylic acid; *Eudragit*

4. Chemical Name and CAS Registry Number

Copolymers synthesized from dimethylaminoethyl methacrylate and other neutral methacrylic esters [None]

5. Empirical Formula and Molecular Weight:

Molecular weight range: $\geq 100,000$

6. Structural Formula

Basic Structure:

Variations:

Type E: R_1, $R_3 = -CH_3$
$\qquad R_2 = -CH_2CH_2N(CH_3)_2$
$\qquad R_4 = -CH_3$, $-C_4H_9$

Type L and S: R_1, $R_3 = -CH_3$
$\qquad R_2 = -H$
$\qquad R_4 = CH_3$

Type RL and RS: $R_1 = -H$, $-CH_3$
$\qquad R_2 = -CH_3$, $-C_2H_5$
$\qquad R_3 = -CH_3$
$\qquad R_4 = -CH_2CH_2N(CH_3)_3^+Cl^-$

Type E30D: R_1, $R_3 = -H$, $-CH_3$
$\qquad R_2$, $R_4 = -CH_3$, $-C_2H_5$

Type L30D: R_1, $R_3 = -H$, $-CH_3$
$\qquad R_2 = -H$
$\qquad R_4 = -CH_3$, $-C_2H_5$

7. Commercial Availability

USA
Röhm Tech Inc.

UK
Dumas Chemicals (Tunbridge Wells) Ltd.

8. Method of Manufacture

Polymerization of acrylic and methacrylic acids or their esters; e.g., butyl ester or dimethylaminoethyl ester.

9. Description

Polymethacrylates are film coatings and matrix structures based on polymeric methacrylates. They are synthetic cationic and anionic polymers of dimethylaminoethylmethacrylates, methacrylic acid and methacrylic acid esters in varying ratios.

Type E—A cationic polymer based on dimethylaminoethylmethacrylate and other neutral methacrylic acid esters available as 12.5% ready-to-use solution in isopropanol/acetone (60:40); light yellow in color with the characteristic odor of the solvents; solvent-free granules contain $\geq 98\%$ dried weight content. Type L (easily soluble in intestinal fluid) is 50% methacrylic acid and Type S (barely soluble in intestinal fluid) is 30% methacrylic acid; both are anionic polymers of methacrylic acid and methacrylic acid ester in different ratios available as 12.5% solution in isopropanol without plasticizer (L 12.5, S 12.5); and as 12.5% ready-to-use solution in isopropanol with 1.25% dibutylphthalate as plasticizer (L 12.5 P, S 12.5 P); colorless, with the characteristic odor of the solvent.

Type RS (5% trimethylammoniummethacrylate chloride) and Type RL (10% trimethylammoniummethacrylate chloride) are copolymers of acrylic and methacrylic acid esters containing some quaternary ammonium groups, available as 12.5% ready-to-use solution in isopropanol and acetone (60:40). Not more than a slightly yellow in color, usually clear or slightly turbid, it has the characteristic odor of solvents. Solvent-free granules contain $\geq 98\%$ of the dried weight.

Type E30D and *Eudragit* L30D: By means of emulsion polymerization, an aqueous dispersion (30% dried resin) of a milky white, low viscosity liquid with a weak aromatic odor is produced.

Eudragit E30D is an acrylic acid ethyl ester: methacrylic acid methyl ester (70:30) copolymer.

Eudragit L30D is a methacrylic acid: acrylic acid methyl ester (50:50) copolymer.

10. Pharmacopeial Specifications

Test	NF
Identification	+
Loss on drying	$\leq 5.0\%$
Residue on ignition	$\leq 0.1\%$
Arsenic	≤ 2 ppm
Heavy metals	$\leq 0.002\%$
Monomers	$\leq 0.3\%$

	Assay and Viscosity Requirements				
	Methacrylic acid dried basis (%)		Viscosity (cps)		
Type	Min	Max	Min	Max
A	46.0	50.6	50	200
B	27.6	30.7	50	200
C	46.0	50.6	100	200

USP reference standards are available for types A, B, and C. (Designation of types A, B, and C should not be confused with trade name designations of Eudragits.)

11. Typical Properties

Density: D_{20}^{20}; Type E 12.5: 0.81 g/ml; Type L 12.5P: 0.845 g/cm³; Type S 12.5P: 0.845 g/ml; Type RL 12.5: 0.825 g/cm³; Type RS 12.5: 0.825 g/ml.

Solubility: Type E—Soluble in polar organic solvents, such as alcohols (ethanol, isopropanol), acetone, esters, chloroform, etc. Insoluble in water, petroleum, ether, etc., and saliva. Swells and dissolves in acidic media. Type L—Soluble in polar organic solvents, such as alcohols (ethanol, isopropanol), acetone and mixtures of these with esters, chloroform, etc. Insoluble in water, petroleum, ether, etc. Does not swell at pH<5.7; soluble at pH>6. Type S—Soluble in polar organic solvents, such as alcohols (ethanol, isopropanol), acetone and mixtures of these with esters, chloroform, etc. Insoluble in water, petroleum, ether, etc. Does not swell at pH<6.5; soluble at pH>7. Types RL and RS—Soluble in isopropanol and ethanol in combination with acetone or methylene chloride; also in methanol, chloroform, trichlorethylene, ethyl acetate and glycol monomethyl ether. Barely soluble in pure isopropanol or carbon tetrachloride. Insoluble in petroleum ether or light petroleum. Swells in aqueous media: the amount of water absorbed depends on the pH of the solution and the type (RL swells more than RS due to its higher concentration of hydrophilic quaternary groups). Types E30D and L30D—Miscible with water in all proportions.

pH: Type E30D—7.5 to 8.5; Type L30D—2.0 to 3.0

Viscosity: Type RL—5 to 15 cps (12.5% solution in isopropanol and acetone (60:40)). Type RS—5 to 15 cps.

Refractive index: n_D^{20}; Type E 12.5: 1.38; Type L 12.5: 1.39; Type S 12.5: 1.39; Type RL 12.5: 1.383; Type RS 12.5: 1.383.

Alkali value (mg KOH/g of dried substance): Type E—180; Type RL—27; Type RS—13.5.

Acid value: Type L: 315; Type S: 190.

12. Stability and Storage Conditions

Dry powder forms appear to be stable at room temperature. Dispersions are stable for about one year after manufacturing if stored at room temperature in tight containers. The dispersions are sensitive to extreme temperatures.

13. Incompatibilities

Incompatibilities occur with acid and/or alkaline conditions, depending upon which polymer is being used. Types L30D and E30D are incompatible with soluble electrolytes, pH changes, organic solvents, extremes of temperature, finely divided pigments and severe shearing gradients, all of which may cause coagulation of the dispersion. Type L30 dispersion is also incompatible with magnesium stearate.

14. Safety

Acute toxicity studies have been performed in rats, rabbits and dogs. No toxic effects were observed with Types L30D, E, L, S, RS, and RL at doses of dry lacquer substance ranging from 6–28 g/kg of body weight over a two-week period. Chronic toxicity studies were performed in rats over a period of 3 months. No significant changes were found in the animal organs. Types E30D and L30D showed no mutagenic activity by the Ames test.

15. Handling Precautions

The usual precautions must be employed when volatile solvents are used.

16. Regulatory Acceptance

NF XVI. In the U.S. supporting documents for Eudragit have been filed with the FDA. Types E30D and L30D have been accepted by the Federal Health Authority (BGA, Berlin) and the Swiss IKS, and have been applied for elsewhere.

17. Applications in Pharmaceutical Formulation or Technology

Binder—*Eudragit* E has been used as a granulation binder in concentrations between 5 and 20%.

Film former—*Eudragit* E is used as a film coating agent, soluble in gastric fluid. *Eudragit* L and S are employed as film coating agents resistant to gastric fluid with different solubilities (L<pH 6, S>pH 7). *Eudragit* RL and RS form water-insoluble film coats for delayed-release products. Permeability is dependent upon pH. *Eudragit* RL film coats are more permeable than those of *Eudragit* RS.

Eudragit L 100-SS is available as a redispersible powder, an alternative to *Eudragit* L30D for enteric film coating.

18. Related Substances

—

19. Comments

For spray coating, the lacquer solutions and dispersions must be thinned with suitable solvents. Suitable plasticizers are glyceryl triacetate and phthalic acid esters, polyethylene glycols, triacetin and dibutyl phthalate, citric acid esters.

Water vapor permeability (film thickness about 25 μm):

　Type E 12.5 and E 100 — 350 g H_2O/m²/d

　Type L 12.5P and S 12.5P — 150 g H_2O/m²/d

Water vapor absorption (film thickness about 25 μm)

　Type RL 12.5 — 450 g/m²/d

　Type RS 12.5 — 250 g/m²/d

20. References

1. K. Lehmann, Acrylic coatings in controlled release tablet manufacture, *Mfg. Chem. Aerosol News,* 44: 36-38 May (1973).
2. K. Lehmann, Polymer coating of tablets—a versatile technique, *Mfg. Chem. Aerosol News,* 45: 48-50 May (1974).
3. K. Lehmann and D. Dreher, The use of aqueous synthetic polymer dispersions for coating pharmaceuticals, *Drugs Made in Germany,* XVI: 126-136 (1973); *Pharmaceutical Industry,* 34: 894-899 (1972).
4. K. Lehmann, Acrylic resin coatings for drugs, *Drugs Made in Germany,* XI: 34-41 (1968).
5. K. Lehmann, and D. Dreher, Permeable acrylic resin coatings for the manufacture of depot preparations of drugs, Part 2. Coating of granules and pellets and preparation of matrix tablets, *Drugs Made in Germany,* XII: 59-71 (1969).
6. K. Lehmann, Enteric and retard coatings of pharmaceutical preparations with aqueous acrylic resin dispersions, *Acta Pharmaceutica Technologica,* 21 (4): 255-260 (1975).
7. K. Lehmann, Acrylic coatings in controlled release tablet manufacture. Part 2, *Mfg. Chem. Aerosol News,* 44: 39-41, June (1973).
8. B.H. Lippold and B.C. Lippold, Release of carbutamide from drugs with polymethacrylic acid derivatives, *Pharm. Ind.,* 36 (6): 432-437 (1974).

9. B.C. Lippold, and B.H. Lippold, Sorption of sulfon-amides by derivatives of poly(methacrylic acid), *Pharmazie,* 29 (8): 534-540 (1974).

10. C.F. Lerk, W.J. Bolink, K. Zuurman, Active substance-release from a drug preparation with a constant release rate, *Pharm. Ind.,* 38 (6): 561-566 (1976).

11. R. Gurny, P. Guitard, P. Buri, Determination of water vapor permeability for various methacrylate copolymer compounds, *Acta Pharm. Technol.,* 23 (1): 29-38 (1977).

12. K. Lehmann, H.M. Boessler, D. Dreher, Controlled drug release from small particles encapsulated with acrylic resins, *Acta Pharm. Suec.,* 13: Suppl., 37-38 (1976)

13. R. Gurny, P. Guitard, P. Buri, J. Sucker, Realization and theoretical development of controlled-release drug forms using methacrylate films—3. Preparation and characterization of controlled-release drug forms, *Pharm. Acta Helv.,* 52 (8): 182-187 (1977).

USA: E. A. Holstills*; A. Bruno**; D. Hovermale**; J. Mollica**
UK: J. S. Wilde*

Polyoxyethylene Alkyl Ethers

1. Nonproprietary Name
BP: Cetomacrogol 1000

2. Functional Category
BP: Nonionic emulsifying agent (cetomacrogol 1000)

3. Synonyms
Macrogol ethers; *Texofor A series; Empilan KB, KM series; Cremophor A* series; *Volpo* series; *Ethylan C* series; *Brij* series; *Renex* series; *Flurafac* series; *cyclogol 1000* series

4. Chemical Names and CAS Registry Number
Polyethylene glycol ethers of *n*-alkanols, e.g., cetomacrogol 1000 is polyethylene glycol 1000 monocetyl ether [9004-95-9]

5. Empirical Formula   Molecular Weight
—   —

6. Structural Formula
General formula:
$$CH_3(CH_2)_x(O-CH_2-CH_2)_yOH$$
where $(x + 1)$ is the number of carbon atoms in the alkyl chain, typically:

12 lauryl	(dodecyl)
14 myristyl	(tetradecyl)
16 cetyl	(hexadecyl)
18 stearyl	(octadecyl)

and y is the number of ethylene oxide groups in the hydrophilic chain, typically 10–60.
The products tend to be mixtures of polymers of slightly varying molecular weights, and the numbers quoted are average.
For example, in cetomacrogol 1000, x is 15 or 17, and y is 20–24.
Note: Two systems of nomenclature are used for the polyoxyethylene ethers. The number 10 in the name Texofor A10 refers to the approximate polymer length in oxyethylene units (i.e., y). The number 1000 in the name cetomacrogol 1000 refers to the average molecular weight of the polymer chain.

7. Commercial Availability
USA

Alcolac, Inc.
Bage, Inc.
BASF Wyandotte Corp.
Conoco Chemicals Co., Div. Conoco, Inc.
Emery Industries
GAF Corp.
Glyco, Inc.
Henkel KGaA
ICI Americas, Inc.
Lanatex Products, Inc.
Lippo Chemicals, Inc.
Mazer Chemicals, Inc.
Quad Chemical - Lonza Specialty Chemicals
Sandoz Colors & Chemicals
Sherex Chemical Co.
Surfactants, Inc.

UK

A.B.M. Chemicals, Ltd.
Albright & Wilson, Ltd.
Blagden Campbell Chemicals Ltd.
Croda Chemicals Ltd.
Diamond Shamrock Europe Ltd.
Honeywell-Atlas, Ltd.
Pechiney Ugine Kuhlmann, Ltd.
Witco Chemical, Ltd., Cyclo Div.

8. Method of Manufacture
By condensation of linear fatty alcohols with ethylene oxide. The reaction is controlled so that the required ether is formed with the polyethylene glycol of the desired molecular weight.

9. Description
Liquid, paste or solid waxy substances; colorless, white or creamy with a slight odor.
Cetomacrogol 1000: A cream-colored, waxy, unctuous mass which melts on heating to a clear, brownish-yellow liquid; almost odorless.

10. Pharmacopeial Specifications
Cetomacrogol 1000:

Test	BP
Identification	+
Acid value	≤ 0.5
Alkalinity	+
Hydroxyl value	40.0–52.5
Melting point	$\geq 38°C$
Refractive index (at 60°C)	1.448–1.452
Saponification value	≤ 1.0
Water	$\leq 1.0\%$ w/w

11. Typical Properties

Name	Density at 20°C (g/cm³)	Solubility Water	Ethanol	Fixed oils	Other	Viscosity at 25°C or at pour point	MPt or pour point (°C)	Water content (%)	Acid no.	Hydroxyl no.	Cloud point (1% aq. sol.)	HLB	CMC* (%)	Surface tension of aq. sol. (mN/m) (0.05%)	(0.2%)	Physical form
Texofor A1P series	1.025 (at 60°C)	S	S		S chloroform S xylene		40				Sol at boil	16.2	0.006	42.9	42.3	Solid
AP	0.875	I	S				31				Insol					
A6	0.140	I	S				26				Insol					Solid
A10	0.970	S	S				30				75°C		0.004	36.5	36.7	Solid
A14	0.995	S	S				35				Clouds at boil			36.9	36.6	Solid
A30	1.035	S	S				43				Sol at boil		0.003	46.0	46.0	Solid
A45	1.055	S	S				47				Sol at at boil		0.004	47.5	47.0	Solid
A60	1.065	S	S				48				Sol at at boil		0.003	48.3	48.3	Solid

11. Typical Properties (cont.)

Name	Density at 20°C (g/cm³)	Solubility Water	Ethanol	Fixed oils	Propylene glycol	Viscosity at 25°C or at pour point	MPt or pour point (°C)	Water content (%)	Acid no.	Hydroxyl no.	Cloud point (1% aq. sol.)	HLB	CMC* (%)	Surface tension of aq. sol. (mN/m) (0.05%)	(0.2%)	Physical form
Brij 30	0.95 (at 25°C)	I	S	S	S	30 mN s/m²		1 max	2 max	145-165		9.7				Liquid
35	1.05	S	S	I	S		33	3 max	5 max	40-60		16.9	0.013			Solid
52		I	S	S	I		33	1 max	1 max	160-180		5.3				Solid
56		I	S	I	I		31	3 max	1 max	75-90		12.9				Solid
58		S	S	I	I		38	3 max	1 max	45-60		15.7				Solid
72		I	S	S	I		43	1 max	1 max	150-170		4.9				Solid
76		I	S	I	S		38	3 max	1 max	75-90		12.4				Solid
78		I	S	I	I		38	3 max	1 max	45-60		15.3				Solid
93		I	S	S	S	30 mN s/m²	10	1 max	1 max	160-180		4.9				
97		S	S	I	I	100 mN s/m²	16	3 max	1 max	80-95		12.4				
99		S	S	I	S		33	3 max	1 max	50-65		15.3				

Key S = soluble
  I = insoluble
  D = dispersible
  SH = soluble on heating

* Generally, critical micelle concentrations of nonionic surfactants are extremely low.

Name	Density at 20°C (g/cm³)	Solubility Water	Ethanol	Fixed oils	Many organic solvents	Viscosity at 25°C or at pour point	MPt or pour point (°C)	Water content (%)	Refractive index	Acid no.	Sap no.	Iodine no.	Hydroxyl no.	Cloud point (1% aq. sol.)	HLB	CMC* (%)	Physical form
Renex series 30	1.0	S	S	I	S	60 mN s/m²	14	3 max		1 max			75-85	18.4°C	14.5		Liquid + suspended solid
31	1.0	S	S	I	S	130 mN s/m²	16	3 max		1 max			60-74	99°C	15.4		
36	1.0	D	S	I	S	80 mN s/m²		1 max		1 max			118-133	<32°C	11.4		
Cremophor series A6	(at 60°C) 0.896-0.906	S	S	I			41-43	<1	(at 60°C) 1.4420-1.4424	<1	<3	<1	115-135		10-12		
A11	0.964-0.968	S	S	I			34-36	<1	1.4464-1.4474	<1	<1	<1	70-80		12-14		
A25	1.020-1.028	S	S	I			44-46	<1	1.4512-1.4520	<1	<3	<1	35-45		15-17		
Ethosperse series 1A4	0.95	S	S	S	S	30 mN s/m²		0.5 max		2 max			145-160				
1A12	1.10	S	S	SH	S	1000 mN s/m²		1.0 max		2 max			72-82				
TDA6	0.98	D	S	I	S	80 mN s/m²		1.0 max		1 max			118-133				
S120	1.16	S	S	I	S	460 mN s/m²		1.0 max		0.5 max			385-430				
G26	1.12 (at 38°C)	S	S	I	S	150 mN s/m² (at 38°C)		0.5 max		2 max			133-142				

Key S = soluble
  I = insoluble
  D = dispersible
  SH = soluble on heating

* Generally, critical micelle concentrations of nonionic surfactants are extremely low.

Name	Density at 20°C (g/cm³)	Solubility Water	Ethanol	Fixed oils	Other	Viscosity at 25°C or at pour point	MPt or pour point (°C)	water content (%)	Hydroxyl no.	Cloud point (1% aq. sol.)	HLB	CMC* (%)	Surface tension of aq. sol. (mN/m)	Physical form
Ethylan series D252	0.903 (at 20°C)	I				31 mm²/s (at 20°C)	5	<0.5		Insol	5.6			Liquid
D253	0.930	I				36 mm²/s	3	<0.5		Insol	7.8			Liquid
D254	0.948	I				57 mm²/s	5	3.0		Insol	9.8			Liquid
D256	0.972	S				72 mm²/s	15	<0.5		43	11.4			Liquid
D257	0.974 (at 40°C)	S				26 mm²/s (at 60°C)	21	<0.5		49	12.2			Liquid
D2512	1.001	S				40 mm²/s	29	<0.5		92	14.2			Solid
D2560	—	S				120 mm²/s	45	<0.5		>100	18.6			Solid
Plurafac series RA20	0.9965 (at 20°C)					71 mm²/s (at 25°C)	4	<0.1	69-78				(0.1%, 20°C) 30.7	
RA30	0.976					20-80 mm²/s	-6	<0.1	85-95				28.6	
RA40	0.978					60-80 mm²/s	-27	<0.2	65-75				30.3	
RA340	0.977					70 mm²/s	-23		73				30.5	

Key S = soluble
  I = insoluble
  D = dispersible
  SH = soluble on heating

* Generally, critical micelle concentrations of nonionic surfactants are extremely low.

12. Stability and Storage Conditions

Stable in strongly acidic or alkaline conditions. The presence of strong electrolytes may induce separation of cetomacrogol. The surfactants can undergo autooxidation on storage, resulting in the formation of peroxides and a continual increase in acidity. Keep in an airtight container.

13. Incompatibilities

Discoloration and/or precipitation with sulfonamides, salicylates, phenolic substances, iodides, mercury salts and tannins. Benzocaine and oxidizable drugs. Inactivation of phenolic preservatives due to hydrogen bonding with ether oxygen atoms. Cloud points are depressed by phenols, again due to hydrogen bonding between ether oxygen atoms and phenolic hydroxyl groups. Salts, other than nitrates, iodides and thiocyanates (which cause an increase), also depress cloud points.

14. Safety

In toxicity data from suppliers, for example, for Volpo CS20 (cetomacrogol 1000 BP), information has been given that an acute oral toxicity test with rats gave an LD_{50} of 3.6 ± 0.8 g/kg of body weight. For the Texofor A series, the LD_{50} is greater than 500 mg/kg of body weight. For the Plurafac surfactants, toxicity details are summarized as follows: They show about the same level of oral toxicity as many commonly used surfactants. They have oral LD_{50} values ranging from 2-4 g/kg of body weight. On the basis of these oral LD_{50} values, they are classed as moderately toxic. The percutaneous toxicities of the clear liquid surfactants are reported as >2-6 g/kg of body weight. Except for Plurafac RA-40, they are reported to be only slightly or mildly irritating to the skin. Patch test, rabbit eye irritation and acute oral toxicity (rat) for Brij series are summarized on Table I.

Table I — Safety and Toxicology

Product	No. of reactors/ no. of persons tested (% conc., w/v)	Irritation potential (%)	% tolerated	Conc. % (w/v)	Irritation rating unwashed	Washed after 2 seconds	Acute oral toxicity (Rat) LD50 (g/kg) (Data determined on male and/or female rats)
Brij 30	0/50 (100)	20	—	100	Severely irritant	Mildly irritant	9
				20	Minimally irritant	Nonirritant	
Brij 3058					No data available	See Brij 30 data	
Brij 35	0/50 (60)	100	—	100	Minimally irritant	Practically nonirritant	9
Brij 3558					No data available	See Brij 35 data	
Brij 52	38/100 (60)			60	Practically nonirritant	Nonirritant	22
	11/100 (20)	—	—				
Brij 56	2/200 (60)			60	Mildly irritant	Nonirritant	2.8
	0/199 (20)	—	—				
Brij 58	0/200 (60)	—	—	60	Nonirritant	Nonirritant	3.6
Brij 72	0/200 (60)	—	—	60	Minimally irritant	Nonirritant	>25
Brij 76	0/200 (60)	—	—	60	Practically nonirritant	Nonirritant	2.5
Brij 78	0/200 (60)	—	—	60	Minimally irritant	Nonirritant	2.1
Brij 92	0/200 (60)	—	—	100	Practically nonirritant	Nonirritant	25
Brij 93	1/104 (100)	—	—	100	Nonirritant	Nonirritant	32
Brij 96	0/200 (100)	—	—	100	Mildly irritant	Mildly irritant	2.8
Brij 97	0/104 (100)	—	—	100	Mildly irritant	Mildly irritant	3.6
Brij 98	0/200 (100)	—	—	100	Mildly irritant	Minimally irritant	2.9
Brij 99	0/104 (100)	—	—	100	Minimally irritant	Minimally irritant	2.4
Arlasolve 200	0/204 (100)	—	—	100	Moderately irritant	Mildly irritant	9.7

15. Handling Precautions

Avoid ingestion, inhalation and contact with skin, eyes, nose and mouth.

16. Regulatory Acceptance

BP 1980 (cetomacrogol 1000)

17. Applications in Pharmaceutical Formulation or Technology

Polyoxyethylene ethers are nonionic surface-active agents. Thus, they are used as: emulsifying agents for w/o and o/w emulsions, both pharmaceutical and cosmetic; solubilizing agents for essential oils, perfumery chemicals, vitamin oils and drugs of low water solubility; gelling and foaming agents; e.g., Brij 72 gives a quick-breaking foam, while Brij 97 (and others) gives clear gels at 15-20% concentration; anti-dusting agents for powders; wetting and dispersing (steric stabilization) agents for coarse-particle liquid dispersions; and detergents, especially in shampoos and similar cosmetic cleaning preparations.

18. Related Substances

Polyoxyethylene diethers and mixtures (e.g., polyoxyl 20 Cetostearyl ether NF); polyoxyethylene (mono- and di-) ethers with unsaturated alkyl side chains (e.g., polyoxyl 10 oleyl ether NF); polyoxyethylene ethers with alkylaryl side chains (e.g., nonoxynol 10 NF, octoxynol 9 NF) and related polyethers (e.g., tyloxapol USP)

19. Comments

Polyoxyethylene ethers of various compositions are included in a monograph in the Japanese Pharmacopeia.

20. Specific References

1. J. Schick Martin, *Non-Ionic Surfactants*, Vol. 1, Marcel Dekker, Inc., New York, 1966.

2. E. Azaz, M. Donbrow and R. Hamburger, *Pharm. J.*, 15: 211(1973).

3. P. Mukergee and K. J. M. Mysels, "Critical Micelle Concentrations of Aqueous Surfactant Systems," National Bureau of Standards, Washington, D.C., 1971.

4. D. Guveli, S. S. Davis and J. B. Kayes, *J. Pharm. Pharmacol.*, 26:127S (1974).

5. P. H. Elworthy and W. G. Guthrie, *J. Pharm. Pharmacol.*, 22: 114S (1970).

6. C. McDonald and C. Richardson, The effect of added salts on solubilization by a non-ionic surfactant, *J. Pharm. Pharmacol.*,33: 38–39 (1980).

7. K. A. Walters, P. H. Dugard and A. T. Florence, Non-ionic surfactants and gastric mucosal transport of paraquat, *J. Pharm.Pharmacol.*, 33: 207–213 (1980).

USA: S. T. Anik*; Z. Chowhan**
UK: J. B. Kayes*; W. Lund**; A. Winfield**

Polyoxyethylene Castor Oil Derivatives

1. Nonproprietary Name

NF: Polyoxyl 35 castor oil; polyoxyl 40 hydrogenated castor oil

CTFA: Polyoxyethylene (40 and 60) castor oil derivatives

2. Functional Categories

NF: Wetting and/or solubilizing agent; emulsifying and/or solubilizing agent

Others: Non ionic emulsifying agents; solubilizers; dispersing agents

3. Synonyms

Cremophor EL:	Polyethoxylated castor oil; glycerol polyethyleneglycol ricinoleate
Cremophor RH 40:	Polyethoxylated hydrogenated castor oil; glycerol polyethyleneglycol oxystearate; PEG 40 hydrogenated castor oil
Cremophor RH 60:	PEG 60 hydrogenated castor oil
Emulphor El-719:	Polyoxyethylated vegetable oil
Mapeg; Cremothon	

4. Chemical Name and CAS Registry Number

—

5. Empirical Formula

Cremophors are mixtures of various hydrophobic and hydrophilic components. In *Cremophor EL*, the hydrophobic constituents comprise about 83% of the whole and are esters of ricinoleic acid with glycerol/polyglycol ethers with some unchanged castor oil. The hydrophilic part (17%) consists of glycerol/polyglycol ethers and polyglycols.

About 75% of the components of *Cremophor RH 40* are hydrophobic. They are fatty acid esters of glycerol/polyglycol and of polyglycols. The hydrophilic portion is of polyglycols and glycerol ethoxylates.

6. Structural Formula

—

7. Commercial Availability

USA

BASF
MAZER

UK

BASF
Blagden Campbell
GAF

8. Method of Manufacture

Cremophor EL is produced by reacting 1 mole of castor oil with 35 to 40 moles of ethylene oxide.

Cremophor RH 40 is produced by reacting 1 mole of hydrogenated castor oil with 40 to 45 moles of ethylene oxide.

Cremophor RH 60 is produced by reacting 1 mole of hydrogenated castor oil with 60 moles of ethylene oxide.

9. Description

Cremophor EL: A pale yellow, oily liquid, which is clear at temperatures above 26°C. It has a slight but characteristic odor.

Cremophor RH 40: A white, semisolid paste at room temperature. It liquefies at 30°C. The odor is very faint and characteristic. It has a slight taste in aqueous solution.

Cremophor RH 60: A white paste at room temperature. It has little taste or odor in aqueous solution.

Emulphor El-719: A clear yellow to light brown liquid at 25°C.

10. Pharmacopeial Specifications

Polyoxyl 35 castor oil

Test	NF
Identification	+
Specific gravity	1.05-1.06
Viscosity (capillary viscometer)	650-850 cps at 25°C
Water	≤3.0%
Residue on ignition	≤0.3%
Heavy metals	≤0.001%
Acid value	≤2.0%
Hydroxyl value	65-80
Iodine value	25-35
Saponification value	60-75

Polyoxyl 40 hydroginated castor oil

Test	NF
Identification	+
Congealing temperature	20-30°C
Water	≤3.0%
Residue on ignition	≤0.3%
Acid value	≤2.0%
Hydroxyl value	60-80
Iodine value	≤2.0
Saponification value	45-69

11. Typical Properties

Cremophors

Acid number (Ph.Eur. Vol. III method):
EL: ≤2.0
RH 40: ≤1.0
RH 60: ≤1.0

Cloud point (1% solution):
EL: 72.5°C
RH 40: 95.6°C

Critical micelle concentration (from plots of surface tension versus concentration):
EL: ~0.009%
RH 40: ~0.039%

Density:
EL: 1.05-1.06 g/cm³ (25°C)

HLB:
EL: 12-14
RH 40: 14-16
RH 60: 15-17

Hydroxyl number (Ph.Eur. Vol. III, method A):
EL: 65-78
RH 40: 60-80
RH 60: 50-70

Iodine number (Ph.Eur. Vol. III method):
EL: 28-32
RH 40: ≤1
RH 60: ≤1

Melting point:
EL: Residual solids liquefy at 19-20°C
RH 40:   ~30°C
RH 60:   ~40°C

pH (Ph.Eur. method—10% solution):
EL: 6-8
RH 40:   6-7
RH 60:   6-7

Refractive index:
EL: ~1.471 (25°C)
RH 40:   1.453-1.457 (60°C)

Saponification number (Ph.Eur. Vol. III method):
EL: 65-70
RH 40:   50-60
RH 60:   40-50

Solidifying point:
RH 40:   21-23°C

Solubility/miscibility:
Water: EL, RH—soluble. the solubility decreases with a rise in temperature.
Ethanol: EL, RH—soluble*
Chloroform: EL, RH 40—soluble
Cremophor EL and RH grades are miscible on heating with fatty acids (e.g., oleic and stearic), fatty alcohols (e.g., Lauryl and Stearyl) and some oils of animal and vegetable origin (e.g., castor oil and olive oil).
EL and RH types are miscible with all other *Cremophor* grades.
Other solvents: EL soluble in propan-1-ol, propan-2-ol and ethyl acetate.
RH soluble in propan-1-ol and propan-2-ol*.

Surface tension (ring method; 0.1% w/v solution):
EL: 40.9 mN/m
RH 40:   43.0 mN/m
Note: Owing to the heterogenous nature of *Cremophors*, large aging effects are apparent, and sufficient time must be allowed to reach a reasonably stable state of quasi-equilibrium.

Viscosity:
EL: 650-800 mN s/m^2 (25°C)
RH 40:   20-40 mN s/m^2 (30% aqueous solution, 25°C)

Water content:
EL: ≤3% (Karl Fischer)
RH 40:   ≤2%
RH 60:   ≤2%

---

*If anhydrous alcohols are used, *Cremophor RH 60* may not completely dissolve. Solution can be effected by the addition of 0.5-1.0% of water.

12. Stability and Storage Conditions

Cremophor EL can be sterilized by heating in an autoclave for 30 minutes at 120°C. In this process the product may acquire a deeper shade which, however, has no significance. If *Cremophor RH* grades are heated for a long period, they may separate into solid and liquid phases on cooling. The product can be restored to its original form by homogenization.
Aqueous solutions of *Cremophor RH 40* withstand sterilization at 120°C, but this may cause a slight decrease in the pH value.
Solutions of *Cremophor RH 40* in aqueous alcohols are stable. Store in a tightly closed container protected from light.

Prolonged storage only recommended in full containers. The method of manufacture used for the *Cremophor RH* grades ensures that they are near-sterile; however, microbial contamination and growth can occur once the container is opened.

13. Incompatibilities

Cremophors should not be used in strongly acidic or alkaline solutions, as the ester components may hydrolyze.
In aqueous solution, *Cremophor EL* is stable towards most electrolytes in the concentrations normally employed. It is, however, incompatible with mercuric chloride.
Some organic substances may cause precipitation at certain concentrations, especially compounds containing phenolic hydroxyl groups, e.g., phenol, resorcinol and tannins.
Cremophors RH 40 and 60 are largely unaffected by the salts that cause hardness in water.

14. Safety

The following information has been summarized from data sheets obtained from the *Cremophors'* manufacturer and is based on their current knowledge and experience.
Acute Toxicity: Average lethal dose (LD$_{50}$) values with a 7-day postobservation period.

Animal	Route Administration	Approx. LD$_{50}$ per kg of body weight		
		EL (ml)	RH 40 (g)	RH 60 (g)
Rat	Oral	> 6.4	>16.0	>16.0
Rabbit	Oral	>10.0	—	—
Cat	Oral	>10.0	—	—
Rabbit	Percutaneous	2.5 (max.	—	—
Rat	Percutaneous	4.0 applicable)	—	—
Mouse	Intraperitoneal	—	> 6.4	>12.5
Mouse	Intravenous	—	>12.0	—

Subacute toxicity:
(a) Oral administration to beagle dogs over four weeks: EL: no clinically detectable damage except for soft faeces after daily doses of 0.5, 1, 2.5 and 5.3 ml/per kg of body weight. clinical-chemical and pathological-histological tests showed no pathological change caused by *Cremophor EL*. RH 40: No clinical symptoms of injury when feed contained 1%, 3% and 9%.
(b) Oral administration to rats over four weeks: RH 40: no symptoms of poisoning from intake of feed containing 3.2% and 6.4%.
Chronic toxicity: In feeding tests carried out for six months in rats and dogs, *Cremophor RH 40* was tolerated and there were no visible symptoms of poisoning or marked changes in food intake, body weight or the characteristics of blood, urine and various organs in animals given the EL grade. Concentrations administered were:

	rats	dogs
EL:	< 1%	<1%
RH 40:	<10%	<5%

Inhalation toxicity: Rats have inhaled, for eight hours, air saturated with the volatile components of EL and RH 40 grades without injury. In humans, no irritation of mucous membranes of the respiratory tract is caused by the application of aerosols which contain RH 40.

Compatibility with the skin and mucous membranes:
Skin—Human: Swab tests have shown the RH grades to be compatible. Rabbit: Undiluted EL grade applied to the backs and ears, for more than 20 hours, caused slight or insignificant inflammation that disappeared rapidly.
Eyes—Rabbit: EL undiluted (0.05 ml): slight reddening of the conjunctiva, which disappeared within a few hours. EL (50% aqueous solution): slight irritation with lachrymation, which disappeared rapidly. EL (30% aqueous solution): no irritating effect. RH 40 (30% aqueous solution): no inflammation. RH 60 (50% aqueous solution): no inflammation.

Sensitization:
Guinea pigs: EL (50% in acetone): repeated application to skin by brush caused an inflammatory reaction at the site, but no sensitization. EL (0.1% solution in 0.9% sodium chloride solution): intracutaneous injection (0.05 or 0.1 ml) repeated ten times on subsequent days caused no sensitization of the skin. RH 40 (20% and 50% in acetone): brushed ten times on skin did not cause sensitization. No indication of sensitization when maximization test* applied.
*(Magnusson and Kligman, *J. invest. Derm.*, 52, 268-276 (1969)).

Teratogenic studies:
Using the FDA guidelines for reproduction studies for the safety evaluation of drugs for human use (Food and Drug Administration, Washington, DC, January, 1966), there were no teratogenic or embryotoxic effects after the administration of EL and RH 40 grades under the following conditions:
(a) to pregnant NMRI mice: EL, orally in daily doses of 5 and 10 ml/kg of body weight; RH 40, orally in daily doses of 5 g and 10 g/kg of body weight, from the 6th to the 15th day *post coitum.*
(b) to pregnant Sprague-Dawley rats, when the feed included: EL (5% and 10%) from the 6th to the 20th day *post coitum*; RH 40 (5% and 10%) from zero to the 20th day *post coitum.*

Effect on absorption: The surface-active properties of *Cremophors* may affect the rate at which drugs are absorbed through the skin. For this reason the makers recommend that preparations which contain RH grades should be subjected to pharmacological and clinical tests before they are adopted for practical use.

Parenteral administration: There have been reports of anaphylactic reactions in animals and humans after parenteral administration of pharmaceutical products containing *Cremophor EL*. The possibility cannot be precluded that similar reactions could occur in preparations which contain *Cremophor RH 40*. No such reactions have been observed on oral administration. In rats, RH 40 administered intravenously during four weeks was tolerated locally at a daily dose which exceeded 300 mg/kg of body weight and tolerated generally at a dose exceeding 900 mg/kg of body weight.

15. Handling Precautions

Avoid ingestion, inhalation and contact with skin, eyes, nose and mouth.

16. Regulatory Acceptance

Cremophor EL, which was listed under the name *Glycerine Polyethyleneglycol Ricinoleate* (E484) in Appendix II of the EEC Directive regarding Additives for Feeding Stuffs (70/524/EEC), has been transferred to Appendix I. This means that *Cremophor EL* may now be used in all EEC countries as an additive in the production of animal feeding stuffs.

17. Applications in Pharmaceutical Formulation or Technology

Cremophor EL is of value as an emulsifier and solubilizer, and is particularly suitable for the production of liquid preparations. Volatile oils, fat-soluble vitamins and other hydrophobic substances can be emulsified or dissolved in an aqueous medium with *Cremophor EL*. In 1 ml of a 25% *Cremophor EL* solution in water, it is possible to incorporate: approximately 10 mg of vitamin A palmitate; approximately 10 mg of vitamin D; approximately 120 mg of vitamin E Acetate; approximately 120 mg of vitamin K_1.
To solubilize fat-soluble vitamins, the active ingredient(s) should first be dissolved in *Cremophor EL*. The water should then be added very slowly, with vigorous stirring. As the water is added, the viscosity increases, reaching a maximum at a water content of approximately 40%. Solubilization can be facilitated by heating to approximately 60°C for a short time and in some cases adding polyethylene glycols and/or propylene glycol.
The taste of *Cremophor EL* can be masked by a banana flavor.
Cremophor EL has been used as a solvent in proprietary injections of diazepam, propanidid and alfaxolone with alfadolone acetate. It is also used in the production of glycerin suppositories.
In veterinary practice, *Cremophor EL* can be used to emulsify cod liver oil and also oils and fats incorporated into animal feeding stuffs.
Cosmetic application of the EL grade is mainly as a solubilizer for perfume bases and volatile oils in vehicles containing 30 to 50% alcohol (ethanol or propanol). It can replace castor oil in hand lotions.
Cremophor RH 40: An advantage of the RH 40 grade over the EL grade is that it is almost tasteless. In aqueous alcoholic or completely aqueous solutions, RH 40 can be used to solubilize vitamins, essential oils and certain drugs.
Using 1 ml of a 25% solution of *Cremophor RH 40* in water, it is possible to solubilize: approximately 88 mg of vitamin A palmitate; approximately 160 mg of vitamin A propionate. Other materials which can be solubilized by RH 40 are: alfadolone; alfaxolone; hexachlorophane; hexetidine; methotrimeprazine; miconazole; propanidid; thiopentone.
In aerosol vehicles which include water, the addition of *Cremophor RH 40* improves the solubility of the propellant in the aqueous phase. This enhancement applies both to dichlorodifluoromethane and to propane/butane mixtures.
Foam formation in solutions of RH 40 in aqueous ethanol can be suppressed by the addition of small amounts of polypropylene glycol 2000.
Cremophor RH 40 is also used as an emulsifier of fatty acids and alcohols.

18. Related Substances

Cremophor RH 410 is a mixture of 90% *Cremophor RH 40* with 10% water.
Cremophor RH 455 is a mixture of 90% *Cremophor RH 40*, 5% propylene glycol and 5% water.
At room temperature, *Cremophors* RH 410 or 455 are viscous, slightly opalescent liquids.
As well as the EL and RH types, other *Cremophors* of different chemical types are manufactured, e.g., *Cremophor A* series—reaction products of ethylene oxide with a saturated fatty alcohol. *Cremophor S* series—reaction products of ethylene oxide with stearic acid.

19. Comments

—

20. References

1. D. Dye and J. Watkins, Suspected anaphylactic reaction to Cremophor EL, *Brit. Med. J.* 1: 1353 (1980).
2. D. Blatchley, Allergy to Diazepam, *Brit. Med. J.*, 1: 287, (1977).
3. N. E. Webb, Method of solubilization of selected drug substances, *Bull. Parenteral Drug Assn.*, 30: 7 (1976).
4. T. J. Macek, Preparation of parenteral dispersions, *J. Pharm. Sci.*, 52: 694 (1962).
5. U. Schaeppi and R. S. Phelan, "Emulphor-(620) Vehicle: Blood Pressure Effects of I.V. Infusion in Dogs and Rhesus Monkeys," sponsored by Dept. of HEW, Report No. MRI-CC-9-72-42, Sep. 29, 1972.
6. U. Schaeppi, R. W. Fleischman, D. McCracken, M. Ethier and Y. Luthra, "Emulphor (EL-620) Vehicle for CCNU and Methyl CCNU Toxicity of I.V. Infusion in Two Dogs and Two Monkeys," sponsored by Dept. of HEW, Report No. MRI-CC13-73-49, Nov. 2, 1973.

USA: J. H. Lazarus*; Z. Chowhan**
UK: S. S. Davis*

Polyoxyethylene Sorbitan Fatty Acid Esters

1. Nonproprietary Names

NF: Polysorbates 20, 40, 60 and 80
BP/EP: Polysorbates 20, 60 and 80

2. Functional Category

NF: Wetting and/or solubilizing agent; emulsifying and/or solubilizing agent
BP/EP: Non-ionic surface-active agents

3. Synonyms

Polyethylene oxide sorbitan esters, *Tweens, Sorlates, Monitans, Crillets*

4. Chemical Names and CAS Registry Number

Polysorbate 20—Sorbitan, monododecanoate, poly(oxy-1, 2-ethanediyl) derivs.; polyoxyethylene 20 sorbitan monolaurate. [9005-64-5]
Polysorbate 21—Polyoxyethylene 4 sorbitan monolaurate. [None]
Polysorbate 40—Sorbitan, monohexadecanoate, poly(oxy-1,2-ethanediyl) derivs.; polyoxyethylene 20 sorbitan monopalmitate. [9005-66-7]
Polysorbate 60—Sorbitan, monooctadecanoate, poly(oxy-1,2-ethanediyl) derivs.; polyoxyethylene .20 sorbitan monostearate. [9005-67-8]
Polysorbate 61—Polyoxyethylene 4 sorbitan monostearate. [None]
Polysorbate 65—Sorbitan, trioctadecanoate, poly(oxy-1,2-ethanediyl) derivs.; polyoxyethylene 20 sorbitan tristearate. [9005-71-4]
Polysorbate 80—Sorbitan, mono-9-octadecanoate, poly-(oxy-1,2-ethanediyl) derivs.; (Z); polyoxyethylene 20 sorbitan monooleate. [9005-65-6]
Polysorbate 81—Sorbitan, tri-9-octadecenoate, poly(oxy-1,2-ethanediyl) derivs.; polyoxyethylene 5 sorbitan monooleate. [None]
Polysorbate 85—Sorbitan, tri-9-octadecenoate, poly(oxy-1,2-ethanediyl) derivs.; polyoxyethylene 20 sorbitan trioleate. [9005-70-3]

5. Empirical Formulae* and Molecular Weight*

Empirical Formulae*	Molecular Weight*
Polysorbate 20: $C_{58}H_{114}O_{26}$	1126
Polysorbate 21: $C_{26}H_{50}O_{10}$	522
Polysorbate 40: $C_{62}H_{122}O_{26}$	1282
Polysorbate 60: $C_{64}H_{126}O_{26}$	1310
Polysorbate 61: $C_{32}H_{62}O_{10}$	606
Polysorbate 65: $C_{100}H_{194}O_{28}$	1842
Polysorbate 80: $C_{64}H_{125}O_{26}$	1309
Polysorbate 81: $C_{54}H_{120}O_{21}$	1104
Polysorbate 85: $C_{100}H_{188}O_{28}$	1836

*Formulae and weights are approximate.

6. Structural Formula

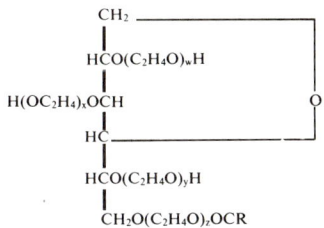

Polyoxyethylene sorbitan
monoester

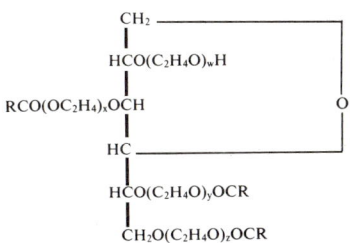

Polyoxyethylene sorbitan triester

$w+x+y+z = 20$ Polysorbate 20, 40, 60, 65, 80 and 85)
$w+x+y+z = 5$ (Polysorbate 81)
$w+x+y+z = 4$ (Polysorbate 21 and 61)

7. Commercial Availability

USA

Bage, Inc.
Croda Chemicals, Inc.
Durkee Industrial Foods/SCM Corp.
Emery Industries
Glyco, Inc.
Hodag Chemical Corp.
ICI Americas, Inc.
Lanetex Products, Inc.
Lippo Chemicals, Inc.
Mazer Chemicals, Inc.
Quad Chemical-Lonza Specialty Chemicals
Ruger Chemical Co.
Sandoz Colors & Chemicals
Surfactants, Inc.
United States Biochemicals Corp.

UK

Atlas Chemical Indust. (UK), Ltd.
Blagden Campbell Chemical, Ltd.
Croda Chemicals, Ltd.

8. Method of Manufacture

These surfactants are prepared starting from sorbitol by: 1) elimination of a water, forming a sorbitan (a cyclic sorbitol anhydride); 2) partial esterification of the sorbitan with a fatty acid, such as oleic or stearic acid, yielding a hexitan ester (i.e., a *Span*); and 3) chemical addition of ethylene oxide in the presence of a catalyst to yield a polysorbate (the polyoxyethylene derivative). A sample schematic diagram follows:

CH$_2$OH
|
HCOH
|
HCOH
|
HCOH
|
HCOH
|
CH$_2$OH

SORBITOL

1,4 SORBITAN

CH$_2$OH
|
CHOH

HO   OH

CH$_2$OOCC$_{17}$H$_{33}$
|
CHOH

HO   OH

SORBITAN MONO-OLEATE

(a *Span*)

CH$_2$(OC$_2$H$_4$)$_w$OCC$_{17}$H$_{33}$

CH(OC$_2$H$_4$)$_x$OH

HO(OC$_2$H$_4$)$_y$ (OC$_2$H$_4$)$_z$OH

POLYSORBATE 80

(a *Tween*)

Note: All *Spans* and *Tweens* are actually *mixtures*, with one particular *Span* or *Tween* predominating.

9. Description

Polysorbates have a characteristic odor and a warm, somewhat bitter taste. Their colors and physical forms at 25°C are as follows:

Polysorbate Type	Color and Form at 25°C
Polysorbate 20	Yellow oily liquid
Polysorbate 21	Yellow oily liquid
Polysorbate 40	Yellow oily liquid
Polysorbate 60	Yellow oily liquid
Polysorbate 61	Tan solid
Polysorbate 65	Tan solid
Polysorbate 80	Yellow oily liquid
Polysorbate 81	Amber liquid
Polysorbate 85	Amber liquid

10. Pharmacopeial Specifications

Test	NF	BP/EP
Identification		
Polysorbate 20	+	+
Polysorbate 40	+	Not official
Polysorbate 60	+	+
Polysorbate 80	+	+
Saponification value		
Polysorbate 20	40-50	40-50
Polysorbate 40	41-52	Not official
Polysorbate 60	45-55	45-55
Polysorbate 80	45-55	45-55
Hydroxyl value		
Polysorbate 20	96-108	96-108
Polysorbate 40	89-105	Not official
Polysorbate 60	81-96	81-96
Polysorbate 80	65-80	65-80
Water		
Polysorbate 40	3.0%	Not official
Polysorbate 20, 60 and 80	3.0%	3.0%
Residue on ignition		
Polysorbate 20, 40, 60 and 80	0.25%	—
Arsenic		
Polysorbate 20, 40, 60 and 80	1 ppm	—
Heavy Metals		
Polysorbate 40	0.001%	Not official
Polysorbate 20, 60 and 80	0.001%	10 ppm

Test	NF	BP/EP
Acid value		
Polysorbate 40	2.2	Not official
Polysorbate 20, 60 and 80	2.2	2.0
Iodine value		
Polysorbate 20	—	5.0
Polysorbate 40	—	Not official
Polysorbate 60	—	5.0
Polysorbate 80	—	18-24
Reducing substances		
Polysorbate 40	—	Not official
Polysorbate 20, 60 and 80	—	+
Sulfated ash		
Polysorbate 40	—	Not official
Polysorbate 20, 60 and 80	—	0.2%
Specific gravity		
Polysorbate 20	—	1.10 (approx.)
Polysorbate 40	—	Not official
Polysorbate 60	—	1.10 (approx.)
Polysorbate 80	1.06-1.09	1.08 (approx.)
Viscosity at 25°C		
Polysorbate 20	—	400 cps (approx.)
Polysorbate 40	—	Not official
Polysorbate 60	—	—
Polysorbate 80	300-500 centistokes	400 cps (approx.)

11. Typical Properties

Chemical:

	Hydroxyl Number	Saponification Number	Percent Water	Acid Number
Polysorbate 20	96-108	40-50	3.0	2.0
Polysorbate 21	225-255	100-115	3.0	3.0
Polysorbate 40	90-105	41-52	3.0	2.0
Polysorbate 60	81-96	45-55	3.0	2.0
Polysorbate 61	170-200	95-115	3.0	2.0
Polysorbate 65	44-60	88-98	3.0	2.0
Polysorbate 80	65-80	45-55	3.0	2.0
Polysorbate 81	134-150	96-104	3.0	2.0
Polysorbate 85	39-52	80-95	4.8-5.2	2.0

Note: The pH of *Tweens* ranges from 6.0-8.0 (5% solution).

Physical:

| | Solubility | | | | Specific | | |
	H2O	EtOH	Veg. Oil	Mineral Oil	Gravity @ 25°C	Viscosity (cps)	HLB #
Polysorbate 20	L	L	U	U	1.1	400	16.7
Polysorbate 21	D	L	U	U	1.1	500	13.3
Polysorbate 40	L	L	U	U	1.08	500	15.6
Polysorbate 60	L	L	U	U	1.1	600	14.9
Polysorbate 61	D	LW	LWT	LW	1.06	solid	9.6
Polysorbate 65	D	L	D	L	1.05	solid	10.5
Polysorbate 80	L	L	U	U	1.08	425	15.0
Polysorbate 81	D	L	LT	L	—	450	10.0
Polysorbate 85	D	L	LT	U	1.00	300	11.0

Note: Abbreviations: D = dispersible; L = soluble; T = turbid; U = insoluble; W = in the warm. Both the fire point and the flash point for all polysorbates listed above are approximately 149°C.

12. Stability and Storage Conditions

Polysorbates are stable to electrolytes as well as to weak acids and bases. There is gradual saponification by strong acids and bases. The oleic acid esters are sensitive to oxidation. Preserve in a tight container protected from light, and store in cool conditions.

13. Incompatibilities

Discoloration and/or precipitation occurs with various substances, especially with phenols, tannins, tars and/or tar-like compounds.

14. Safety

Polysorbates are well tolerated, practically non-irritating and of very low toxicity.

15. Handling Precautions

Avoid ingestion, inhalation and contact with skin, nose, and mouth.

16. Regulatory Acceptance

	NF XVI	BP/EP
Polysorbate 20	Yes	Yes
Polysorbate 21	—	—
Polysorbate 40	Yes	—
Polysorbate 60	Yes	Yes
Polysorbate 61	—	—
Polysorbate 65	—	—
Polysorbate 80	Yes	Yes
Polysorbate 81	—	—
Polysorbate 85	—	—

17. Applications in Pharmaceutical Formulation or Technology

Use	Concentration (%)
Emulsifiers	
Used alone in water-in-oil emulsions	1-15
Used in combination with hydrophilic emulsifiers in oil-in-water emulsions	1-10
Used to increase the water-holding properties of ointments	1-10
Solubilizers	
For poorly soluble active constituents in lipophilic bases	1-10
Wetting Agents	
For insoluble active constituents in lipophilic bases	0.1-3

18. Related Substances

None

19. Comments

Tweens 20, 60 and 80 are obtainable in a specially deodorized form as *Tween* 20 SD, 60 SD, and 80 SD.

20. Specific References

1. J. Blanchard, Effect of polyols on interaction of preservatives with Polysorbate 80, *J. Pharm. Sci.*, 69:(2), 169 (1980).
2. L.V. Allen, Jr., R. S. Levinson, C. Robinson and A. Lau, Effect of surfactant on tetracycline absorption across everted rat intestine, *J. Pharm. Sci.*, 70:(30), 269 (1981).
3. Z. T. Chowhan and R. Pritchard, Effect of surfactants on percutaneous absorption of naproxen I: Comparison of rabbit, rat and human excised skin, *J. Pharm. Sci.*, 67:(9), 1272-1274 (1978).
4. "Atlas products for Cosmetics and Pharmaceuticals", ICI United States Inc., 1977.

USA: J. J. Tagman*; A. Bruno **; Z. Chowhan**
UK: J. B. Kayes*

Polyoxyethylene Stearates

1. Nonproprietary Names

Table I

Name	Synonyms	Commercial Names & Source
PEG-6 Stearate	Polyethylene Glycol 300 Monostearate	*Cerasynt 616*
	Polyoxyethylene (6) Monostearate	*Kessco PEG 300 Monostearate*
		Lipal 300S
		Lipo PEG 3-S
		Protamate 300 DPS
		Polystate C
PEG-8 Stearate	Polyoxyl 8 Stearate	*Cerasynt 660*
	Macrogol Stearate 400	*Emerest 2640*
	Polyoxyethylene 8 Stearate	*Grocor 400*
		Hodog 40-S
	Polyoxyethylene Glycol 400 Stearate	*Kessco PEG-400 Monostearate*
		Myrj 45
		Pegosperse 400 MS
		Protamate 400 DPS
Polyoxyl 40 Stearate NF	Polyoxyethylene Glycol 2000 Monostearate	*Emerest 2672*
		Lipal 395
	Polyoxyethylene (40) Monostearate	*Myrj 52*
		Myrj 52-S
	Polyoxyl 40 Stearate BP	*Pegosperse 1750 MS*
	Macrogol Stearate 2000	*Protomate 2000, DPS*
Polyoxyethylene 50 Stearate NF	Polyethylene Glycol 50 Monostearate	*Atlas G-2153*
		Lipal 505
	Polyoxyethylene (50) Monostearate	*Myrj 53*
PEG-12 Stearate	Polyethylene Glycol 600 Monostearate	*Kessco PEG 600 Monostearate*
	Polyoxyethylene (12) Monostearate	*Lipo-PEG 6-S*
		Pegosperse 600 MS
		Protamate 600 DPS
PEG-20 Stearate	Polyethylene Glycol 1000 Monostearate	*Cerasynt 840*
		Kessco PEG 1000 Monostearate
	Polyoxyethylene (20) Monostearate	*Lipo-PEG 10-S*
		Pegosperse 1000 MS
		Protomate 1000 DPS
PEG-100 Stearate	Polyethylene Glycol 100 Monostearate	*Myrj 59*
	Polyoxyethylene (100) Monostearate	
PEG-12 Distearate	Polyethylene (12) Distearate	*Kessco PEG 600 Distearate*
	Polyethylene Glycol 600 Distearate	*Protamate 600 DS*
PEG-32 Distearate	Polyethylene Glycol 1540 Distearate	*Kessco PEG 1540 Distearate*
	Polyoxyethylene (32) Distearate	
PEG-150 Distearate	Polyethylene Glycol 6000 Distearate	*Kessco PEG 6000 Distearate*
	Polyoxyethylene (150) Distearate	*Kessco X-221*
		Protamate 6000DS

2. Functional Category

NF: Wetting and/or solubilizing agent; emulsifying and/or solubilizing agent

Others: Non-ionic emulsifier; solubilizer

3. Synonyms

See Table I.

4. Chemical Names and CAS Registry Number

Poly(oxy-1,2-ethanediyl), α-hydro-ω-hydroxy-octadecanoate Polyethylene glycol monostearate [9004-99-3]

Poly(oxy-1,2-ethanediyl)-α-(1-oxooctadecyl)-ω-hydroxy-polyethylene glycol monostearate [9004-99-3]

5. Empirical Formula

Table II

$$CH_3(CH_2)_{16}\overset{\displaystyle O}{\overset{\|}{C}}O(CH_2CH_2O)_nH$$

		Average (n) =
PEG-6	— Stearate	6
PEG-8	— Stearate	8
PEG-40	— Stearate	40
PEG-50	— Stearate	50
PEG-12	— Stearate	12
PEG-20	— Stearate	20
PEG-100	— Stearate	100

(mixture of palmitates and stearates)

$$R-\overset{\displaystyle O}{\overset{\|}{C}}-(OC_2CH_2)_n-O-\overset{\displaystyle O}{\overset{\|}{C}}-R$$

		Average (n) =
PEG-12	— Distearate	12
PEG-32	— Distearate	32
PEG-150	— Distearate	150

$$R-\overset{\displaystyle O}{\overset{\|}{C}} —\text{ Stearoylradical (mixture of palmitates and stearates)}$$

Molecular Weight: There are two systems used to indicate the approximate molecular weight. In one system, the number after PEG (see Table I) refers to the approximate length in oxyethylene units. In the other system (see synonyms in Table I), the larger number refers to the average molecular weight of the polymer chain.

6. Structural Formula

See Table II.

7. Commercial Availability

USA

Armak

Diamond Shamrock Corp.

Emery Indust.

Glyco

Gross & Co., A. Millmaster Onyx Group, Kewanee Indust., Inc.

Hodag Chemical Corp.

ICI United States, Inc.

Lippo Chemicals, Inc.

Malmstrom

PVO

Protameen Chemicals, Inc.

Van Dyk & Co.

UK

ABM Chemical Industries (UK), Ltd.
Atlas Chemical Indust. (UK), Ltd.
Blagden Campbell Chemicals, Ltd.
Croda Chemicals Ltd.
Lankro Chemicals Ltd.

8. Method of Manufacture

Polyoxyethylene stearates are made by the direct reaction of fatty acids with ethylene oxide. One of the reactions involved is shown below:

$$RCOOH + n[CH_2-CH_2] \xrightarrow{} RCOO\,(C_2H_4O)_nH$$
$$\underset{O}{\diagdown}$$

Fatty Acid   Polyoxyethylene
(Stearic Acid)   Fatty Acid

9. Description

PEG-6 Stearate: soft solid; PEG-8 Stearate: waxy cream; PEG-40 Stearate: waxy solid, with a faint, bland, fat-like odor, off-white to light tan in color; PEG-50 Stearate: solid, with a bland, fat-like odor to odorless; PEG-12 Stearate: pasty solid; PEG-20 Stearate: waxy solid; PEG-100 Stearate: solid; PEG-12 Distearate: paste; PEG-32 Distearate: solid; PEG-150 Distearate: solid

10. Pharmacopeial Specifications

Polyoxyethylene 40 Stearate

Test	NF
Identification	+
Acid value	≤2
Congealing range	37-47°C
Heavy metals	≤0.001%
Arsenic	≤3 ppm
Hydroxyl value	25-40
Free Polyethylene Glycols	17%-27%
Water	≤3.0%
Saponification value	25-35
Average polymer length	~40 oxyethylene units

Polyoxyethylene 50 Stearates

Test	NF
Identification	+
Acid value	≤2
Saponification value	20-28
Hydroxyl value	23-35
Free Polyethylene Glycols	17-27%
Water	≤3.0%
Arsenic	≤3 ppm
Heavy metals	≤0.001%
Average polymer length	~50 oxyethylene units

11. Typical Properties

Name	M.P. (°C)	HLB	Solubility Water	Alcohol	Mineral Oil
PEG-6 Stearate	28-32	9.7	DH	S	S
PEG-8 Stearate	28-33	11.1	D	S	I
PEG-40 Stearate	38-46	16.9	S	S	I
PEG-50 Stearate	c 45°	17.9	S	S	I
PEG-12 Stearate	c 37°	13.6	S	S	I
PEG-20 Stearate	c 41°	15.6	S	S	I
PEG-100 Stearate	44	18.8	S	S	I
PEG-12 Distearate	c 39°	10.6	DH	S	—
PEG-32 Distearate	c 45°	14.8	S	S	—
PEG-150 Distearate	c 55°	18.4	S	I	—

D = Dispersible   I = Insoluble
S = Soluble   c = Approx.
DH = Dispersible (with heat)

Name	Acid Value	Sap. No.	Ester Value	Hydroxyl No.	Iodine No.	Water	Free Eth. Oxide
PEG-6 Stearate	5.0 max	95-110	—	—	0.5 max	—	100 ppm max
PEG-8 Stearate	5.0 max	82-102	80-102	68-94	1.0 max	1.5% max	100 ppm max
PEG-12 Stearate	8.5 max	62-78	60-75	55-75	1.0 max	1.0% max	100 ppm max
PEG-20 Stearate	5.0 max	40-50	35-50	36-52	1.0 max	1.5% max	100 ppm max
PEG-100 Stearate	—	9-17	—	15-18	—	—	100 ppm max
PEG-12 Distearate	10.0 max	93-102	85-105	20 max	1.0 max	1.0% max	100 ppm max
PEG-32 Distearate	10.0 max	50-62	45-58	20 max	0.25 max	1.0% max	100 ppm max
PEG-150 Distearate	10.0 max	15-25	7.0-17	15.0 max	0.1 max	1.0% max	100 ppm max

The methods of analysis for the indicated values are shown below:

    Acid value—AOCS Cd 3-63
    Saponification no.—AOCS Cd 3 - 25
    Ester value/sap value/acid value/hydroxyl no.—AOCS Tx la - 66
    Iodine no.—AOCS Tg la - 64
    Water—FCC, 2nd Edition, p. 977
    Free ethylene oxide—CTFA H-81

    AOCS—American Oil Chemists Society
    FCC—Food Chemical Codex
    CTFA—Cosmetic, Toiletry and Fragrance Association, Inc.

12. Stability and Storage Conditions

These compounds are generally stable to electrolytes, as well as weak acids or bases. Strong acids and bases will cause gradual hydrolysis. Store in a tight container at room temperature.

13. Incompatibilities

These compounds are unstable in hot alkaline solutions due to hydrolysis, and will also saponify with strong acids or bases. Discoloration or precipitation will occur with salicylates, phenolic substances, iodine salts and salts of bismuth, silver and tannins. Complexation with preservatives may also occur. Levels of over 5% may cause a decrease in the antimicrobial activity of tetracycline, bacitracin, chloramphenicol, phenoxymethylpenicillin and sodium penicillin.

14. Safety

In general, all of these compounds are well-tolerated and are practically non-toxic.

The acute oral toxicity, primary skin and acute eye irritation for these compounds have been evaluated on various animals. The acute oral toxicity was carried out on rats, and the materials were found to be non-toxic. The primary skin tests were performed on rabbits, and they were not found to be primary skin irritants. The acute eye test was also carried out on rabbits, and the materials were not found to be eye irritants.

15. Handling Precautions

Materials that exceed the 100 ppm limit for free ethylene oxide may present an explosion hazard when stored in a closed container. This is due to the release of ethylene oxide to the container headspace, where it may build up to a level which exceeds the explosion limit.

16. Regulatory Acceptance

NF XVI

17. Application in Pharmaceutical Formulation or Technology

The materials are generally used as emulsifiers in o/w type creams and lotions. Their hydrophilicity or lipophilicity depends on the number of ethylene oxide units present: the larger the number, the greater the hydrophilic properties. They can be blended with other surfactants to obtain any hydrophile-lipophile balance for lotions or ointment formulations. They are particularly useful for emulsifying when astringent salts or other strong electrolytes are present.

Use	Concentration
Emulsifier for o/w creams or lotions	0.5-10%
Auxiliary emulsifier for o/w	
intravenous fat emulsion	0.5-5%
Suppository component	1-10%
Tablet lubricant	1-2%

18. Related Substances

—

19. Comments

—

20. Specific References

1. W. B. Satkowski, S. K. Huang and R. L. Liss, *Polyethylene esters of fatty acids in non-ionic surfactants,* Martin J. Schick, ed., Marcel Dekker, Inc., New York, 1967, Vol. 1, p. 142.
2. "General Characteristics of Atlas Surfactants." ICI United States, Inc., Wilmington, Delaware 19897. Bulletin O-I (LG-60).
3. *Guide to the physiological suitability of Atlas Surfactants.* ICI United States, Inc., Wilmington, Delaware 19897. 1974.
4. O .G. Fitzhugh, A. R. Bourke, A. A. Nelson and J. P. Frawley, Chronic oral toxicities of four stearic acid emulsifiers, *Toxicol. and Appl. Pharmacol.,* 1: 315-331 (1959).
5. B. L. Oser and M. Oser, Nutritional studies on rats containing high levels of parti ester emulsifiers, *J. Nutr.,* 60:367-390; *ibid.,* 60:489-505; *ibid.,* 61: 149-166; *ibid.,* 61, 235-252 (1956 and 1957).
6. P. J. Culver, C. S. Wilcox, C. M. Jones and R. S. Rose, Jr., Intermediary metabolism of certain polyoxyethylene derivatives in man; *J. Pharmacol. Exp. Therap.,* 103: 337 (1951).
7. D. Chakravarty, J. L. Lach and S. M. Blaug, *Drug Standards,* 25: 137 (1957).
8. E. Ullmann and B. Moser, *Arch. Pharm.,* 295: 136-43 (1962).
9. K. Thoma, E. Ullmann and G. Zelfel, *Arch. Pharm.,* 295: 670-8 (1962).
10. I. Cohn, S. Singleton, Q. L. Hartwig and M. Atik, *J. Am. Med. Assoc.,* 183: 755 (1963).
11. T. J. Smith and Nephew, Ltd., Fr. 1: 395,184.
12. K. Thoma, E. Ullmann and O. Fickel, *Arch. Pharm.,* 303 (4), 289-296 and 297-304 (1970).
13. J. Maly, *Acta Fac. Pharm. Univ. Comeniana,* 17, 181-5 (1969).
14. D. Duchene, A. Djiane and F. Puisieux, *Ann. Pharm. Fr.,* 28:(4), 289-98 (1970).

USA: P. Reisberg*; P. Nadkarni*; C. Fox*; J. Mollica**; Z. Chowhan**

UK: J. B. Kaye*

Polyvinyl Alcohol

1. Nonproprietary Name
USP: Polyvinyl alcohol

2. Functional Category
USP: Suspending and/or viscosity-increasing agent

3. Synonym
—

4. Chemical Names and CAS Registry Number
Ethenol, homopolymer
Vinyl alcohol polymer [9002-89-5]

5. Empirical Formula   Molecular Weight
$(C_2H_4O)_n$

High viscosity: 200,000 (avg)
Medium viscosity: 130,000 (avg)
Low viscosity: 30,000 (avg)

6. Structural Formula
$$---CH_2-CH-CH_2-CH-CH_2-CH---$$
$$OHOHOH$$

7. Commercial Availability

USA

E.I. du Pont de Nemours & Co.
ICN/KK Labs, Inc.
Monsanto Co.
Sonoco Products Co.

UK

British Traders and Shippers Ltd.
Degussa Ltd.
Hoechst (UK) Ltd.
The Nippon Syn. Chem. Ind. Co. Ltd.

8. Method of Manufacture
Prepared from polyvinyl acetates by replacement of acetate groups with hydroxy groups. The alcoholysis proceeds most rapidly in a methanol and methyl acetate mixture in the presence of catalytic amounts of alkali or mineral acids. The polyvinyl acetate is about 88% hydrolyzed.

9. Description
White to cream-colored granular powder or granules. Odorless.

10. Pharmacopeial Specifications

Test	USP
Viscosity	85.0-115.0% of label in cps at 20°C of a 4% (w/w) aqueous solution
pH (1 in 25 solution)	5.0-8.0
Loss on drying	≤5.0%
Residue on ignition	≤2.0%
Water-insoluble substances	≤0.1%
Saponification values	+
Hydrolysis value	+

11. Typical Properties
Refractive index: 1.49-1.53
Melting point: 228°C
Specific heat: 0.4 cal/g/°C
Specific gravity: 1.19-1.27
Solubility: Essentially soluble in hot or cold water. Partially soluble in some polyhydroxy compounds, certain amines and amides.

12. Stability and Storage Conditions
Slow degradation at 100° C. Rapid degradation at 200°C. Stable to light. Decomposes in strong acid. Softens or dissolves in weak acids and alkalis. Resistant to most organic solvents.

13. Incompatibilities
Incompatible with most inorganic salts, especially sulfates and phosphates. Phosphates will cause 5% polyvinylalcohol to precipitate from aqueous solution.

14. Safety
Nontoxic when applied to eyes or skin. No irritation up to 10%. Acceptable in cosmetics up to 7%. Not cleared by FDA to be taken internally. Aqueous solutions (5%) of polyvinylalcohol injected subcutaneously to rats of six different polyvinylalcohol polymers have been found to cause anemia and infiltrate various organs and tissues. Elvanols 71-30 and 70-05 both caused hypertension and other associated changes. (Hall, C. E. and Hall, O., *Lab. Invest.*, 12, 671 (1963).

15. Handling Precautions
—

16. Regulatory Acceptance
USP XX

17. Applications in Pharmaceutical Formulation or Technology
Topical ophthalmic dosage forms

18. Related Substances
—

19. Comments
—

20. Specific References
1. N. Krishna and F. Brow, *Amer. J. Ophthalmol.*, 57: 99 (1964).
2. T. F. Patton and J. R. Robinson, *J. Pharm. Sci.*, 64: 1312 (1975).
3. Monsanto Technical Bulletin, number 6082B.
4. A. O. Okhamfe and P. York, Moisture permeation mechanism of some aqueous based film coats, *J. Pharm. Pharmacol.*, 34 Supp. 53P (1982).

USA: M. J. Akers*; J. Mennonna**; D. Hovermale**; J. Mollica**

Potassium Citrate

1. Nonproprietary Names

USP: Potassium citrate
BP/EP: Potassium citrate

2. Functional Category

BP: Systemic alkalinizing substance
Others: Alkalizer, gastric antacid, expectorant

3. Synonyms

Citrate of potash

4. Chemical Names and CAS Registry Number

USP: Tripotassium citrate monohydrate [6100-05-6] 1,2,3-propanetricarboxylic acid-2-hydroxy-tripotassium salt, monohydrate
BP/EP: Tripotassium-2-hydroxypropane-1,2,3-tricarboxylate monohydrate

5. Empirical Formula   Molecular Weight

$C_6H_5K_3O_7 \cdot H_2O$ 324.42

6. Structural Formula

$$CH_2—COOK$$
$$|$$
$$HO—C—COOK \cdot H_2O$$
$$|$$
$$CH_2—COOK$$

7. Commercial Availability

USA

Alba Chemical, Inc.
Atomergic Chemetals Corp.
Cyclo Chemicals Corp.
Gallard-Schiesinger Chemical Mfg. Corp.
HEXCEL Corp., Specialty Chemicals Div.
ICN K & K Labs. Inc.
May & Baker, Ltd.
McKesson Chemical Co.
Miles Laboratories, Inc./Citro-tech Products/
     Industrial Mktg. Dept.
Pfaltz & Bauer, Inc.
Pfizer, Inc.-Chemical Div.
Sturge Ltd., John & E.
Thompson-Hayward Chemical Co.
Uhe Co., George
United States Biochemicals Corp.

8. Method of Manufacture

Potassium citrate, monohydrate is produced by adding potassium bicarbonate or carbonate to a solution of citric acid until effervescence ceases. The resulting solution is filtered and evaporated to dryness.

9. Description

Transparent crystals or a white, granular powder. It is odorless and has a cooling, saline taste.

10. Pharmacopeial Specifications

Test	USP	BP
Potency (assay)	99-100.5%	99-101%
(dried at 180° for 4 hours)	$C_6H_5K_3O_7$	$C_6H_5K_3O_7$
Identification	+	+
Alkalinity or acidity	+	+
Loss on drying	3-6%	—
Clarity & color of solution	—	—
Heavy metals	0.001%	≤10 ppm
Tartrate	+	—
Sodium	—	+
Chloride	—	≤50 ppm
Oxalate	—	≤400 ppm
Sulfate	—	+
Readily carbonizable substances	—	+
Water	—	≥4%; ≤7%

11. Typical Properties

Solubility: Very soluble in water (167 g/100 cm³); insoluble in alcohol; slightly soluble in glycerol.
Crystal structure: Prismatic
Melting point: 230°C (loses water at 180°C)
Density: 1.98 g/cm³
pH of aqueous solution: Approximately 8.5

Academy HPE Laboratory Project Data
Potassium Citrate, Granular

Method	Lab No.	Results
% Consolidation BTD-6	8	Volume: 9.0%
% Consolidation BTD-6	8	Weight: 6.0%

Supplier: Pfizer

12. Stability and Storage Conditions

Store in a tight container.

13. Incompatibilities

Aqueous solutions are slightly alkaline and will react with acidic substances. Alkaloidal salts may be precipitated from their aqueous or hydro-alcoholic solutions. Calcium and strontium salts will cause precipitation of the corresponding citrates.

14. Safety

—

15. Handling Precautions

—

16. Regulatory Acceptance

USP XXI; BP 1980

17. Applications in Pharmaceutical Formulation or Technological Use

Use	Concentration
Buffer for solutions	0.3-2%
Sequestering agent	0.3-2%

18. Related Substances

—

19. Comments

—

20. Specific References

—

USA: J. Cooper*; G. E. Amidon**

Potassium Sorbate

1. Nonproprietary Names

NF: Potassium sorbate
BP: Potassium sorbate

2. Functional Categories

NF: Antimicrobial preservative
BP: Antimicrobial preservative.
Others: Mycostatic, fungistatic

3. Synonym

2,4-Hexadienoic acid potassium salt

4. Chemical Names and CAS Registry Number

2,4-Hexadienoic acid (E,E)-potassium salt
Potassium (E,E)-sorbate
Potassium sorbate [590-00-1] and [24634-61-5]

5. Empirical Formula

$C_6H_7KO_2$

Molecular Weight

150.22

6. Structural Formula

7. Commercial Availability

USA

American Hoechst Corporation
Ashland Chemical Co.
Biotech Products Div.
Miles Laboratories, Inc.
Monsanto Industrial Chemicals Co.
Pfizer, Inc./Chemicals Division

UK

Hoechst (U.K.), Ltd.
Pfizer, Ltd.

8. Method of Manufacture

Potassium sorbate is prepared from sorbic acid and potassium hydroxide (U.S. Patent 3,173,948).

9. Description

White crystals or powder with (faint) characteristic odor. Melts at 270°C with decomposition.

10. Pharmacopeial Specifications

Test	NF	BP
Identification	+	+
Acidity or alkalinity	+	+
Loss on drying	≤1.0%	—
Heavy metals	≤0.001%	≤10 ppm
Assay	98.0-101.0%	99.0-101.0%
Arsenic	—	≤2 ppm
Water	—	≤1.0%
Aldehyde (as C_2H_4O)	—	≤0.15%

11. Typical Properties

Solubility (20°C): Water: 58.2%; alcohol: 6.5%.
Soluble in propylene glycol; very soluble in acetone, chloroform, ether, fats and oils.
Density of crystals: 1.363 g. Melting point: 270°C approximately, melts with decomposition.

12. Stability and Storage Conditions

Protect from light and excessive heat. Store in an airtight container.

13. Incompatibilities

—

14. Safety

Sorbic acid is an irritant to the eyes and the skin. Consequently, the same precautions should be observed with potassium sorbate. It is safe for oral use. Acceptable daily intake is up to 25 mg/kg of body weight.

15. Handling Precautions

—

16. Regulatory Acceptance

NF XVI; BP Addendum, 1982

17. Applications in Pharmaceutical Formulation or Technology

Same as sorbic acid, but potassium sorbate is more soluble in water.

18. Related Substances

Sorbic acid has the same pharmaceutical properties and uses as potassium sorbate. It is less soluble in water.

19. Comments

Antimicrobial activity depends on the pH and is effective only below pH 6.5.

20. Specific References

See sorbic acid

USA: J. Cooper*; C. D. Yu*; J. B. D'Silva**
UK: M. C. Allwood**

Povidone

1. Nonproprietary Name
USP: Povidone
BP: Povidone

2. Functional Category
USP: Tablet binder; suspending and/or viscosity-increasing agent
BP: Pharmaceutical excipient

3. Synonyms
Polyvidone; polyvinylpyrrolidone; PVP; *Kollidon*; *Plasdone*

4. Chemical Names and CAS Registry Number
2-Pyrrolidinone, 1-ethenyl-, homopolymer
1-Vinyl-2-pyrrolidinone-polymer [9003-39-8]

5. Empirical Formula and Molecular Weight
$(C_6H_9NO)_n$
It is produced as a series of products having mean molecular weights ranging from about 10,000 to about 700,000.

6. Structural Formula

7. Commercial Availability
USA
BASF Wyandotte Corp.
GAF Corp.
UK
BASF UK Ltd.
Becpharm Ltd.
Blagden Campbell Chem. Ltd.
GAF Great Britain Ltd.

8. Method of Manufacture
The synthesis of povidone consists of six steps. Acetylene and formaldehyde are reacted in the presence of highly active copper acetylide catalyst to form butynediol, which is hydrogenated to butanediol and then cyclodehydrogenated to form butyrolactone. Pyrrolidone is produced by reacting butyrolactone with ammonia. This is followed by a vinylation reaction in which pyrrolidone and acetylene are reacted under pressure. The monomer, vinylpyrrolidone, is finally polymerized in the presence of a combination of catalysts to produce povidone.

9. Description
A white to creamy white, odorless or almost odorless, hygroscopic powder.

SEM: KY-39
Excipient: Povidone (K29-32)

Supplier: GAF
Lot no: 82A-3

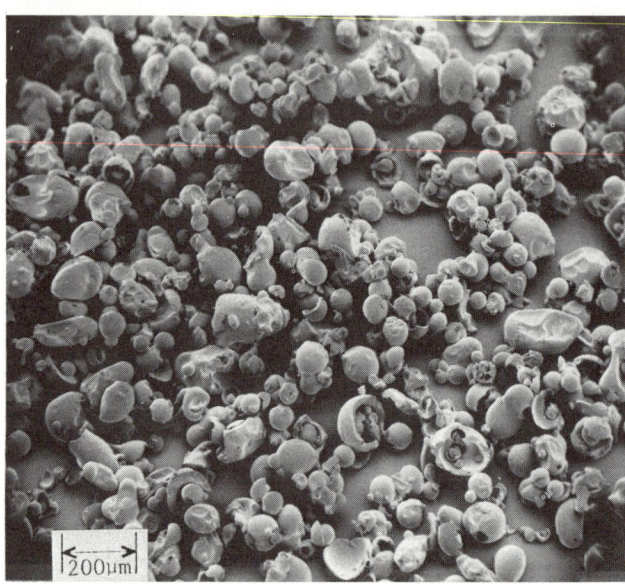

Magnification: 60×   **Voltage:** 5 kV

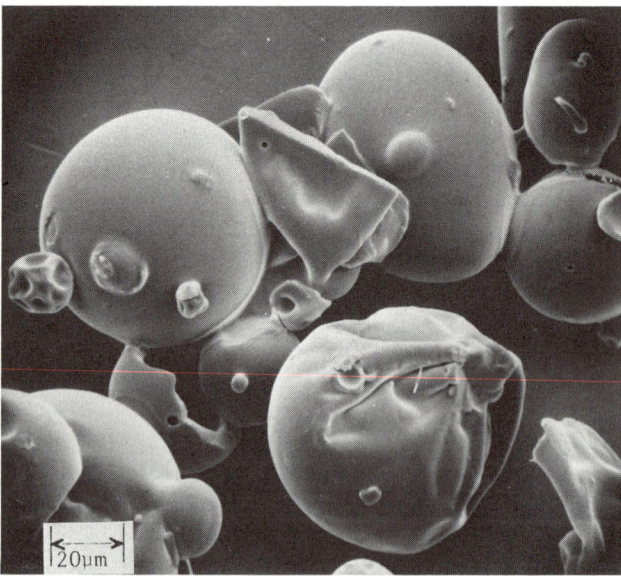

Magnification: 600×   **Voltage:** 10 kV

SEM: KY-40
Excipient: Povidone (C-30)

Supplier: GAF
Lot no.: 82A-4

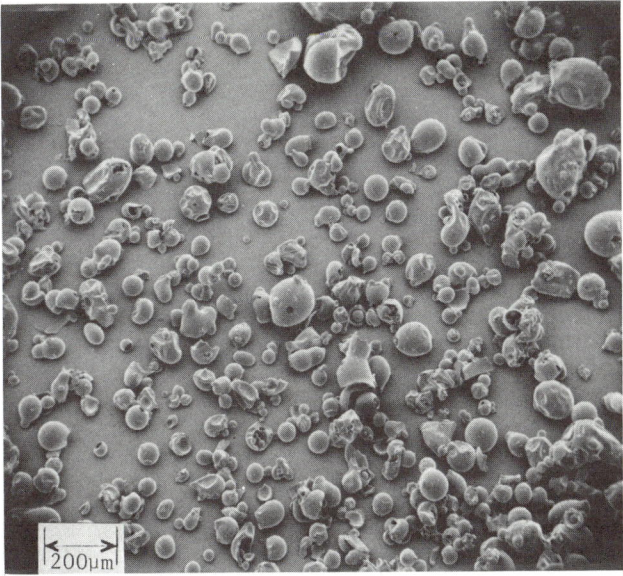

Magnification: 60× **Voltage:** 10 kV

SEM: KY-41
Excipient: Povidone (C-15)

Supplier: GAF
Lot no.: 82A-1

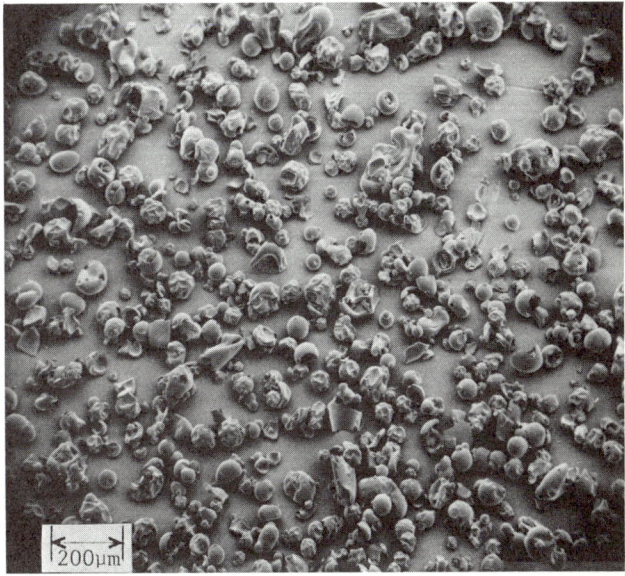

Magnification: 60× **Voltage:** 5 kV

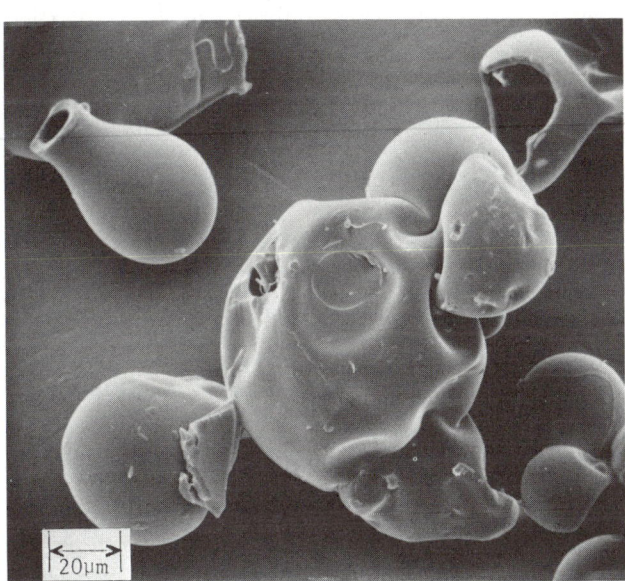

Magnification: 600× **Voltage:** 10 kV

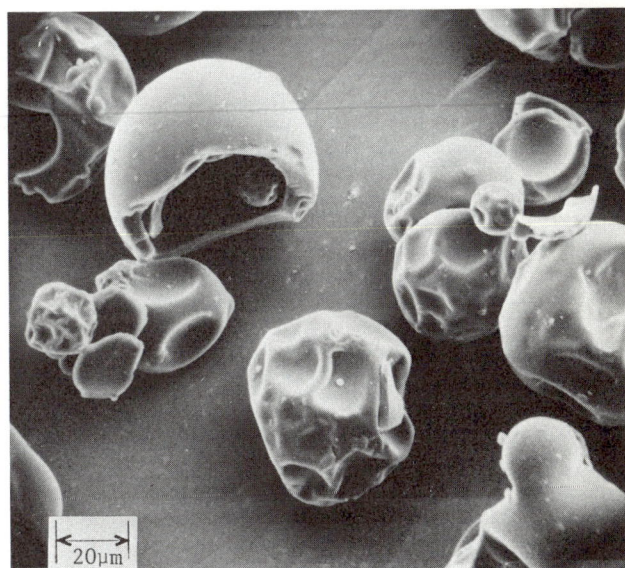

Magnification: 600× **Voltage:** 10 kV

SEM: KY-42

Excipient: Povidone (K26-28)

Supplier: GAF
Lot no.: 82A-2

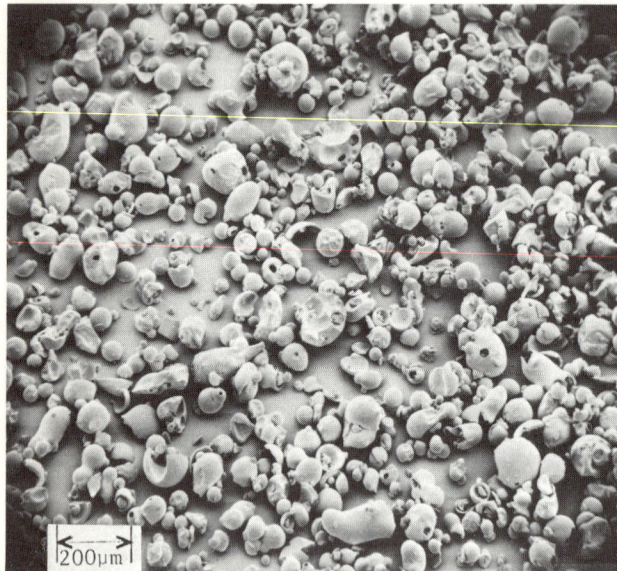

Magnification: 60× **Voltage**: 5 kV

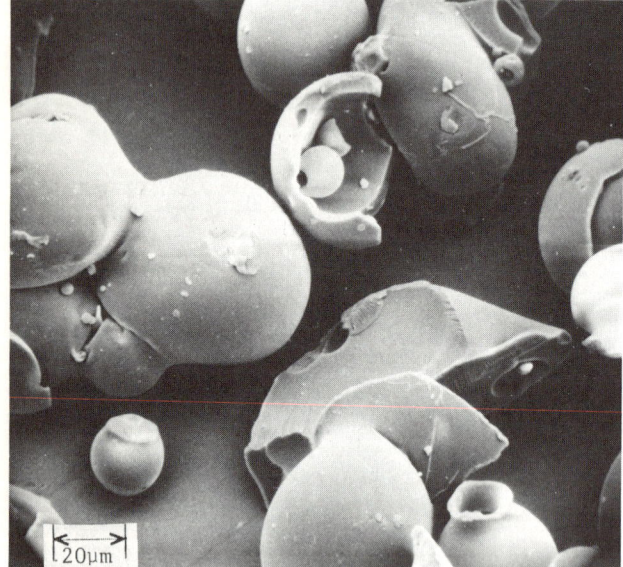

Magnification: 600× **Voltage**: 10 kV

10. Pharmacopeial Specifications

Test	USP	BP
Identification	+	+
pH (1 in 20 solution)	3.0 to 7.0	—
Water	≤5.0%	≤5.0%
Residue on ignition	≤0.1%	—
Lead	≤10 ppm	—
Heavy metals	—	≤10 ppm
Aldehydes	≤0.2% as C_2H_4O	≤0.2% as C_2H_4O
Vinylpyrrolidinone	≤0.2%	≤0.2%
Nitrogen content (assay)	11.5–12.8%	11.5 to 12.8%
Clarity and color of solution	—	+
K-Value (declared as 15 or less)	85.0–115.0%	—
K-Value (declared as 15 or more)	90.0 to 108.0%	—
Sulfated ash	—	<0.1%

11. Typical Properties

Density (He): between 1.17 and 1.18 g/ml

Bulk volume: 2.3 ml/g [Kollidon 25]; 3.2 ml/g [Plasdone K 30]

Tapped volume: 1.9 ml/g [Kollidon 25]; 2.5 ml/g [Plasdone K30]

Hygroscopicity: Povidone is hygroscopic, significant amounts of moisture being absorbed at low relative humidities (See Fig. 26-SD-8 and Fig. 26-SD-9 for sorption-desorption isotherms).

K-Value: K-value refers to the average molecular weight relationship described for several grades. USP requires that the k-value range of povidone be labeled in the title.

K-value	Average Molecular Weight
15	about 10,000
30	about 40,000
60	about 160,000
90	about 360,000

Softening point: ~150° C

Solubility: Readily soluble in water, up to 60%. Freely soluble in many organic solvents, including monohydric (ethanol, methanol) and polyhydric alcohols, acids, esters, ketones, methylene chloride, chloroform, ethylene dichloride, butylamine, pyridine and di- and triethanolamine. Essentially insoluble in ethers, hydrocarbons, carbon tetrachloride, ethyl acetate and mineral oil.

Viscosity: The viscosity of solutions containing 10% or less povidone is essentially the same as that of water. Solutions more concentrated than 10% become more viscous, depending upon the concentration and the molecular weight of the polymer employed.

Academy HPE Laboratory Project Data

	Method	Lab #	Results
Moisture Content			
GAF C-15	MC-3	1	5.31%
GAF K29-32	MC-3	1	4.43%
GAF C30	MC-3	1	3.36%
GAF K26-28	MC-15	15	4.50%

Academy HPE Laboratory Project Data

	Method	Lab #	Results
Bulk/Tap Density			
GAF C15	BTD-1	1	B:0.467 g/ml T:0.568 g/ml
GAF K29-32	BTD-1	1	B:0.368 g/ml T:0.472 g/ml
GAF C30	BTD-1	1	B:0.316 g/ml T:0.410 g/ml
GAF C15	BTD-7	14	B:0.490 g/ml T:0.570 g/ml
GAF K29-32	BTD-7	14	B:0.400 g/ml T:0.479 g/ml
GAF C30	BTD-7	14	B:0.350 g/ml T:0.420 g/ml
GAF	BTD-6	8	VOLUME: 14.5% WEIGHT: 14.0%
Solubility			
(Water) C-15	SOL-2	1	1×10^3 mg/ml
(Alcohol) C-15	SOL-2	1	1×10^3 mg/ml
(n-Hexane) C-15	SOL-1	1	0.012 mg/ml
(Water) K-29-32	SOL-2	1	1×10^3 mg/ml
(Alcohol) K-29-32	SOL-2	1	1×10^3 mg/ml
(n-Hexane) K-29-32	SOL-1	1	0.016 mg/ml
(Water) C30	SOL-2	1	1×10^3 mg/ml
(Alcohol) C-30	SOL-2	1	1×10^3 mg/ml
(n-Hexane) C-30	SOL-1	1	0.010 mg/ml
Average Flow Rate			
GAF C15	FLO-1	14	20 g/sec.
GAF C30	FLO-1	14	Poor flow
GAF K29-32	FLO-1	14	16 g/sec.
EMC Plot (USP)	EMC-1	15	Fig:15-EMC-6
COM Plot (K29-32)	COM-7	12	Fig:12-COM-38
COM Plot (USP)	COM-2	21	Fig:21-COM-33
COM Plot (C15)	COM-4,5,6	29	Fig:29-COM-17
COM Plot (K29-32)	COM-4,5,6	20	Fig:20-COM-18
COM Plot (C30)	COM-4,5,6	29	Fig:29-COM-19
SDI Plot (C15)	SDI-2		Fig:26-SDI-8
SDI Plot (C30)	SDI-2	26	Fig:26-SDI-9
SDI Plot (K29-32)	SDI-2	26	Fig:26-SDI-10

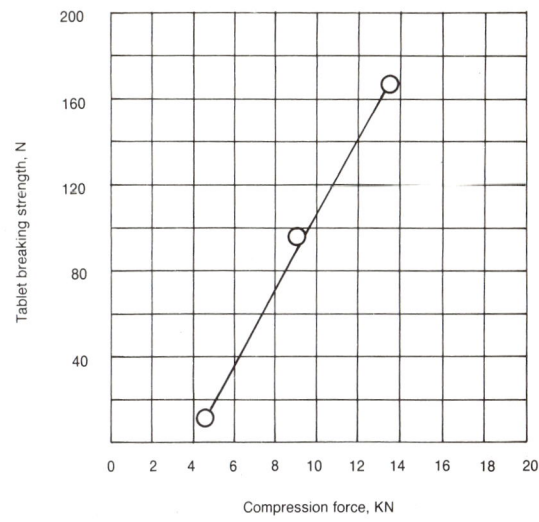

Povidone USP, K 29-32 (GAF, Lot #G90920B-76)
Tablet weight: 500 mg

Figure: 12-COM-38   **Method:** COM-7

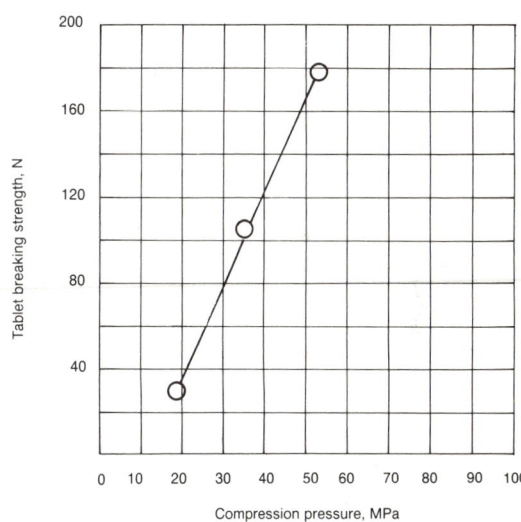

Povidone USP (Domtar, Canada, Lot #G80908C)
Tablet weight: 500 mg

Figure: 21-COM-33   **Method:** COM-2

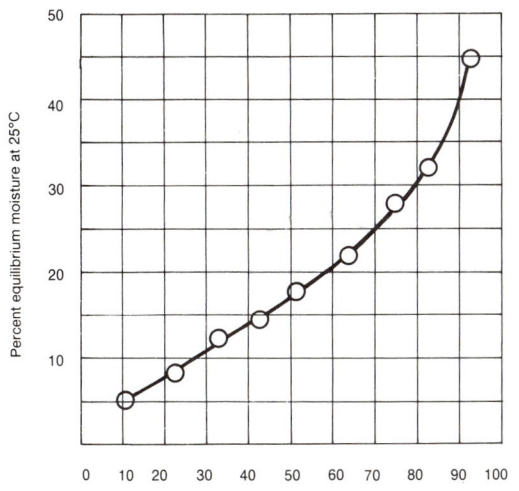

Povidone USP (GAF, Lot #690429B)

Figure: 15-EMC-6   **Method:** EMC-1

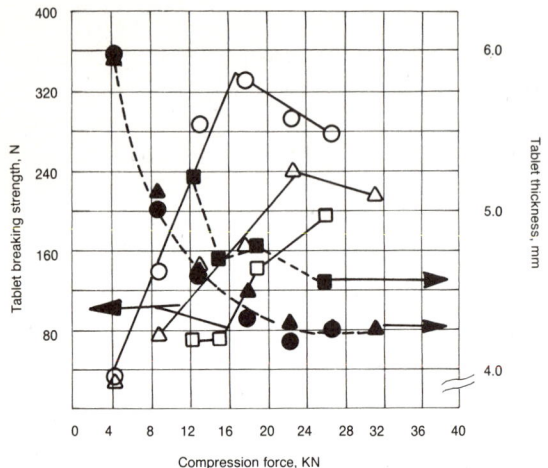

Povidone C 15 (GAF, Lot #G-453)

○ ● : Unlubricated, Carver laboratory press (COM-5)
△ ▲ : Lubricated, Carver laboratory press (COM-6)
□ ■ : Lubricated, Instrumented Stokes model F—Single punch press (COM-4)

Figure: 29-COM-17   **Methods:** COM-4,5,6

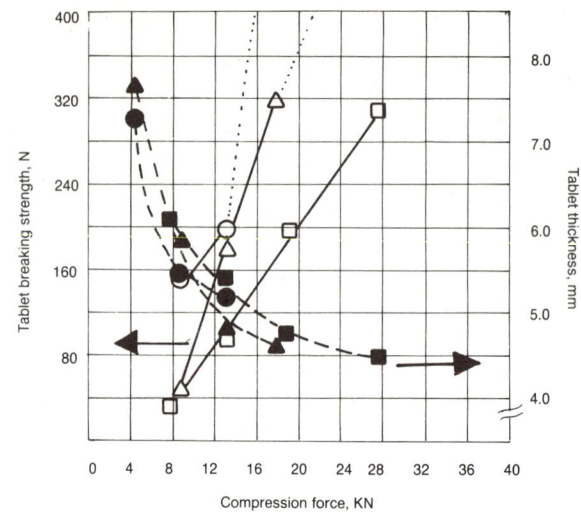

Povidone C-30 (GAF, Lot #G80905A-105)

○ ● : Unlubricated, Carver laboratory Press (COM-5)
△ ▲ : Lubricated, Carver laboratory Press (COM-6)
□ ■ : Lubricated, instrumented Stokes model F—Single punch punch press (COM-4)

Figure: 29-COM-19   **Methods:** COM-4,5,6

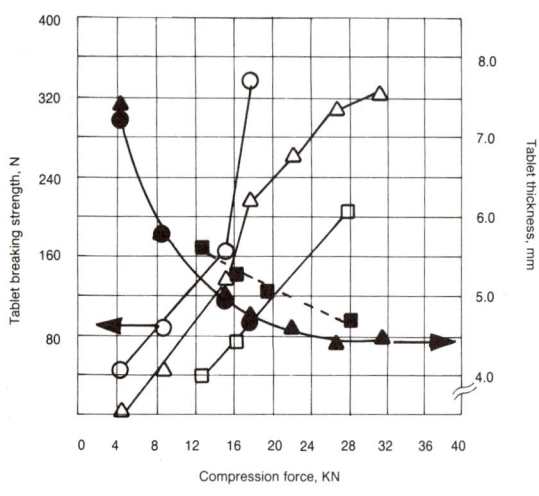

Povidone K 29-32 (GAF, Lot #G-90920B-79)

○ ●: Unlubricated, Carver laboratory press (COM-5)
△ ▲: Lubricated, Carver laboratory press (COM-6)
□ ■: Lubricated, instrumented Stokes model F—Single punch press (COM-4)

Figure: 29-COM-18   **Methods:** COM-4,5,6

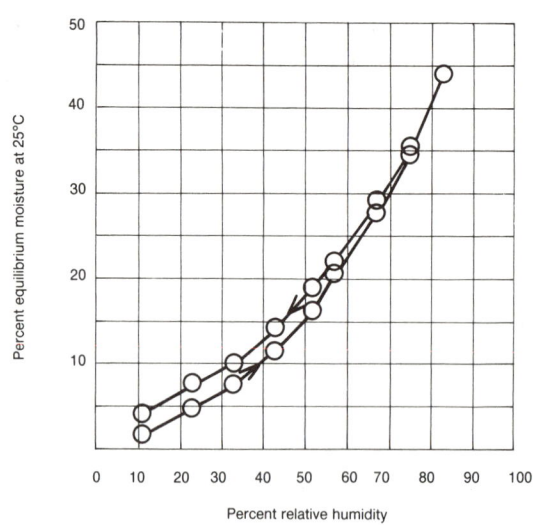

Povidone C-15 (GAF, Lot #G-453)

Figure: 26-SDI-8   **Method:** SDI-2

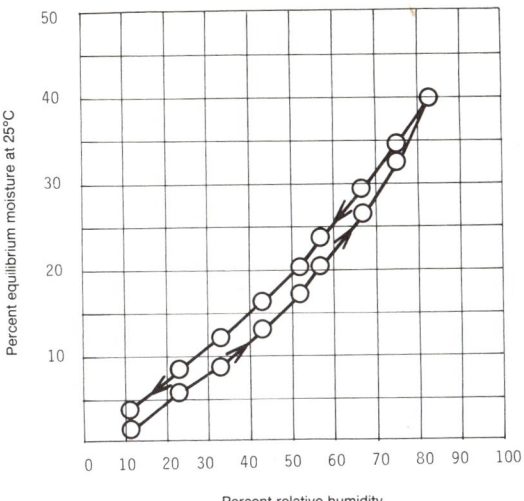

Povidone C-30 (GAF, Lot #G80905A-105)

Figure: 26-SDI-9 **Method:** SDI-2

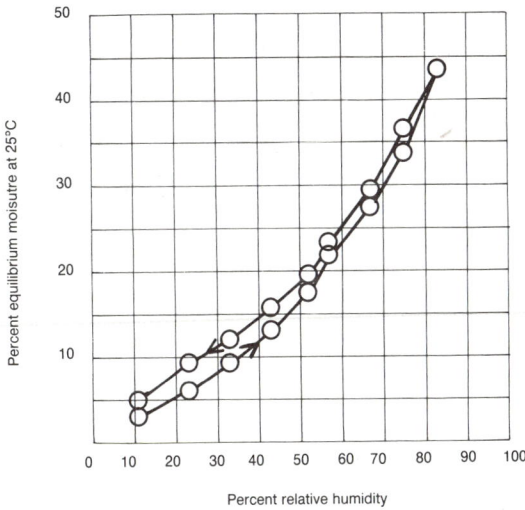

Povidone K 29-32 (GAF, Lot #G90920B-76)

Figure: 26-SDI-10 **Method:** SDI-2

12. Stability and Storage Conditions

Povidone darkens to some extent on heating at 150° C, with reduction in water solubility. It is stable to a short cycle of heat exposure around 110-130° C. Steam sterilization of an aqueous solution does not alter its properties. Aqueous solutions are susceptible to mold growth, and hence require suitable preservatives. Povidone can be stored under ordinary conditions without undergoing decomposition or degradation. However, since the powder is hygroscopic, it should be stored in a moisture-proof, tight container.

13. Incompatibilities

Povidone is compatible in solution and with a wide range of inorganic salts, natural and synthetic resins and other chem-

icals. It forms molecular adducts in solution with sulfathiazole sodium, sodium salicylate, salicylic acid, phenobarbital, tannin and possibly other compounds.

14. Safety

Chemically, povidone is inert and non-toxic. The acute oral toxicity in rats and guinea pigs is above 100 g/kg. Prolonged administration of therapeutic doses are well tolerated without injury. It has no irritant effect on the skin and causes no sensitization. It does not irritate the mucous membrane of rabbit eyes, is not antigenic and does not interfere in antibody formation. It is well tolerated by the upper respiratory tract in inhalation studies.

15. Handling Precautions

No restrictions specified.

16. Regulatory Acceptance

USP XXI; BP 1980

17. Applications in Pharmaceutical Formulation or Technology

Use	Concentration
Carrier for drugs	10–25% solution
Dispersing agent	up to 5% solution
Suspending or viscosity builder	up to 5% solution
Tablet binder; tablet diluent; coating agent	0.5–5% solution

Povidone is used in the form of a solution as a binder in tablet granulations. It is also added to powder blends in dry form and granulated in situ by the addition of water, alcohol or water-alcohol.

18. Related Substances

Crospovidone NF. Special related substances, such as Plasdone K and C and Polyclar H and L, are available from GAF for special use.

19. Comments

For accurate standardization of solutions, the water content must be determined before use and taken into account for calculation. Molecular adduct formation properties may be used as an advantage for solid solutions, slow release solids and parenteral formulations.

20. Specific References

1. "Polyvinylpyrrolidone—Physical, chemical, physiological and functional properties," GAF Technical Bulletin, 9642-079.
2. "Polyvinylpyrrolidone," BASF Bulletin B, 359e.
3. J. A. Plaizier–Vercammen and R. E. DeNeve, Interaction of povidone with aeromatic compounds III: Thermodynamics of binding equilibria and interaction forces in buffer solutions at varying pH values and varying dielectric constant, *J. Pharm. Sci.*, 71 (5):552-556 (1982).
4. Z. T. Chowhan, A. A. Amaro and Y. P. Chow, Tablet-to-tablet dissolution variability and its relationship to homogeneity of a water-soluble drug, *Drug Development and Industrial Pharmacy*, 8 (2):145-168 (1982).
5. J. C. Callahan, G. W. Cleary, M. Elefant, G. Kaplan, T. Kensler and R. A. Nash, Equilibrium moisture content of pharmaceutical excipients, *Drug Development and Industrial Pharmacy*, 8 (3):335-369 (1982).

USA: D. M. Patel*; W. D. Walkling**; Z. Chowhan**

Propane

1. Nonproprietary Name
NF: Propane

2. Functional Category
USP: Aerosol propellant

3. Synonyms
—

4. Chemical Names and CAS Registry Number
Propane; dimethylmethane; propyldihydride [74-98-6]

5. Empirical Formula   Molecular Weight
C_3H_8 44.10

6. Structural Formula

```
      H  H  H
      |  |  |
  H—C—C—C—H
      |  |  |
      H  H  H
```

7. Commercial Availability

USA

Aeropres Corporation
Diversified Chemical and Propellant Company
Exxon Company
Industrial Hydrocarbons, Inc.
Phillips Chemical Company
Shell Chemical Company

UK

Air Products, Ltd.
Calor Group, Ltd.

8. Method of Manufacture
See butane

9. Description
Propane is a liquefied gas and exists as a liquid at room temperature when contained under its own vapor pressure or as a gas when exposed to room temperature and atmospheric pressure. It is essentially a clear, colorless, odorless, liquid, but may have a slight ethereal odor.

10. Pharmacopeial Specifications

Test	NF
Identification	+
Water	$\leq 0.001\%$
High-boiling residues	≤ 5 ppm
Acidity of residue	+
Sulfur compounds	+
Assay	$\geq 98.0\%$ C_3H_8

11. Typical Properties
Boiling point: −43.7°F; − 42.1°C
Vapor pressure: (psig at 70°F.) 110.0; (psig at 130°F.) 256
Liquid density (g/cm³ at 70°F.): 0.50
Vapor density (g/cm³ at boiling point): 0.241
Kauri-butanol value: 25
Solubility: Soluble in ethanol; insoluble in water
Viscosity: 0.102 (cps at 68°F)
Flammability in air: lower limit (v/v %) 2.2; upper limit (v/v %) 9.5; flash point (°F)−156

12. Stability and Storage Conditions
Store in tight containers. Do not expose to excessive heat.

13. Incompatibilities
See butane

14. Safety
Asphyxiant. Threshold limit value: 1,000 ppm. Propane is highly flammable and explosive.

15. Handling Precautions
Proper protective measures when using propane include: wearing rubber gloves, safety glasses and protective clothing.
Emergency measures: Fire: Stop the flow of gas. If possible, apply powder extinguisher at the flashing point. Use water to keep containers cool. Leakage: By forced ventilation, maintain the concentration of the gas below the range of the explosive mixture. See butane.

16. Regulatory Acceptance
NF XVI

17. Applications in Pharmaceutical Formulation or Technology
See butane

18. Related Substances
Isobutane; propane

19. Comments
Store cylinders outdoors, avoiding direct sunlight or heat radiation. Provide adequate ventilation. Avoid fire and provide spark-resistant electrical fittings. See butane.

20. Specific References
1. British Standards (BS) 4250: Specification for commercial butane and propane.
2. BS 3960: Non refillable liquefied gas containers, part 1.
3. BS 5045: Transportable gas containers, part II.
4. "Threshold Limit Values for 1979". Guidance Note EH 15/79 from the Health and Safety Executive. Pub. H.M.S.O. ISBN 0-11-883193-3
5. "Dangerous properties of industrial materials," 4th ed., N. Irving Sax. Pub., Van Nostrand Reinhold Co., New York, 1975. ISBN 0-442-27368-1.
6. British Aerosol Manufacturers Association, "A guide to safety in aerosol manufacture," 1st Ed., 1977.

USA: J.J. Sciarra*
UK: P. J. Davies*

Propylene Glycol

1. Nonproprietary Names

USP: Propylene glycol
BP/EP: Propylene glycol

2. Functional Category

USP: Humectant; solvent; plasticizer
Others: Inhibitor of fermentation and mold growth; hygroscopic agent; disinfectant; stabilizer for vitamins; water-miscible cosolvent.

3. Synonyms

1,2-Propanediol; propane-1,2-diol; methyl glycol; methyl ethylene glycol; 1,2-dihydroxypropane

4. Chemical Names and CAS Registry Number

1,2-Propanediol [57-55-6]
Propane-1,2-diol

5. Empirical Formula   Molecular Weight

$C_3H_8O_2$ 76.09

6. Structural Formula

$$CH_3CH - CH_2OH$$
$$\quad\quad |$$
$$\quad\quad OH$$

7. Commercial Availability

USA

Ashland Chemical Co.
Bage, Inc.
Dow Chemical Co.
Fanning Corp., The
McKesson Chemical Co.
Mobay Chemical Corp.
Neal & Co., M.F.
Olin Chemicals Corporation
Pfaltz and Bauer, Inc.
Quad Chemical - Lonza Specialty Chemicals
Ruger Chemical Co.
Stoney-Mueiler, Inc.
Thompson-Hayward Chemical Co.
Union Carbide Corp., Specialty Chemicals & Plastics Div.

UK

Carless Chemicals Ltd.
Dow Chemical Co., Ltd.
K&K Greeff Fine Chemicals, Ltd.
Shell Chemicals (UK), Ltd.
Union Carbide, Ltd.

8. Method of Manufacture

Propylene is converted to chlorohydrin by chlorine water and hydrolyzed to 1,2-propylene epoxide. With further hydrolysis, 1,2-propylene epoxide is converted to propylene glycol.

9. Description

A clear, colorless, viscous and practically odorless liquid having a sweet, slightly acrid taste resembling glycerol.

10. Pharmacopeial Specifications

Test	USP	BP/EP
Identification	+	+
Solubility	—	+
Specific gravity	1.035-1.037	—
Relative density	—	1.036-1.040
Distilling range	185°-189°C	—
Acidity	+	+
Water	≤0.2%	—
Residue on ignition	≤3.5 mg/50 g	—
Chloride	0.007%	≤50 ppm
Sulfate	0.006%	≤70 ppm
Arsenic	≤3 ppm	—
Heavy metals	≤5 ppm	≤5 ppm
Refractive index	—	1.431-1.433
Oxidizing substances	—	+
Reducing substances	—	+
Sulfated ash	—	≤0.01%
Assay	≥99.5%	—

11. Typical Properties

Autoignition temperature: 421°C (780°F)
Boiling point: 188°C (389°F)
Flash point: 99°C (210°F)
Freezing point: −59°C
Heat of combustion: 431.0 kcal/mol
Specific rotation $[\alpha]_D^{20}$: −15.0° for *l*-form
Solubility: Miscible with water, acetone, alcohol, glycerin and chloroform; soluble in a ratio of 1:6 ether; immiscible with light mineral oil; immiscible with fixed oils, but will dissolve some essential oils
Surface tension: 40.1 dyne/cm at 25°C
Vapor density: 2.62
Vapor pressure: 0.07 mm at 20°C
Viscosity: 0.581 poise at 20°C

12. Stability and Storage Conditions

Under ordinary conditions, propylene glycol is stable in well-closed containers, but at high temperatures in the open it tends to oxidize, giving rise to products such as propionaldehyde, lactic acid, pyruvic acid and acetic acid. It is chemically stable when mixed with glycerin, water or alcohol. Propylene glycol withstands autoclave sterilization in sealed containers. Store in a well-closed container. Protect from light. Absorbs moisture when exposed to moist air.

13. Incompatibilities

Incompatible with oxidizing reagents such as potassium permanganate.

14. Safety

Probably as a consequence of its metabolism and excretion, propylene glycol is less toxic than other glycols. Some local irritation is produced upon application to mucous membranes or upon subcutaneous or intramuscular injection. Hypersensitivity to 38% propylene glycol applied topically has been reported.

15. Handling Precautions

There is a moderate hazard of fire and explosion when propylene glycol is exposed to heat or flame.

16. Regulatory Acceptance

USP XXI; BP/EP 1980

17. Applications in Pharmaceutical Formulation or Technology

Function	Dosage form	Concentration
Solvent or co-solvent	Oral solutions	10-25%
	Parenterals	10-60%
	Topical preparations	5-80%
	Aerosol solutions	10-30%
Humectant	Topicals	~15%
Preservative	Solutions; semisolids	15-30%

18. Related Substances

Propylene glycol monostearate; NF; emulsifying agent

19. Comments

Propylene glycol has become widely used as a solvent, extractant and preservative. It is a better general solvent than glycerin and dissolves a wide variety of compounds, such as corticoids, phenols, sulfa drugs, barbiturates, vitamins (A and D), most alkaloids and many local anesthetics. As an antiseptic it is similar to ethanol, and against mold growth it is similar to glycerin and only slightly less effective than ethanol. Propylene glycol is acceptable to the Food and Drug Administration for use in foods and cosmetics. The Council on Pharmacy and Chemistry of the American Medical Association has also considered it a harmless ingredient for pharmaceutical products. No ill effects from its industrial use have been reported.

20. Specific References

1. C. D. Yu and J. S. Kent, Effect of propylene glycol on subcutaneous absorption of a benzimidazole hydrochloride, *J. Pharm. Sci.,* 71 (4): 476-478 (1982).
2. M. P. Feffer and D. R. Harken, Effect of dosing volume on intramuscular absorption rate of aminoglycosides, *J. Pharm. Sci.,* 70: 449 (1981).
3. J. S. Kent, R. V. Tomlinson, C. M. Ackley and J. Hsu, Volume and concentration effects on absorption parameters of a substituted benzimidazole anthelmintic after subcutaneous injection, *Drug Develop. & Indust. Pharm.,* 7: 261 (1981).
4. J. I. Wells, D. A. Bhatt and K. A. Khan, Improved wet massed tablet using plasticized binder, *J. Pharm. Pharmacol.,* 34 Suppl.: 46P (1982).

USA: P. S. Tsai*; R. A. Lipper**
UK: H. C. Worthington*; W. Lund

Propylene Glycol Alginate

1. Nonproprietary Name
FCC: Propylene glycol alginate

2. Functional Category
Pharmaceutical stabilizer; emulsifier; thickening agent; suspending agent

3. Synonyms
Hydroxypropyl alginate; *Kelcoloid S, LVF*, and *HVF*

4. Chemical Name and CAS Registry Number
Propylene glycol ester of alginic acid [9005-37-2]

5. Empirical Formula
$(C_9H_{14}O_7)_n$

6. Structural Formula
—

7. Commercial Availability
USA
Kelco Co.

UK
Alginate Industries (UK), Ltd.
Kello International
Ubichem Ltd.

8. Method of Manufacture
The propylene glycol esters of alginic acid vary in composition according to the degree of esterification and the percentages of free and neutralized carboxyl groups in the molecule.

9. Description
White to yellowish, fibrous or granular powder that is practically odorless and tasteless.

10. Pharmacopeial Specifications

11. Typical Properties
Propylene glycol alginate dissolves in water, in solutions of dilute organic acids, and, depending upon the degree of esterification, in hydro-alcoholic mixtures containing up to 60% w/w alcohol to form stable viscous colloidal solutions at a pH of $\simeq 3$. The viscosity of a 1% solution can vary from 21 cps for *Kelcoloid S* to 400 cps for *Kelcoloid HVF*. Propylene glycol alginate is most stable in the pH range of 3–6. In alkaline solutions, the ester is rapidly saponified.

12. Stability and Storage Conditions
Store in a tightly closed container. Propylene glycol alginates gradually become insoluble when stored at elevated temperatures for extended periods of time.

13. Incompatibilities
Degradation occurs in the alkaline pH range.

14. Safety
The incorporation of 5–15% propylene glycol alginate in the diet of purebred dogs for 1 year caused no harmful effects. Numerous studies have attested to the high level of safety of alginates in food use. Allergy tests conducted with propylene glycol alginate have shown it is not an allergen.

15. Handling Precautions
None. Propylene glycol alginate has been shown to possess no eye or skin irritation properties.

16. Regulatory Acceptance
CFR 172.858

17. Applications in Pharmaceutical Formulations or Technology
Propylene glycol alginate is used as a stabilizer, suspending, gelling and emulsifying agent in the concentration range of 1–5% depending on the system under study and the grade or type of alginate product employed.

18. Related Substances
—

19. Comments
Formulation aid for slightly acidic media (pH 3-6).

20. Specific References
None.

USA: R. Dusel*; J. McGinity**

Propylparaben

1. Nonproprietary Names

NF: Propylparaben
BP/EP: Propyl hydroxybenzoate

2. Functional Category

NF: Antimicrobial preservative
BP/EP: Antimicrobial preservative

3. Synonyms

Propyl chemosept; propyl parasept; *Betacide P; Nipagin M; Propyl Aseptoform; Propyl Parasept; Propylparaben; Protaben M; Tegosept M; Solbrol P*

4. Chemical Names and CAS Registry Number

4-Hydroxybenzoic acid propyl ester
Propyl-*p*-hydroxybenzoate [94-13-3]
Propyl-4-hydroxybenzoate

5. Empirical Formula   Molecular Weight

$C_{10}H_{12}O_3$ 180.20

6. Structural Formula

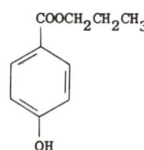

7. Commercial Availability

USA

Beta Chemical Corporation
Greeff & Company, Inc., R.W.
Inolex Personal Care Division
Mallinckrodt, Inc.
Napp Chemicals
Nipa Laboratories, Inc.
Protameen Chemicals, Inc.
Tenneco Chemical, Inc.

UK

BDH Chemicals, Ltd.
Bofors (Great Britain) Co., Ltd.
Bush, Boake, Allen, Ltd.
NIPA Laboratories, Ltd.

8. Method of Manufacture

Propylparaben is prepared by the esterification of *p*-hydroxybenzoic acid with *n*-propanol.

9. Description

Propylparaben is a white, crystalline, odorless, tasteless powder.

SEM-MF-11
Excipient: Propylparaben
Supplier: Bate Chemical Co., Ltd.

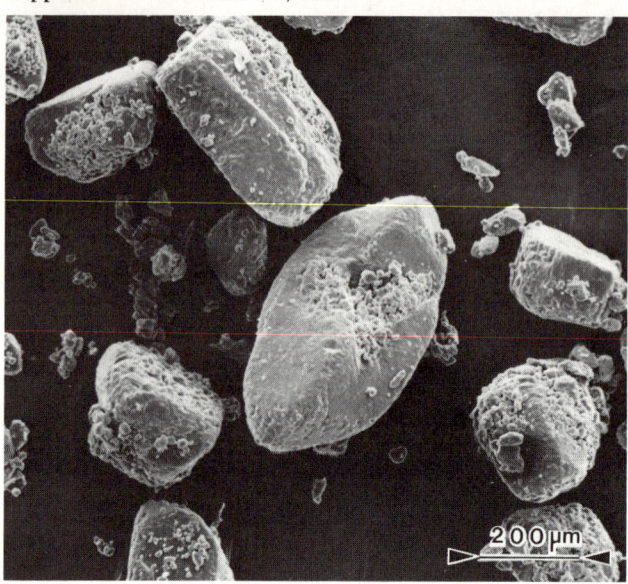

Magnification: 60X

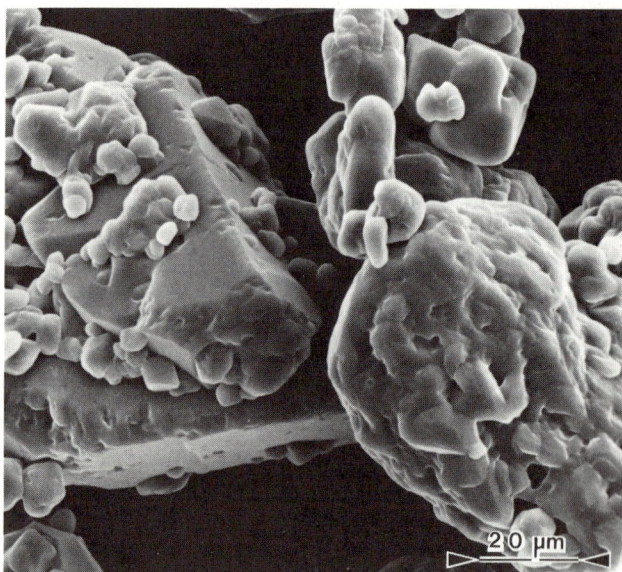

Magnification: 600X

10. Pharmacopeial Specifications

Test	NF	BP/EP
Identification	+	+
Melting range	95°-98°C	95°-98°C
Acidity	+	+
Loss on drying	≤0.5%	—
Residue on ignition	≤0.05%	—
Assay	99.0-100.5%	99.0-101.0%
Sulfated ash	—	≤0.1%
Clarity and color of solution	—	+

11. Typical Properties

Solubility: Very slightly soluble in cold water (0.05% w/v at 25°C; 0.3% w/v at 80°C); readily soluble in ethanol (50% w/v), propylene glycol (25% w/v), acetone or diethyl ether.

Moderately soluble in benzene or carbon tetrachloride; slightly soluble in natural fats and oils.

pKa value: 8.4 (22°C)
Oil/water partition coefficients: liquid paraffin, 0.5; arachis oil, 80.0
Boiling point: 295°C
Flash point: 140°C
Refractive index: 1.5049 (at 14°C, sodium light)
Specific gravity: 1.232 at 14°C

Academy HPE Laboratory Project Data

	Method	Lab #	Results
Solubility (water)	SOL-8	30	0.04%

12. Stability and Storage Conditions

Propylparaben should be stored in a well-closed container. Aqueous solutions at pH 3-6 can be sterilized at 120°C for 20 minutes without decomposition. Aqueous solutions at pH 3-6 are stable (less than 10% decomposition) for up to about four years at room temperature. Aqueous solutions at pH 8 or higher are subject to rapid hydrolysis (10% or more after about 60 days at room temperature).

Predicted Rate Constant and Half-Life of Hydrolysis at 25°C

Concentration of HCl (N)	Rate constant $k \pm \sigma^*$ (hr^{-1})	Half-life $t^{1/2} \pm \sigma^*$ (day)
0.1	$(1.255 \pm 0.042) \times 10^{-4}$	230 ± 7.6
0.01	$(1.083 \pm 0.81) \times 10^{-5}$	$2,670 \pm 200$
0.001	$(8.41 \pm 0.96) \times 10^{-7}$	$34,300 \pm 3,900$
0.0001	$(2.23 \pm 0.37) \times 10^{-7}$	$130,000 \pm 22,000$

* indicates the standard error

Some pharmaceutical preparations containing parabens require autoclave sterilization under pressure at 121.5°C for 20 minutes. Predicted results are shown below:

Concentration of HCl (N)	Rate constant $k \pm \sigma^*$ (hr^{-1})	Predicted residual % after sterilization
0.1	$(4.42 \pm 0.10) \times 10^{-1}$	86.30 ± 0.30
0.01	$(4.67 \pm 0.19) \times 10^{-2}$	98.46 ± 0.06
0.001	$(2.96 \pm 0.24) \times 10^{-3}$	99.90 ± 0.01
0.0001	$(7.8 \pm 1.1) \times 10^{-3}$	99.97 ± 0.004

* indicates the standard error

13. Incompatibilities

The antimicrobial properties of propylparaben are reduced in the presence of non-ionic surfactants. Adsorption of propylparaben to plastics has been reported, with the amount adsorbed dependent upon the type of plastic. Propylparaben is discolored in the presence of iron and is subject to hydrolysis by weak alkalis and strong acids.

14. Safety

In rare instances, propylparaben can elicit skin sensitization and induce cutaneous allergic responses. Allergy from ingestion or parenteral administration has not been reported. Propylparaben (5% in propylene glycol) causes no primary irritation. The acute and chronic oral toxicity of propylparaben is low.

15. Handling Precautions

Avoid inhalation, ingestion and contact with skin, eyes, mouth and nose.

16. Regulatory Acceptance

NF XVI; BP/EP 1980

17. Applications in Pharmaceutical Formulation or Technology

Propylparaben (0.05 to 0.25%) alone or in combination with other esters of *p*-hydroxybenzoic acid or with other antimicrobial agents is used as a preservative in pharmaceutical preparations. Propylparaben [0.02% together with methylparaben (0.18%)] has been used for preservation of various parenterals. As a rule, the preservative effect is increased in combination with other *p*-hydroxybenzoate esters or by the addition of 2-5% propylene glycol.

18. Related Substances

Butylparaben; ethylparaben; methylparaben. Sodium propyl hydroxybenzoate (BP), the sodium salt of propylparaben, may be used instead of propylparaben because of its better water solubility, provided the pH of the preserved preparation does not rise.

Molecular weight: 202.20

Solubility:	Water	50 g/100 g solvent
	Ethanol (96%)	2 g/100 g solvent

19. Comments

The following tabulation lists the minimal concentration (% in water) of methylparaben required to inhibit growth.

Aerobacter aerogenes ATCC 8308	0.10
Aspergillus niger ATCC 10254	0.02
Bacillus cereus var. *mycoides* ATCC 6462	0.0125
Bacillus subtilis ATCC 6633	0.025
Candida albicans ATCC 10231	0.0125
Escherichia coli ATCC 9637	0.01
Penicillium digitatum ATCC 10030	0.0063
Pseudomonas aeruginosa	0.20
Rhizopus nigricans ATCC 6227A	0.0125
Saccharomyces cerevisiae ATCC 9763	0.0125
Staphylococcus aureus ATCC 6538P	0.05

The effectiveness decreases with increasing pH due to the formation of phenolate anion.

20. Specific References

1. S. M. Blaug and D. E. Grant, Kinetics of degradation of parabens, *J. Soc. Cosmet. Chem.*, 25:495 (1974).
2. T. R. Aalto *et al.*, *p*-Hydroxybenzoic acid esters as preservatives, *J. Am. Pharm. Assoc. Sci. Ed.*, 42:449 (1953).
3. J. Schimmel and M. N. Slotsky, Preservation of Cosmetics. In: "Cosmetics, Science and Technology," 2nd Ed., Vol. III, M. S. Balsam and E. Sagarin, Eds., Wiley–Interscience, New York, 1974, pp. 391–470.
4. H. Sokol, Recent developments in the preservation of pharmaceuticals, *Drug Standards*, 20:89 (1952).
5. C. Matthews *et al.*, *p*-Hydroxybenzoic acid esters as preservatives, *J. Am. Pharm. Assoc.*, 45:260(1956).
6. E. L. Richardson, Preservatives: Frequency of use in cosmetic formulas as disclosed to FDA, *Cosmetics and Toiletries*, 92:85-88 (1977).
7. A. Kamada, N. Yata, K. Kubo and M. Arakawa, Stability of *p*-hydroxybenzoic acid esters in acidic medium, *Chem. Pharm. Bull.*, 21:(9), 2073-76 (1973).
8. K. Kakemi, H. Sezaki, E. Arakawa, K. Kimura and K. Ikeda, Interactions of parabens and other pharmaceutical adjuvants with plastic containers, *Chem. Pharm. Bull.*, 19:2523-29 (1971).

USA: M. Rieger*, P. Kotwal**, Z. Chowhan**
UK: M. C. Allwood**

Saccharin

1. Nonproprietary Names

NF: Saccharin
BP: Saccharin

2. Functional Category

USP: Sweetening agent
BP: Sweetening agent

3. Synonyms

Gluside; *Saccharinose*; *Saccharol*; benzosulfimide; *o*-sulfobenzoic acid imide.

4. Chemical Names and CAS Registry Number

1,2-Benzisothiazol-3(2*H*)-one,1,1-dioxide
1,2-Benzisothiazolin-3-one 1,1-dioxide [81-07-2]

5. Empirical Formula   Molecular Weight

$C_7H_5NO_3S$ 183.18

6. Structural Formula

7. Commercial Availability

USA

Alba Chemical, Inc.
American International Chemical, Inc.
Atomergic Chemetals Corp.
Boots Co., Ltd.
Chemical Dynamics Corp.
Conray Chemicals, Inc.
Delamar, Inc.
Greeff & Co., R. W.
ICC Industries, Inc.
Ingredients International, Inc.
Maruzen Fine Chemicals, Inc.
Neal & Co., M. F.
Pfaltz and Bauer, Inc.
Reisman Corp, H.
Ruger Chemical Co.
Sherwin-Williams Co., Chemicals, Div.
Tri-K Industries, Inc.
Uhe Co., George
United States Biochemicals Corp.

UK

British Saccharin Sales Co.

8. Method of Manufacture

Saccharin is made from toluene by the following series of reactions: Toluene is reacted with chlorosulfonic acid to form orthotoluene sulfonyl chloride; orthotoluene sulfonyl chloride is reacted with ammonia to form the sulfonamide; the methyl group is then oxidized with dichromate, yielding orthosulfamyl benzoic acid which, when heated, forms the cyclic imide, saccharin.

9. Description

White crystals or a white crystalline powder. Odorless or has a faint aromatic odor. In dilute solution, saccharin is approximately 500 times as sweet as sucrose.

SEM-MF-18
Excipient: Saccharin

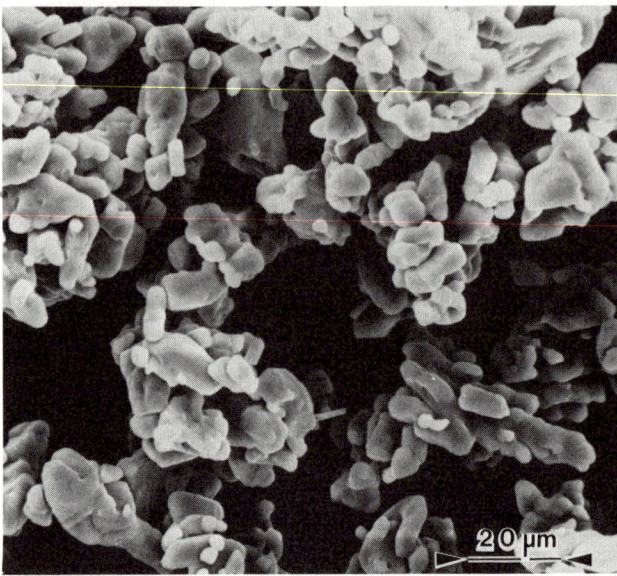

Magnification: 600×

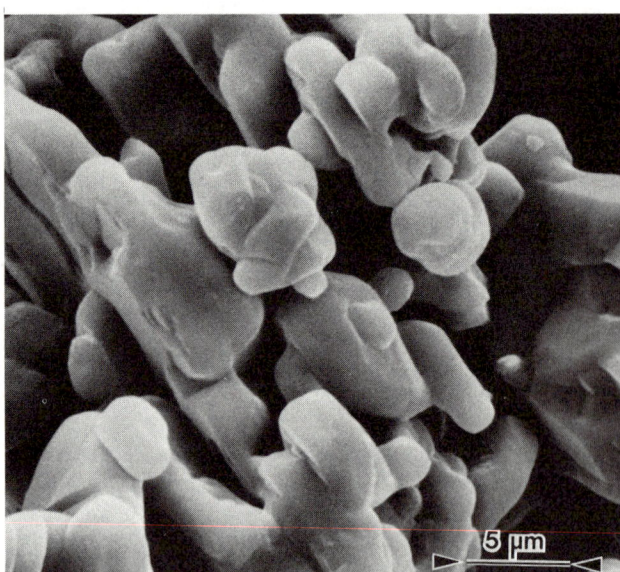

Magnification: 2,400×

10. Pharmacopeial Specification

Test	NF	BP
Identification	+	+
Loss on drying	≤1.0%	≤1.0%
Residue on ignition	≤0.2%	—
Sulfated ash	—	≤0.2%
Toluene sulfonamides	≤0.0025%	—
Arsenic	≤3 ppm	≤2 ppm
Heavy metals	≤0.001%	≤10 ppm
Assay	98.0%-101.0%	≥99.0%
Melting range	226-230°C	226-230°C

Test	NF	BP
Selenium	≤0.003%	—
Readily carbonizable substances	+	+
Benzoic and salicylic acids	+	–
Related substances	—	+

11. Typical Properties

Academy HPE Laboratory Project Data

	Method	Lab #	Results
Moisture content	MC-9	5	0.10%

Density: 0.828g/cm^3

Dissociation constant: pKa = 1.6 (25°C)

Solubility: 1 g/290 ml water; 1 g/31 ml alcohol; 1 g/25 ml boiling water. Slightly soluble in chloroform and ether. Readily dissolved by a dilute solution of ammonia, an alkali hydroxide solution and an alkali carbonate solution (with the evolution of carbon dioxide).

Ultraviolet absorption: In 0. 01N sodium hydroxide-E 1%, 1 cm @ 234 nm = 351; E 1%, 1 cm @ 268 nm = 89; inflection @ 284 nm.

12. Stability and Storage Conditions

Stable. Store in a well-closed container.

13. Incompatibilities

No citations in the literature

14. Safety

Photosensitization or sensitivity reactions have been attributed to saccharin on rare occasions. Erythema of the face due to photosensitivity caused by saccharin has been reported. Urticaria occurred in a woman following the ingestion of food containing saccharin. Experiments in rats have indicated that tumors of the bladder could be produced by 5% saccharin in the diet over 2 years (equivalent to 175 g daily in humans). The FDA recommends limiting adult daily consumption to ≤1 g. Further experiments in rats suggested that a contaminant of commercial saccharin, *o*-toluene sulfonamide, might account for co-carcinogenic effects. Surveys and tests among diabetic patients have not shown any significant incidence of bladder tumors, although saccharin has been in use since the 19th century.

15. Handling Precautions

No restrictions specified

16. Regulatory Acceptance

NF XVI; BP 1980

17. Application

Sweetening agent. 60 mg is equivalent to 30 g of sucrose. It is used as a sweetening agent in vehicles, canned foods, beverages and diets of diabetics to replace sucrose.

18. Related Substances

Saccharin sodium

19. Comments

None

20. Specific References

1. H. J. Kingley (letter), *Cent. Afr. J. Med.,* 12, 243 (1966).

2. R. Miller *et al.,* A case of episodic urticaria due to saccharin ingestion, *J. Allergy & Clin. Immunol.,* 53:240 (1974).

3. *Medical News,* FDA endorses proposal that intake of saccharin should be limited, *J. Am. Med. Assoc.,* 217:412 (1971).

4. *Medical News,* Rat study raises doubts about saccharin study," *ibid.,* 219:990 (1973).

5. R. M. Hicks, *et al.,* Cocarcinogenic action of saccharin in the chemical induction of bladder cancer; and Impurities in saccharin and bladder cancer, *Nature,* London, 243:347, 424 (1973).

6. A. Beringer, *Wien. Med. Wschr.,* 123:41 (1971), per *Int. Pharm. Abstr.,* 11:52 (1972).

USA: S. N. Pagay*; J. Cooper**; J. Mennona**

UK: P.C. Record*

Saccharin Sodium

1. Nonproprietary Names
USP: Saccharin sodium
BP: Saccharin sodium

2. Functional Category
USP: Sweetening agent
BP: Sweetening agent

3. Synonyms
Soluble saccharin; sodium *o*-benzosulfimide; soluble gluside

4. Chemical Names and CAS Registry Numbers
1,2-Benzisothiazol-3(2*H*)-one-1,1-dioxide, sodium salt
1,2-Benzisothiazolin-3-one-1,1-dioxide, sodium salt
dihydrate [6155-57-3] anhydrous [128-44-9]

5. Empirical Formula   Molecular Weight
$C_7H_4NNaO_3S$ 205.16
$C_7H_4NNaO_3S \cdot \frac{2}{3}H_2O$ (84%)   217.24
$C_7H_4NNaO_3S \cdot 2H_2O$ (76%)   241.19

6. Structural Formula

·2H$_2$O   76% saccharin sodium (dihydrate)

·⅔H$_2$O   84% saccharin sodium

7. Commercial Availability
USA
Alba Chemical, Inc.
American International Chemical, Inc.
Atomergic Chemetals Corp.
Boots Co., Ltd.
Chemical Dynamics Corp.
Conray Chemicals, Inc.
Dolamar, Inc.
Greeff & Co., R.W.
ICC Industries, Inc.
Ingredients International, Inc.
Maruzen Fine Chemicals, Inc.
Neal & Co., M.F.
Pfaltz and Bauer, Inc.
Reisman Corp., H.
Ruger Chemical Co.
Sherwin-Williams Co., Chemicals Div.
Tri-K Industries, Inc.
Uhe Co., George
United States Biochemicals Corp.
UK
British Saccharin Sales Co.

8. Method of Manufacture
Saccharin is produced by the oxidation of *o*-toluene-sulfonamide by potassium permanganate in a solution of sodium hydroxide. Acidification of the solution precipitates the saccharin, which is then dissolved in water at 50°C and neutralized by addition of sodium hydroxide. Rapid cooling of the solution initiates the crystallization of the saccharin sodium from the liquors.

9. Description
A white, odorless or faintly aromatic, efflorescent, crystalline powder with an intensely sweet taste. Both forms of saccharin sodium (76% and 84%) are identical in their appearance.

10. Pharmacopeial Specifications

Test	USP	BP
Identification	+	+
Water	≤15.0%	3–15% w/w
Benzoate and salicylate	+	—
Arsenic	≤3 ppm	≤2 ppm
Selenium	≤0.003%	—
Alkalinity	+	—
Toluenesulfonamides	≤0.0025%	—
Heavy metals	≤0.001%	≤10 ppm
Readily carbonizable substances	+	—
Free acid or alkali	—	+
Melting point of isolated saccharin	—	≥226°C
Related substances	—	+
Assay	98.0–101.0% (anhydrous)	≥99.0% (anhydrous)

11. Typical Properties
Density (84% saccharin sodium): a) Particle—1.67 g/cm³; b) bulk—0.82 g/cm³; c) tapped—0.92 g/cm³
Melting point: No melting point; decomposes upon heating.
Moisture content: 9.00% (HPE Laboratory Project, Method MC-3, Lab #5); loss on drying (vacuum drying for 24 hours at 110°C): 5.5% by weight (⅔H$_2$O: 84%); 14.5% by weight (2H$_2$O: 76%). During drying, water evolution occurs in two distinct phases, as indicated by thermogravimetric analysis and the endothermic transitions shown by differential scanning calorimetry.
pH: 6.6 (10% aqueous solution).
Solubility (84% and 76% saccharin sodium):

Solvent	Solubility (g/100 ml)	
	25°C	60°C
Water	83.3	—
Ethanol (100%)	0.98	—
Ethanol (96%)	approximately 2	—
Propylene glycol	29	—
Propane-2-ol	insoluble	—
Buffer solutions:		
pH 2.2 (phthalate)	87	152
pH 4.0 (citrate-phosphate)	83	145
pH 7.0 (citrate-phosphate)	83	152
pH 9.0 (borate)	83	145

Specific surface area: 0.25 m²/g (Quantasorb) (84% and 76% saccharin sodium)

Academy HPE Laboratory Project Data			
	Method	Lab #	Results
Moisture Content	MC-3	5	9.00%

12. Stability and Storage Conditions

Store in an airtight container (efflorescent).

13. Incompatibilities

No citations in the literature.

14. Safety

Estimated acceptable temporary daily intake: up to 2.5 mg/ kg of body weight.

15. Handling Precautions

No restrictions specified.

16. Regulatory Acceptance

USP XXI; BP 1980; under "Artificial Sweeteners" in *Food Regulations 1969* (SI 1969: 1817); permitted in food in England and Wales.

17. Applications in Pharmaceutical Formulation or Technology

As a sweetening agent (about 0.01%); as a sugar substitute in preparations for diabetics.

18. Related Substances

Saccharin NF XV; BP 1980; Saccharin calcium USP XX.

19. Comments

Subject of monographs in pharmacopeias in the following countries: Argentina, Austria, France, Germany, Hungary, India, Japan, Mexico, Netherlands, Nordic, Portugal, Spain, Switzerland, Turkey, Yugoslavia.

20. Specific References

1. FDA endorses proposal that intake of saccharin should be limited, *J. Amer. Med. Assoc.*, 217: 412 (1971).
2. Rat study raises doubts about saccharin's safety, *J. Amer. Med. Assoc.*, 219: 990 (1972).
3. R. M. Hicks *et al.*, Co-carcinogenic action of saccharin in the chemical induction of bladder cancer, *Nature*, 243: 347 (1973).
4. R. M. Hicks *et al.*, Impurities in saccharin and bladder cancer, *Nature*, 243: 424 (1973).
5. A. Beringer, Ist die anwendung der susstoffe bei diabetikern gefahrlich, *Wien. Med. Wschr.*, 132: 41 (1973).
6. Saccharin in the balance, *Br. Med. J.*, 3: 185 (1973).
7. Saccharin: review of safety issues, Council on Scientific Affairs, *J. Amer. Med. Assoc.*, 254: 2622-4 (1985).

USA: S. N. Pagay*; J. Cooper*; D. Hovermale**
UK: P. C. Record*

Sesame Oil

1. Nonproprietary Names
NF: Sesame oil
BP/EP: Sesame oil

2. Functional Category
NF: Solvent and oleaginous vehicle

3. Synonyms
Oleum sesami; benne oil; gingelly oil (gingili oil); teel oil

4. Chemical Names and CAS Registry Number
Sesame oil

5. Empirical Formula   Molecular Weight
—   —

6. Structural Formula
A typical analysis of refined sesame oil indicates the composition of the acids, present as glycerides, to be: saturated: palmitic acid, 9.1%; stearic acid, 4.3%; arachidic acid, 0.8%; unsaturated: oleic acid, 45.4%; linoleic acid, 40.4%. Sesamine, a complex cyclic ether, and sesamiline, a glycoside, are present in small amounts.

7. Commercial Availability
USA
Carnilli, Albert & Laloue
Fanning Corp., The
Ingredients International, Inc.
Janca's Jojoba Oil & Seed Co.
Lippo Chemicals, Inc.
Polyesther Corp.
Ruger Chemical Co.
S.S.T. Corp.
Tri-K Industries, Inc.
Vitamins, Inc.
Welch, Holme & Clark Co.
UK
E.J.R. Lovelock, Ltd.

8. Method of Manufacture
Sesame oil is obtained from the seeds of one or more cultivated varieties of *Sesamum indicum* (pedaliaceae) by expression or extraction. It is subjected to a refinement process to obtain refined sesame oil for pharmaceutical use.

9. Description
The refined oil is a clear, pale yellow liquid with a slight, pleasant odor and a bland taste.

10. Pharmacopeial Specifications

Test	NF	BP/EP
Identification	+	+
Specific gravity	0.916–0.921	—
Heavy metals	≤0.001%	—
Solidification range of fatty acids	20°–25°C	—
Iodine value	103–116	104–120
Saponification value	188–195	187–195
Unsaponifiable	≤1.5%	≤1.8% w/w
Cottonseed oil	+	—
Acid value	—	≤0.6
Peroxide value	—	≤5.0
Refractive index	—	1.472–1.476
Relative density	—	0.915–0.923
Alkaline impurities	—	+
Foreign fixed oils	—	+
Free fatty acids	+	—

11. Typical Properties
Solidification: ~ −5° C
Solubility: Slightly miscible in alcohol; soluble with carbon disulfide, chloroform, ether, and petroleum ether.

Solubility at 25°C:
Water: Insoluble
Ethanol: Slightly soluble
Propylene glycol: —
Hexane: Soluble

Academy HPE Laboratory Project Data

	Method	Lab No.	Results
Viscosity	V15-2	30	43.37
Specific gravity	DE-5	30	0.914

12. Stability and Storage Conditions
Stable. It should be kept in a well-filled, airtight container protected from light. Excess exposure to heat should be avoided. Sesame oil does not readily turn rancid. It is more stable than most other fixed oils.

13. Incompatibilities
No citations in the literature.

14. Safety
Practically nontoxic to humans when ingested orally. Probable oral LD_{50} in humans is above 15 g/kg of body weight. Contact dermatitis is a possible safety consideration.

15. Handling Precautions
No restrictions specified.

16. Regulatory Acceptance
NF XVI; BP/EP 1980

17. Applications in Pharmaceutical Formulation or Technology

Use	Concentration
Solvent and vehicle in parenteral products for intramusclar administration	As required
Manufacture of iodized oil, liniments, ointments, and plasters	As required

18. Related Substances
Corn oil; cottonseed oil; peanut oil

19. Comments
Sesame oil is sterilized by maintaining it at 150°C for one hour, or by aseptic filtration.

20. Specific References
1. K. Hirano, T. Ichihashi and H. Yamada, Studies on the absorption of practically water-insoluble drugs following injection V; subcutaneous absorption in rats from solutions in water immiscible oils, *J. Pharm. Sci.*, 71 (5):495 (1982).

USA: A. Rahman*; D. Sanvordeker**; N. B. Batuyios**

Shellac

1. Nonproprietary Name
NF: Shellac

2. Functional Category
USP: Coating agent

3. Synonyms
Lacca; lac; dewaxed orange shellac; orange shellac; refined bleached shellac; regular bleached shellac; pharmaceutical glaze

4. Chemical Names and CAS Registry Number
Shellac; lacca, lac [9000-59-3]

5. Empirical Formula   Molecular Weight
Undefined   Undefined

Composition: Shellac is a refined natural product. The main component (about 95%) of shellac is a resin, which on mild basic hydrolysis gives a mixture of aliphatic and alicyclic hydroxyacids. The composition of the hydrolysate is variable, but in general there are about 50% aliphatic and 5-10% of alicyclic acids. Aleuritic acid and shellolic acid are the major aliphatic and alicyclic components, respectively. Shellac also contains about 5-6% wax and a small amount of pigment.

6. Structural Formula
Aleuritic acid
$$CH_2OH-(CH_2)_5-(CHOH)_2-(CH_2)_7-COOH$$
Shellolic acid

7. Commercial Availability
Many different grades of shellac are available. The main division is into orange shellac and bleached shellac. Whereas the latter can be further divided into regular bleached shellac and refined (wax-free) bleached shellac, there are many grades of orange shellac which differ in color, wax content, amount of alcohol-insoluble matter and details of the extraction process used. Shellac can also be obtained commercially in pharmaceutical glazes in which the appropriate grade of shellac has been dissolved in ethanol.

USA
Colony Import & Export Corp.
Mantrose-Haeuser Co., Millmaster Onyx Group

UK
A. F. Suter & Co., Ltd.
Angelo Rhodes, Ltd.
Batewell, Ltd.
Hicks Bros (Produce), Ltd.
M. Hamburger & Sons, Ltd.
Thew, Arnott & Co., Ltd.
William Ransom and Son, Ltd.

8. Method of Manufacture
Lac is a resinous substance prepared from a secretion that encrusts the bodies of a scale insect, *Laccifer lacca* (Coccidae), which lives on the sap of the stems of various trees. Most commercial shellac is produced in India and Thailand; smaller amounts come from Burma and Malaya. Secretions are found most abundantly on the smaller branches and twigs which are broken off and constitute "sticklac." After scraping the twigs and soaking in water, the water-soluble components are removed by treatment with dilute alkali. The resulting water-insoluble materials, which retain a second coloring matter—the yellow erythrolaccin—are dried and then constitute "seed lac." Shellac is obtained from seed lac by either "handmade" or "machine-made" methods. In the handmade method, seed lac is melted in a bag suspended over a fire. Shellac is squeezed out and, when sufficiently cooled, is stretched into large sheets and broken into flakes. Alternatively, the molten shellac is poured into circular molds which on cooling becomes commercial button shellac. Machine-made shellac is prepared from seed lac by a process using steam heat or by a solvent-extraction process using hot ethanol. Shellacs produced by the heat and the solvent-extraction processes cannot usually be differentiated by chemical tests although they differ physically. In the USA particularly, "bleached shellac" is widely available. This form is prepared by dissolving lac in hot soda solution, followed by bleaching with chlorine or sulfurous acid, precipitating with acid, collecting, washing and "pulling" under water into sticks.

9. Description
Thin, hard, brittle, transparent, pale lemon-yellow to brownish-orange flakes of varying sizes and shapes, also available as a powder. Odorless, or with a faint odor; tasteless.

10. Pharmacopeial Specifications

NF	Acid value (on dried basis)	Loss on drying	Wax
Orange shellac	Between 68 and 76	≤2.0%	≤5.5%
Dewaxed orange shellac	Between 71 and 79	≤2.0%	≤0.2%
Regular bleached shellac	Between 73 and 89	≤6.0%	≤5.5%
Refined bleached shellac	Between 75 and 91	≤6.0%	≤0.2%

Test	NF
Identification	+ (see above)
Loss on drying	+
Arsenic	≤1.5 ppm
Heavy metals	≤0.001%
Acid value	+ (see above)
Wax	+ (see above)
Rosin	+

11. Typical Properties
Alcohol (95%)-insoluble matter: ≤1.0%
Ash: ≤1.0%
Density: 1.035-1.140
Saponification value: 185-210
Hydroxyl value: 230-280
Melting range: 115-120°C
Iodine value: 10-18

Refractive index (20°C): 1.5210-1.5272
Solubility: In ether, 13-15%; in benzene, 10-20%; in petroleum ether, 2-6%. Sparingly soluble in oil of turpentine. Insoluble in water; soluble in aqueous solutions of ethanolamines, alkalis or borax.

Solvent	Solubility, mg/ml	
	25°C	**37°C**
Water	Insoluble	Insoluble
Ethanol	500	500
Propylene glycol	100	500
Hexane	Insoluble	Insoluble
Isooctane	Insoluble	Insoluble

A comprehensive listing of electrical, mechanical, optical and thermal properties may be found in References 1 and 2.

12. Stability and Storage Conditions

After long storage, shellac becomes less readily soluble in alcohol, less fluid on heating, and darker in color. It is recommended that supplies of shellac be used within four months of purchase. It is important that shellac be stored in a well-closed container at temperatures below 27°C and that wax-containing grades are mixed before use to assure uniform distribution of wax.

13. Incompatibilities

Shellac is chemically reactive with aqueous alkalis, organic bases, alcohols and agents which esterify hydroxyl groups. It should therefore be used with caution in the presence of such compounds.

14. Safety

In pharmaceutical applications there are no reports of safety hazards. Shellac which complies with pharmacopeial requirements is nontoxic, and there have been no substantiated cases of allergic reactions or sensitization.

15. Handling Precautions

Avoid ingestion, inhalation and contact with eyes and nose.

16. Regulatory Status

NF XVI

17. Applications in Pharmaceutical Formulation or Technology

Alcoholic solutions containing about 35% shellac are used for the enteric coating of tablets or beads (see section 19). Alcoholic solutions containing about 40% shellac have been used to apply one or two sealing coats to protect tablet cores from moisture.

18. Related Substances

—

19. Comments

Since shellac is insoluble in acidic conditions but soluble at higher pH's, it would appear to be a suitable enteric coating material. However, in practice, delayed disintegration and drug release may occur *in vivo* because shellac is insoluble in the slightly acid environment of the upper intestine. Further, studies using the USP disintegration test for enteric-coated tablets have indicated that there is a marked increase in the disintegration time over a six-month storage period for shellac-coated tablets. It is likely that this effect is due to the polymerization of shellac which occurs over storage periods of this duration.

20. Specific References

1. G. S. Misra *et al.*, Shellac. In: "Encycl. Polym. Sci. Technol.," Vol. 12, 1970, pp. 419-440.
2. J. Martin, Shellac. In: "Encycl. of Chem. Tech.," 2nd Ed., Vol. 18, 1969, pp. 21-32.
3. H. S. Cockeram *et al.*, The physical and chemical properties of shellac, *J. Soc. Cos. Chem.*, 12: 316 (1961).
4. P. Yates and G. F. Field, Lac-I. The structure of shellolic acid, *Tetrahedron*, 26: 3135 (1970).
5. P. Yates, P. M. Burke and G. F. Field, Lac-II. The stereochemistry of shellolic and epishellolic acids, *Tetrahedron*, 26: 3159 (1970).
6. G. T. Luce, Disintegration of tablets enteric coated with CAP, *Manuf. Chem. Aerosol News*, 49: (7), 50 (1978).

USA: R. C. Vasavada*; R. O. Zimmerer, Jr.**
UK: J. W. Kennerley**

Colloidal Silicon Dioxide

1. Nonproprietary Name
NF: Colloidal silicon dioxide

2. Functional Category
NF: Suspending and/or viscosity-increasing agent; glidant and/or anticaking agent
Others: Flow conditioning agent; tablet disintegrant

3. Synonyms
Colloidal silica; fumed silica; light anhydrous silicic acid; silicic anhydride; silicon dioxide fumed; *Aerosil*; *Cab-O-Sil*; *Syloid*

4. Chemical Name and CAS Registry Number
Silica [7631-86-9]

5. Empirical Formula   Molecular Weight
SiO_2 60.08

6. Structural Formula

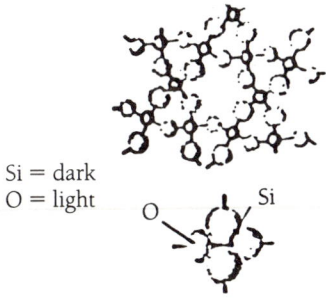

Si = dark
O = light

7. Commercial Availability
USA
Atomergic Chemetals
Cabot Corporation
Degussa, Inc.
E. I. DuPont & Co.
W. R. Grace & Co.

UK
Bush, Beach & Segner Bayley
J. Crosfield & Sons Ltd.
Croxton and Garry Ltd.

8. Method of Manufacture
Colloidal silicon dioxide is prepared by the hydrolysis of a silicon compound, such as silicon tetrachloride, at 1110°C using a vapor phase process.

9. Description
Submicroscopic, light, loose, bluish-white, odorless, tasteless, non-gritty, amorphous powder.

SEM: KY-43
Excipient: Silicon Dioxide (Aerosil A-200)
Manufacturer: Degussa   Lot No. 87A-1 (04169C)

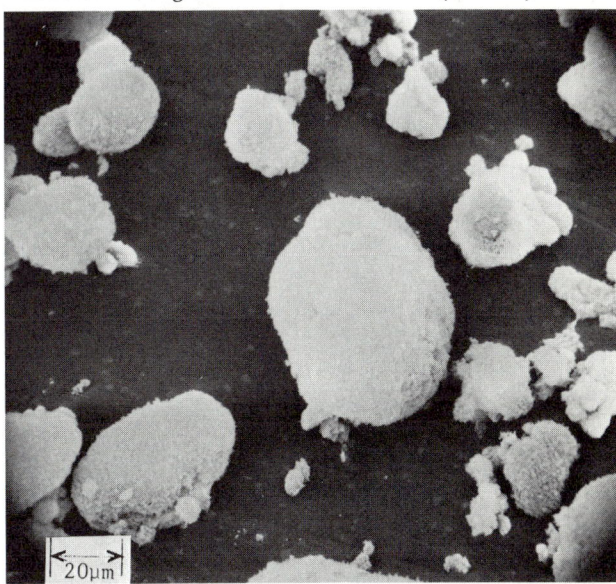

Magnification: 600X   **Voltage:** 20 kV

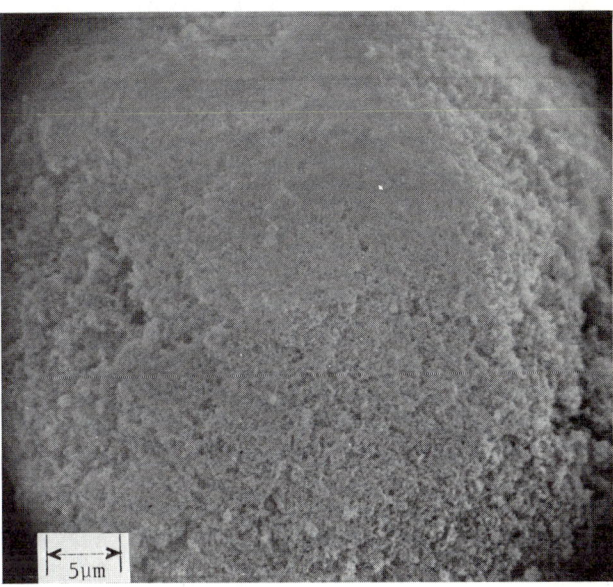

Magnification: 2400X   **Voltage:** 20kV

SEM-UK-1
Excipient: Aerosil-200
Manufacturer: Degussa   **Lot No.** 512 H

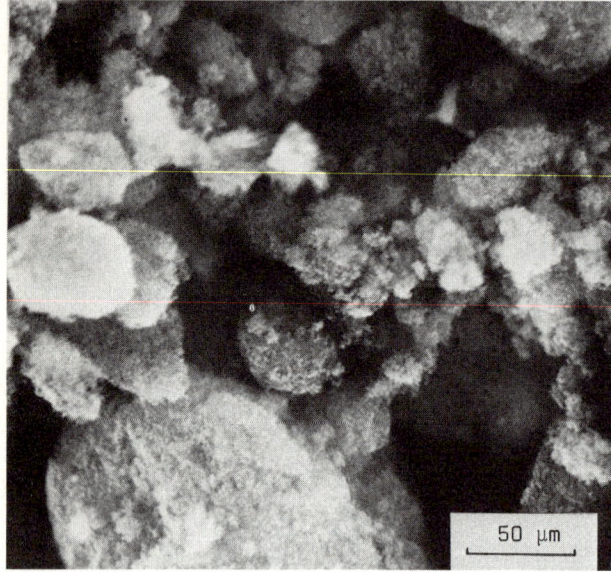

Magnification: 360×

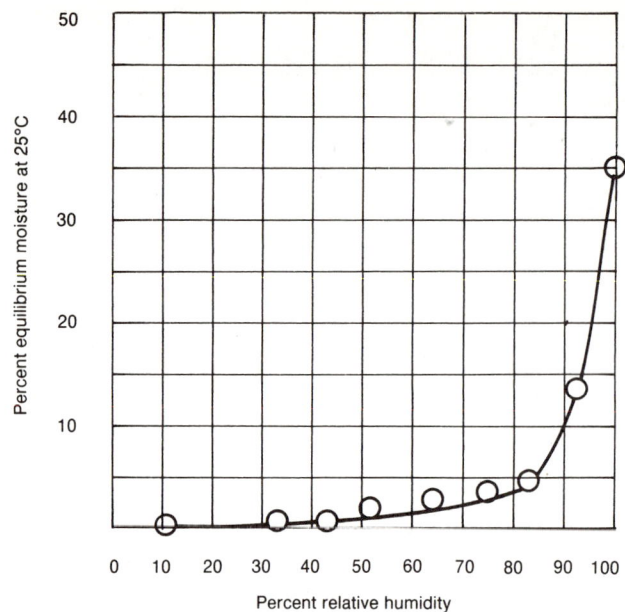

Colloidal Silicon Dioxide, NF, *Cab-O-Sil* M5 (Cabot, Lot #1L 288)

Figure: 2-EMC-8   **Method:** EMC-1

10. Pharmacopeial Specifications

Test	NF
Identification	+
pH (1 in 25 aqueous dispersion)	3.5-4.4
Loss on drying	≤2.5%
Loss on ignition	≤2.0%
Arsenic	≤8 ppm
Assay limits (ignited at 1000°C for 2 hrs)	99.0-100.5%

11. Typical Properties

Academy HPE Laboratory Project Data

	Method	Lab #	Results
Moisture content	MC-20	2	0.60%
Bulk/Tap density (Aerosil A-200)*	BTD-4	1	B:0.029g/cm³ T:0.040g/cm³
	BTD-7	14	B:0.042g/cm³ T:0.069g/cm³
(Cab-O-Sil M5)	BTD-6	8	Not measurable
Particle size dist.	PSD-1	1	Not measurable
Density (Syloid)	DE-4	36	2.0647
EMC Plot (Cab-O-Sil M5)	EMC-1	2	Fig:2-EMC-8
SDI Plot (Aerosil A-200)	SDI-2	26	Fig:26-SDI-11
PSD Plot (Aerosil A-200)	PSD-8	33	Fig:33-PSD-3

Suppliers: Buffalo Solvent, Degussa*

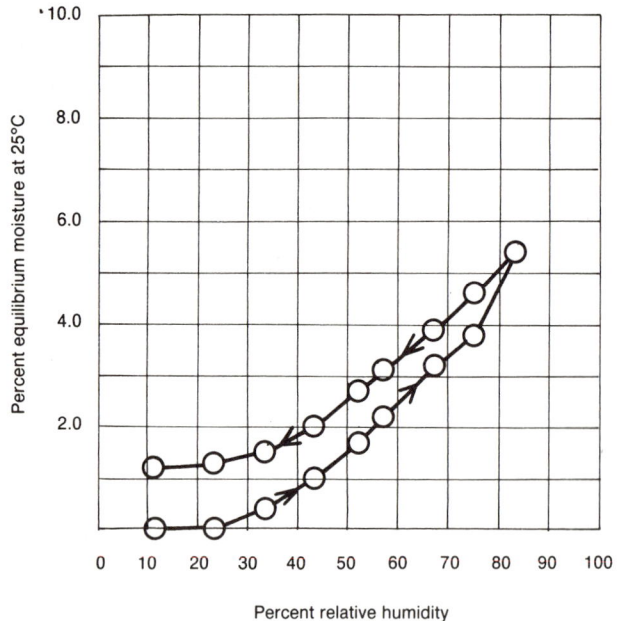

Silicon Dioxide (Degussa, *Aerosil* A-200, Lot #0146 9C)

Figure: 26-SDI-11   **Method:** SDI-2

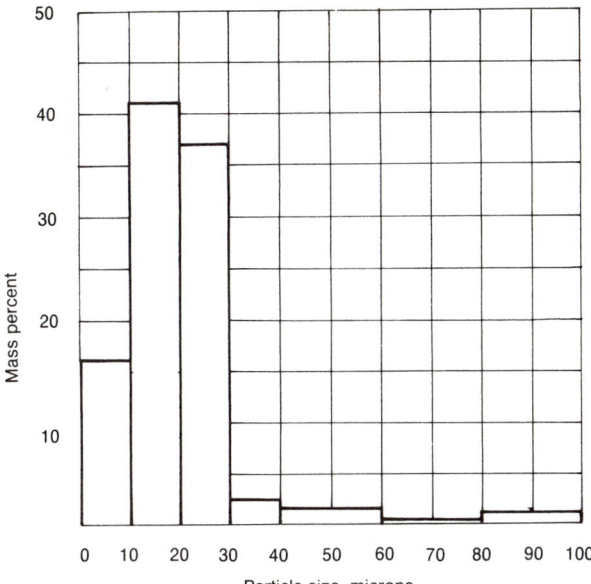

Silicon Dioxide (Degussa, *Aerosil* A-200)

Figure: 33-PSD-3   **Method:** PSD-8

Density: Particle: 220 g/l; Compacted bulk: 50-120 g/l
Flowability: 35.52% (Carr compressibility index). See R. L. Carr, *Brit. Chem. Eng.*, 15:1541 (1970).
Moisture content: 3.8% (Karl Fischer—at equilibrium with ambient laboratory RH)

Moisture sorption profile:
4% at 54% RH.
8% at 72% RH.
18% at 78% RH.

Particle size: 7-16 nm
Solubility: Insoluble in purified water; forms a colloidal dispersion; Soluble in hot solutions of alkali hydroxide; Insoluble in acids, except Hydrofluoric; Insoluble in organic solvents.
Specific surface area: Stroehlein apparatus, single point: 200-400 m²/g; BET method: 50-380 m²/g
Commercial grades and their properties: Several grades of Cab-O-Sil and Aerosil are produced by varying the manufacturing process. These modifications do not affect the silica content, specific gravity, refractive index, color or amorphous form. However, particle size, surface areas and bulk densities are affected. The physical properties of Cab-O-Sil and Aerosil are given in Tables I and II, respectively.

Table I (Cab-O-Sil)

Grade	BET Surface Area m²/gm	Density g/l	Nominal Particle Diameter (nm)	pH (4% in water)
M-5	200 ± 25	36.8 Max.	14	3.6-4.3
MS-7	200 ± 25	72.0 ± 8	14	3.6-4.3
MS-75	255 ± 15	72.0 ± 8	11	3.6-4.3
HS-5	325 ± 25	36.8 Max.	8	3.6-4.3
EH-5	390 ± 40	36.8 Max.	7	3.6-4.3
S-17	400 ± 20	72.0 ± 8	7	3.6-4.3

Table II (Aerosil)

Grade	BET Surface Area m²/g	Average Primary Particle Size (nm)	Bulk Density g/l	Moisture Content (%)	pH (4% aq. dispersion)
Aerosil 130	130 ± 25	16	Apx. 60	<1.5	3.6-4.3
Aerosil 200	200 ± 25	12	Apx. 60	<1.5	3.6-4.3
Aerosil 300	300 ± 30	7	Apx. 60	<1.5	3.6-4.3
Aerosil 380	380 ± 30	7	Apx. 60	<1.5	3.6-4.3
Aerosil 0	200 ± 25	12	Apx. 60	<1.5	3.6-4.3
Aerosil OX50	50 ± 15	40	Apx. 80	<1.5	3.8-4.5
Aerosil TT600	200 ± 50	40	Apx. 60	<2.5	3.6-4.2
Aerosil MOX80	80 ± 30	30	Apx. 60	<1.5	3.6-4.2
Aerosil MOX170	170 ± 30	15	Apx. 60	<1.5	3.6-4.2
Aerosil LK84	170 ± 30	—	Apx. 60	<1.5	3.6-4.3
Aerosil R972	120 ± 30	16	Apx. 60	<0.5	3.5-4.1*

*In water: acetone or methanol = 1:1

12. Stability and Storage Conditions

Colloidal silicon dioxide is hygroscopic, but absorbs large quantities of water without liquefying. Store in a well-closed container.

13. Incompatibilities

The use of silicon dioxide as an excipient may have clinical consequences only for diethylstilbestrol preparations.

14. Safety

Prolonged inhalation of the dust can cause fibrosis of the lung (silicosis). However, no such incidence has been reported. Intraperitoneal and subcutaneous applications may produce local tissue reactions and/or granulomas. Colloidal silicon dioxide should not be admnistered parenterally.

15. Handling Precautions

Protect the mouth and eyes from dust and avoid excessive inhalation. The working area should be well ventilated.
Risk of ignition is minimized by electrical grounding of equipment.

16. Regulatory Acceptance

NF XVI

17. Applications in Pharmaceutical Formulation and Technology

Drying agent for hygroscopic materials. Absorbent dispersing agent for liquids in powders or suppositories.
Glidant and anti-adherent in tabletting processes and encapsulation (0.1-0.5%).
Thixotropic thickening and suspending agent in gels and semi-solid preparations (2-10%). The degree of viscosity increase depends on the polarity of the liquid (polar liquids

generally require greater concentration than non-polar liquids). In ointments, viscosity is largely independent of temperature.

Emulsion stabilizer (1-5%).

In aerosols, it promotes particulate suspension, eliminates hard settling and minimizes clogging of the spray nozzle (0.5-2%).

18. Related Substances

—

19. Comments

The incidence of microbial contamination in samples is very low.

20. Specific References

1. Aerosil in pharmaceuticals and cosmetics, *Bulletin No. 49*, Degussa, Germany.
2. "Cab-O-Sil properties and functions," Cabot Corporation, Boston, Massachusetts.
3. Aerosil—Manufacture, Properties & Application, *Bulletin No. 11*, Degussa, Germany.
4. Aerosil for improving the flow behavior of powder substances, *Bulletin No. 31*, Degussa, Germany.
5. Aerosil as a thickening agent for liquid systems, *Bulletin No. 23*, Degussa, Germany.
6. Absorption of pharmaceutically active substances in Aerosil, *Bulletin No. 19*, Degussa, Germany.
7. Hans Johansen and Niels Moller, Solvent deposition of drugs on excipients, *Arch. Pharm. Chemi. Sci.*, 5: 33 (1977).
8. K. Y. Yang, R. Glemza and C. I. Jarowski, Effects of amorphous silicon dioxides on drug dissolution, *J. Pharm. Sci.*, 68:(5), 560-565 (1979).
9. J. C. Callahan, G. W. Cleary, M. Elefant, G. Kaplan, T. Kensler and R. A. Nash, Equilibrium moisture content of pharmaceutical excipients, *Drug Develop. and Indust. Pharm.*, 8:(3), 355-369 (1982).

USA: D. Harpaz*, F. Groves**, Z. Chowhan**
UK: A. Selkirk*

Sodium Alginate

1. Nonproprietary Names

NF: Sodium alginate
BP: Sodium alginate

2. Functional Category

NF: Suspending and/or viscosity-increasing agent
Others: Disintegrating agent; tablet binder

3. Synonyms

Alginic acid; sodium salt; algin; sodium polymannuronate *Satialgine S20; Album S 160 and S 15/600; Kelgin, Kelcosol, Keltone, Kelco-gel LV, HV; Sodium Alginate, Type S-11*

4. Chemical Name and CAS Registry Number

Sodium alginate is the purified carbohydrate product extracted from brown seaweed by the use of dilute alkali. It consists chiefly of the sodium salt of alginic acid, a polyuronic acid composed of β-D-mannuronic acid residues linked so that the carboxyl group of each unit is free while the aldehyde group is shielded by a glycosidic linkage. [9005-38-3]

5. Empirical Formula

$(C_6H_7O_6Na)_n$

6. Structural Formula

7. Commercial Availability

USA

Edward Mendell Co., Inc.
Gallard-Schlesinger
George Uhe Co. Inc.
Kelco Co.
Meer Corporation

UK

Alginate Industries Ltd.
British Ceca Co.
Chemical Exchange (UK) Ltd.
Croxton and Garry

8. Method of Manufacture

Sodium alginate is prepared by the neutralization of purified alginic acid with sodium bicarbonate.

9. Description

Sodium alginate occurs as a white or buff powder which is odorless and tasteless. The powder may be coarse or fine.

10. Pharmacopeial Specifications

Test	NF	BP
Identification	+	+
Assay	90.8-106.0%	—
Microbial limits	≤200 per gram *Salmonella* species and *E coli* absent	—
Loss on drying	≤15% by weight	≤22.0%
Sulfated ash	—	30.0-35.0%
Ash	18-24%	—
Lead	≤0.001%	≤10 ppm
Arsenic	≤1.5 ppm	≤3 ppm
Heavy metals	≤0.004%	—
Iron	—	≤400 ppm

11. Typical Properties

Academy HPE Laboratory Project Data			
	Method	Lab #	Results
Moisture Content	MC-8	18	19.25%

Viscosity Method	Conc.	Visco-meter	Spindle	Factor	Results
VIS-3	2.0%	RVF	2	40	2160cps[a]
VIS-3	2.0%	RVF	3	100	2050cps[a]
VIS-3	2.0%	HBT	2	160	2000cps[b]
VIS-3	2.0%	HBT	1	40	3040cps[b]
VIS-3	3.0%	RVF	2	100	9850cps[b]
VIS-3	3.0%	RVF	3	100	8350cps[b]
VIS-3	3.0%	HBT	2	160	8640cps[b]
VIS-3	3.0%	HBT	3	400	7200cps[b]

Supplier: Mendell[a]; Algum[b]

Sodium alginate is slowly soluble in water, forming a viscous, colloidal solution. It is insoluble in alcohol and in hydro-alcoholic solutions in which the alcohol content is greater than 30% by weight. It is also insoluble in other organic solvents and in acids where the pH of the resulting solution falls below 3.0. Various grades of sodium alginate are available yielding aqueous solutions of varying viscosities within a range of 20 to 400 centipoises in 1% solution at 20°C. Solutions are sterilized by autoclaving. Some decrease in viscosity occurs following sterilization. The extent of this loss depends on the presence of other substances added to the solution. A 1% solution in distilled water has a pH of approximately 7.2.

12. Stability and Storage Conditions

Since sodium alginate is hygroscopic, the moisture content at equilibrium is a function of the relative humidity. Dry storage stability is excellent when the powder is stored in a well-closed container at temperatures of 25°C or less. Solutions are most stable at a pH between 4 and 10. Viscosity decreases for sodium alginate solutions above a pH of 10. Solutions should not be stored in metal containers. Preparations for external use may be preserved by the addition of chlorocresol (0.1%), chloroxylenol (0.1%), or esters of *p*-hydroxybenzoic acid, or, if the medium is acidic, benzoic acid may be used.

13. Incompatibilities

Sodium alginate is incompatible with acridine derivatives, crystal violet, phenylmercuric nitrate and acetate, calcium salts, alcohol in concentrations greater than 5%, and heavy metals. High concentrations of electrolytes cause an increase in viscosity until salting-out of the sodium alginate occurs. Salting-out occurs if more than 4% of sodium chloride is present.

14. Safety

No satisfactory data have been reported in the literature concerning the acute oral toxicity (LD_{50}) of sodium alginates. The incorporation of 5 to 15% sodium alginate in the diet of purebred beagle dogs for one year caused no harmful effects. Administration of 5 g/kg of body weight to rats within a 24-hour period caused no mortalities nor signs of toxicity. The effect of degraded and undegraded sodium alginate on the colon of guinea pigs indicated that sodium alginate did not cause ulcerative colitis in either its degraded or undegraded form. Numerous studies have attested to the high level of safety of sodium alginate in foods. Allergy tests conducted with sodium alginate have shown that the material is not allergenic.

15. Handling Precautions

None. Sodium alginate has not been shown to possess any eye or skin irritation properties.

16. Regulatory Acceptance

NF XVI; BPC 1973

17. Applications in Pharmaceutical Formulations or Technology

Use	Concentration (%)
Pastes and creams	5-10%
Stabilizer in emulsions	1-3%
Suspending agent	1-5%
Tablet disintegrant	2.5-10%
Tablet binder	1-3%

18. Related Substances

Calcium sodium alginate

19. Comments

Sodium alginate is also used as a hemostatic agent in surgical dressings. It has been reported that sodium alginate could be sterilized by ethylene oxide without loss of viscosity.

20. Specific References

1. Literature issued by Kelco Company, San Diego, CA.
2. Literature issued by Edward Mendell Co., Carmel, NY.
3. D. Coats and G. Richardson, *Can. J. Pharm. Sci.*, 9: 60 (1974).
4. K. A. Khan and C. T. Rhodes, *Pharm. Acta Helv.*, 47: 41 (1972).

USA: R. Dusel*; J. McGinity*; M. R. Harris*;
W. A. Vadino*; J. Cooper**

Sodium Ascorbate

1. Nonproprietary Name
USP: Sodium ascorbate

2. Functional Category
Antioxidant

3. Synonyms
Ascorbin; L-Ascorbic acid; monosodium salt

4. Chemical Names and CAS Registry Number
L-ascorbic acid, monosodium salt, monosodium L-ascorbate [134-03-2]

5. Empirical Formula
$C_6H_7NaO_6$

Molecular Weight
198.11

6. Structural Formula

7. Commercial Availability

USA
Atomergic Chemetals Corp.
Gallard-Schlesinger Chemical Mfg. Corp.
Hoffmann-LaRoche, Inc.
Ingredients International, Inc.
Pfaltz and Bauer, Inc.
Pfizer, Inc.-Chemical Div.
Reisman Corp., H.
Ruger Chemical Co.
S.S.T. Corp.
Takeda-Fallek Sales, Inc.
Uhe Co., George

UK
Pfizer Ltd.
Roche Products Ltd.

8. Method of Manufacture
An equivalent amount of sodium bicarbonate is added to a solution of ascorbic acid in water. Following the cessation of effervescence, the addition of isopropanol precipitates the sodium ascorbate.

9. Description
White or slightly yellow crystalline powder; practically odorless.

No. SEM: KY-11
Excipient: Sodium ascorbate USP, Powder-M
Manufacturer: Pfizer   **Lot No.:** 9B-1 (C92220-C4025)

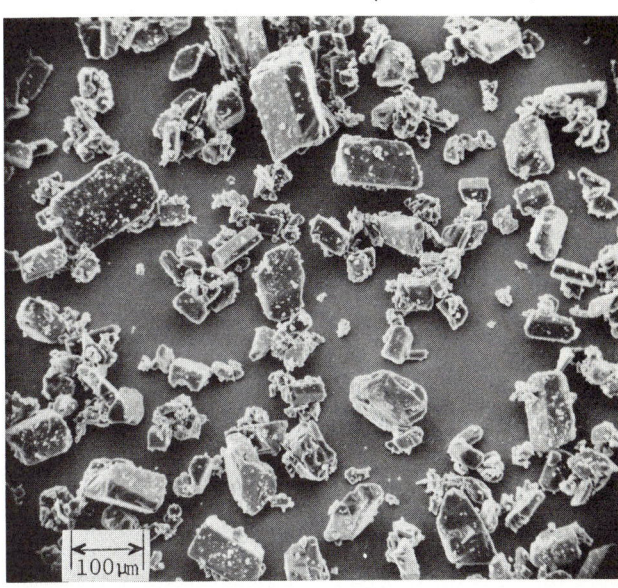

Magnification: 120×   **Voltage:** 20 kV

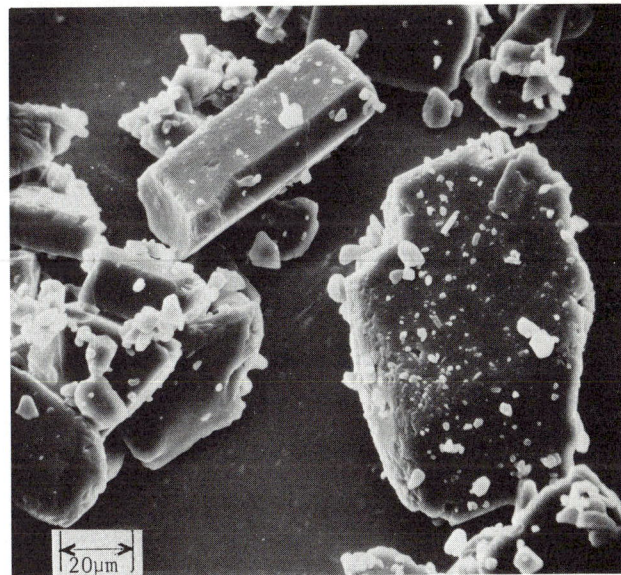

Magnification: 600×   **Voltage:** 20 kV

10. Pharmacopeial Specifications

Test	USP
Identification	+
pH (1 in 10 solution)	7.0-8.0
Specific rotation	+103° to +108°
Loss on drying	≤0.25%
Heavy metals	≤0.002%
Assay	99.0–101.0%

11. Typical Properties
Solubility: Water: 0.62 g/ml (25°C); Alcohol: very slight; chloroform: insoluble; ether: insoluble.
Decomposition: 218°C

12. Stability and Storage Conditions

Relatively stable in air; gradually darkens upon exposure to light.

13. Incompatibilities

Oxidizing agents; heavy metal ions (especially copper and iron); methenamine; sodium nitrite; sodium salicylate; theobromine salicylate

14. Safety

No adverse effects in concentrations when employed as an antioxidant.

15. Handling Precautions

—

16. Regulatory Acceptance

USP XXI

17. Applications in Pharmaceutical Formulation or Technology

Antioxidant

18. Related Substances

Ascorbic acid

19. Comments

—

20. Specific References

—

USA: J. Cooper*; B. Rasadi**
UK: E. Cole*

Sodium Benzoate

1. Nonproprietary Names
NF: Sodium benzoate
BP/EP: Sodium benzoate

2. Functional Category
USP: Antimicrobial preservative
BP: Antimicrobial preservative
Others: Bacteriostatic agent

3. Synonyms
Benzoate of soda

4. Chemical Names and CAS Registry Number
Sodium benzoate [532-32-1]
Benzoic acid
Sodium salt

5. Empirical Formula

Empirical Formula	Molecular Weight
$C_7H_5NaO_2$	144.11

6. Structural Formula

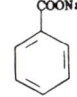

7. Commercial Availability

USA
Aceto Chemical Co.
American International Chemical, Inc.
Atomergic Chemetals Corp.
Bentex Chemicals, Inc.
Groeff & Co., R. W.
Ingredient Technology Corp. Flavor & Fragrance Div.
Kalama Chemical, Inc.
Mallinckrodt, Inc.
McKesson Chemical Co.
Pfaltz and Bauer, Inc.
Pfizer, Inc.-Chemical Div.
Ruger Chemical Co.
Tenneco Chemicals, Inc.
Thompson-Hayward Chemical Co.
Tri-K Industries, Inc.

UK
Carless Chemicals, Ltd.
Hopkin & Williams
Koch-Light Laboratories, Ltd.
Kodak, Ltd.

8. Method of Manufacture
Sodium benzoate is prepared by treatment of benzoic acid with either sodium carbonate or sodium bicarbonate.

9. Description
White granular or crystalline powder. Odorless, or with faint odor of benzoin. Taste is sweetish, astringent and saline.

SEM-MF-15: Excipient: Sodium benzoate
Supplier: Bush, Boake, Allen Corp.

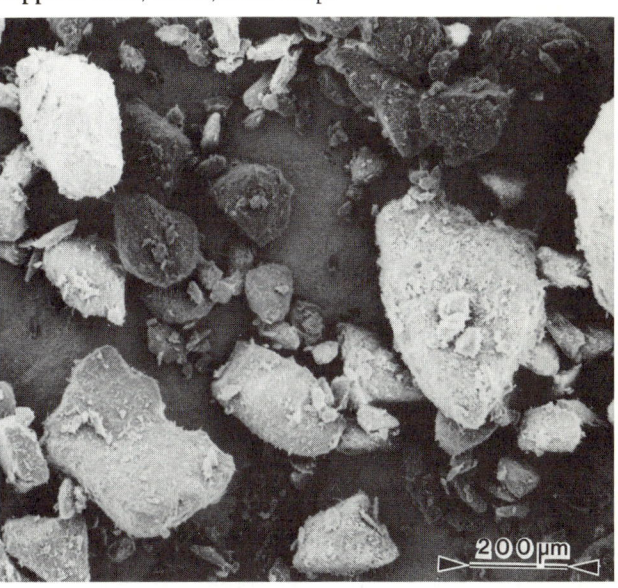

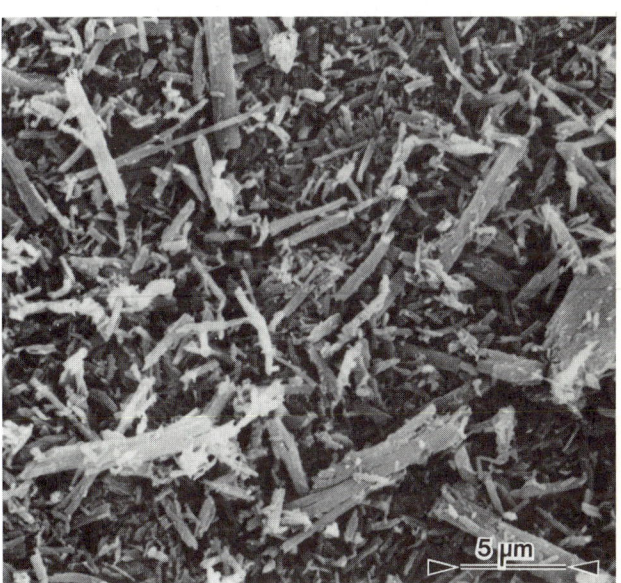

Magnification: 2,400×

10. Pharmacopeial Specifications

Test	NF	BP
Identification	+	+
Water	≤1.5%	—
Loss on drying	—	≤2.0%
Heavy metals	≤0.001%	10 ppm
Arsenic	≤3 ppm	—
Chloride	—	≤200 ppm
Total Chlorine	—	300 ppm
Alkalinity	+	—
Acidity or alkalinity	—	+
Assay range	99.0-100.5%	−100.5%
Color and clarity of solution	—	+

11. Typical Properties

pH (aqueous solution at 25°C): 8.0
Colligative: Sodium chloride equivalent = 0.40; freezing point depression (1.0% w/v) = 0.24°; 2.25% w/v aqueous solution is isotonic
Density: 1.15 g/cm³ (at 24°C)
Solubility[a]: Water, 25°C: 1.8; water, boiling: 1.4; ethanol, 25°C: 75; ethanol, (95%), 25°C: 50

[a]Solubilities are expressed as milliliters of solvent required to dissolve one gram of sodium benzoate.

12. Stability and Storage Conditions

Store in a tightly sealed container.

13. Incompatibilities

Sodium benzoate is incompatible with ferric salts, calcium salts and salts of heavy metals, including silver, lead and mercury.

14. Safety

Ingested benzoate is conjugated with glycine in the liver to yield hippuric acid, which is excreted in the urine. For sodium benzoate: rat (oral) LD_{50} = 4,100 mg/kg; rat (intravenous) LD_{50} = 1,714 ± 124 mg/kg. The World Health Organization's acceptable daily intake of total benzoates, calculated as benzoic acid, has been estimated as up to 5 mg/kg of body weight. Symptoms of systemic toxicity to benzoates resemble those of salicylates. Whereas oral administration of the free acid form may cause severe gastric irritation, benzoate salts are well tolerated in gram quantities (e.g., sodium benzoate given in six grams *p.o.* as a liver function test).

15. Handling Precautions

Avoid excessive inhalation of this compound.

16. Regulatory Acceptance

NF XVI; BP/EP 1980

17. Applications in Pharmaceutical Formulation or Technology

Antifungal and bacteriostatic preservative in concentrations of approximately 0.1%.

18. Related Substances

Benzoic acid

19. Comments

Preservative efficiency is best seen in slightly acidic solutions.

20. Specific References

1. E. R. Garrett and O. R. Woods, The optimum use of acid preservatives in oil-water systems: Benzoic acid in peanut oil-water," *J. APhA Sci. Ed.,* 42:736-739 (1953).
2. M. Grayson, Ed., "Encyclopedia of Chemical Technology," 3rd ed., Vol. 3, John Wiley and Sons, New York, 1978, pp. 778-792.
3. J. Nishijo and I. Yonetani, Interaction of theobromine with sodium benzoate, *J. Pharm. Sci.,* 71:354-356 (1982).

USA: R. Lipper*; J. Cooper*; J. B. D'Silva**
UK: M. C. Allwood; B. Crowshaw; J. Emerson

Sodium Bicarbonate

1. Nonproprietary Names
USP: Sodium bicarbonate
BP/EP: Sodium bicarbonate

2. Functional Category
USP: Alkalizing agent
BP: Antacid; systemic alkalinizing substance
Others: Buffering agent

3. Synonyms
Sodium hydrogen carbonate, sodium acid carbonate, baking soda

4. Chemical Names and CAS Registry Number
Carbonic acid monosodium salt [144-55-8]
Monosodium carbonate

5. Empirical Formula   Molecular Weight
$NaHCO_3$ 84.01

6. Structural Formula

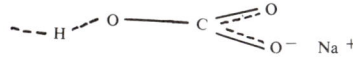

7. Commercial Availability
USA
Allied Chemical Corp.
Ashland Chemical Co.
Bage, Inc.
Baker Chemical Co., J. T.
Church & Dwight Co.
Mallinckrodt, Inc.
McKesson Chemical Co.
Pfaltz and Bauer, Inc.
Ruger Chemical Co.
Stauffer Chemical Co.
Thompson-Hayward Chemical Co.

UK
Allen & Sons (Chemicals), Ltd., Frederick
B.D.H. Chemicals, Ltd.
Dunn Bros. (Manchester), Ltd.
Hopkin & Williams
Imperial Chemical Industries plc
Koch-Light Laboratories, Ltd.
C. Page & Co., Ltd.

8. Method of Manufacture
Manufactured by the ammonia-soda or "Solvay" process: $NaCl + NH_3 + CO_2 + H_2O \rightarrow NaHCO_3 + NH_4Cl$; or by passing carbon dioxide gas into a saturated solution of sodium carbonate.

9. Description
An odorless, white crystalline powder with a saline, slightly alkaline taste.
A variety of particle-size grades of powder and granules are available.

SEM-MF-8
Excipient: Sodium bicarbonate
Supplier: Merck Frost-Canada

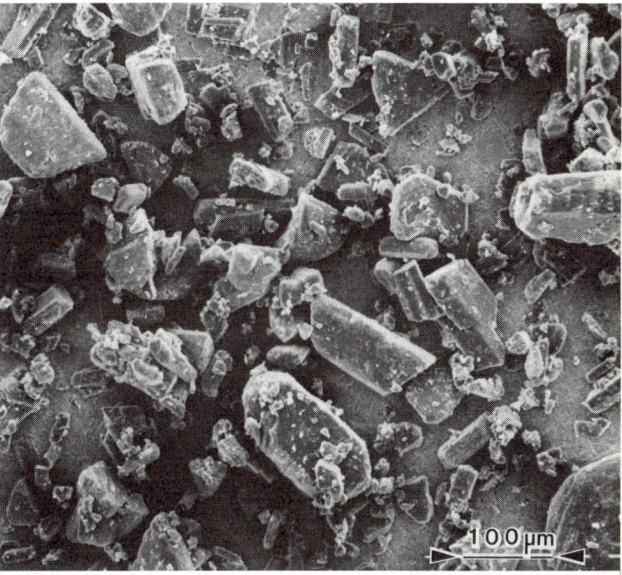

Magnification: 120✕

SEM-MF-8
Excipient: Sodium bicarbonate
Supplier: Merck Frost-Canada

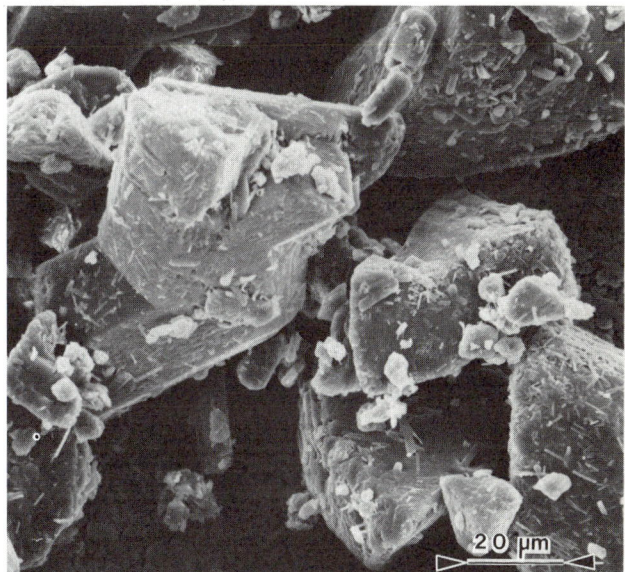

Magnification: 600✕

10. Pharmacopeial Specifications

Test	USP	BP/EP
Identification	+	+
Loss on drying	≤0.25%	–
Insoluble substances	+	–
Clarity and color of solution	–	+
Normal carbonate	+	–
Carbonate (5% solution): pH	–	≤8.6
Ammonia	+	–
Arsenic	≤3 ppm	≤2 ppm
Heavy metals	≤5 ppm	≤10 ppm
Ammonium	–	+
Calcium	–	+
Chloride	–	≤150 ppm
Sulfate	–	≤150 ppm
Assay limits	99.0-100.5%	99.0-101.0%

11. Typical Properties

Carbon dioxide yield: Approximately 52% by weight
Crystal form: Monoclinic prisms
Density: 2.159 g/cm^3
Freezing point depression: 0.396°C (1% w/v solution)
Hygroscopicity: At relative humidities below approximately 80%, the moisture content is less than 1%. Above 85% relative humidity, it rapidly absorbs excessive amounts of water, and may start to decompose.
Melting point: 270°C with decomposition.
Neutralization capacity: 20 parts of sodium bicarbonate will neutralize approximately 16.7 parts of citric acid or 17.9 parts of tartaric acid.
Osmotic pressure: A solution containing 1.39% w/v is iso-osmotic with serum.
pH: 8.3 (0.1 M solution)
Refractive index: 1.3344 (1% w/v aqueous solution at 20°C)
Solubility: Water: 1 part in 11 parts (20°C); 1 part in 4 parts (100°C); ethanol (96%; 20°C): insoluble; ether (20°C): practically insoluble.

12. Stability and Storage Conditions

Upon heating at 250°C to 300°C., sodium bicarbonate decomposes and is converted into anhydrous sodium carbonate. However, the process is both time and temperature-dependent commencing at about 50°C. The conversion is 90% complete within 75 minutes at 93°C. The reaction proceeds via surface-controlled kinetics, and when sodium bicarbonate crystals are heated for a short period of time, very fine needle-shaped crystals of anhydrous sodium carbonate appear on the surface. At ordinary temperatures, aqueous solutions slowly decompose with the formation of the carbonate; the decomposition is accelerated by agitation or heat. Aqueous solutions stored in glass containers may develop deposits of small glass particles. Sediments of calcium carbonate with traces of magnesium and other metals have been found in injections sterilized by autoclaving; this sedimentation is retarded by the inclusion of disodium edetate (0.01 to 0.02%). Solutions to be sterilized by autoclaving are first treated in the final container with carbon dioxide gas for 1 minute; the sealed container is then autoclaved but not opened until at least two hours after it has cooled to ambient temperature. Store in a well-closed container.

13. Incompatibilities

Reacts with acids, acidic salts and many alkaloidal salts, with the evolution of carbon dioxide. It can intensify the darkening of salicylates. Heating or agitating the aqueous solution partially converts it into normal carbonate, with the evolution of carbon dioxide. In powder mixtures, atmospheric moisture or water of crystallization from another ingredient is sufficient for sodium bicarbonate to react with compounds such as boric acid or alum. In liquid mixtures containing bismuth subnitrate, sodium bicarbonate reacts with the acid formed by hydrolysis of the bismuth salt.

14. Safety

Extracellular fluid, including plasma, normally contains approximately 142 mmol (142 meq) of sodium per liter. Hyponatremia is indicated with a sodium concentration of less than 137 mmol per liter, with symptoms of fatigue, muscle weakness, diarrhea, abdominal cramps, confusion, hypotension, weakened pulse, cyanosis, pitting edema, oliguria and convulsions. Hypernatremia may occur when the sodium concentration is more than 147 mmol per liter; its symptoms are restlessness, weakness, thirst, reduced salivation and lacrimation, swollen tongue, skin flushing, pyrexia, dizziness, headache, oliguria, hypotension, tachycardia, delirium, hyperpnea and respiratory arrest. While hyponatremia is not usually associated with sodium bicarbonate, hypernatremia could be a risk if an excessive amount of sodium bicarbonate is administered by injection. There is likely to be less hazard if sodium bicarbonate is administered orally, unless renal function is impaired.

15. Handling Precautions

Low hazard. Adopt usual precautions for particulate solids.

16. Regulatory Acceptance

USP XXI; BP 1980; GRAS list

17. Applications in Pharmaceutical Formulations or Technology

Use	Concentration (%)
Isotonic injection/infusion solution	1.4
Source of carbon dioxide in effervescent tablets and granules	25-50
Buffering of weak acids in tablets to increase dissolution and reduce gastric irritation	10-40
Included in some injections (e.g., nicotinic acid) to form the more soluble sodium salt	

18. Related Substances

Other metal carbonates and bicarbonates can be used for producing carbon dioxide in effervescent tablets and for buffering purposes.

19. Comments

Monographs for sodium bicarbonate appear in most pharmacopeias.

20. Specific References

1. D. N. Travers and R. C. White, The mixing of micronised sodium bicarbonate with sucrose crystals, *J. Pharm. Pharmacol.* 23: 260S, 261S (1971).

2. E. Shefter, A. Lo and S. Ramalingham, A kinetic study of the solid state transformation of sodium bicarbonate to sodium carbonate, *Drug Dev. Commun.*, 1: 29, 38 (1974).

3. K. A. Javaid and D. E. Cadwallader, Dissolution of aspirin from tablets containing various buffering agents, *J. Pharm. Sci.*, 61: 1370, 1373 (1972).

4. W. D. Mason and N. Winer, Kinetics of aspirin, salicylic acid and salicyluric acid following oral administration of aspirin as a tablet and two buffered solutions, *J. Pharm. Sci.*, 70: 262, 265 (1981).

5. K. D. Rainsford, Gastric mucosal ulceration induced in pigs by tablets but not suspensions or solutions of aspirin, *J. Pharm. Pharmacol.*, 30: 129, 131 (1978).

6. N. R. Anderson, G. S. Banker, and G. E. Peck, Quantitative evaluation of pharmaceutical effervescent systems I: design of testing apparatus, *J. Pharm. Sci.*, 71: 3, 6 (1982).

7. N. R. Anderson, G. S. Banker, and G. E. Peck, Quantitative evaluation of pharmaceutical effervescent systems II: stability monitoring by reactivity and porosity measurements, *J. Pharm. Sci.*, 71: 7, 13 (1982).

8. Effervescent tablets. In: "Pharmaceutical Dosage Forms: Tablets," Vol. 1, H. A. Lieberman and L. Lachman, Eds. R. Mohrle, Marcel Dekker, Publisher (1980).

USA: S. N. Pagay*; P. J. Russo**; Z. Chowhan**
UK: P. Wright*

Sodium Chloride

1. **Nonproprietary Names**

   USP: Sodium chloride
   BP: Sodium chloride

2. **Functional Category**

   USP: Tonicity agent
   Others: Tablet, capsule diluent, control of colloidal properties; cleaning and polishing of capsules.

3. **Synonyms**

   Salt; common salt; rock salt; sea salt; table salt; natural halite.

4. **Chemical Name and CAS Registry Number**

   Sodium chloride [7647-14-5]

5. **Empirical Formula**   **Molecular Weight**

   NaCl   58.44

6. **Structural Formula**

   NaCl

7. **Commercial Availability**

   USA

   J. T. Baker Chemical Company
   Morton Salt Company

   UK

   British Salt, Ltd.
   New Cheshire Salt Works, Ltd.
   Steetley Chemicals, Ltd.
   Charles Tennant & Co., Ltd.

8. **Method of Manufacture**

   Sodium chloride occurs in nature as mineral halite. It is produced by mining (rock salt), by evaporation of brine from underground salt deposits, and from sea water by solar evaporation.

9. **Description:**

   Cubic crystals, granules or powder; colorless; transparent or translucent in large crystals. White, odorless, saline taste.

10. **Pharmacopeial Specifications**

Test	USP	BP
Identification	+	+
Acidity or Alkalinity	+	+
Loss on Drying	≤0.5%	≤1.0%
Heavy Metals	≤5 ppm	≤10 ppm
Arsenic	≤3 ppm	—
Barium	+	+
Iodide and/or Bromide	+	+
Calcium and Magnesium	≤0.005%	≤100 ppm Ca
		≤1 ppm Mg
Iron	≤2 ppm	≤20 ppm
Potassium (for parenteral use)	—	≤0.1%
Sulfate	≤0.015%	≤300 ppm
Sodium Ferrocyanide	—	—

Test	USP	BP
Assay Range	99-101%	≥99.5%
Ammonium	—	≤20 ppm
Phosphate	—	≤2.5 ppm
Clarity and Color of Solution	—	+

SEM-MF-6

Excipient: Sodium Chloride-Powder
Supplier: Mallinckrodt Canada, Ltd. **Lot No.:** N.A.

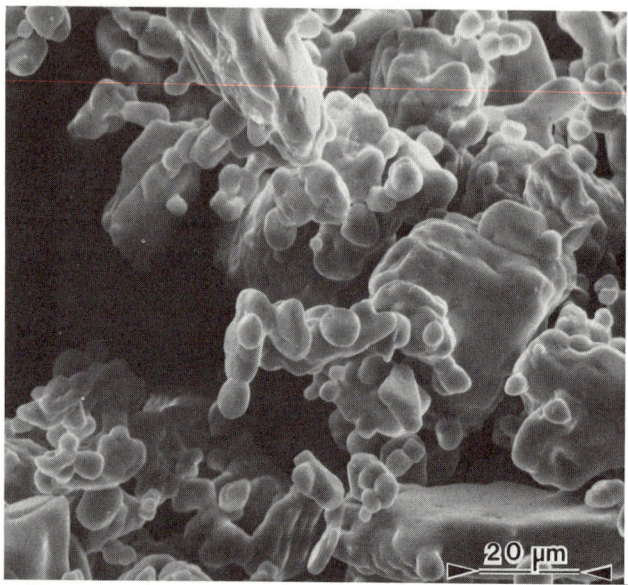

Magnification: 600×

SEM-MF-6

Excipient: Sodium Chloride-Powder
Supplier: Mallinckrodt Canada, Ltd. **Lot No.:** N.A.

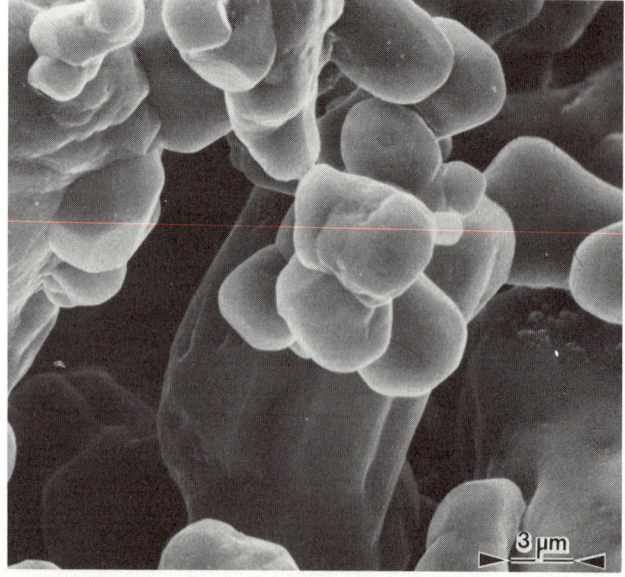

Magnification: 2,400×

SEM-MF-7

Excipient: Sodium Chloride-Granular
Supplier: Van Waters & Rogers, Ltd. **Lot No.**: N.A.

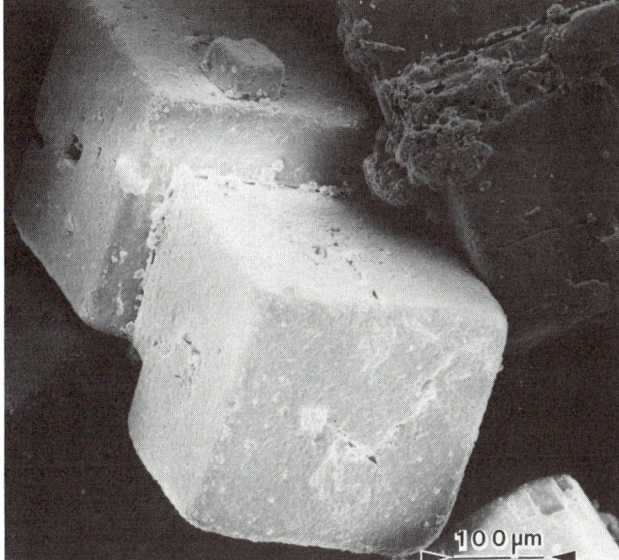

Magnification: 120×

SEM-MF-7

Excipient: Sodium Chloride-Granular
Supplier: Van Water & Rogers, Ltd. **Lot No.**: N.A.

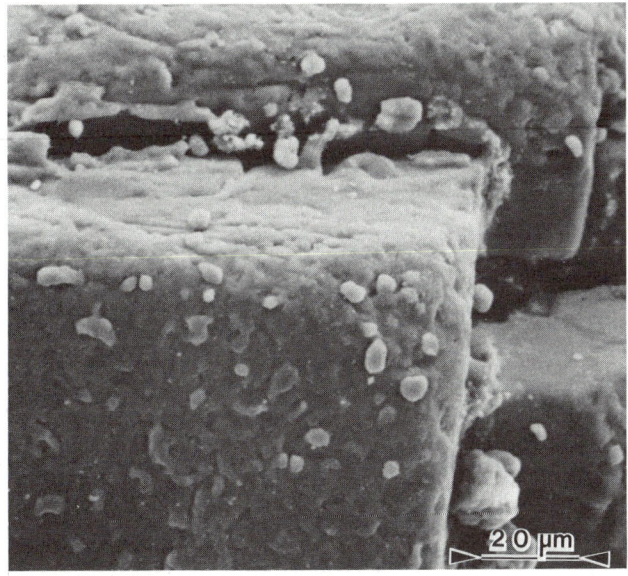

Magnification: 600×

11. Typical Properties

Angle of repose: 30°-40° (powder); 38° (cubic crystals, 30/40 mesh) (tilting table, method Ref. 2); 37° (cubic crystals, 40/60 mesh)
Compaction: By plastic deformation to form tablets (See Ref. 2 for graph of compaction pressure versus tensile strength.)
Crystal lattice: Face-centred cubic

Density: 2.165 g/cm³ (solid); bulk (powder 30/40 mesh): 0.93 g/cm³ (Ref. 2); tapped (500 taps): 1.09 g/cm³ (Ref. 2); 1.20 g/cm³ (saturated solution)
Freezing point depression:

Solution containing sodium chloride (g per 100 g water)	Freezing point depression (°C)
11.69	6.90
17.53	10.82
23.38	15.14
30.39	21.12

Hardness: 2-2.5 Mohs scale (solid); 13-14 kg/mm² Brinell
Lubrication:

$$R \text{ value} \left(\frac{\text{transmitted force}}{\text{axial force}} \right) = 0.95\text{-}0.99 \text{ (powder) (Ref. 2)}$$

Moisture content: 0.05% below 75% RH; hygroscopic above 75% RH
Melting point: 800°C
Osmotic pressure: 0.9% solution is isosmotic with serum.
pH: 6.7-7.3 (solution)
Poisson ratio: 0.30 (powder, 20/40 mesh) (Ref. 3)
Refractive index: 1.5442 (at 589 nm) (solid); 1.343 (at 589 nm) (1 molal solution)
Solubility:
Water: 1 g/2.8 ml (25°C)
        1 g/2.6 ml (100°C)
Ethanol (96%): 1 g/250 ml (20°C)
Glycerol: 1 g/10 ml (20°C)
Vapor pressure: 133.3 N/m² at 865°C (solid); 1759.6 N/m² at 20°C (saturated solution); (equivalent to 75.3% RH)

12. Stability and Storage Conditions

Stable. Store in a well-closed container. Solutions stored in glass containers may cause the separation of glass particles. Solutions are sterilized by autoclaving or bacterial filtration.

13. Incompatibilities

Reacts to form precipitates in solutions with silver, lead and mercury salts. Strong oxidizing agents liberate chlorine from acidified solutions of sodium chloride. Aqueous solutions are corrosive to iron.

14. Safety

LD_{50} (orally) in rats is 3.75 g/kg of body weight. MLD (intravenously) in rats is 2.5 g/kg of body weight. Oral ingestion of overdoses can induce irritation of the gastro-intestinal tract, hypernatremia, convulsions, vomiting and respiratory distress. Death has resulted from its administration as an emetic. Hyperosmotic solutions may act systemically, and a fatal effect has been reported from a saturated solution used as an enema.

15. Handling Precautions

Evolves vapor with eye-irritating properties if heated, in bulk, to high temperatures. Adopt usual precautions for a particulate solid.

16. Regulatory Acceptance

USP XXI; BP 1980

17. Applications in Pharmaceutical Formulation or Technology

Use	Concentration (%)
Means to obtain isotonicity in intravenous or opththalmic solutions.	up to 0.9

Use	Concentration (%)
Tablet diluent and absorbent with direct compression properties (formerly used in hypodermic tablets).	10–80
Water-soluble tablet lubricant.	5
Capsule diluent.	10–80
Controlled flocculation of suspensions.	0–1
Control of micellar properties of surface-active substances.	0–5
Control of viscosity in aqueous detergent systems, especially shampoos.	0–5
Cleaning/polishing capsules.	—
Production of non-lubricated active tablets in an alternate die-fill machine by the use of scavenging salt tablets at the alternate station.	100

18. Related Substances

Domestic salt may contain sodium iodide (as a prophylactic substance against goiter) and agents such as magnesium carbonate, calcium phosphate or starch, which reduce the hygroscopic characteristics and maintain the powder in a free-flowing state. Morton Dendritic salt (food grade), which is porous, can be used as an absorbent for liquid medications and as a tablet diluent in specific formulations.

19. Comments

Monographs for sodium chloride appear in most national pharmacopeias.

20. Specific References

1. D. W. Kaufmann, Ed., Sodium chloride, monograph No. 145, *American Chemical Society*, Van Nostrand Reinhold (1960).

2. E. Shotton and B. A. Obiorah, The effect of particle shape and crystal habit on the properties of sodium chloride, *J. Pharm. Pharmacol.*, 25, 37P, 43P (1973).

3. J. E. Rees and E. Shotton, Some observations on the aging of sodium chloride compacts, *J. Pharm. Pharmacol.*, 22, 17S, 23S (1970).

4. S. Leigh, J. E. Carless and B. W. Burt, Compression characteristics of some pharmaceutical materials, *J. Pharm. Sci.*, 56, 888, 892 (1967).

5. L. Lachman, H. A. Lieberman and J. L. Kanig, Eds., *The Theory and Practice of Industrial Pharmacy*, 2nd Edition, Lea and Febiger, Philadelphia, 1976, pp. 309-320.

6. A. J. Richard, Ultra centrifugal study of effect of sodium chloride on micelle size of fusidate sodium, *J. Pharm. Sci.*, 64, 873, 875 (1975).

7. D. Shah, B. Ecanow and R. Balagot, Coacervate formation by inorganic salts with benzalkonium chloride, *J. Pharm. Sci.*, 62, 1741, 1742 (1973).

8. C. McDonald and C. Richardson, The effect of added salts on solubilization by a non-ionic surfactant, *J. Pharm. Pharmacol.*, 33, 38, 39 (1981).

9. C. McDonald and R. E. Lindstrom, The effect of urea on the solubility of methyl p-hydroxybenzoate in aqueous sodium chloride solution, *J. Pharm. Pharmacol.*, 26, 39, 45 (1974).

10. A. G. Mattha, Rheological studies on Plantago albicans (Psyllium) seed gum dispersions II. Effect of some pharmaceutical additives, *Pharm. Acta Helv.*, 52, 214, 217 (1977).

USA: A. Palmieri, III*; R. A. Lipper**
UK: P. Wright*

Sodium Citrate, Dihydrate and Anhydrous

1. Nonproprietary Names
USP: Sodium citrate
BP/EP: Sodium citrate

2. Functional Category
USP: Buffering agent
BP: Systemic alkalinizing substance

3. Synonyms
Trisodium citrate; citrosodine; citnatin

4. Chemical Names and CAS Registry Number
USP: 1,2,3-propanetricarboxylic acid-2-hydroxy, trisodium salt [68-04-2]
BP: Trisodium 2-hydroxypropane-1,2,3-tricarboxylate-dihydrate [6132-04-3]

5. Empirical Formula / Molecular Weight

Empirical Formula	Molecular Weight
$C_6H_5Na_3O_7$ • Anhydrous	258.07
$C_6H_5Na_3O_7$ • $2H_2O$	294.10

6. Structural Formula

$$
\begin{array}{l}
CH_2 \bullet CO_2\,Na \\
| \\
HOCCO_2Na \qquad \bullet \quad \boxed{2H^2O} \\
| \\
CH_2 \bullet CO_2Na
\end{array}
$$

7. Commercial Availability

USA
Ashland Chemical Co.
HEXCEL Corp., Specialty Chemicals Div.
Hoffmann-LaRoche, Inc.
McKesson Chemical Co.
Miles Laboratories, Inc./Citro-tech
  Products/Industrial Mktg. Dept
Pfaltz and Bauer, Inc.
Pfizer, Inc.-Chemical Div.
Ruger Chemical Co.
Thompson-Hayward Chemical Co.

UK
John & E. Sturge Ltd.
Pfizer Ltd.
Roche Products Ltd.

8. Method of Manufacture
Sodium citrate is produced by adding sodium carbonate to a solution of citric acid until effervescence ceases. The resulting solution is filtered and evaporated to dryness.

9. Description
The dihydrate consists of odorless, colorless or white crystals, or a white crystalline powder with a cooling, saline taste.

SEM: MF-28
Excipient: Sodium citrate, granular, hydrous
Supplier: Pfizer Co., Ltd.

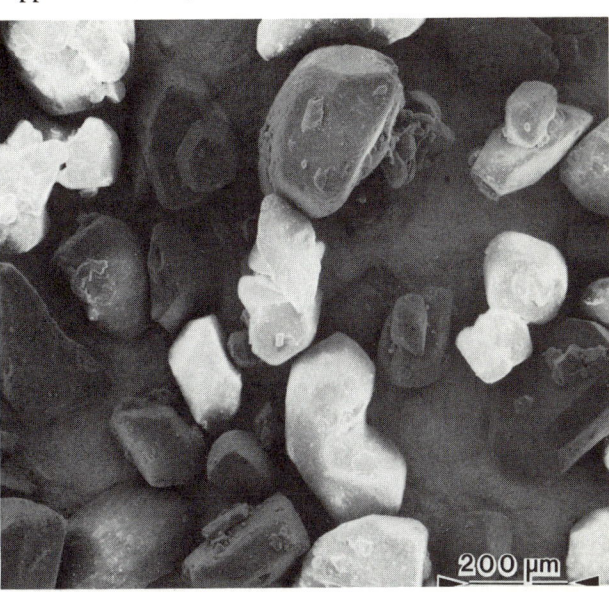

Magnification: 60×

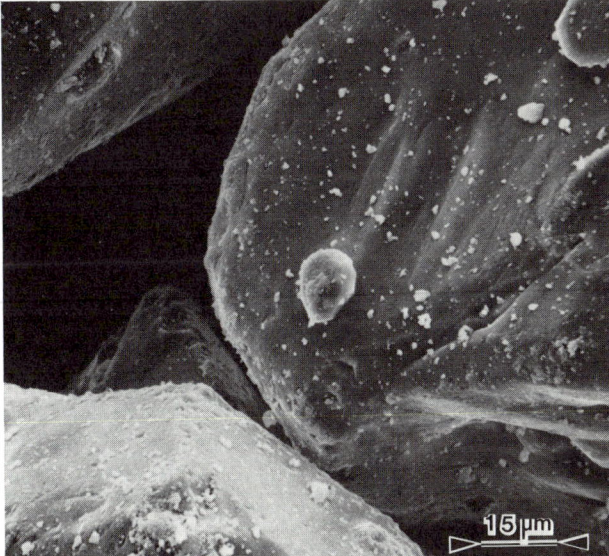

Magnifcation: 600×

10. Pharmacopeial Specifications

Test	USP	BP/EP
Potency (assay)	99-100.5% $C_6H_5Na_3O_7$	99-101% $C_6H_5Na_3O_7$
Identification	+	+
Alkalinity or acidity	—	+
Water, anhydrous	≤ 1.0%	
Water, dihydrate	10%-13%	11-13% w/w
Clarity & color of solution	—	+
Heavy metals	0.001%	≤ 10 ppm
Chloride	—	≤ 50 ppm
Oxalate	—	≤ 400 ppm
Sulfate	—	+
Tartrate	+	—
Readily carbonizable substances	—	+
Alkalinity	+	—

11. Typical Properties

Solubility: Very soluble in water (72 g/100 cm^3). Insoluble in alcohol.

Crystal structure: Monoclinic

Melting point: 150°C (converts to anhydrous form at 150°C)

Density: 1.19 g/cm^3

pH of aqueous solution: Slightly alkaline to litmus; pH approximately 8.

Academy HPE Laboratory Project Data

Method	Lab #	Results
Bulk/tap volume	Anhydrous, Powder	
% Consolidation BTD-6	8	Volume: 14.5%
% Consolidation BTD-6	8	Weight: 13.0%
	Anhydrous, Granular	
% Consolidation BTD-6	8	Volume: 7.0%
% Consolidation BTD-6	8	Weight: 5.0%
	Hydrous, Fine Granular	
% Consolidation BTD-6	8	Volume: 7.5%
% Consolidation BTD-6	8	Weight: 8.0%
	Hydrous, Granular	
% Consolidation BTD-6	8	Volume: 7.5%
% Consolidation BTD-6	8	Weight: 7.0%

Supplier: Pfizer

12. Stability and Storage Conditions

USP: Store in a tight container. BP/EP: Store in a well-closed container.

13. Incompatibilities

Aqueous solutions are slightly alkaline and will react with acidic substances. Alkaloidal salts may be precipitated from their aqueous or hydro-alcohol solutions. Calcium and strontium salts will cause precipitation of their corresponding citrates.

14. Safety

LD$_{50}$ I.P. in rats: 6.0 mmoles/kg.

15. Handling Precautions

No restrictions specified.

16. Regulatory Acceptance

USP XXI; BP/EP 1980.

17. Applications in Pharmaceutical Formulation or Technology

Use	Concentration (%)
Sequestering agent	0.3-2.0
Buffering agent	0.3-2.0

18. Related Substances

Sodium citrate; pentahydrate

19. Comments

None

20. References

1. N. R. Anderson, G. S. Banker and G. E. Peck, Quantitative evaluation of pharmaceutical effervescent systems II: Stability monitoring of reactivity and porosity measurements, *J. Pharm. Sci.*, 71 (1): 7-13 (1982).

USA: A. E. Buckpitt*; G. E. Amidon**

Sodium Lauryl Sulfate

1. Nonproprietary Names

NF: Sodium lauryl sulfate
BP: Sodium lauryl sulphate

2. Functional Category

NF: Emulsifying and/or solubilizing agent; wetting and/or solubilizing agent
BP: Anionic emulsifying agent
Others: Wetting agent, detergent, emulsifying agent

3. Synonym

Dodecyl sodium sulfate; *Avirol 118 Conc*; *Carsonol SLS*; *Conco Sulphate Wa Dry, Wag*; *Cycloryl 31, 580, 583N, 599*; *Detergent 66*; *Duponol C*; *Empicol LZ*; *Emulsifier No 104*; *Maprofix LK, 563*; *Product 75, 161*; *Richonol A Powder*; *Sipon WD*; *Standapol 112 Conc*; *Stepanol WA-100*; *Sulfopon WA-1*; *Sulfotex WALA*; *Tensopol*; *Texapon K12, K1296, V, Z, L-108*

4. Chemical Names and CAS Registry Number

Sulfuric acid monododecyl ester sodium salt
Sodium monododecyl sulfate [151-21-3]

5. Empirical Formula   Molecular Weight

Chiefly $C_{12}H_{25}NaO_4S$ 288.38

6. Structural Formula

$$\left[CH_3-(CH_2)_{10}-CH_2-O-\overset{\displaystyle O}{\underset{\displaystyle O}{\overset{\|}{\underset{\|}{S}}}}-O \right]^{-} Na^{+}$$

A mixture of sodium alkyl sulfates, consisting mainly of sodium lauryl sulfate with residual quantities of sodium chloride and sodium sulfate.

7. Commercial Availability

USA

Alcolac, Inc.
Carson Chemical, Inc.
Continental Chemical Co.
Cyclo Chemicals Corp.
Ideal Chemical and Supply Co.
E. I. DuPont de Nemours & Co.
Proctor and Gamble Co.
Onyx Chemical Co.
Proctor and Gamble Co.
Richardson Co.
Henkel, Inc.
Stepan Chemical Co.

UK

Albright and Wilson, Ltd.
Henkel Chemicals, Ltd.
Millmaster-Onyx
Tensia, Ltd.
Witco Chemicals, Ltd.

8. Method of Manufacture

Following sulfation of lauryl alcohol, the acid is neutralized with sodium carbonate.

9. Description

White or cream-colored to pale yellow crystals, flakes or powder having a smooth feel, a soapy, bitter taste and a faint odor of fatty substances.

SEM-MF-29
Excipient: Sodium lauryl sulfate
Supplier: Canadian Alcolac Ltd.

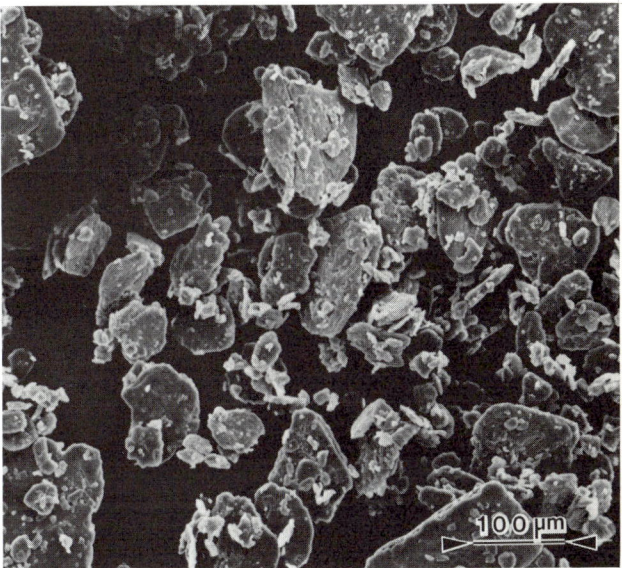

Magnification: 120×

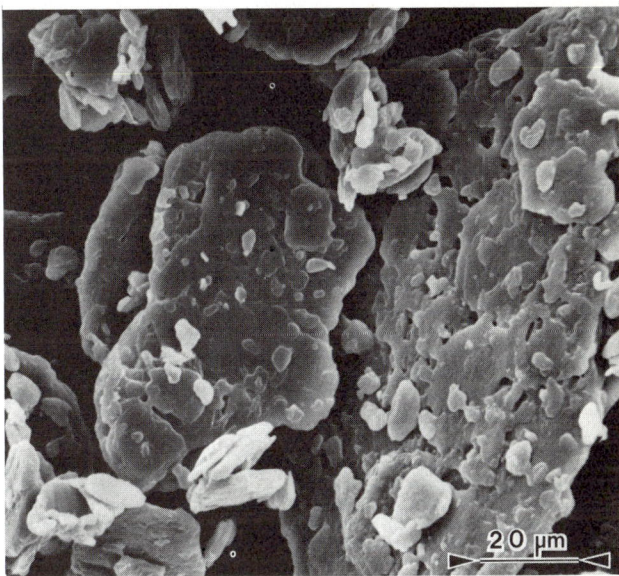

Magnification: 600×

10. Pharmacopeial Specifications

Test	NF	BP
Identification	+	+
Alkalinity	+	+
Heavy metals	≤0.002%	—
Arsenic	≤3 ppm	—
Combined sodium chloride and sodium sulfate	≤8.0%	≤8.0%
Unsulfated alcohols	≤4.0%	—
Non-esterified alcohols	—	≤4.0%
Total alcohols	≥59.0%	
Assay (calculated as $C_{12}H_{25}OSO_3Na$)		≥85%

11. Typical Properties

Acid value: 0

Critical micelle concentration: (at 20°C): 8.2×10^{-3} mol/L (0.23 g/l); (at 37°C): 8.0×10^{-3} mol/L (0.23 g/l); recommended as a test for purity.

Density (at 20°C): 1.07 g/cm^3

HLB value: About 40.

Interfacial tension: 11.8 mN/m (non-aqueous liquid not specified—0.05% solution at 30°).

Melting point: 204-207°C (pure substance).

Microbiological properties: Sodium lauryl sulfate has a bacteriostatic action against gram-positive bacteria, but is ineffective against many gram-negative organisms. It potentiates the fungicidal actions of certain substances (sulfanilimide, sulfathiazole).

Moisture content: ≤5%; not hygroscopic.

pH: 7-9.5 (1% aqueous solution).

Solubility: Freely soluble in water, giving an opalescent solution. Partly soluble in alcohol. Practically insoluble in chloroform, ether and light petroleum.

Spreading coefficient: −7.0 (0.05% solution at 30°C).

Surface tension: 25.2 mN/m (0.05% solution at 30°C). 5.1 mN/m (45×10^{-3} mol/L). 6.50 mN/m (40×10^{-3} mol/L).

Wetting time (Draize Test): 118 sec. (0.05% solution at 30°C).

12. Stability and Storage Conditions

Stable at pH 7. Hydrolysis occurs in solution below pH 4, becoming accelerated below pH 2.5. The rate is temperature and concentration dependent. Store in a well-closed container.

13. Incompatibilities

Sodium lauryl sulfate is incompatible with cationic materials and acids below pH 2.5. It causes a loss of activity of cationic surface-active agents, even in concentrations too low to cause precipitation. Unlike soaps, it is compatible with dilute acids and calcium and magnesium ions. It is liable to corrode and perforate tinplate aerosol containers. Sodium lauryl sulfate is incompatible with some alkaloidal salts. It precipitates with lead and potassium salts.

14. Safety

Toxicity: LD$_{50}$ values: (acute)—oral (rats): 1.0 to 2.7 g/kg. Intraperitoneal (rats): 210 mg/kg; (mice): 250 mg/kg. Intravenous: Causes marked toxic effects on lung, kidney and liver of animals. Should not be used in IV preparations for humans. Subcutaneous: The maximum concentration showing no gross irritation was 0.125%.

Skin absorption: Dependent on time, concentration applied and area of application.

Skin irritation: Irritating to the skin in high concentrations; e.g., a single application of 10%, or 2.5% applied daily for eight days, or 1% in hydrophilic ointment applied under occlusion for 16 hours/day for more than three days.

Eye irritation: The maximum concentration tolerated in the Draize test is 20%.

Irritation: Dust is an irritant to the eyes and the upper respiratory tract.

Allergenicity: Sodium lauryl sulfate has not been shown to cause allergenic skin hypersensitivity, but is a primary irritant.

15. Handling Precautions

Causes irritation. Avoid contact with eyes, skin and clothing. Avoid breathing dust. Dust should be removed by exhaust systems, and/or workers should use dust respirators. Wash thoroughly after handling.

16. Regulatory Acceptance

NF XVI; BP 1980

17. Applications in Pharmaceutical Formulation or Technology

Use	Concentration (%)
Wetting agent in dentrifices	1-2
Skin cleanser in topical applications	1
Tablet lubricant	1-2
Solubilizer in concentrations greater than CMC	>0.0025
Anionic emulsifier, forms self-emulsifying bases with fatty alcohols	0.5-2.5
Detergent in medicated shampoos	9-45

18. Related Substances

Magnesium lauryl sulfate (soluble tablet lubricant).

19. Comments

The commercial product is made from a mixture of C_{10} to C_{16} alcohols which contain a majority of lauryl alcohol, and, therefore, the average molecular weight of the commercial product is approximately 302. It is more irritating than the alkyl aryl sulfonates and is a poor foamer in hard water.

20. References

1. S. Ross and A. M. Saberstein, Hemolysis by colloidal electrolytes, *J. Colloid Sci.*, 9:157 (1954).
2. S. L. Sanders, "Proceedings of the 38th Annual Meeting of the Chemical Specialties Manufacturers Association," p. 107 (1951).
3. E. I. DuPont de Nemours and Co., Inc., Material Safety Data Sheet for Duponol® C, Sodium Lauryl Sulfate (1978).
4. E. I. DuPont de Nemours and Co., Inc., Sodium Lauryl Sulfate, Haskell Laboratory Report ES-3606.
5. L. C. Barail, Toxicity of soap and detergents, *Soap and Sanitary Chemicals*, 30:52 (1954).
6. K. S. Birdi, *Anal. Biochem.*, 74(2):620, 622 (1976).
7. R. Vold and K. Mittal, *Anal. Chem.*, 44(4):849, 850 (1972).
8. J. E. Newbury, *Colloid & Polymer Sci.*, 257:773, 775 (1979).
9. J. Kloubec, *J. Col. Int. Sci.*, 41(1):17, 22 (1972).
10. B. R. Vijayendran, *J. Col. Int. Sci.*, 60(2):418, 419 (1977).

USA: N. O. Nuessle*; R. El-Rashidy**
UK: G. G. Liversidge*; J. Fairbrother**

Sodium Metabisulfite

1. Nonproprietary Names
NF: Sodium metabisulfite
BP: Sodium metabisulphite

2. Functional Category
USP: Anti-oxidant
BP: Anti-oxidant

3. Synonyms
Sodium acid sulfite; sodium pyrosulphite

4. Chemical Names and CAS Registry Number
Disulfurous acid, disodium salt, disodium pyrosulfite [7681-57-4]

5. Empirical Formula
$Na_2S_2O_5$

Molecular Weight
190.10

6. Structural Formula

$$Na^+O^--S-O-S-O^-\ Na^+$$

with two $=O$ groups on each S.

7. Commercial Availability

USA

Aldrich Chemical Co.
Allied Chemical Corp.
J. T. Baker Chemical Co.
DuPont De Nemours & Co.
Eastman Organic Chemicals
Fisher Scientific
Mallinckrodt, Inc.
Marathon Morco Co.
MC&B Manufacturing Chemists
Virginia Chemical Co.

UK

Albright & Wilson
William Blythe & Co., Ltd.
May & Baker Ltd.
Pechiney Ugine Kuhlman

8. Method of Manufacture
Sodium metabisulfite is prepared by saturating a solution of sodium hydroxide with sulfur dioxide and allowing crystallization to occur. Hydrogen is passed through the solution to exclude air. Saturating a solution of sodium carbonate with sulfur dioxide and allowing crystallization to occur. Formed when sodium bisulfite undergoes thermal dehydration.

9. Description
Colorless, prismatic crystals or a white to creamy white crystalline powder having the ordor of sulfur dioxide and an acid and saline taste. It crystallizes from H_2O with $7H_2O$.

10. Pharmacopeial Specifications

Test	NF	BP
Identification	+	+
Chloride	≤0.05%	—
Thiosulfate	≤0.05%	+
Arsenic	≤3 ppm	≤4 ppm
Heavy metals	≤0.002%	≤40 ppm
Iron	≤0.002%	—
Acidity	—	+
Assay range (as $Na_2S_2O_5$)	Equiv. to 65-67.4% SO_2	≥95%

11. Typical Properties
Melting point: Sodium metabisulfite melts with decomposition at less than 150°C.
Solubility: Water: 54 g in 100 ml at 20°C, 81.7 g in 100 ml at 100°C. Slightly soluble in alcohol, freely soluble in glycerin. A 1.38% solution in water is iso-osmotic with serum.

12. Stability and Storage Conditions
Sodium metabisulfite is immediately converted to sodium and bisulfite ions ($Na^+HSO_3^-$) in water. Recommended storage—NF: Store in a well-filled, tight container, and avoid exposure to excessive heat. BP: Store in a well-closed container. Upon exposure to air and moisture, sodium metabisulfite is slowly oxidized to sodium sulfate with disintegration of the crystals. Strong acid solutions will liberate sulfur dioxide. Addition of dextrose decreases stability.

13. Incompatibilities
Sodium metabisulfite reacts with sympathomimetics and other drugs which are *o* or *p*-hydroxybenzyl alcohol derivatives to form sulfonic acid derivatives possessing little or no activity. The most important drugs subject to this inactivation reaction are adrenaline and its derivatives. Also incompatible with chloramphenicol due to a more complex reaction. Decomposes in strong acids.

14. Safety
Toxicity: Gastric irritation due to the liberation of sulfurous acid may occur following ingestion. With large doses there may be colic and diarrhea, circulatory disturbances, CNS depression and death. It is oxidized in the body to sulfates and is excreted in the urine. The estimated acceptable daily intake (as SO_2) in man is up to 700 mcg/kg of body weight. The use of sulfiting agents in foods and drug products has been a source of increasing concern. Reactions include nausea, diarrhea, anaphylactic shock, acute asthma attacks and loss of consciousness. Reactions occur mainly in asthmatic patients but can occur in non-asthmatics with no known allergy. See reference 7.

15. Handling Precautions
Avoid contact with skin, nose and mouth.

16. Regulatory Acceptance
NF XVI; BP 1980

17. Applications in Pharmaceutical Formulation or Technology

Use	Concentration %
Anti-oxidant	0.01-1

18. Related Substances

Most substances sold under the name sodium bisulfite are actually the anhydride, sodium metabisulfite, since the latter is less hygroscopic and more stable during storage and shipment.

19. Comments

Sodium metabisulfite is employed as an anti-oxidant in acid preparations; for alkaline preparations, sodium sulfite is usually preferred. Sodium metabisulfite usually contains small amounts of sodium sulfite and sodium sulfate.

20. References

1. G. E. Schumacher and R. N. Hull, Some factors influencing the degradation of sodium bisulfite in dextrose solutions, *Am. J. Hosp. Pharm.*, 23: 245 (1966).
2. T. Higuchi and L. C. Schroeter, Reactivity of bisulfite with a number of pharmaceuticals, *J. Am. Pharm. Assoc.*, 48: 535 (1959).
3. S. F. Halaby and A. M. Mattocks, Absorption of sodium bisulfite from peritoneal dialysis solutions, *J. Pharm. Sci.*, 54: 52 (1965).
4. J. W. Wilkins, Jr., J. A. Greene and J. M. Weller, Toxicity of intraperitoneal bisulfite, *Clin. Pharm. Ther.*, 9:328 (1968).
5. L. C. Schroeter, Sulfurous acid salts as pharmaceutical antioxidants, *J. Pharm. Sci.*, 50:891 (1961).
6. L. C. Schroeter, Oxidation of sulfurous acid salts in pharmaceutical systems, *J. Pharm. Sci.*, 52:888 (1963).
7. D. M. Jamieson et al., Metabisulfite sensitivity: case report and literature review, *Ann. Allergy*, 54:115 (1985).

USA: J. T. Stewart*; J. G. Cooney**; J. C. Boylan**

Sodium Starch Glycolate

1. Nonproprietary Name
NF: Sodium starch glycolate
BP: Sodium starch glycollate

2. Functional Category
USP: Tablet disintegrant
Others: Tablet and capsule disintegrant

3. Synonyms
Sodium carboxymethyl starch; *Explotab*; *Primojel*

4. Chemical Names and CAS Registry Number
Starch carboxymethyl ether, sodium salt

5. Empirical Formula   Molecular Weight
—   —

6. Structural Formula

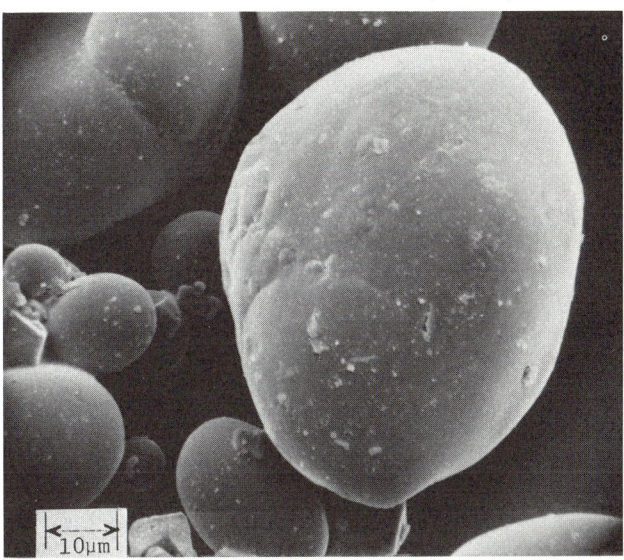

SEM: KY-47
Excipient: Sodium carboxymethyl starch (*Primojel*)
Manufacturer: Generichem **Lot no.**: 89A-1 (FXR-23)

Magnification: 1,200×   **Voltage**: 10 kv

7. Commercial Availability
USA

Avebe America, Inc.
Edward Mendell Co., Inc.
Generichem Corporation

UK

Forum Chemicals Ltd.
Kingsley & Keith
Royal Scholten-Honig
Tunnel Avebe Starches, Ltd.

8. Method of Manufacture
Sodium starch glycolate is prepared synthetically by U.S. Patent 3,034,911.

9. Description
White to off-white, odorless, tasteless, free-flowing powder. Microscopic: oval or spherical granules, 30-100 μm in diameter with some less-spherical granules ranging from 10-35 μm in diameter.

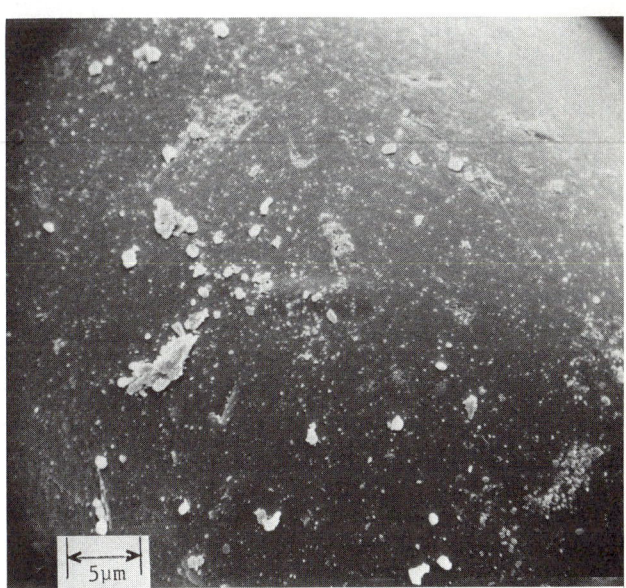

Magnification: 2,400×   **Voltage**: 10 kv

SEM: KY-48
Excipient: Sodium carboxymethyl starch (*Explotab*)
Manufacturer: Mendell **Lot no.:** 89A-2 (C-178)

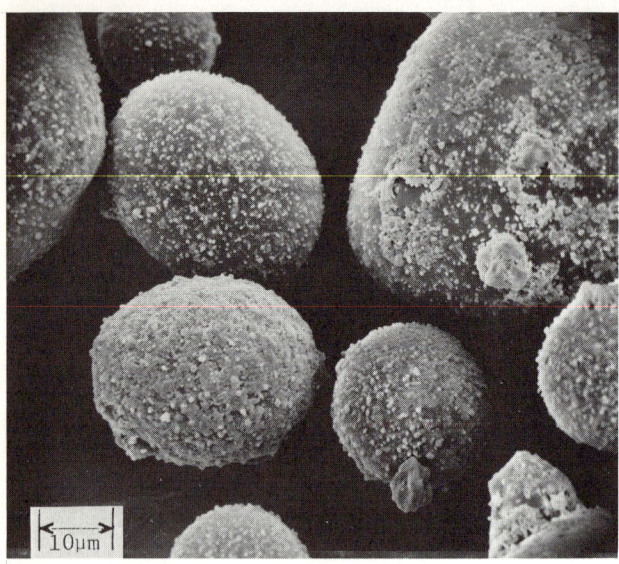

Magnification: 1,200×   **Voltage:** 10 kv

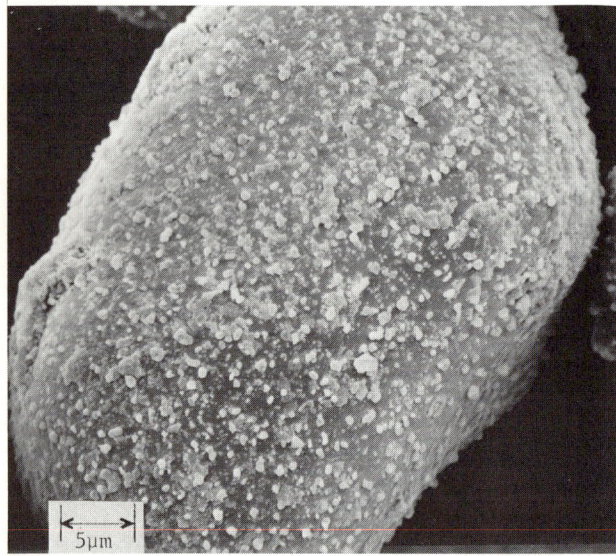

Magnification: 2,400×   **Voltage:** 10kv

10. Pharmacopeial Specifications

Test	NF	BP
pH/acidity or alkalinity	5.5-7.5 (lg in 30 ml)	5.5-7.5 (2% w/v dispersion)
Loss on drying	≤10.0%	≤10.0%

10. Pharmacopeial Specifications

Test	USP	BP
Heavy metals	≤0.002%	≤20 ppm
Sodium chloride	≤10.0%	10.0%
Iron	≤0.002%	≤20 ppm
Microbial limits	Absence of *Salmonella* species and *Escherichia coli*	
Sodium glycolate	—	≤2%
Assay range (washed and dried)	2.8% to 4.2% sodium	2.8% to 4.5% sodium
Identification	+	+

11. Typical Properties

Academy HPE Laboratory Data			
	Method	Lab #	Results
Moisture content	MC-23	21	3.12%[b]
Moisture content	MC-22	2	1.20%[c]
Bulk/Tap density	BTD-1	1	B: 0.794 g/cm³[a]
Bulk/Tap density			T: 1.000 g/cm³[a]
Bulk/Tap density	BTD-7	14	B: 0.850 g/cm³[a]
Bulk/Tap density			T: 1.000 g/cm³[a]
Bulk/Tap density	BTD-6	8	Volume: 8.0%[c]
Bulk/Tap density			Weight: 7.0%[c]
Particle size dist.	PSD-5A	21	< 44µm: 71.0%[b] 44-74µm: 26.0% 74-149µm: 3.0%
Solubility (Water)	SOL-1	1	Gels[a]
Solubility (Alcohol)	SOL-1	1	2.08%[a]
Solubility (n-Hexane)	SOL-1	1	0.010%[a]
Particle friability	PF-1	36	0.037%[a]
Average flow rate	FLO-1	14	13 g/sec.[a]
Compression (at 38-186 MN/m²)	COM-2	21	No compacts formed[b]
Compression (at 500 & 1,000 lbs.)	COM-7	12	No compacts formed[a]
EMC Plot	EMC-1	2	Fig: 2-EMC-9[c]
PSD Plot	PSD-5A	21	Fig: 21-PSD-3[b]
SI Plot	SI-1	13	Fig: 13-SI-10[a]
COM Plot	COM-5,6	29	Fig: 29-COM-16[a]

Suppliers: Generichem[a]; Kingsley & Keith[b]; Mendell[c]

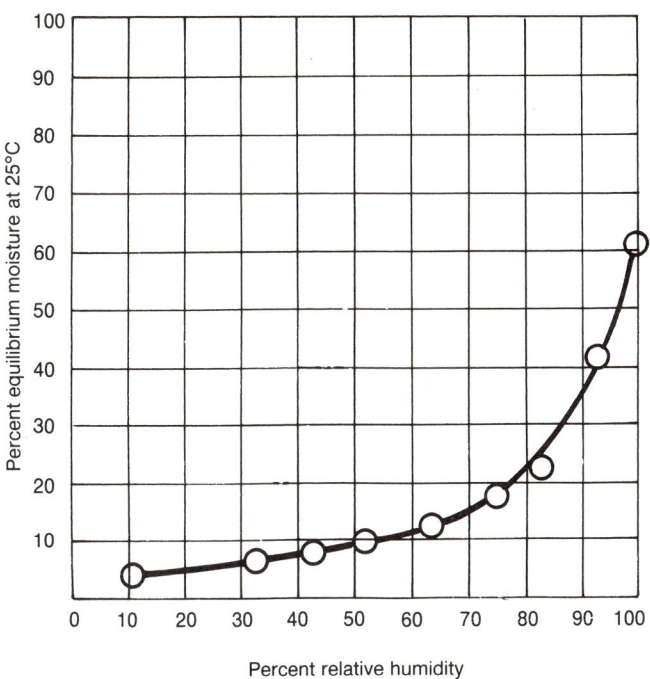

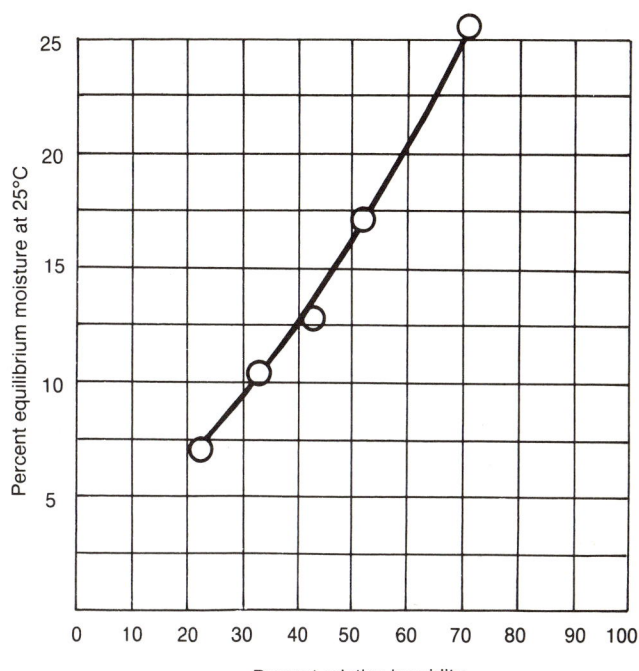

Sodium starch glycolate, NF, *Explotab* (Mendell, Lot #959)
Figure: 2-EMC-9   **Method:** EMC-1

Sodium carboxymethyl starch (Generichem, Lot #KYR 8)
Figure: 13-SI-10   **Method:** SI-1

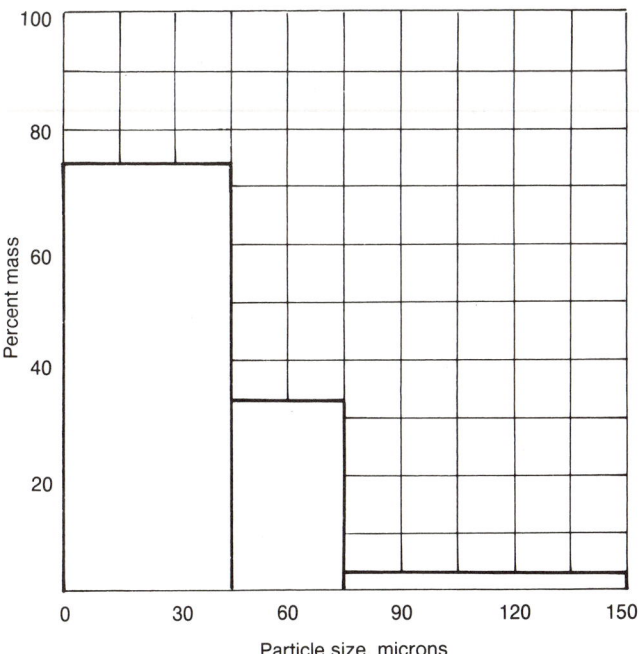

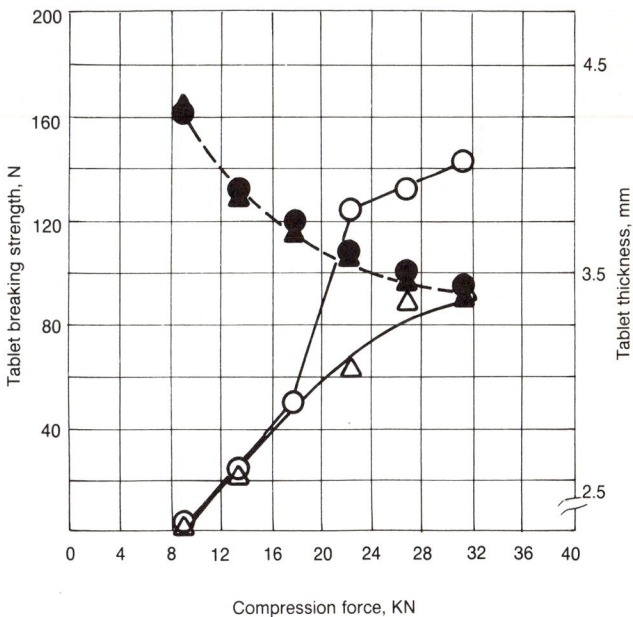

Sodium carboxymethyl starch (Kingsley & Keith, Canada, Lot #070)
Figure: 21-PSD-3   **Method:** PSD-5A

Sodium carboxymethyl starch (Generichem, Lot #KRY 8)
○ ● : Unlubricated, Carver Laboratory Press (COM-5)
▲ △ : Lubricated, Carver Laboratory Press (COM-6)
Figure: 29-COM-16   **Method:** COM-5,6

Ash: 15% (max.)

Particle size: All particles pass 125 μm sieve (#I15 mesh).

Degree of substitution: Approx. 0.25.

Swelling capacity: In water, sodium starch glycolate swells up to 300 times its volume.

Density: (He)-1.5 g/cm³

Bulk volume: 1.4 g/cm³; pH: 5.5-7.5; Sodium chloride: 5% (max.); viscosity [2% solution, Brookfield: 25 cps (max.)].

Solubility: At 2% w/v, it disperses in cold water and settles in the form of a highly saturated layer. Insoluble in organic solvents.

12. Stability and Storage Conditions

Stable. Store in a well-closed container to protect it from wide variations in humidity and temperature that may cause caking. It has a long shelf-life stability.

13. Incompatibilities

No citations found.

14. Safety

—

15. Handling Precautions

No restrictions specified.

16. Regulatory Acceptance

NF XVI; BP 1980 (Addendum 1982)

17. Applications in Pharmaceutical Formulation or Technology

Use	Concentration
Tablet/capsule disintegrant (Wet granulation or direct compression)	2-10.0%

18. Related Substances

Starch, USP; Pregelatinized starch, USP.

19. Comments

With the use of sodium carboxymethyl starch as a disintegrant, compression pressure had no apparent affect on the disintegration time. Tablets containing sodium carboxymethyl starch, when stored at elevated temperatures and high humidity, increased in disintegration time and decreased in dissolution rate.

20. Specific References

1. E. Cid and F. Jaminet, Influence of adjuvants on the dissolution rate and stability of acetylsalicylic acid in compressed tablets, *J. Pharm. Belg.*, 26: 38-48 (1971)
2. E. Cid and F. Jaminet, Influence of particle size of acetylsalicylic acid (Aspirin) on the dissolution rate of tablets, *Farmaco Ed. Prat.*, 27: 298-304 (1972).
3. R. A. Khan and C. T. Rhodes, Effect of disintegrant concentration on disintegration and compression characteristics of two insoluble direct compression systems, *J. Pharm. Sci.*, 8: 77-80 (1973).
4. K. Kolaroki *et al.*, Evaluation of starch sodium glycolate (Primogel) as a disintegrating substance for tablets, *Farm. Pol.*, 30: 989-92 (1974).
5. K. A. Khan and C. T. Rhodes, Effect of compaction pressure on the dissolution efficiency of direct compression systems, *Pharm. Acta Helv.*, 49: 258-61 (1974).
6. E. Mendell, Evaluation of carboxymethyl starch as a tablet disintegrant, *Pharm. Acta Helv.*, 49: 248-50 (1974).
7. J. F. Bavitz *et al.*, Disintegrability characteristics of three selected tablet excipients, *Drug Dev. Commun.*, 1: 331-47 (1974-1975).
8. K. A. Khan and C. T. Rhodes, Disintegration properties of calcium phosphate dibasic dihydrate tablets, *J. Pharm. Sci.*, 64: 166-68 (1975).
9. J. M. Newton and F. W. Razzo, Interaction of formulation factors and dissolution fluid and the *in vitro* release of drug from hard gelatin capsules, *J. Pharm. Pharmacol.*, 27: 78P (1975).
10. K. A. Khan and C. T. Rhodes, Water-sorption properties of tablet disintegrants, *J. Pharm. Sci.*, 64: 447-51 (1975).
11. K. A. Khan and D. J. Rooke, Effect of disintegrant type upon the relation between compressional pressure and dissolution efficiency, *J. Pharm. Pharmacol.*, 28: 633-6 (1976).
12. C. A. Farley and W. Lund, Suspending agents for extemporaneous dispensing: Evaluation of alternatives to tragacanth, *Pharm. J.*, 216: 562-6 (1976).
13. A. J. Torode *et al.*, "Pharmaceutical preparations in tablet form," Ger. Offen. Patent No. 2605656.
14. K. A. Kahn and C. T. Rhodes, Compressional properties of some directly compressed formulations containing dibasic calcium phosphate dihydrate, *Pharm. Acta Helv.*, 52: 222-26 (1977).
15. M. H. Rubenstein and E. J. Price, *In vivo* evaluation of the effect of five disintegrants on the bioavailability of furosemide from 40 mg tablets, *J. Pharm. Pharmacol.*, 29: 5P (1977).
16. J. Estere *et al.*, Effects of distinegrating agents on the dissolution of phenylbutazone tablets, *Cienc. Ind. Farm.*, 10: 215-27 (1978).
17. C. Caramella *et al.*, The influence of disintegrants on the characteristics of coated acetylsalicylic acid tablets, *Farmaco. Ed. Prat.*, 33: 498-507 (1978).
18. P. P. Bhatia *et al.*, Disintegration/compressibility of tablets using CLD and other excipients, *Drug Cosmet. Ind.*, 122: 38-9, 42, 44, 46, 52, 171-5 (1978).
19. M. Jacob *et al.*, Compatibility trials for various drugs and excipients for tablet use, *J. Pharm. Belg.*, 34: 96-8 (1979).
20. A. G. Stewart, The release of a model low-dose drug (riboflavine) from hard gelatin capsule formulations, *J. Pharm. Pharmacol.*, 31: 1-6 (1979).
21. R. F. Shangraw, J. W. Wallace and F. M. Bowers, Morphology and functionality in tablet excipients for direct compression: Part II, *Powder Technology*, 5 (10): 44-60 (1981).
22. K. A. Khan and C. T. Rhodes, Water sorption properties of tablet disintegrants, *J. Pharm. Sci.*, 64 (3): 447-451 (1975).
23. K. A. Khan and C. T. Rhodes, Disintegration properties of calcium phosphate dibasic dihydrate tablets, *J. Pharm. Sci.*, 64 (3): 166-168 (1975).
24. S. T. Horhota, J. Burgio, L. Lonski and C. T. Rhodes, Effect of storage at specified temperature and humidity on properties of three directly compressible tablet formulations, *J. Pharm. Sci.*, 65 (12): 1741-1749 (1976).

USA: J. Appino*; I. Pahigianis**; Z. Chowhan**

Sorbic Acid

1. Nonproprietary Names
NF: Sorbic acid
BP: Sorbic acid

2. Functional Category
USP: Antimicrobial preservative
BP: Antimicrobial preservative

3. Synonyms
2,4-Hexadienoic acid (*E,E*); 2-propenylacrylic acid; (*E,E*)-sorbic acid

4. Chemical Names and CAS Registry Number
(E,E)-2,4-hexadienoic acid [22500-92-1] and sorbic acid [110-44-1]

5. Empirical Formula   Molecular Weight
$C_6H_8O_2$ 112.13

6. Structural Formula

$$H_3C-CH=CH-CH=CH-COOH$$

7. Commercial Availability
USA

American International Chemical, Inc.
Chemical Dynamics Corp.
ICN K & K Labs, Inc.
Monsanto Co.
Pfizer, Inc.-Chemical Div.
Ruger Chemical Co.
Tri-K Industries, Inc.
United States Biochemicals Corp.

UK

Hoechst UK, Ltd.
Pfizer Ltd.

8. Method of Manufacture
The naturally occurring sorbic acid is extracted as the lactone (parasorbic acid) from the berries of mountain ash (*Sorbus aucuparia L.* (Rosaceae)). There are various methods for synthetic preparation: condensation of crotonaldehyde and ketene in the presence of boron trifluoride; condensation of crotonaldehyde and malonic acid in pyridine solution; and from 1,1,3,5-tetraalkoxyhexane.

9. Description
White to yellow-white crystalline powder, tasteless, faint characteristic odor.

SEM-MF-25
Excipient: Sorbic acid
Supplier: Pfizer Co., Ltd.
Sorbic Acid: 2A

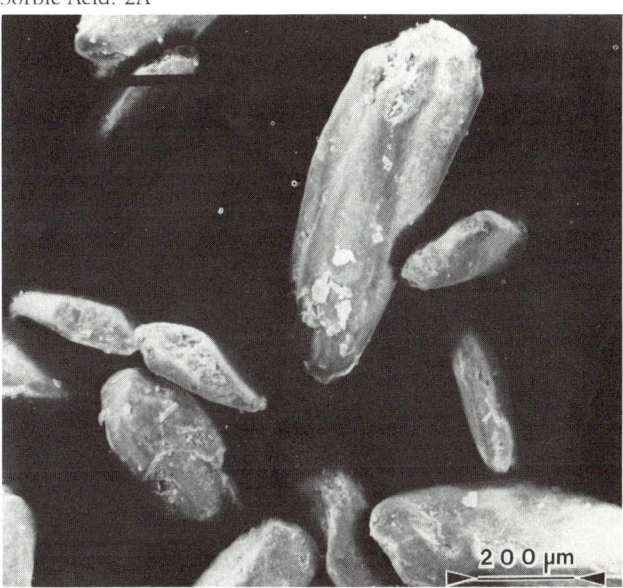

Magnification: 60×

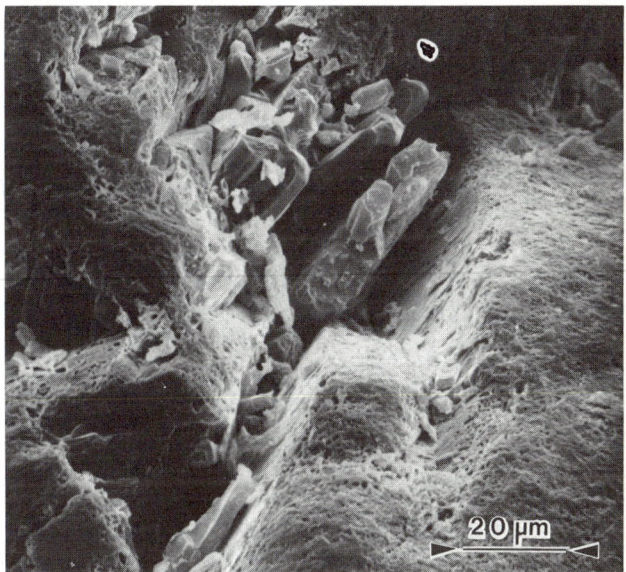

Magnification: 600×

10. Pharmacopeial Specifications

Test	NF	BP
Identification	+	+
Melting range	132-135°C	133-137°C
Water	≤0.5%	≤0.5%
Residue on ignition	≤0.2%	—
Heavy metals	≤0.001%	≤10 ppm
Arsenic	—	≤2 ppm
Sulfated ash	—	≤0.2%
Assay range	99.0-101.0%	≥99%
Aldehyde	—	≤0.15% of C_2H_4O

11. Typical Properties

pKa value: 4.76

Solubility: Water: 0.25% at 30°C, 3.8% at 100°C; propylene glycol: 5.5% at 20°C; absolute ethanol or methanol: 12.9%; 20% ethanol: 0.29%; glycerol: 0.31%; acetone: 9.2%; glacial acetic acid: 11.5%

Volatility: Sublimes above 80°C

Antibacterial activity: Bacteria 2,000-4,000 μg/ml MIC value (pH below 6.0 only) Yeasts/Fungi 800-1,200 μg/ml MIC value

12. Stability and Storage Conditions

Sorbic acid is sensitive to oxidation, especially in aqueous solution, but also in solid form (particularly in the presence of light). Sorbic acid can be stabilized by phenolic antioxidants such as propyl gallate (0.02%). Store in a tight container, protected from light, at a temperature not exceeding 15°C (BP), or avoid exposure to excessive heat (NF).

13. Incompatibilities

Some loss of activity occurs in the presence of non-ionic surfactants and in plastics. Oxidizing agents will cause oxidation which is catalyzed by heavy metal salts. Propylene and glycols improve antimicrobial activity.

14. Safety

Allergic reactions and irritation after continuous application to skin have been reported in the literature. LD_{50} orally in rats: 7.36 g/kg.

15. Handling Precautions

Sorbic acid dust is an eye and respiratory irritant. Use appropriate protective equipment.

16. Regulatory Acceptance

NF XVI; BP 1982

17. Applications in Pharmaceutical Formulation or Technology

Preservative (in liquids and semi-solids), 0.05%-0.2%. In view of the limited stability and activity against bacteria, sorbic acid is frequently used in combination with other antimicrobials or with glycols where synergistic effects appear to take place.

18. Related Substances

Potassium sorbate is frequently used instead of sorbic acid because of its higher water solubility (58.2% at 20°C). For antibacterial activity, potassium sorbate must have an acid pH. See monograph.

19. Comments

None

20. References

1. R. Woodford, E. Adams, *Amer. Perfumer and Cosmetics,* 85: 25 (1970).
2. T. Eklund, *J. Appl. Bacteriol.,* 54: 383 (1983).
3. A. D. Worth, *J. Appl. Bacteriol.,* 43(2): 215 (1977).
4. E. M. Saiban, R. R. M. Harman, *Br. J. Dermatol.,* 99: 583 (1978).
5. T. P. Radus, G. Gys, *J. Pharm. Sci.,* 72: 221 (1983).

USA: M. Tuckerman*; C. D. Shively**; J. C. Boylan**
UK: M. C. Attwood*

Sorbitan Esters (Sorbitan Fatty Acid Esters)

1. Nonproprietary Names

NF: Sorbitan monolaurate
Sorbitan monooleate
Sorbitan monopalmitate
Sorbitan monostearate
BP: Sorbitan monolaurate
Sorbitan monooleate
Sorbitan monostearate
USAN: Sorbitan sesquioleate
Sorbitan trioleate
Sorbitan tristearate
INN: Sorbitan laurate
Sorbitan oleate
Sorbitan palmitate
Sorbitan stearate
CTFA: Sorbitan dioleate
Sorbitan laurate
Sorbitan oleate
Sorbitan palmitate
Sorbitan sesqui-isostearate
Sorbitan sesquistearate
Sorbitan tri-isostearate
Sorbitan trioleate

2. Functional Category

NF: Wetting and/or solubilizing agent; emulsifying and/or solubilizing agent
BP: Non-ionic surface active agent

3. Synonyms

Arlacel C; Arlacel 20; Arlacel 40; Arlacel 60; Arlacel 80; Arlacel 83; Arlacel 85; Armotan ML; Armotan MO; Armotan MS; Capmul O; Capmul S; Crill 1; Crill 2; Crill 3; Crill 4; Crill 35; Crill 43; Crill 45; Emsorb 2500; Emsorb 2503; Emsorb 2505; Emsorb 2507; Emsorb 2510; Emsorb 2515; Emsorb 2518; Emsorb 2519; Glycomul L; Glycomul LC; Glycomul O; Glycomul P; Glycomul S; Glycomul SOC Special; Glycomul TO; Glycomul TS; Hodag SMS; Hodag SSO; Liposorb; Liposorb O; Liposorb P; Liposorb S; Liposorb SC; Liposorb SQO; Liposorb TO; Liposorb TS; Protachem; Protachem SML; Protachem SMO; Protachem SMP; Protachem SMS; Protachem SOC; Protachem STO; Sorbester P12; Sorbester P16; Sorbester P17; Sorbester P18; Sorbester P37; Sorbester P38; Span 20; Span 40; Span 60; Span 65; Span 80; Span 85.

4. Chemical Names and CAS Registry Number

Sorbitan, esters, monododecanoate; or
Sorbitan, monolaurate [1338-39-2 or 5959-89-7]
Sorbitan, esters, mono-9-octadecenoate, (Z)-; or
Sorbitan, monooleate [1338-43-8 or 5938-38-5]
Sorbitan, esters, monohexadecanoate; or
Sorbitan, monopalmitate [1338-40-5 or 26266-57-9]
Sorbitan, esters, mono-octadecanoate; or
Sorbitan, monostearate [1338-41-6]
Sorbitan, esters, sesqui-isooctadecanoate; or
Sorbitan, sesqui-isostearate [none]
Sorbitan, esters, sesqui-9-octadecenoate, (Z)-; or

4. Chemical Names and CAS Registry Number

Sorbitan, sesquioleate [8007-43-0]
Sorbitan, esters sesqui-octadecanoate; or
Sorbitan, sesquistearate [none]
Sorbitan, esters, tri-isooctadecanoate; or
Sorbitan, tri-isostearate [54392-27-7]
Sorbitan, esters, tri-9-octadecenoate, (Z, Z, Z)-; or
Sorbitan, trioleate [1338-44-9 or 26266-58-0]
Sorbitan, esters, tri-octadecanoate; or
Sorbitan, tristearate [7281-30-3 or 26658-19-5]

5. Empirical Formula / Molecular Weight

Sorbitan monolaurate:
Approx. $C_{18}H_{34}O_6$ — Approx. 346
Sorbitan monooleate:
Approx. $C_{24}H_{44}O_6$ — Approx. 429
Sorbitan monopalmitate:
Approx. $C_{22}H_{42}O_6$ — Approx. 403
Sorbitan monostearate:
Approx. $C_{24}H_{46}O_6$ — Approx. 431
Sorbitan sesqui-isostearate:
Approx. $C_{33}H_{63}O_{6.5}$ — Approx. 564
Sorbitan sesquioleate:
Approx. $C_{33}H_{60}O_{6.5}$ — Approx. 561
Sorbitan sesquistearate:
Approx. $C_{33}H_{63}O_{6.5}$ — Approx. 564
Sorbitan tri-isostearate:
Approx. $C_{60}H_{114}O_8$ — Approx. 964
Sorbitan trioleate:
Approx. $C_{60}H_{108}O_8$ — Approx. 958
Sorbitan tristearate:
Approx. $C_{60}H_{114}O_8$ — Approx. 964

6. Structural Formula

$R_1 = R_2 = OH$, $R_3 = R$ for sorbitan monoesters,
$R_1 = OH$, $R_2 = R_3 = R$ for sorbitan diesters,
$R_1 = R_2 = R_3 = R$ for sorbitan triesters,
where R = $(C_{11}H_{23})$ COO for laurate,
$(C_{17}H_{33})$ COO for oleate,
$(C_{15}H_{31})$ COO for palmitate,
$(C_{17}H_{35})$ COO for stearate.
The sesqui-esters are mixtures of equimolar monoesters and diesters.

7. Commercial Availability

USA

Armak Co.
Capital City Products Co.
Croda Chemicals, Inc.
Glyco Inc.
Hodag Chemical Corp.
ICI Americas, Inc.
Lippo Chemicals, Inc.
Malmstrom Chemical
Protameen Chemicals, Inc.

UK

Atlas Chemical Industries Ltd.
Blagden Campbell Chemicals Ltd.
Croda Chemicals Ltd.

8. Method of Manufacture

Sorbitol is dehydrated to form a hexitan (1,4-sorbitan), which is then esterified with the desired fatty acid.

9. Description

Liquid or solid, creamy to amber substances with a more or less distinctive odor and taste.

10. Pharmacopeial Specifications

Test	NF	BP
Identification:	+	+
Acid value:		
Sorbitan monolaurate	≤8	4.0-7.0
Sorbitan monooleate	≤8	5.0-8.0
Sorbitan monopalmitate	≤8	No monograph
Sorbitan monostearate	≤10	5.0-10.0
Hydroxyl value:		
Sorbitan monolaurate	330-358	330-358
Sorbitan monooleate	190-215	193-209
Sorbitan monopalmitate	275-305	No monograph
Sorbitan monostearate	235-260	235-260
Iodine value:		
Sorbitan monooleate	62-76	—
Saponification value:		
Sorbitan monolaurate	158-170	158-170
Sorbitan monooleate	145-160	149-160
Sorbitan monopalmitate	140-150	No monograph
Sorbitan monostearate	147-157	147-157
Water:		
Sorbitan monalaurate	≤1.5%	—
Sorbitan monooleate	≤1.0%	—
Sorbitan monopalmitate	≤1.5%	—
Sorbitan monostearate	≤1.5%	—
Assay for fatty acids:		
Sorbitan monolaurate	55.0-63.0%	—
Sorbitan monooleate	72.0-78.0%	—
Sorbitan monopalmitate	63.0-71.0%	—
Sorbitan monostearate	68.0-76.0%	—
Assay for polyols:		
Sorbitan monolaurate	39.0-45.0%	—
Sorbitan monooleate	25.0-31.0%	—
Sorbitan monopalmitate	32.0-38.0%	—
Sorbitan monostearate	27.0-34.0%	—
Residue on ignition	≤0.5%*	—
Heavy metals	≤0.001%*	—
Arsenic	—	≤3 ppm**
Sulphated ash	—	≤0.25%**

*For all of the four sorbitan esters listed in NF
**For all of the three sorbitan esters listed in BP

11. Typical Properties

Name	Surface tension in water (1%) (dynes/cm)	HLB +1	Viscosity (25°C) (cP)	Melting point range (°C)
Span 20	28	8.6	4250	Liquid
Arlacel 20	—	8.6	3000	Liquid
Span 40	36	6.7	—	44-47
Arlacel 40	—	4.7	—	ca. 48
Span 60	46	4.7	—	50-53
Arlacel 60	—	4.7	—	51-54
Span 65	48	2.1	—	48-53
Span 80	30	4.3	1000	Liquid
Arlacel 80	—	4.3	1900	Liquid
Arlacel 83	—	3.7	1500	Liquid
Span 85	32	1.8	210	Liquid
Arlacel 85	—	1.8	275	Liquid
Arlacel C	—	3.7	1000	Liquid

Solubility: Sorbitan esters are generally soluble or dispersible in oil. They are also soluble in most organic solvents. In water they are generally insoluble but dispersible.

12. Stability and Storage Conditions

Gradual soap formation through strong acids or bases, but stable in weak acids or bases. Preserve in a well-closed container.

13. Incompatibilities

No citations in the literature.

14. Safety

Sorbitan esters are well-tolerated when taken orally, with very low levels of toxicity. They are practically irritation-free topically.

Product	Patch Tests (Schwartz) On Human Subjects — No. reactors /No. of persons tested (conc., % w/v)	Irritation to Rabbit Eye — Irritation rating (conc., % w/v)	Oral Toxicity LD$_{50}$ (g/kg. rat)
Arlacel 20	0/50 (100)	Nonirrit. (30)	36
Arlacel 40	0/50 (50)	Nonirrit. (30)	>16
Arlacel 60	0/50 (50)	Nonirrit. (30)	>16
		Min. irrit. (100)	
Arlacel 80	0/50 (100)	Nonirrit. (75)	>16
		Nonirrit. (30)	
Arlacel 83	0/50 (100)	Nonirrit. (100)	>40
		Nonirrit. (30)	
Arlacel 85	2/50 (100)	Nonirrit. (30)	>40
	0/49 (5)		
Span 20	0/50 (100)	Nonirrit. (30)	41
Span 40	0/50 (50)	Nonirrit. (30)	>16
Span 60	0/50 (50)	Nonirrit. (30)	31
Span 65	1/201 (40)	Nonirrit. (40)	>16
Span 80	0/50 (100)	Nonirrit. (30)	>40
Span 85	0/50 (100)	Nonirrit. (100)	>40
		Nonirrit. (30)	

15. Handling Precautions

No restrictions specified.

16. Regulatory Acceptance

NF XVI: Sorbitan monolaurate; sorbitan monooleate; sorbitan monostearate; sorbitan monolaurate. BP 1980: Sorbitan monloaurate; sorbitan monooleate; sorbitan monostearate

17. Applications in Pharmaceutical Formulation or Technology

Use	Concentration (%)
Emulsifiers	
Used alone in water-in-oil emulsions	1-15
Used in combination with hydrophilic emulsifiers in oil-in-water emulsions	1-10
Used to increase the water-holding properties of ointments	1-10
Solubilizers	
For poorly soluble, active constituents in lipophilic bases	1-10
Wetting Agents	
For insoluble, active constituents in lipophilic bases	0.1-3

18. Related Substances

Polysorbates (Tweens). These products are polyoxyethylene derivatives of sorbitan esters. The hydrophilic properties of these derivatives are predominant because of the presence of polyoxyethylene chains. Polysorbates are oil-in-water emulsifying agents, and are used in the preparation of emulsions, creams, ointments and suppository bases. Polysorbates 20, 60 and 80 are listed in NF, BP 1980 and EP, while polysorbate 40 is listed in the NF only. Polysorbates are well-tolerated when taken orally, with very low levels of toxicity. They are practically irritation-free topically.

19. Comments

Parenteral acceptability: The following is a list of sorbitan esters which have been used in parenteral products (Source: "Physician's Desk Reference").

Sorbitan ester	Conc. (w/v)	Adm. route
Span 20	0.01%	I.M.
Span 40	0.05%	I.M.
Span 85	0.02%	I.M.

20. Specific References

1. K. Konno, T. Jinno and A. Kitahara, Solubility, critical aggregating or micellar concentration and aggregate formation of non-ionic surfactants in non-aqueous solutions, *J. Colloid Interface Sci.*, 49: 383 (1974).
2. A. Vissers, Sorbitan derivatives as surfactants in modern food technology, *Afinidad*, 32: 635 (1975) — in Spanish.
3. K. L. Mittal, ed., "Micellization, Solubilization, and Microemulsions," Vol. 1, Part III, Plenum Press, New York, 1977.
4. C. W. Whitworth and Y. Pongpaibul, The influence of some additives on the stability of aspirin in an oleaginous suppository base, *Can. J. Pharm. Sci.*, 14: 36 (1979).
5. E. Suzuki *et al.*, Studies on methods of particle size reduction of medicinal compounds. VIII. Size reduction by freeze-drying and the influence of pharmaceutical adjuvants on the micrometric properties of freeze-dried powders, *Chem. Pharm. Bull.*, 27: 1214 (1979).

USA: C. Yu;* J. Mullins**
UK: J.B. Kayes*

Sorbitol

1. Nonproprietary Names

NF: Sorbitol
BP 1980: Sorbitol; Sorbitol Solution (70%); Sorbitol for parenteral use
USP: Sorbitol Solution

2. Functional Category

USP: Sweetening agent; humectant; tablet and capsule diluent
BP: Pharmaceutical aid

3. Synonyms

D-Glucitol, D-sorbitol, sorbite, sorbol

4. Chemical Names and CAS Registry Number

1, 2, 3, 4, 5, 6 - Hexanehexol
D-Sorbitol
D-Glucitol [50-70-4]

5. Empirical Formula   Molecular Weight

$C_6H_{14}O_6$ 182.17

6. Structural Formula

$$
\begin{array}{c}
CH_2OH \\
| \\
HCOH \\
| \\
HOCH \\
| \\
HCOH \\
| \\
HCOH \\
| \\
CH_2OH
\end{array}
$$

7. Commercial Availability

USA
Atomergic Chemetals Corp.
EM Laboratories, Inc.
Gallard-Schlesinger
ICI United States, Inc.
Lonza, Inc.
Merck & Co.
Pfizer Chemicals Div.
Toyomenka (America), Inc.
Tri-K Industries, Inc.

8. Method of Manufacture

Sorbitol was first isolated from the juice of Mountain Ash berry (*Sorbus americana, S. decora*) in 1872 by the French chemist, Joseph Boussingault. Today, it is prepared by high-pressure hydrogenation with copper-chromium or nickel catalyst or by electrolytic reduction of glucose and corn syrup. If cane or beet sugars are used as a source, the disaccharide is hydrolyzed to dextrose and fructose prior to hydrogenation.

9. Description

White or almost colorless, crystalline, odorless, hygroscopic powder. Also available as granules, flakes and pellets to prevent caking. Pleasant, cooling, sweet taste (50-60% the sweetness of sucrose).

10. Pharmacopeial Specifications

Test	NF	BP	Parenteral use, BP	Solution USP	Solution BP
Identification	+	+	+	+	+
Water	≤1.0%	≤1.5%	+	29.0–31.0%	—
Residue on ignition	≤0.1%	—	—	≤0.1%	—
Sulfated ash	—	≤0.1%	≤0.1%	—	≤0.1%
Chloride	≤0.005%	≤50 ppm	≤50 ppm	≤0.005%	≤50 ppm
Sulfate	≤0.010%	≤100 ppm	≤100 ppm	0.010%	≤100 ppm
Arsenic	≤3 ppm	≤1 ppm	≤1 ppm	≤2.5 ppm	≤1 ppm
Heavy metals	≤0.001%	≤5 ppm	≤5 ppm	≤0.001%	≤5 ppm
Lead	—	—	≤2 ppm	—	—
Reducing sugars	+	+	+	+	+
Total sugars	+	—	—	—	—
Acidity or alkalinity	—	+	+	—	+
Specific optical rotation	—	+4.0°–+7.0°	+13°–+16°	—	—
Clarity and color of solution	—	+	+	—	+
Nickel	—	≤1 ppm	≤1 ppm	—	≤1 ppm
Assay range	91.0–100.5%	98.0–101.0%	98.0–101.0%	≥64.0% w/w	68.0–72.0% w/w
Specific gravity	—	—	—	≥1.285	—
Relative density	—	—	—	—	≥1.290
Refractive index	—*	—	—	1.455–1.465 at 20°C	1.457–1.462

11. Typical Properties

Melting point: 110-112°C (anhydrous); 97.7°C (monohydrate); 93°C (monohydrate, metastable form).

Solubility: Very soluble in water, soluble in warm alcohol and glycerin, and slightly soluble in hydrocarbons. Additional solubility data are given in Table I.

Table I—Solubility of Sorbitol in Hydro-alcoholic Solutions (5)

% Ethanol v/v in Water	% Sorbitol w/v at 25°C
0	94
11	88
20	83
41	70
62	47
82	12
90	3

Approximate upper solubility limit for elixirs would be 50-55% for sorbitol and 9-18% for ethanol. Solubility of sucrose and sorbitol combinations in water at 25°C was also reported by M. Barr *et al.*[6] Sorbitol may be substituted, gram for gram, for sucrose to prepare 70% w/v to 90% w/v syrups.

Moisture content: ≤1.0% (NF XV), USP XX Method I [921], p. 1279 (K. Fischer), and usually not more than 1 or 2%.

Equilibrium moisture content: Data presented in Table II.

Table II—Equilibrium Moisture Content of Crystalline

% Relative Humidity	% Water at Equilibrium
11	0.7
23	0.8
33	1.4
43	1.2
52	1.8
64	2.7
75	28.4
83	36.0
93	50.8

Relative humidities greater than 50% at 25°C should be avoided when sorbitol is added to direct-compression tablet formulas. Sorbitol is classified as a very hygroscopic powder.

True density: 1.49 g/ml.

Negative heat of solution: −26.5 calories/g.

Physical properties: Physical properties of five grades of Sorbitol NF in solid state are presented in Table III. In addition, some physical properties of sorbitol in water are presented in Table IV.

Supplier: ICI Americas Inc., Lot No. 2405JI

Table III—Physical Properties of Five Grades of Sorbitol NF/FCC

Testing Parameter	(Granular) Type S-6921 Lot No. G96251	(Tablet Type) Type S-6929 Lot No. G87151	(Coarse Powder) Type S-6926 Lot No. G99241	(60 mesh) Type S-6930 Lot No. G8Y181	(Fine Powder) Type S-6924 Lot No. G8X151
Density (20 gm. sample)					
Loose bulk	0.77 g/ml	0.50 g/ml	0.72 g/ml	0.68 g/ml	0.53 g/ml
Tapped (consolidated)	0.85 g/ml	0.70 g/ml	0.85 g/ml	0.81 g/ml	0.69 g/ml
Particle size distribution (20 gm sample—Alpine Air Jet Sieve A200LS)					
on 30 mesh	15%	0%	0%	0%	0%
thru 30 mesh on 60 mesh	48%	33%	33%	0%	2%
thru 60 mesh on 120 mesh	20%	45%	41%	59%	11%
thru 120 mesh	17%	22%	26%	41%	87%
Flowability	Excellent flow (16 sec.)	Hindered flow (31 sec.)	Excellent flow (16 sec.)	Good flow (22 sec.)	Poor flow (0 sec.)
Compression characteristics	Poorly Compressible (Lubricant required)	Compressible (No lubricant required)	Poorly Compressible (Lubricant required)	Poorly Compressible (Lubricant required)	Moderately Compressible (No lubricant required)
Moisture content (Loss on drying: 105° C - 4 hours)	0.9%	0.7%	0.5%	0.5%	0.8%
Melting point (hot stage microscope)	94-96° C	95-96° C	94-96° C	95-96° C	93-94° C

Samples Supplied by Pfizer Chemical Division, New York 10017
Test Data furnished by Purdue Frederick Research Center, Yonkers, New York, 10701

Table IV—Some Physical Properties of Sorbitol in Water

% Solids w/w	% Solids w/v	Density at 25° C	Viscosity in cps at 25° C	Refractive index at 25° C	Freezing Point (° C)
10	11.	1.034	1.2	1.348	−1.1
20	21.2	1.073	1.7	1.365	−3.8
30	33.5	1.114	2.5	1.383	−8.0
40	45.1	1.155	4.4	1.400	−13.0
50	59.4	1.197	9.1	1.418	−26.0
60	74.3	1.240	26.0	1.437	0
70*	90.6	1.293	110.0	1.458	0
80	106.	1.330	900.0	1.478	0

*BP Sorbitol Solution

Academy HPE Laboratory Project Data

	Method	Lab #	Results
Moisture Content			
Crystalline	MC-3	25	0.8333%[b]
Crystalline USP	MC-3	10	0.700%[a]
Tablet type	MC-3	33	0.45%[b]
Tablet type	MC-4	33	0.10%[b]
Coarse	MC-3	33	0.23%[b]
Coarse	MC-4	33	0.00%[b]
Density (bulk/tap):			
Tablet type	BTD-1	1	B:0.505 g/ml[b]
			T:0.641 g/ml[b]
Tablet type	BTD-7	14	B:0.570 g/ml[b]
			T:0.680 g/ml[b]
Coarse	BTD-1	1	B:0.667 g/ml[b]
			T:0.833 g/ml[b]
Coarse	BTD-7	14	B:0.700 g/ml[b]
			T:0.780 g/ml[b]
Solubility			*mg/ml*
Chrystalline			
Tablet type: Water	SOL-2	1	3.77×10³[b]
Alcohol	SOL-2	1	18.00[b]
n-Hexane	SOL-1	1	0.00[b]
Coarse: Water	SOL-2	1	3.50×10³[b]
Alcohol	SOL-2	1	17.50[b]
n-Hexane	SOL-1	1	0.011[b]
EMC Plot (USP)	EMC-1	10	Fig:10-EMC-4[a]
COM Plot (Cryst. tabl.)	COM-3	20	Fig:20-COM-4[b]
COM Plot (Coarse cryst.)	COM-3	20	Fig: 20-COM-5[b]

Supplier: ICI Amer.[a], Pfizer[b]

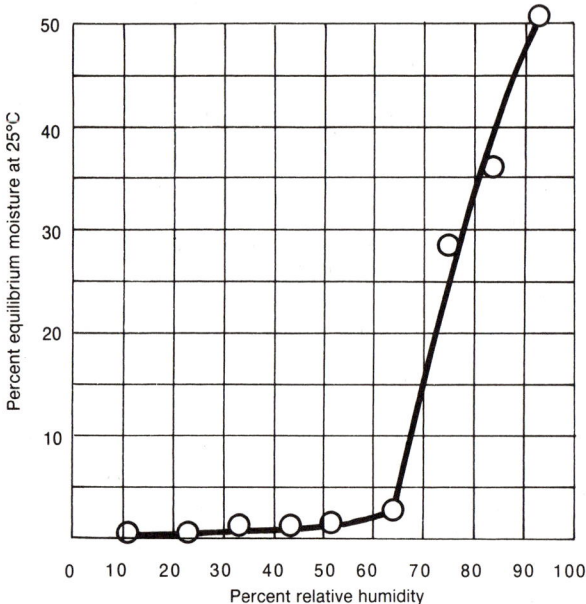

Sorbitol, USP (ICI, Lot No. 2404JI)
Figure: 10-EMC-4   Method: EMC-1

12. Stability and Storage Conditions

Sorbitol is relatively chemically inert and compatible with most excipients. It is stable in air in the absence of catalysts and in cold, dilute acids and bases. Sorbitol does not darken or decompose at elevated temperatures or in the presence of amines. It is non-flammable, non-corrosive and non-volatile. In high concentrations, sorbitol is a stabilizer for labile vitamins and antibiotics.

Sorbitol solutions may be stored in glass, plastic, aluminum and stainless steel containers. It will react with iron oxide and become discolored. Sorbitol will form water-soluble chelates with many di- and trivalent metal ions in strongly acidic and alkaline solutions. Sorbitol solutions, although highly resistant to microbial attack, should be preserved.

Since it is hygroscopic, it should be stored in a tightly-sealed container.

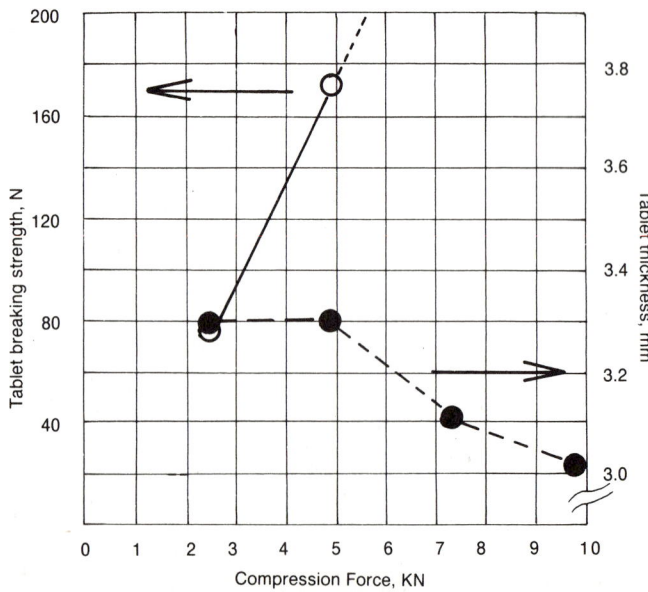

Sorbitol, tablet type, crystalline, USP (Pfizer, Lot. No. 95-1). Mean tablet weight: 500 mg.   Minimum compressional force for compaction: 2.45 KN. Compressional force resulting in capping: 14.7 KN.
Figure: 20-COM-4   Method: COM-3

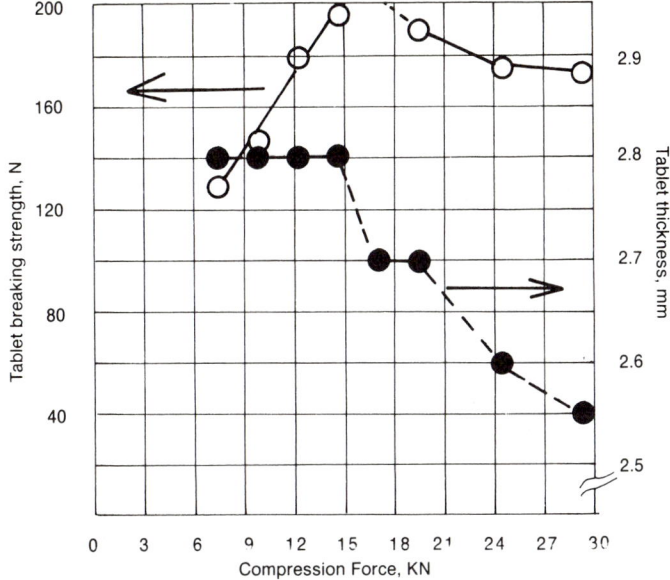

Sorbitol crystalline, coarse, USP (Pfizer, Lot No. G92051-S6926). Mean tablet weight: 500 mg. Minimum compressional force for compaction: 7.35 KN. Compressional force resulting in capping: 19.6 KN. 1% Magnesium stearate required as lubricant.

Figure: 20-COM-5   Method: COM-3

13. Incompatibilities

Addition of liquid polyethylene glycols with vigorous agitation to Sorbitol Solution USP will produce a waxy, water-soluble gel mass with a melting point of 35-40° C.

14. Safety

Sorbitol occurs naturally in many edible fruits and berries. Its caloric value is 3.99 calories/gram. Unlike sucrose, it is absorbed more slowly from the GI tract. Sorbitol is considered non-irritating to local tissues following oral surgery. It is metabolized in the liver to fructose and glucose. When ingested in large amounts (30 grams per day), it produces a laxative effect. Excessive amounts may cause flatulence, abdominal distention and diarrhea. Small quantities of unchanged sorbitol are often found in urine and feces.

Sorbitol is better tolerated by diabetics than sucrose, and is widely used in many non-sugar liquid vehicles. Nevertheless, it is not considered to be unconditionally safe for diabetics. It is not permitted in peritoneal dialysis solutions in the United States and Canada, where it has been replaced by mannitol. Many uremic patients do not metabolize sorbitol sufficiently to avoid cumulative serum levels. Sorbitol is generally considered to be more irritating than mannitol.

15. Handling Precautions

No restrictions specified.

16. Regulatory Acceptance

NF XV; BP 1980

In the United States, there is no official limit on daily dosage. However, according to the FAO/WHO, the acceptable daily intake in man should not exceed 150 mg per kg of body weight (9 grams per day). Sorbitol is a permitted sweetener in West Germany.

17. Applications in Pharmaceutical Formulation or Technology

Use	Concentration (%)
Substitute for glycerin and propylene glycol	25-90
Humectant	3-15
Vehicle for oral and topical liquids	25-90
Prevention of "cap locking" in syrups and elixirs	15-30
Non-sugar sweetener	25-90
Viscosity agent	25-90
Binder and moisture-control agent in tablets	3-10
Plasticizer for gelatin and cellulosic films	5-20
Diluent for injectables	below 10-25
Vehicle for DSS, tetracyclines, ascorbic acid, B-complex, vitamins and iron salts	25-90

18. Related Substances

Mannitol, xylitol, other sugar alcohols.

19. Comments

None

20. Specific References

1. "Tetracycline syrup suspension," LS-99, publication ICI United States Inc., Wilmington, DE 19897.
2. G. R. Sabatini and J. J. Gulesich, Formulation of a stable and palatable oral suspension of Procaine Penicillin G, *J. Am. Pharm. Assoc.*, pr. ed., 17, 806 (1956).
3. J. Swintoski and R. J. Ferlauto, Stabilization of Procaine Penicillin G suspensions, *J. Am. Pharm. Assoc., sc. ed.*, 45, 43 (1956).
4. C. E. Alford, "Stable aluminum hydroxide suspension," U.S. Patent No. 2,999,790, issued 9/12/61.
5. M. E. Barr, S. R. Kohn and L. F. Tice, Solubility of sorbitol in hydroalcoholic solutions, *Am. J. Pharm.*, 129, 102 (1957).
6. R. G. Daoust and M. J. Lynch, Sorbitol in pharmaceutical liquids, *Drug Cosm. Ind.*, 90, June, 689 (1962).
7. M. P. Rabinowitz *et al.*, GLC Assay of sorbitol as cyclic n-butylboronate, *J. Pharm. Sci.*, 63, 1601 (1974).
8. W. C. Griffin, R. W. Behrens and S. T. Cross, Hygroscopic properties of polyols, *J. Soc. Cosm., Chem.*, 1 (1950).
9. C. J. Salivar, "Aqueous calcium tetracyline antibiotic composition," U.S. Patent No. 2,903,395, issued 9/8/59.
10. F. J. Bandelin and J. V. Tuschhoff, Stability of ascorbic acid in various liquid media, *J. Am. Pharm. Assoc.*, sc. ed., 44, 241 (1955).
11. B. D. Parikh and F. V. Lofgren, Stability study of an oral multivitamin liquid preparation, *Drug Standards*, 25, 56 (1958).
12. S. Lindvall and N. S. E. Anderson, Studies on an iron-sorbitol hematinic, *Br. J. Pharmacology*, 17, 358 (1961).
13. B. F. Chow *et al.*, Absorption of B_{12} enhanced by sorbitol, *Am. J. Clin. Nutrition*, 6, 30 (1958).

20. Specific References

14. J. J. Herndon *et al.*, Iron absorption and metabolism, *J. Nutrition*, 64, 615 (1958).
15. R. H. Barry, M. Weiss, J. B. Johnson, E. Deritter, Stability of phenylpropanolamine hydrochloride in liquid formulations containing sugars, *J. Pharm. Sci.*, 71(1), 116-118 (1982).
16. A. M. Molokhia, M. A. Moustafa and M. W. Goudl, Effect of storage conditions on the hardness disintegration and drug release from some tablet bases, *Drug Develop. and Ind. Pharm.* 8(2), 283-292 (1982).

USA: R. Nash*, R. A. Frable**, Z. Chowhan**

Starch

1. Nonproprietary Names

NF: Starch
BP/EP: Starches

2. Functional Category

USP: Tablet and/or capsule diluent; tablet disintegrant
Others: Glidant

3. Synonyms

Amylum; corn starch; maize starch; potato starch; rice starch; wheat starch, *Aytex P, Melojel, Paygel 55, Purity 5, Purity 21*

4. Chemical Name and CAS Registry Number

Starch [9005-25-8]

5. Empirical Formula

$(C_6H_{10}O_5)n$—where n is from 300 to 1,000

Molecular Weight

Variable

6. Structural Formula

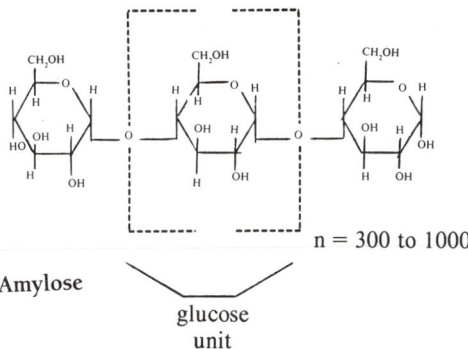

n = 300 to 1000

Amylose

glucose unit

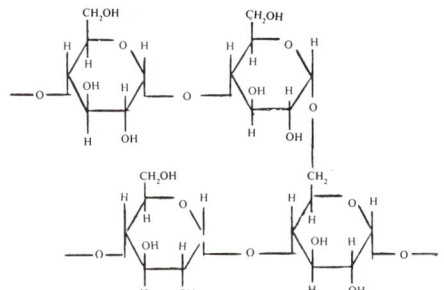

Segment of Amylopectin Molecule

7. Commercial Availability

USA

Anheuser Busch, Inc.
Colorcon, Inc.
Corn Products, Unit of CPC North America
Generichem Corp.
Hubinger
National Starch & Chemical Corp.
Ruger Chemical Co.
Staley Mfg. Co., A.E.
Starchem Corporation
United States Biochemicals Corp.

UK

B. D. H. Chemicals, Ltd.
C. P. C. United Kingdom, Ltd.
J. & W. Starches
Laing National, Ltd.
L. J. Rickards & Co., Ltd.
Tunnel Refineries, Ltd.

8. Method of Manufacture

Starch is extracted from plant sources through a sequence of processing steps involving coarse milling, repeated water washing, wet sieving and centrifugal separations to isolate the starch from other plant and seed materials. The wet starch is then dried, milled and packaged for market.

9. Description

Fine, white, odorless, tasteless powder comprised of very small spherical or ovoid granules whose size and shape are characteristic for each botanical variety. (See NF XV and BP 1980 for detailed description.)

Approximate ranges of granule diameter are:

	BP/EP	NF
Rice	2-10 μm	—
Corn	2-32 μm	up to 35 μm
Wheat	2-45 μm	5-50 μm
Potato	10-100 μm	10-100 μm

SEM:KY-20
Excipient: Corn starch
Manufacturer: Anheuser Busch   **Lot no.:** 96A-3 (67)

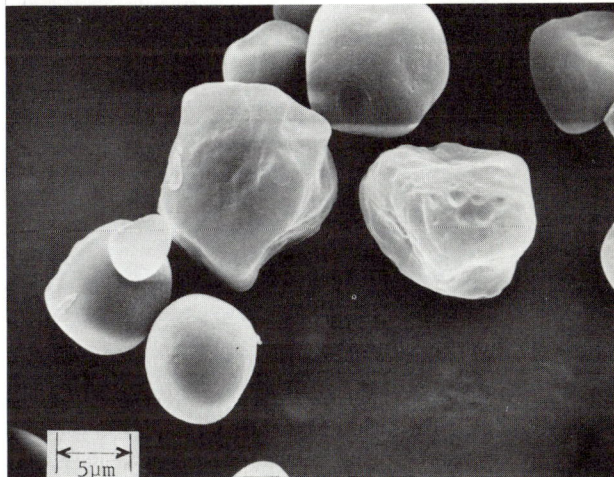

Magnification: 2,400×   **Voltage:** 20 kV

SEM:KY-21
Excipient: Corn starch
Manufacturer: Stalev   **Lot no.:** 96A-4 (G77912)

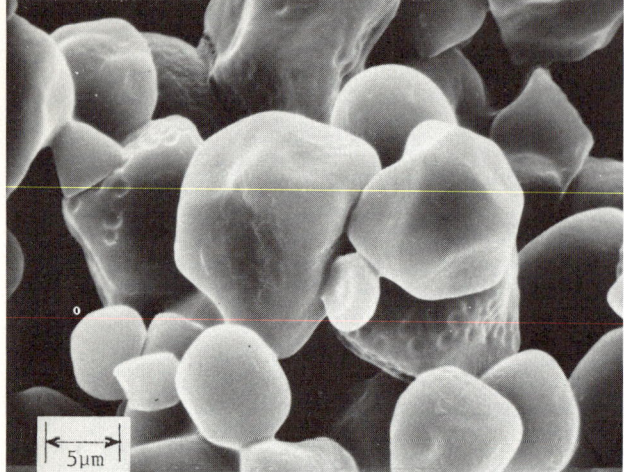

Magnification: 2,400×   **Voltage:** 20 kV

SEM:KY-44
Excipient: Wheat starch (Aytex P)
Manufacturer: Henkel   **Lot no.:** 96A-2 (2919D)

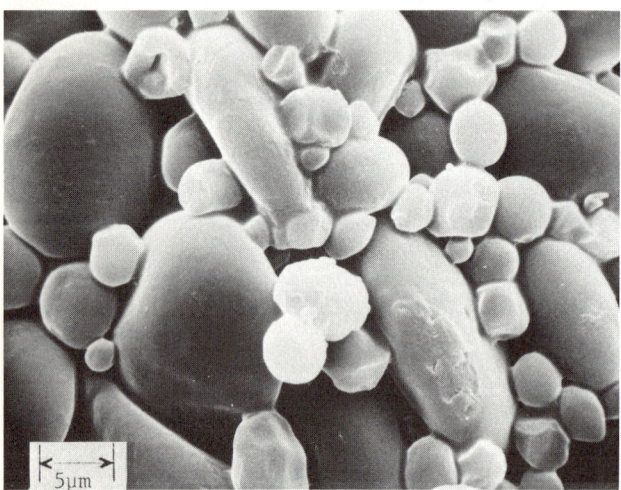

Magnification: 2,400×   **Voltage:** 20 kV

SEM:KY-45
Excipient: Wheat starch (Paygel 55)
Manufacturer: Henkel   **Lot no.:** 96A-1 (2917D)

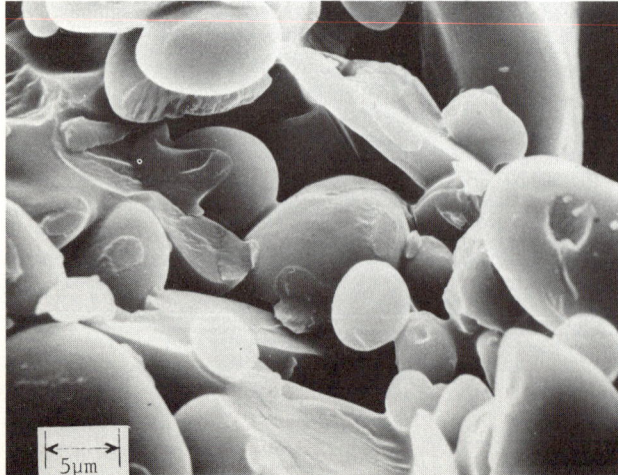

Magnification: 2,400×   **Voltage:** 20 kV

SEM:KY-46
Excipient: Potato starch
Manufacturer: Starchem   **Lot no.:** 96A-5 (1179)

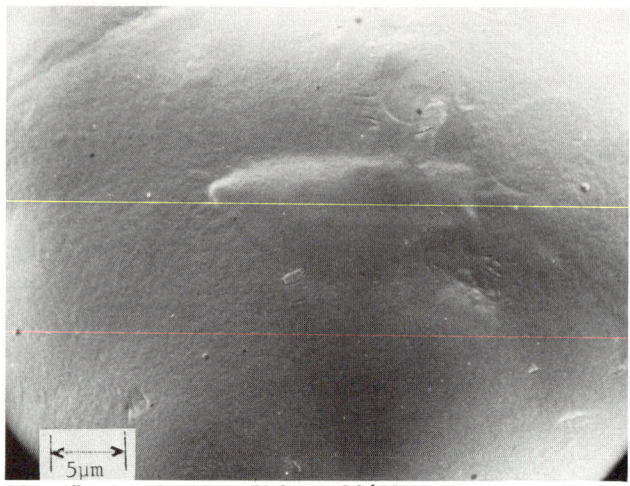

Magnification: 2,400×   **Voltage:** 20 kV

SEM:MF-2
Excipient: Rice starch
Supplier: Matheson, Coleman & Bell

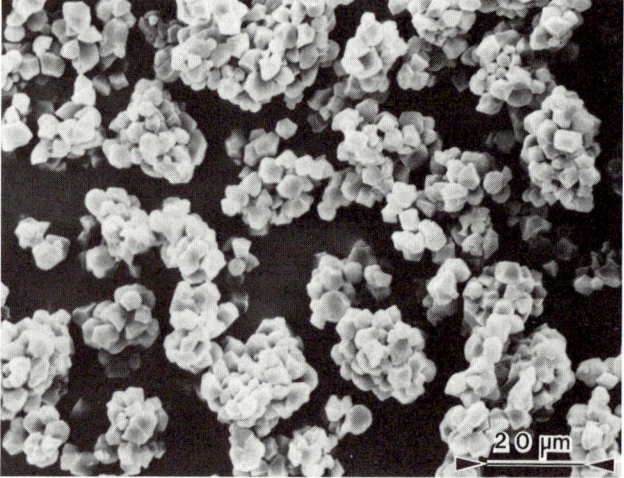

Magnification: ×600

SEM:MF-2
Excipient: Rice starch
Supplier: Matheson, Coleman & Bell

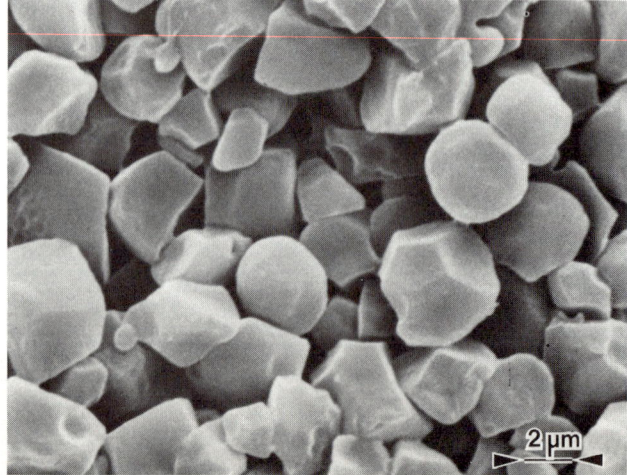

Magnification: 3,000×

10. Pharmacopeial Specifications

Test	NF	BP/EP
Identification	+	+
Microbial limits	+	−
Salmonella	Absent	
E. coli	Absent	
Acidity	−	+
pH (20% slurry)		
Corn starch	4.5-7.0	−
Wheat starch	4.5-7.0	−
Potato starch	5.0-8.0	−
Rice starch	−	−
Foreign matter	−	+
Loss on drying	≤14.0%	≤15% (maize,
corn, rice,		wheat, rice)
wheat, potato		≤20% (potato)
Residue on		
ignition	≤0.5%	−
Sulphated ash	−	≤0.6% (maize,
corn, potato,		wheat, potato)
wheat, rice		≤0.8% (rice)
Iron	≤0.002%	−
Oxidizing substances	≤0.002%	−
Sulfur dioxide	≤0.008%	−
Deformed granules	−	+

11. Typical Properties

Academy HPE Laboratory Project Data

	Method	Lab #	Results
Corn Starch			
NF	MC-20	2	7.10%[a]
	MC-15	14	9.80%[b]
	MC-15	34	9.90%[b]
	MC-15	34	9.86%[c]
Starch 1500	MC-15	14	9.83%[c]
Purity 21	MC-15	34	9.95%[a]
Melojel	MC-15	34	12.49%[a]
Purity 5	MC-15	34	6.98%[a]
Bulk/tap density	BTD-1	1	B:0.490 g/[b]cm³
			T:0.769 g/[b]cm³
	BTD-1	1	B:0.515 g/[c]cm³
			T:0.758 g/[c]cm³
		1	B:0.521 g/[a]cm³
			T:0.806 g/[a]cm³
		1	B:0.485 g/[a]cm³
			T:0.694 g/[a]cm³
		1	B:0.535 g/[a]cm³
			T:0.820 g/[a]cm³
		14	B:0.570 g/[b]cm³
			T:0.670 g/[b]cm³
		14	B:0.540 g/[e]cm³
			T:0.680 g/[e]cm³
	BTD-6	8	VOLUME:9.5%[d]
			WEIGHT:10.0%[d]
Solubility (at 25°C)	SOL-1	1	*mg/ml*
(Water)		1	0.063[b]
(Alcohol)		1	0.030[b]
(*n*-Hexane)		1	0.005[b]
(Water)		1	0.084[c]
(Alcohol)		1	0.020[c]
(*n*-Hexane)		1	0.011[c]

	Method	Lab #	Results
Purity 21 (Water)		1	0.034[a]
(Alcohol)		1	0.012[a]
(*n*-Hexane)		1	0.004[a]
Melojel (Water)		1	0.020[a]
(Alcohol)		1	0.010[a]
(*n*-Hexane)		1	0.002[a]
Purity 5 (Water)		1	0.062[a]
(Alcohol)		1	0.014[a]
(*n*-Hexane)		1	0.000[a]
Particle size dist.	PSD-6	23	≤74 µm:100%[a]
	PSD-6	23	≤74 µm:100%[a]
	PSD-6	23	≤74 µm:100%[a]
EMC plot	EMC-1	2	Fig:2-EMC-10[a]
SDI plot	SDI-1	14	Fig:14-SDI-7[b]
SDI plot (Starch 1500)	SDI-1	14	Fig:14-SDI-8[d]
Wheat Starch			
Moisture content			
(*Paygel 55*)	MC-15	14	7.50%[f]
(*Paygel 55*)	MC-15	34	7.67%[f]
(*Aytex P*)	MC-15	14	7.94%[f]
(*Aytex P*)	MC-15	34	8.32%[f]
Particle size	PSD-2	5	58 µm
Potato Starch			
Moisture content	MC-29	23	15.30%[g]
	MC-15	34	15.85%[g]
Particle size	PSD-6	23	≤74 µm:100%[g]

Suppliers: National[a]; Anheuser[b]; Staley[c]; Hubinger[d]; Colorcon[e]; Henkel[f]; Star[g].

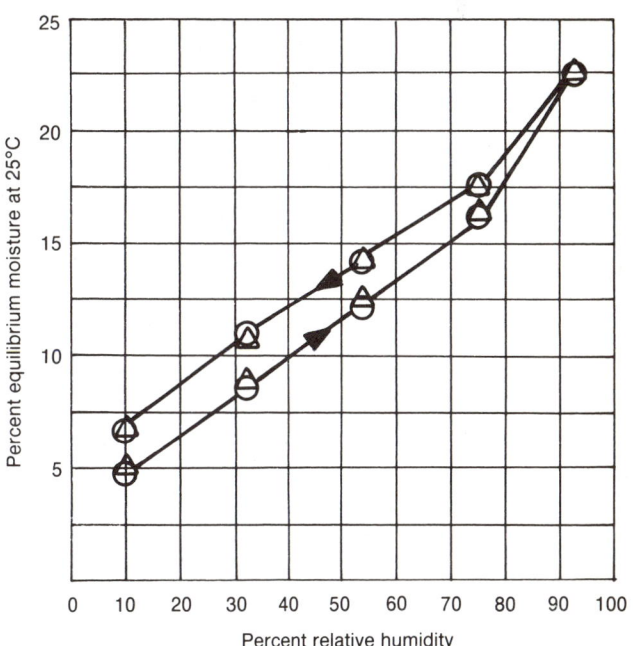

○ : Starch, wheat, Paygel 55 (Henkel Corp., Lot #2917D)
△ : Starch, wheat, Aytex P (Henkel Corp., Lot #2919D)
Figure: 14-SDI-9 **Method:** SDI-1

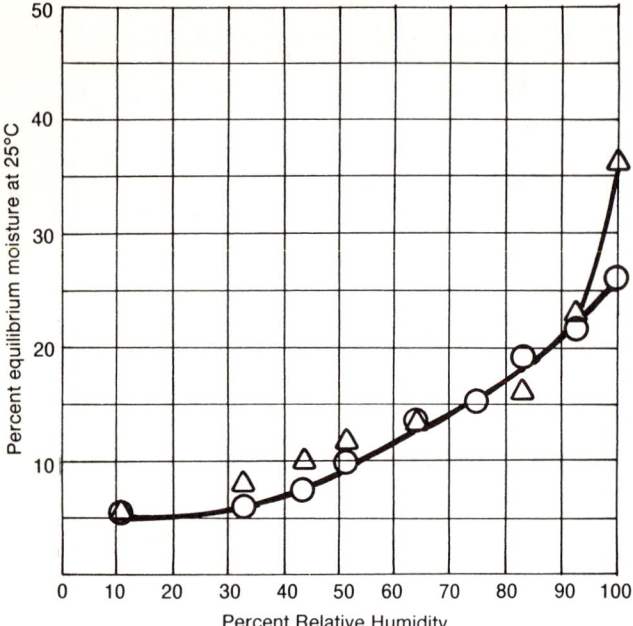

O : Corn starch USP (National, Lot #421)
△ : Pregelatinized starch USP (National, Lot #HJW 103)
Figure: 2-EMC-10   **Method:** EMC-1

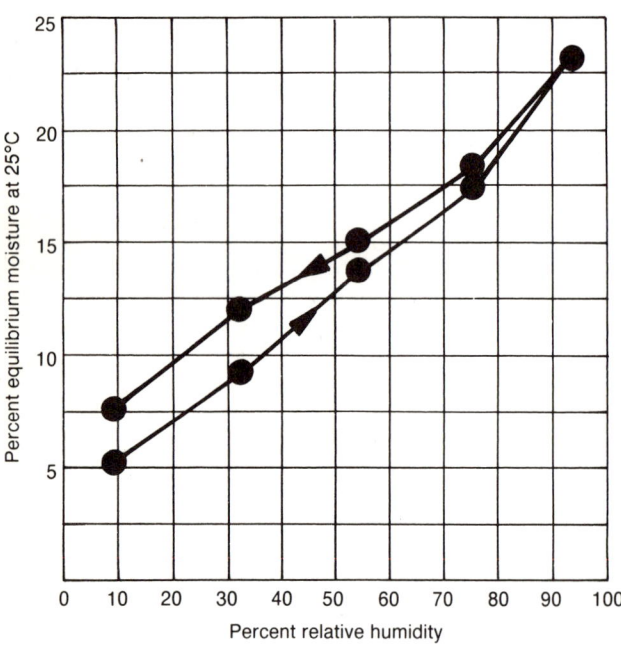

Starch, corn (Anheuser Busch, Lot #67)
Figure: 14-SDI-7   **Method:** SDI-1

Density: Bulk — maize: 0.462 g/ml (Swiss catalogue method); tapped — maize: 0.658 g/ml (Engelsmann volumeter); particle — maize: 1.478 g/cm³ (air pycnometer).
Solubility:
McIlvaine's citric acid-phosphate buffer, at both 25° and 60° C:

    at pH 2: < 1 in 1000
        pH 4: < 1 in 1000
        pH 7: < 1 in 1000
        pH 8: < 1 in 1000

Purified water: < 1 in 1000 at 25°C
Ethanol (96 per cent):   < 1 in 1000 at 25°C
Chloroform: < 1 in 1000 at 25°C
Equilibrium moisture content: All starches rapidly absorb atmospheric moisture. Approximate equilibrium moisture content values at 50% relative humidity are: Corn—11%; wheat—13%; rice—14%; potato—18%. Sorption isotherm data reveal that, between 30% and 80% RH, corn starch is the least hygroscopic form, while potato starch is the most hygroscopic. Corn starch as marketed usually contains 10-14% moisture.
Swelling temperature: Maize 65°C; potato 64°C; wheat 55°C
Gelatinization temperature: Maize 73°C; potato 72°C; wheat 63°C.
Particle size distribution: range: Potato 20-180 μm; maize 10-25 μm; wheat 10-40 μm.
Weight (median diameter): Maize 17 μm; wheat 23 μm.
Specific surface area: Maize 0.6-0.75 m²/g.
Flowability: Compressibility index: Maize 30%; poor flow; cohesive. (R. L. Carr, *British Chem. Eng.*, 1970, 15: 1541-1549).
Compression characteristics: See below graph of tensile strength versus upper punch force. Tablet machine—Manesty F; speed: 50 min⁻¹; weight: 490-510 mg. Strength test—Diametral compression between flat-faced rams. Upper ram stationary, lower moving at 66 μms⁻¹.
pH of aqueous preparation. Maize: 5.5-6.5 (2%) at 25°C.
Rheological properties: Viscosity of aqueous preparation (2% at 25°C): 13.0 mNs/m² (13.0 cP) at rate of shear 676.3/s (maize)—using Haake Rotovisco RV3; head—DMK 50.

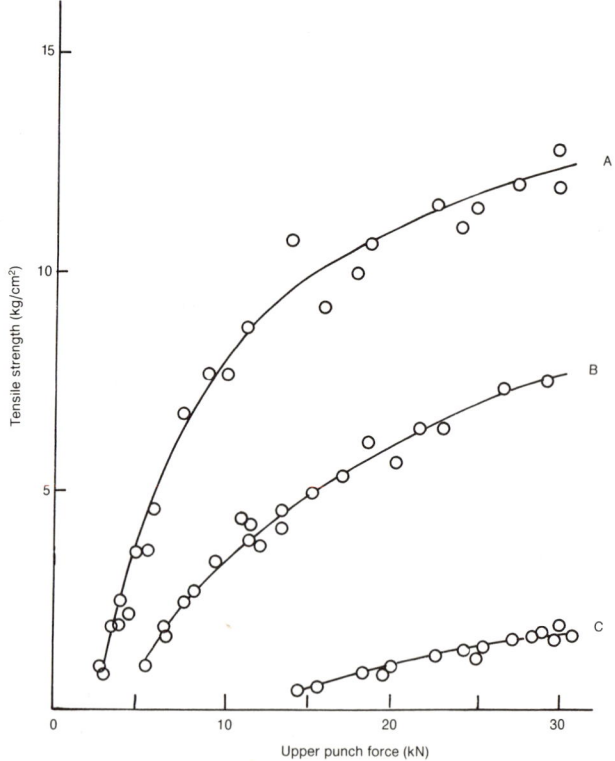

Acceleration 250 rpm/min., maximum speed 250 rpm. Rotor—NV viscosity sensor system (damping factor = 10.)

A. Potato starch   B. Maize Starch   C. Wheat starch
Tensile strength of compacts of different starches

12. Stability and Storage Conditions

Uncooked dry starch is quite stable during storage if protected from high humidity. It should be stored in a cool, dry location in an air-tight container. When used as a diluent or disintegrant in solid dosage forms, it is considered inert under normal storage conditions. Cooked starch solutions or pastes, however, are physically unstable, and are readily attacked by microorganisms to form a wide variety of starch derivatives and "modified starches" with unique physical properties.

13. Incompatibilities

None in most applications.

14. Safety

Starch is an edible food substance, and is recognized as safe for general use.

15. Handling Precautions

As an industrial chemical, starch presents the hazard of a dust explosion common to any fine organic powder when exposed to an open flame or spark source in finely-dispersed form. Store in a clean, dry, well-ventilated room.

16. Regulatory Acceptance

Corn starch, wheat starch and potato starch—NF XVI; BP/EP 1980; rice starch—BP/EP 1980

17. Applications in Pharmaceutical Formulation or Technology

Diluent: Starch is a suitable diluent for the preparation of standardized triturates of colorants or potent drugs to facilitate subsequent mixing or blending processes in manufacturing operations. It also has utility in dry-filled capsule formulations for volume adjustment of the fill matrix.

Tablet formulations: Freshly prepared starch paste (5-25% w/w) is a widely used binder for tablet granulations. Selection of the amount required in a given system can be determined through optimization studies, using parameters such as granule friability, tablet friability, hardness, disintegration rate and drug dissolution rate. Starch is the most commonly used tablet disintegrant at levels of 3-15%. Unmodified starch does not compress well, however, and tends to increase tablet friability and capping if used in high concentrations. In granulated formulas, about half the total starch content is included in the granulation mixture, and the balance as part of the final blend with the dried granulation.

18. Related Substances

Pregelatinized starch, NF—A starch that has been chemically or mechanically processed to rupture all or part of the granules in the presence of water and is then subsequently dried. Sterilizable maize starch, BP—Maize starch that has been chemically or physically treated so that it does not gelatinize on exposure to moisture or steam sterilization. It contains magnesium oxide, in a proportion not greater than 2.2%. Pregelatinized maize starch, BP—Starch prepared by heating an aqueous slurry of maize starch and removing the water from the resulting paste. Soluble starch, BPC 1973—Potato or maize starch which has been chemically treated to destroy the gelatinizing power of the starch. Starch 1500—Starch that has been mechanically processed to rupture some of the granules in the presence of water, and then subsequently dried. This material meets the requirements of NF for pregelatinized starch.

19. Comments

Whereas the NF specifies that starch be produced from maize, wheat or potato, the BP 1980 also permits starch to be produced from rice. In tropical and subtropical countries where other starches are not available, the BP 1980 permits the use of tapioca starch, subject to additional requirements. End linkages are supplemented by branches occurring about every 20-30 anhydroglucose units. The starches from different plant sources differ in terms of the amylose/amylopectin ratio. Corn starch, for example, contains about 27% amylose, potato starch about 22%, and tapioca starch about 17%, while waxy maize starch is nearly 100% amylopectin with no amylose content. These variables modify the physical properties such that the various types of starch may not be interchangeable for a given pharmaceutical application. Starch grains swell instantaneously by about 5-10% in mean diameter in water at 37°C. Polyvalent cations produce more swelling than monovalent ions, but pH has little effect.

20. Specific References

1. "Corn Starch," Corn Industries Research Foundation, Inc., 1958.
2. Technical Data Sheets, Colorcon Inc., West Point, PA.
3. Technical Service Bulletins, National Starch & Chemical Corp., Bridgewater, NJ.
4. J. T. Ingram and W. Lowenthal, Mechanism of action of starch as a tablet disintegrant, *J. Pharm. Sci.*, 55: 1065 (1966).
5. N. R. Patel and R. E. Heppenen, Mechanism of action of starch as disintegrating agent in aspirin tablets, *J. Pharm. Sci.*, 55: 1065 (1966).
6. A. M. Sakr *et al.*, *Mfg. Chem.*, 44: 37 (1973).
7. J. A. Radley, Ed., Starch products, *Appl. Sci.* (1976).
8. W. Lowenthal, *Pharm. Acta. Helv.*, 48: 589-609 (1973).
9. D. E. Wurster, G. E. Peck and D. O. Kildsig, A comparison of the moisture adsorption-desorption properties of corn starch, U.S.P., and directly compressible starch, *Drug Develop and Indust. Pharm.*, 8 (3): 343-354 (1982).
10. J. C. Callahan, G. W. Cleary, M. Elefant, G. Kaplan, T. Kensler, R. A. Nash, Equilibrium moisture content of pharmaceutical excipients, *Drug Develop. and Indust. Pharm.*, 8 (3): 355-369 (1982).
11. R. F. Shangraw, J. W. Wallace and F. M. Bowers, Morphology and functionality in tablet excipients for direct compression: Part II, *Pharm. Technology*, 5 (10): 44-60 (1981).
12. Z. T. Chowhan, A. A. Amaro and Y. P. Chow, Tablet to tablet dissolution variability and its relationship to the homogeneity of a water soluble drug, *Drug Develop. and Indust. Pharm.*, 8 (2): 145-168 (1982).
13. E. M. Rudnic, C. T. Rhodes, S. Wells and P. Bernardo, Evaluation of the mechanism of disintegrant action, *Drug Develop. and Indust. Pharm.*, 8 (1): 87-109 (1982).
14. N. Kitamori and T. Makino, Improvement in pressure dependent dissolution of trepibuton tablets by using intragranular disintegrants, *Drug Develop. and Indust. Pharm.*, 8 (1): 125-139 (1982).
15. P. York, Studies of the effect of powder moisture content on drug release from hard gelatin capsules, *Drug Devel. Indust. Pharm.*, 6(6): 605-627 (1980).

USA: J. F. Millar*; B. Farhadieh**; B. Kim**; Z. Chowhan**
UK: G. Rowley*

Maize Starch, Sterilizable

1. Nonproprietary Name

USP: Absorbable dusting powder
BP: Sterilizable maize starch

2. Functional Category

BP: Lubricant for surgeons' gloves; vehicle for medicated dusting powders.

3. Synonyms

Modified starch dusting powder; starch-derivative dusting powder; sterilizable maize starch; double-dressed, white maize starch; *Jalan* D 17 maize starch; *Bio-Sorb*.

4. Chemical Name and CAS Registry Number

—

5. Empirical Formula   Molecular Weight

—   —

6. Structural Formula

$(C_6H_{10}O_5)_n$

7. Commercial Availability

UK
CPC (UK), Ltd.
J & W Starches
Laing National, Ltd.
Surgikos, Ltd.

8. Method of Manufacture

Cross-linking of the branched and straight-chain polymers in maize starch is achieved either by physical means or by treatment with phosphorus oxychloride or epichlorhydrin.

9. Description

White, free-flowing powder; ordorless. Particles are polyhedral, sometimes rounded.

10. Pharmacopeial Specifications

Test	USP	BP
Identification	+	+
Stability to autoclaving	+	—
Sedimentation	+	+
pH (1 in 10 suspension)	10.0-10.8	—
Alkalinity (10% w/v suspension)	—	pH 9.5-10.8
Loss on drying	≤12%	≤15%
Residue on ignition	≤3%	—

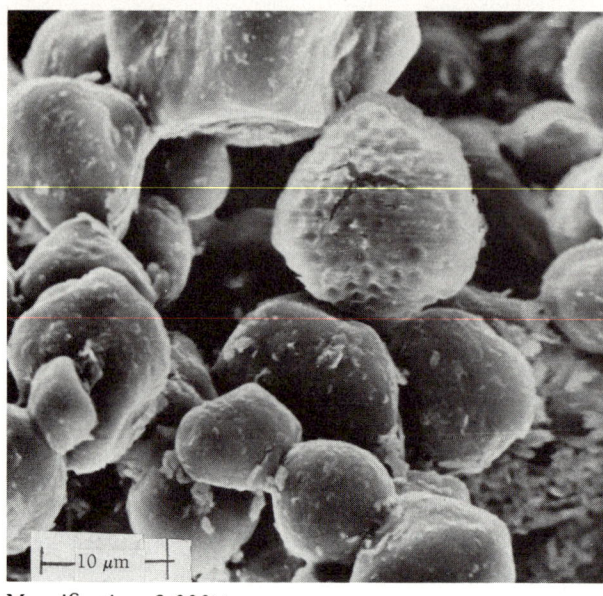

SEM: MF−1A
Excipient: Maize starch, sterilizable
Manufacturer: Biosorb

Magnification: 2,000×

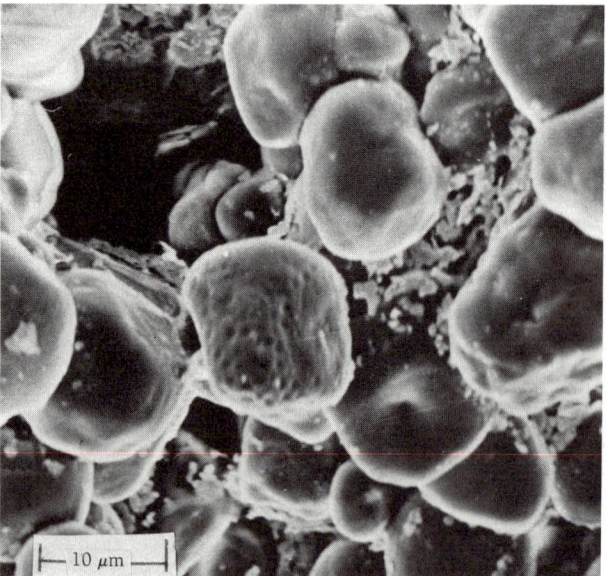

SEM: MF−1B
Excipient: Maize starch, sterilizable
Manufacturer: J & W Starches, Ltd.

Magnification: 2,000×

SEM: MF−1C
Excipient: Maize starch, sterilizable
Manufacturer: CPC, Ltd.

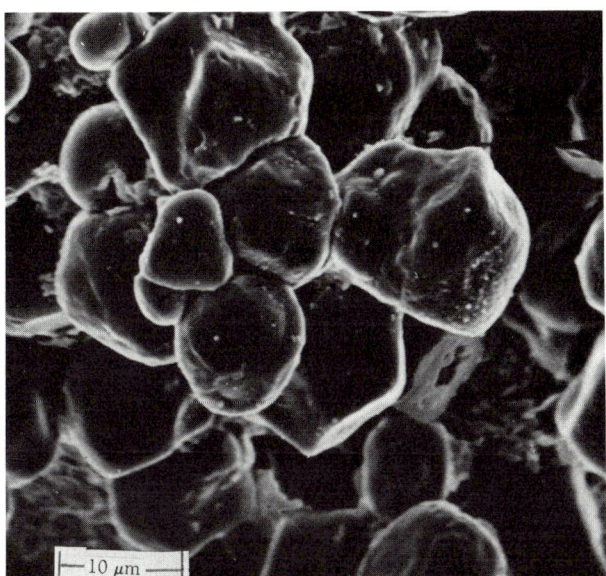

Magnification: 2,000×

Test	USP	BP
Heavy metals	≤0.001%	—
Magnesium oxide	≤2.0%	≤2.2%
Chloride	—	≤350 ppm
Sulphate	—	≤0.2%
Formaldehyde	—	+
Acid-insoluble ash	—	≤0.3%
Ash	—	≤3.5%

11. Typical Properties

Density: Particle: 1.48 g/cm³; bulk: 0.47 - <u>0.55</u>* - 0.59 g/cm³; tapped: 0.64 - <u>0.77</u> - 0.83 g/cm³
Flowability: 24 - <u>27</u> - 30% (Carr index)-see Carr, R.L., *Brit. Chem. Eng.*, 15: 1541 (1970).
Moisture content: 10 - <u>13</u> - 15% (Loss on drying)
Particle size distribution: Range: 6 - 25 μm; weight median diameter: 16 μm

These data are obtained using image shearing microscopy, particle size micrometer and analyzer (Fleming Instrument Type 526).

Solubility (at 25° C): Water - less than 1 in 10,000; ethanol (96 percent) - less than 1 in 1,000; chloroform - 1 in 3,500
Specific surface area: 0.50 - <u>0.80</u> - 1.15 m²/g (Stroehlein apparatus, single point).

*Underlined numbers are average values.

12. Stability and Storage Conditions

Store in a well-closed container. It may be kept in sealed paper packets.

13. Incompatibilities

No citations in the literature.

14. Safety

Tissue reactions and peritonitis at operation sites have been attributed to contamination with surgical glove powders containing modified maize starch. Inhalation of starch dust can cause slight (reversible) local or systemic effects.

15. Handling Precautions

Provide adequate ventilation; moderate fire and explosion hazard; avoid storage near oxidizing agents.

16. Regulatory Acceptance

USP XXI; BP 1980

17. Applications in Pharmaceutical Formulation or Technology

Lubricant, e.g., for surgeons' gloves. Vehicle for medicated dusting powders. May be sterilized by heating at 150° - 160°C for 1 hour, or by spreading in thin layers and autoclaving at 115° - 118°C for 30 minutes.

18. Related Substances

None

19. Comments

Variability in certain properties was noted for batches obtained from different suppliers. Major differences were in pH values.

20. References

1. J. C. Kelsey, *Mon. Bull. Minist. Health*, 21: 17 (1962).
2. C. T. Greenwood, *Adv. Cereal Sci. Technol.*, 1: 119 (review) (1976).
3. F. Berkhout, Manufacture of maize starch. In: *Starch Production Technology*, J. A. Radley, ed., 1976, p. 109.
4. J. A. Radley, Miscellaneous uses of starch. In: *Industrial Uses of Starch and Derivatives*, J. A. Radley, ed., 1976, p. 1.
5. C. T. Greenwood, *Adv. Carbohyd. Chem. Biochem.*, 22: 483 (1967).
6. El Saadany and M. A. Raouf, *Staerke*, 28: 208 (English) (1976).

UK: G. Rowley*

Pregelatinized Starch

1. Nonproprietary Names

NF: Pregelatinized starch
BP: Pregelatinized maize starch

2. Functional Category

BP: Pharmaceutical aid
NF: Tablet binder; tablet and/or capsule diluent; tablet disintegrant
Others: Binder; color extender

3. Synonyms

Compressible starch; *Starch 1500; National 1551*

4. Chemical Name and CAS Registry Number

—

5. Empirical Formula

—

6. Structural Formula

—

7. Commercial Availability

USA

Colorcon, Inc.
National Starch & Chemical Corp.

UK

Colorcon, Ltd.
CPC (UK), Ltd.
J&W Starches, Ltd.
Laing National, Ltd.

8. Method of Manufacture

Fully pregelatinized: Starch pastes, precooked at 62-72°C, containing up to 42% by weight of potato, wheat, or corn starch, are first dried. Chemical additives which may be included in the paste are gelatinization aids (salts or bases) and surface-active agents added to control rehydration or minimize stickiness during drying. Pastes may be spray-dried, roll-dried, or extruded or drum-dried. The dried material in the latter case is processed to produce the desired particle size range.

Partially pregelatinized: Suspensions of ungelatinized starches may be spread on hot drums where partial gelatinization and subsequent drying takes place.

9. Description

Moderately coarse to fine, white to off-white powder. It is odorless and has a slight characteristic taste. Examination of fully pregelatinized starch in a cold water slurry under a polarizing microscope reveals no significant number of ungelatinized granules which show polarization crosses. Examination of samples suspended in glycerin show characteristic forms depending on the method of drying in manufacture: irregular chunks (drum drying), thin plates Partially pregelatinized starch consists of a mixture of ungelatinized starch grains along with agglomerates of starch grains held together with gelatinized starch and having a diameter of up to 420 μm.

10. Pharmacopeial Specifications

Test	NF	BP
Identification	+	+
pH (10% slurry)	4.5-7.0	—
Loss on drying	≤14%	≤15%
Residue on ignition	≤0.5%	—
Iron	≤0.002%	—
Oxidizing substances	+	—
Sulfur dioxide	≤0.008%	—
Microbial limits		
Salmonella spp.	Negative	—
E. coli	Negative	Negative
Protein	—	0.3 - 0.5% w/w
Sulfated ash	—	≤0.5%
Acidity or alkalinity	—	pH 5.5 - 8.0 (20% dispersion)

11. Typical Properties

Solubility: Insoluble in organic solvents. Slightly soluble to soluble in cold water, depending on the degree of pregelatinization. Fully pregelatinized starch conforms to the completeness of solution test in USP. Pastes are prepared by sifting material into water while agitating in the absence of heat. Cold water-soluble matter (partially pregelatinized starches) is 10 - 20%.

Particle size distribution: Partially pregelatinized—screen analysis: through US #100: 90% minimum; retained on US #40: 0.5% maximum. Range: 30 - 150μm; Weight, median diameter: 52 μm (Coulter Counter/Alpine airjet sieve)

Specific surface area: 0.210 m²/g, 0.220 m²/g, (Quantasorb 10.51% N_2 or He); 0.27 - 0.49 m²/g (Ströhlein apparatus, N_2)

Flowability: Carr's Compressibility Index: 18-23% (Typically 19; fair to passable flow)

Rheological properties: Viscosity of aqueous preparation (2%) at 25°C: 8-10 mNs/m² (CP) at a shear rate of 676.3/second using the Haake Rotovisco RV3 Head-DMK 50. Acceleration = 250 rpm/min, maximum speed 250 rpm; Roto-NV viscosity sensor system, damping factor = 10.

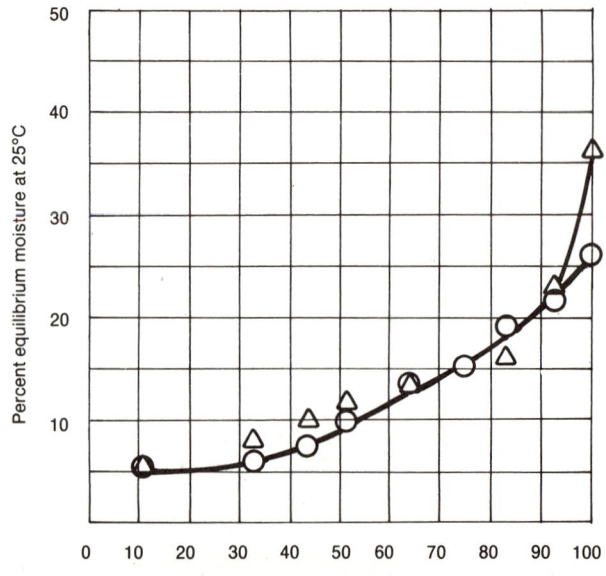

O   Corn starch, USP (National, Lot #421)
△ Pregelatinized starch, USP (National, Lot #HJW103)
Figure: 2-EMC-10 **Method:** EMC-1

Academy HPE Laboratory Project Data

	Method	Lab #	Results
Corn NF	MC-22	2	7.0%[a]
Sta-Rx 1500	MC-15	14	11.30%[b]
Corn	MC-15	34	11.12%[b]
Corn	MC-15	34	8.94%[a]
Wheat (Paygel 90)	MC-15	14	6.60%[c]
Bulk/Tap Density	BTD-7	14	B:0.650g/cm^{3} [b]
			T:0.820 g/cm^{3} [b]
Particle size dist.	PSD-2	5	68μm[a]
(Starch 1500)	PSD-2	5	80μm[b]
EMC Plot (Corn)	EMC-1	2	Fig:2-EMC-10[a]
SDI Plot			
(Wheat-Paygel 90)	SDI-1	14	Fig:14-SDI-8[c]

Suppliers: National[a]; Colorcon Ltd.[b]; Henkel[c]

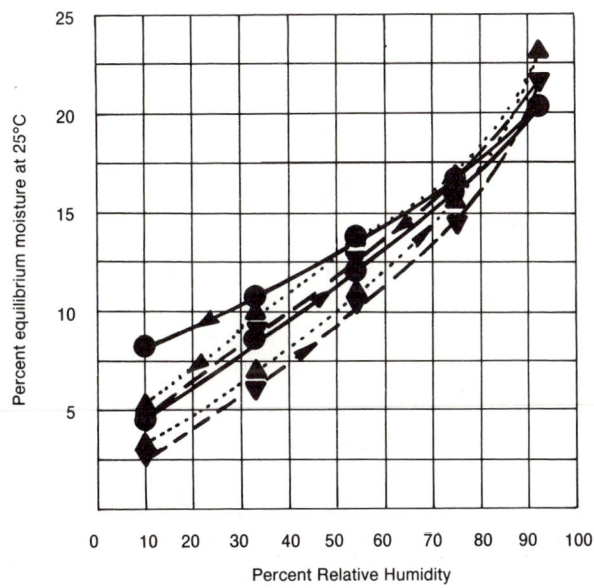

● Starch, corn, Sta-Rx (Staley, Lot #977912)
▲ Starch, wheat, pregelatinized, paygel 90 (Henkel Corp., Lot #289D)
▼ Starch, corn, Sta-Rx 1500 (Colorcon, Lot #904014)

Figure: 14-SDI-8 **Method:** SDI-1

12. Stability and Storage Conditions
Stable. Store in a well-closed container in a cool, dry place.

13. Incompatibilities
Representative of starch

14. Safety
Human and animal feeding studies have shown pregelatinized starch to be harmless.

15. Handling Precautions
No restrictions specified

16. Regulatory Acceptance
NF XVI; BP 1980

17. Applications in Pharmaceutical Formulation or Technology

Use	Concentration (%)*
Tablet binder (wet granulation)	5-10
Tablet binder (direct compression)	5-20
Tablet disintegrant	5-10
Diluent (hard gelatin encapsulation)	5-75

*Partially Pregelatinized Starch

18. Related Substances
See starch monograph.

19. Comments
Partially pregelatinized starch: Avoid the addition of more than 0.5% of magnesium stearate as a lubricant in direct compression formulations because of softening effect. *Starch 1500* is partially pregelatinized starch. *National 1551* is fully pregelatinized starch.

20. Specific References

1. Abdel M. Sakr, Hassan M. Elsabbagh and Kamla M. Emara, *Arch. Pharm. Chem., Sci. Ed.*, 2: 14-24 (1974).
2. Krishna S. Manudhane, Avinash M. Contractor, Hyo Y. Kim and Ralph F. Shangraw, *J. Pharm. Sci.*, 58: 616-620 (1969).
3. G. K. Bolhuis and C. F. Lerk, *Pharm. Weekblad*, 108: 469-481 (1973).
4. J. M. Esnard, J. Clerc, H. Tebbi, D. Duchene, J. Levy and F. Puisieux, *Ann. Pharm. Franc.*, 31: 103-116 (1973).
5. H. Hess, *Pharm. Tech.*, 2, 36-57 (1978).
6. Thelma W. Underwood and Donald E. Cadwallader, *J. Pharm. Sci.*, 61: 239-243 (1972).
7. Joseph B. Schwartz, Ellwood T. Martin and Eugene J. Dehner, *J. Pharm. Sci.*, 64: 328-332 (1975).
8. G. M. Irwin, G. J. Dodson and L. J. Ravin, *J. Pharm. Sci.*, 59: 547-550 (1970).
9. G. C. Cole and G. May, *J. Pharm. Pharmac.*, 27: 353-358 (1977).
10. L. E. Small and L. L. Augsburger, *J. Pharm. Sci.*, 66: 504-509 (1977).
11. L. E. Small and L. L. Augsburger, *Drug Dev. & Ind. Pharm.*, 4: 345-372 (1978).
12. K. T. Jaiyeoba and M. S. Spring, *J. Pharm. Pharmac.*, 32: 1-5 (1980).
13. J. E. Rees and P. J. Rue, *Drug Dev. & Ind. Pharm.*, 4: 131-156 (1978).
14. J. A. Radley, *Industrial uses of starch and derivatives*. In: "Starch Products," J. A. Radley, ed., Applied Science, 1976.
15. R. L. Carr, *Brit. Chem. Eng.* 15: 1541-1549 (1970).
16. Technical Data Sheet, STA-RX Starch, Colorcon Inc.
17. D. E. Wurster, G. E. Peck and D. O. Kildsig, *Drug Develop. & Indust. Pharm.*, 8:(3), 343-345 (1982).
18. J. C. Callahan, G. W. Cleary, M. Elefant, G. Kaplan, T. Kensler and R. A. Nash, *Drug Develop. & Indust. Pharm.*, 8:(3), 355-369 (1982).
19. R. W. Chilankurti, C. T. Rhodes and J. B. Schwartz, *Drug Develop. & Indust. Pharm.*, 8:(1), 63-86 (1982).
20. E. M. Rudnik, C. T. Rhodes, S. Welch and P. Bernardo, *Drug Develop. & Indust. Pharm.*, 8(1), 87-109 (1982).

USA: N. G. Lordi*; M. J. Groves**; Z. Chowhan**
UK: G. Rowley*; J. E. Hogan**

Stearic Acid

1. Nonproprietary Names
NF: Stearic acid
BPC: Stearic acid

2. Functional Category
USP: Tablet and/or capsule lubricant; emulsifying and/or solubilizing agent
Others: Tablet lubricant; emulsion adjunct

3. Synonyms
Octadecanoic acid; *Proiscol Wax*; *Pristerene 4900* and *4901*; *Stearinsaeure*; *Octadecan Saeure*; "stearin" is a misnomer; *Emersol 132*; *Diadem*; *Hydrofol Acid 1870, 1865, 1855*; *Crosterene SB4010, 4020, 2100*; *SA4310*

4. Chemical Name and CAS Registry Number
Stearic acid [57-11-4]
Octodecanoic acid

5. Empirical Formula   Molecular Weight
$C_{18}H_{36}O_2$ 284.47

6. Structural Formula
$CH_3(CH_2)_{16}COOH$

7. Commercial Availability
USA
Ashland Chemical Co.
J.T. Baker Chemical Co.
Croda Chemicals, Inc.
Emery Industries
Sherex Chemical Co.
Witco Chemical Corp.

UK
Croda Chemicals Ltd.
Procter and Gamble Ltd.
Unichema Chemicals Ltd.

8. Method of Manufacture
Hydrolysis of fat by continuous exposure to counter-current stream of high-temperature water and fat in a high-pressure chamber. (Colgate-Emery high-pressure process.) Further purification by steam distillation and high vacuum. Distillates are then separated by selective solvents (Emery process).

9. Description
Stearic acid is a mixture of stearic acid ($C_{18}H_{36}O_2$) and palmitic acid ($C_{16}H_{32}O_2$). The content of stearic acid is not less than 40.0%. The content of palmitic acid is not less than 40%, and the sum of the two is not less than 90%. Hard, white or faintly yellowish, somewhat glossy and crystalline solid, or white (or yellowish white) powder. Its odor and taste are slight, suggesting tallow. Stearic acid is derived from edible sources unless it is labeled for external use, in which case it is exempt from the requirement that it be prepared from edible sources.

No. SEM: KY-49
Excipient: Emersol 153—stearic acid 95%
Manufacturer: Emery Lot no.: 18895

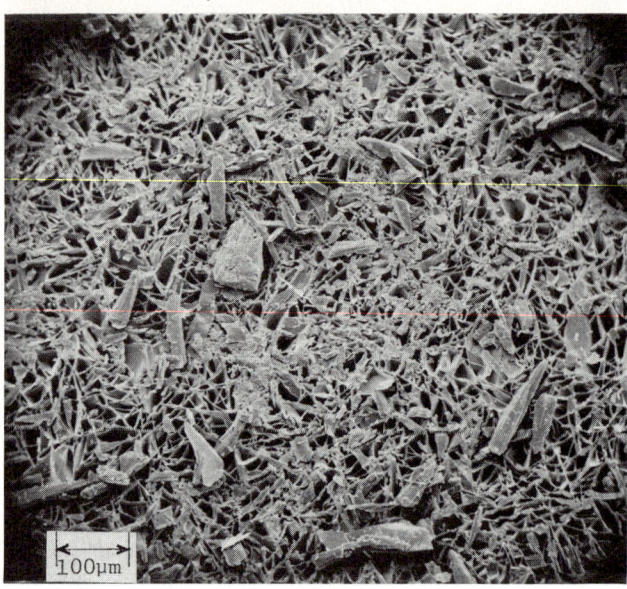

Magnification: 120× **Voltage:** 10 kV

No. SEM: KY-50
Excipient: Emersol 6332—stearic acid—food grade
Manufacturer: Emery Lot no.: 18895

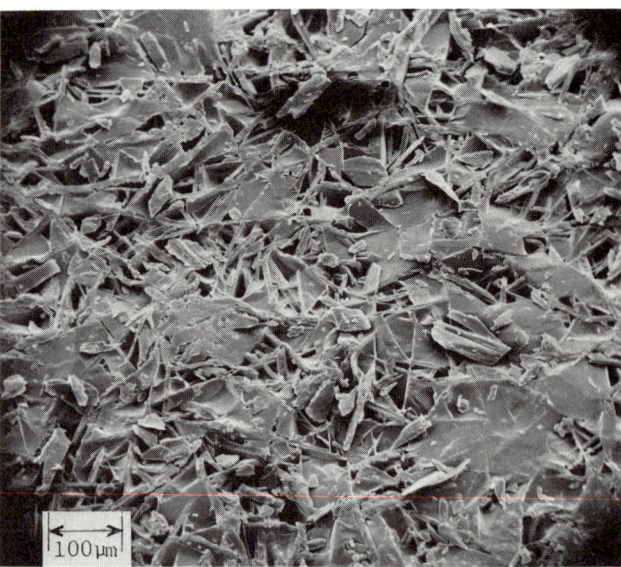

Magnification: 120× **Voltage:** 10kV

No. SEM: KY-51
Excipient: Stearic acid USP (Hydrofol Acid 1655)
Manufacturer: Sherex Chem. Co. **Lot no.:** 9303-M639-521

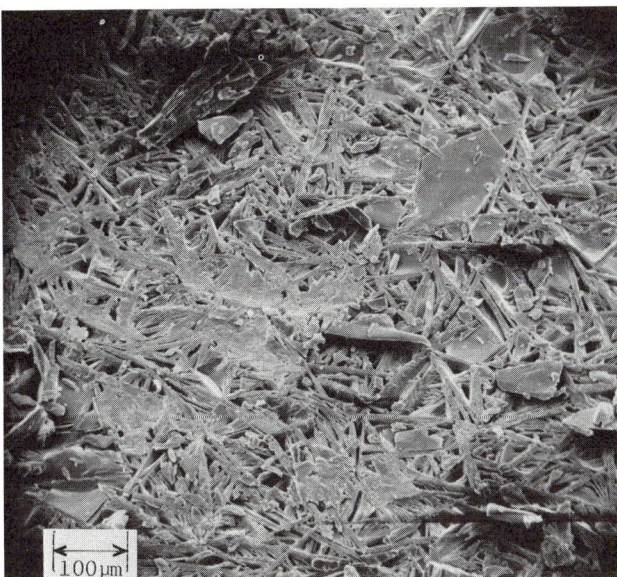

Magnification: 120×; **Voltage:** 10kV;

No. SEM:KY-52
Excipient: Stearic acid (Hydrofol Acid 1870)
Manufacturer: Sherex Chem. Co. **Lot no.:** 9227-M635-421

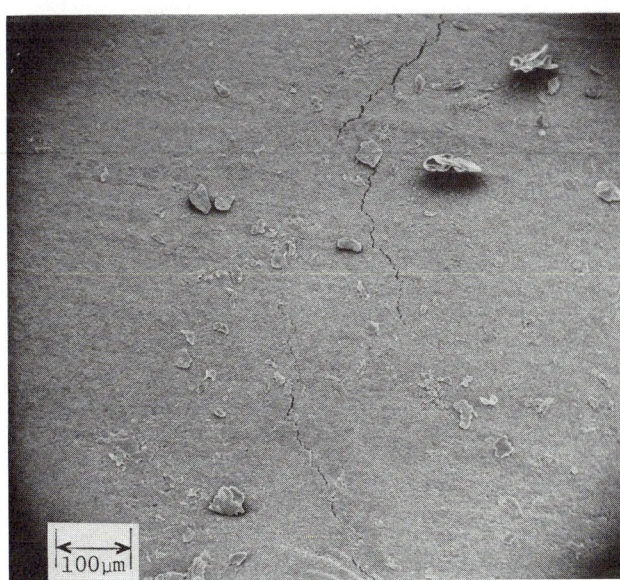

Magnification: 120× **Voltage:** 10kV

10. Pharmacopeial Specifications

Test	NF	BPC
Congealing temperature	Not lower than 54°C	—
Residue on ignition	≤0.1%	—
Heavy metals	≤0.001%	—
Mineral acid	+	+

Test	NF	BPC
Neutral fat or paraffin	+	+
Iodine value	≤4	≤4
Assay	(1) $C_{18}H_{36}O_2$≥40%	
	(1)+(2) $C_{16}H_{32}O_2$≥40% ≥90%	
Acid value	—	200-210
Melting point	—	≥54°C
Sulfated ash	—	≤0.1%

11. Typical Properties

Acid value: 206-209
Boiling point: 383°C
Melting point: (a) 59-64°C
(b) 51-62.5°C
(c) 63-69.2°C
Refractive index: d_4^{20} = 0.847; d^{70} = 0.847; n_D^{20} = 1.4337; n_D^{80} = 1.4229
Solubility: Almost insoluble in water; 1:21 in alcohol; 1:5 in benzene; 1:2 in chloroform; 1:6 in carbon tetrachloride; 1:3 in ether.
Density: (Bulk) 0.847 g/cm³
Moisture content: Almost zero
Saponification value: 200-220
(See Tables I and II)

Academy HPE Laboratory Project Data

	Method	Lab #	Results
Solubility:			
Water 25°C	SOL-6	23	<0.001 g/ml[a]
Water 37°C	SOL-6	23	<0.001 g/ml[a]
Alcohol 25°C	SOL-6	23	0.048 g/ml[a]
Alcohol 37°C	SOL-6	23	0.064 g/ml[a]
Prop. glycol 25°C	SOL-6	23	0.025 g/ml[a]
Prop. glycol 37°C	SOL-6	23	0.025 g/ml[a]
Hexane 25°C	SOL-6	23	0.050 g/ml[a]
Hexane 37°C	SOL-6	23	0.167 g/ml[a]
Water 25°C	SOL-6	23	<0.001 g/ml[c]
Water 37°C	SOL-6	23	<0.001 g/ml[c]
Alcohol 25°C	SOL-6	23	0.116 g/ml[c]
Alcohol 37°C	SOL-6	23	0.320 g/ml[c]
Prop. glycol 25°C	SOL-6	23	0.025 g/ml[c]
Prop. glycol 37°C	SOL-6	23	0.025 g/ml[c]
Hexane 25°C	SOL-6	23	>0.099 g/ml[c]
Hexane 37°C	SOL-6	23	>0.267 g/ml[c]
Water 25°C	SOL-6	23	<0.001 g/ml[b]
Water 37°C	SOL-6	23	<0.001 g/ml[b]
Alcohol 25°C	SOL-6	23	0.049 g/ml[b]
Alcohol 37°C	SOL-6	23	0.066 g/ml[b]
Prop. glycol 25°C	SOL-6	23	0.800-1.250 g/ml[b]
Prop. glycol 37°C	SOL-6	23	0.800-1.250 g/ml[b]
Hexane 25°C	SOL-6	23	2.500 g/ml[b]
Hexane 37°C	SOL-6	23	2.500 g/ml[b]
Density:			
Hydrofol Acid 1655	DE-3	36	0.8864 g/ml[c]
Emersol 153	DE-3	36	0.8745 g/ml[b]
Hydrofol Acid 18%	DE-3	36	0.9859 g/ml[c]
Emersol 6332	DE-3	36	0.8789 g/ml[b]

Suppliers: Baker[a]; Emery[b]; Sherex[c]

Table I — Approximate Specifications of Commercial Grades of Stearic Acid

Grades of Stearic Acid	Titer, °C Min	Titer, °C Max	Iodine value Min	Iodine value Max	Acid value Min	Acid value Max	Saponification value Min	Saponification value Max	Moisture %
Commercially pure, 97%	66	69	0.5	1.0	196	200	197	201	0.2
Commercially pure, 90%	65	68	0.7	1.0	196	200	197	201	0.2
Triple pressed	54.5	56	—	0.5	205	210	206	212	0.5
Double pressed	54	54.5	5.0	7.0	205	211	206	212	—
Single pressed	53	54	5.0	10.0	207	210	207	211	—
Hydrogenated tallow	57	60	—	2	200	206	201	207	—

NOTE: All require 0.5% unsaponifiability

Table II — Specifications of Stearic Acid and Palmitic Acid—Emery Chemical Company

	Titer, °C	Iodine value Max.	Color—% trans. 440/550 nm/Min.	Acid value	Sapon. value
Emersol 110 Stearic Acid	52.8-53.5	8-12	60/94	205-210	206-211
Emersol 120 Stearic Acid,[1,5]	53.7-54.7	5-7	88/89	205-210	206-211
Emerson 132 U.S.P. Lily Stearic Acid[1,5,8]	54.5-55.5	0.5	93/99	205-210	207-211
Emersol 140 Palmitic Acid[3]	53.4-55.5	2	93/99	209-214	210-215
Emersol 142 Palmitic Acid[4]	55.7-57.2	1	93/99	213-218	213-219
Emersol 144 Palmitic Acid[5]	59-62	0.5	93/99	216-219	217-220
Emersol 146 Palmitic Acid	53.9-55	2	93/99	207-213	208-214
Emersol 150 Stearic Acid[1,2]	63.9-65	1	93/99	197-202	198-203
Emersol 153 Stearic Acid[5]	67-69	1.0	80/97	196-199	197-200
Emery 400 Stearic Acid	52 minimum	7-10	1/29	193-209	195-211
Emery 404 Stearic Acid	53.5-54.5	6-9	1/50	197-209	199-211[7]
Emery 410 Stearic Acid	56.1-60	4-7	40/86	195-209	197-207
Emery 420 Stearic Acid	57.2-60	2	71/97	200-207	201-208
Emery 421 Stearic Acid	59.5-61.5	1	90/99	200-207	201-208
Emery 422 Stearic Acid	55.8-57	1	90/99	203-209	204-210

[1]Also available in powdered grades. Sieve test: 99.5% min. through No. 30 U.S. Standard Sieve; 98% through No. 100
[2]80% minimum stearic content
[3]67% minimum palmitic content
[4]78% minimum palmitic content
[5]Corresponding food-grade products available; see Section 4b
[6]By GLC analysis, ASTM D 1983-64T
[7]Typical property
[8]For external use only—for internal use see Emersol 6332 (4b)

12. Stability and Storage Conditions

Stable in pure form; may contain butylated hydroxytoluene (0.005%) as an anti-oxidant. Store in a well-closed container protected from light and heat.

13. Incompatibilities

Incompatible with most metal hydroxides.

14. Safety

Powder may be irritating, but due to very slight water solubility it is easily removed by neutralization.

15. Handling Precautions

Powdered stearic acid may cause irritation, particularly if a person is sensitive to dermatitis.

16. Regulatory Acceptance

NF XVI; BPC 1973

17. Application in Pharmaceutical Formulation or Technology

Use	Concentration
Tablet lubricant	1-3%
Enteric coating ingredient	—
Ointments and creams	≤5-15%

18. Related Substances

Purified stearic acid, NF, is derived from edible sources, and is a mixture of stearic acid and palmitic acid, together comprising 96% of the total content. Stearic acid content must be at least 90% of the total.

NF Specifications: Congealing temperature, 66-69°F; Iodine value, ≥1.5; Acid value, 195-200 (1 g sample).

Other requirements: Stearic acid meets the requirements for residue on ignition, heavy metals, mineral acid, neutral fat or paraffin and assay for stearic acid listed under the Stearic Acid NF monograph.

19. Comments

—

20. References

1. P. J. Jarosz and E. L. Parrott, Effect of tablet lubricant on axial and radial work of failure, *Drug Develop. and Ind. Pharm.*, 8(3), 445-453 (1982).
2. Z. T. Chowhan, Physical paths of instability, *Pharmaceutical Technology*, 6(9), 47-65 (1982).
3. P. Musikabhumma, M. H. Rubinstein and K. A. Khan, Evaluation of stearic acid and polyethylene glycol 6000 as binders for tabletting potassium phenethicillin, *Drug Develop. and Ind. Pharm.*, 8(2), 169-188 (1982).
4. K. T. Mitrevej and L. L. Augsburger, Adherence of tablets in a rotary tablet press II—Effect of blending time and lubricant concentration, *Drug Develop. and Ind. Pharm.*, 8(2), 237-282 (1982).

USA: T. W. Schwartz*; A. Palmieri, III**; J. Mullins**
UK: J. R. Nixon**

Stearyl Alcohol

1. Nonproprietary Name
NF: Stearyl alcohol

2. Functional Category
USP: Stiffening agent
Others: Component of the oil phase of ointments and emulsions to improve the texture; nonionic emulsifier for water-in-oil emulsion; drug release matrix; emulsion adjunct

3. Synonyms
Stenol, octadecyl alcohol, octadecanol, 1-octadecanol, n-octadecanol; *Alfol 18; n-Octadecyl alcohol; Crodacol S; Lorol C; Laurex 18*

4. Chemical Names and CAS Registry Number
1-Octadecanol
1-Octadecanol [112-92-5]

5. Empirical Formula
$C_{18}H_{38}O$

Molecular Weight
270.48

6. Structural Formula
$CH_3-(CH_2)_{16}-CH_2OH$

7. Commercial Availability

USA
A & S Corporation
Conoco Chemicals Co.
Croda Chemicals Inc.
Fallek Chemical Co.
Henkel Corporation
Kraft Chemical Co.
Madron Products, Ltd.
M. Michel and Company

UK
Albright & Wilson Ltd.
Croda Chemicals Ltd.
Klitco Chemical Co. Ltd.
Madron Products Ltd.

8. Method of Manufacturing
Prepared through the reduction of the corresponding fatty acid; also through the reducing action of lithium aluminum hydride on ethyl stearate.

9. Description
Hard, white, waxy pieces, flakes or granules with a slight characteristic odor and bland taste.

SEM:KY-53
Excipient: Cachalot—stearyl alcohol USP
Manufacturer: M. Michel and Co. Inc. **Lot no.:** S-56

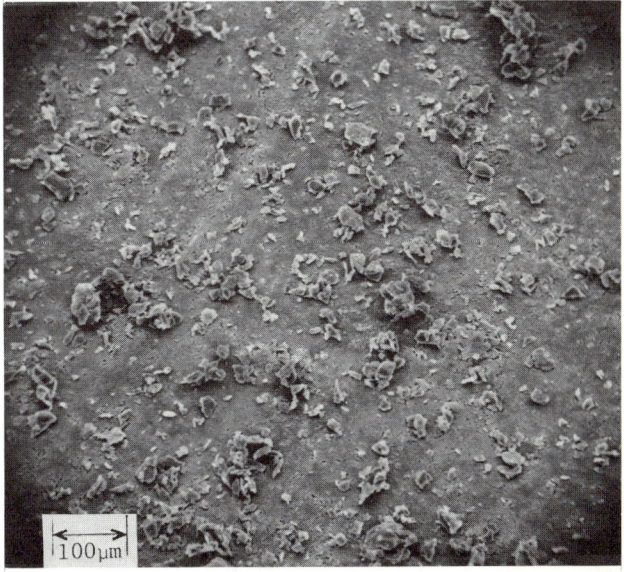

Magnification: 120× **Voltage:** 10 kV

SEM:KY-54
Excipient: Stearyl alcohol 95% USP
Manufacturer: A & S Corp. **Lot no.** 3237

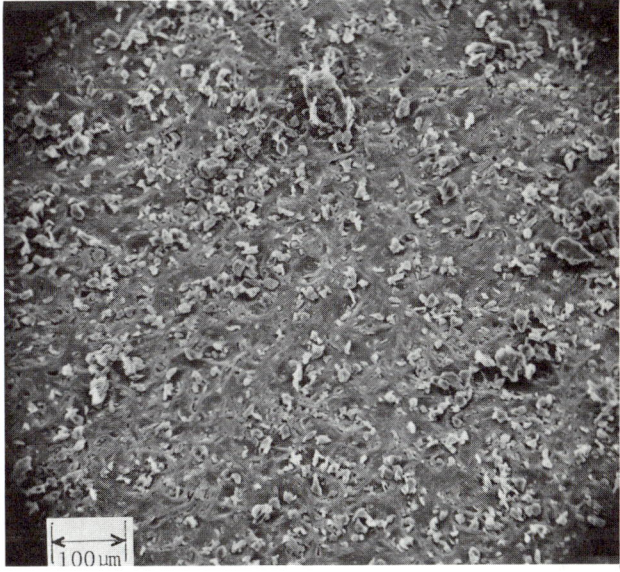

Magnification: 120× **Voltage:** 10kV

SEM:KY-55
Excipient: Crodacol S(70)—stearyl alcohol
Manufacturer: Croda Inc. **Lot no.:** 62978

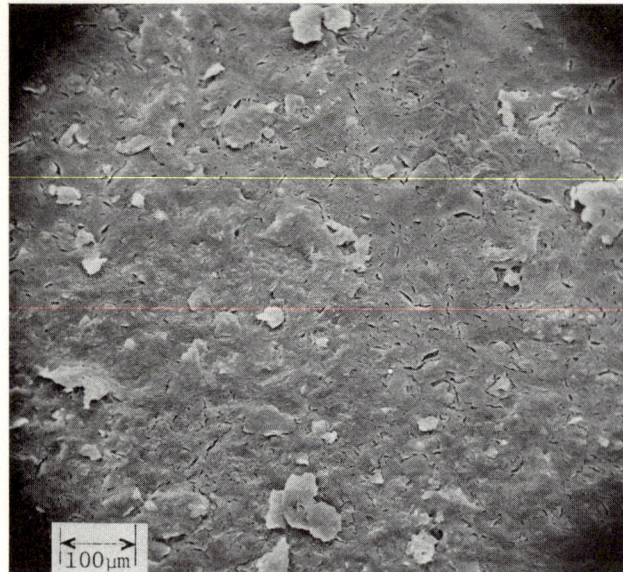

Magnification: 120× **Voltage:** 10 kV

SEM:KY-56
Excipient: Crodacol S(95)—stearyl alcohol USP
Manufacturer: Croda Inc. **Lot no.:** 11679

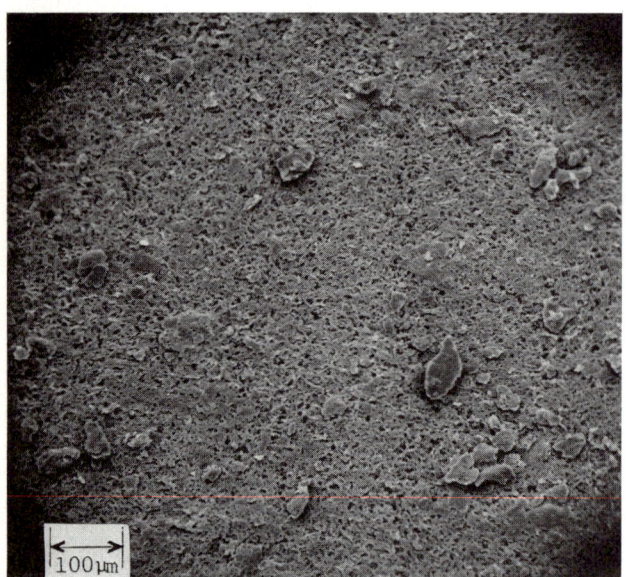

Magnification: 120× **Voltage:** 10 kV

10. Pharmacopeial Specifications

Test	NF
Identification	+
Melting range	Between 55° and 60°C
Acid value	≤2
Iodine value	≤2
Hydroxyl value	Between 195 and 220
Assay	≥90.0% of $C_{18}H_{38}O$, the remainder consisting chiefly of related alcohols

11. Typical Properties

Boiling point: 210.5°C/15 mmHg
Density: 0.8124 g/cm³ @ 50°C
Flash point: (Cleveland) open cup 375°F/191°C
Refractive index: 1.4388 @ 60°C
Saponification value: ≤1
Solidification point: 55° to 57°C
Solubilities:

Acetone	S
Benzene	S
Carbon tetrachloride	M
Cyclohexane	M
95% alcohol	M
Ethyl ether	M
Isopropyl alcohol	S
Kerosene	S
Methanol	M
Light mineral oil	S
VMP naphtha	S
Trichlorethylene	S
Turpentine	S
Water	I

S = Soluble, M = Miscible, I = Insoluble
Vapor pressure: 349.5 @ 760 mm
Viscosity (centipoises): 10.0 @ 60°C

Academy HPE Laboratory Project Data

	Method	Lab No.	Results
Water 25°C	SOL-4	10	0.0000 g/ml
Water 37°C	SOL-4	10	0.00001 g/ml
Alcohol 25°C	SOL-4	10	0.0055 lg/ml
Alcohol 37°C	SOL-4	10	0.0176 lg/ml
Prop. glycol 25°C	SOL-4	10	0.0100 g/ml
Prop. glycol 37°C	SOL-4	10	NA
n-hexane 25°C	SOL-4	10	0.0095 g/ml
n-hexane 37°C	SOL-4	10	0.1481 g/ml

Supplier: A & S Company

12. Stability and Storage Conditions

Stearyl alcohol is stable to acid and alkali. Usually does not go rancid. Preserve in a well-closed container.

13. Incompatibilities

No citations in the literature.

14. Safety

Stearyl alcohol is considered nontoxic, nonirritating and essentially innocuous. However, urticaria-like dermatitis has been reported with its use in topical formulations (Gaul, L. E., *Arch. Derm.*, 99:593 (1969).

15. Handling Precautions

No restrictions specified.

16. Regulatory Acceptance

NF XVI

17. Application in Pharmaceutical Formulations or Technology

Solid dosage forms: Used in the controlled release formulations.

Semi-Solid dosage forms: Used in ointments and creams to increase viscosity and physical stability. Also used to increase the water-holding capacity of petrolatum and in combination with hydrophillic emulsifiers in complex emulsion systems. It functions as an emollient and auxillary emulsifier.

18. Related Substances

Cetostearyl alcohol

19. Comments

None

20. References

1. P. L. Madan *et al.*, *J. Pharm. Sci.*, 63:280 (1974).
2. L. E. Gaul, *Arch. Derm.*, 99:593 (1969).
3. P. L. Madan *et al.*, *J. Pharm. Sci.*, 61:1586 (1972).
4. Hans Schott and Suk Kyu Han, *J. Pharm. Sci.*, 64:658 (1975).
5. L. S. C. Wan and P. K. C. Poon, *Can. J. Pharm. Sci.*, 5:104 (1970).
6. R. R. Egan and Owen Portwood, *Cosmet. Perfum.*, 89:39 (1974).
7. Krishna Kumar *et al.*, *Indian J. Pharm.*, 37:57 (1975).
8. C. M. Prasad and G. P. Srivastava, *Indian J. Hosp. Pharm.*, 8:21 (1971).
9. George E. Mapstone, *Cosmet. Perfum.*, 84:31 (1974).
10. B. W. Barry, *J. Pharm. and Pharmacol.*, 25:131 (1973).

General Product Brochures and Technical Data Sheets from:
1. Conoco Chemicals (Alfol 18 U.S.P.)
2. M. Michel and Company (Cachalot fatty alcohols)
3. Croda, Inc. (Crodacol S)

USA: N. H. Kobayashi*; J. Mullins**

Sucrose

1. Nonproprietary Name

NF: Sucrose
BP/EP: Sucrose

2. Functional Category

USP: Sweetening agent; tablet and/or capsule diluent; coating agent
Others: Demulcent; granulating agent; viscosity-increasing agent; preservative

3. Synonyms

Beet sugar; cane sugar; refined sugar; saccharose; sugar

4. Chemical Names and CAS Registry Number

β-D-Fructofuranosyl α-D-glucopyranoside
Sucrose [57-50-1]

5. Empirical Formula   Molecular Weight

$C_{12}H_{22}O_{11}$ 342.30

6. Structural Formula

α: Axial
β: Equatorial

7. Commercial Availability

USA

Accurate Chemical & Scientific Corp.
Aldrich Chemical Co., Inc.
Alltech Associates, Inc.
American Research Products Co.
American Scientific & Chemical
Amstar Corp., American Sugar Div.
Anachemia Chemicals, Inc.
Apache Chemicals, Inc.
J. T. Baker Chemical Co.
BBL Microbiology Systems, Div. of Becton Dickinson
Biochemical Laboratories, Inc.
Bio-Rad Laboratories
Calbiochem-Behring Corp.
California & Hawaii Sugar Co.
Chem Service, Inc.
Chemical Dynamics Corp.
Delamar, Inc.
Eastern Chemical, Div. of Guardian Chemical Corp.
Eastman Organic Chemicals, Eastman Kodak Co.
EM Laboratories, Inc.
Fischer Scientific Co.
Gallard Schlesinger Chemical Manufacturing Corp.
Gibco Laboratories
Great Western Sugar Co.
Holly Sugar Co.
ICN Nutritional Biochemicals, Life Science Group

Imperial Sugar Co.
Isolab Inc.
La Pine Scientific Co.
Leon Laboratories, Div. of Leon Industries, Inc.
Mallinckrodt, Inc., Specialty Chemicals
MC&B Manufacturing Chemists, Inc.
Miles Laboratories, Inc., Research Products
Pfanstiehl Laboratories, Inc.
P-L Biochemicals, Inc.
Sigma Chemical Co.
Supelco, Inc.
George Uhe Co., Inc.

UK

British Sugar Corp., Ltd.
Hay Lambert Ltd.
Mallinckrodt, Ltd.
Tate & Lyle Refineries

8. Method of Manufacture

Obtained from sugarcane and sugar beet. The juice obtained from these sources is heated to coagulate the water-soluble proteins, which are removed by skimming. The resultant solution is decolorized with charcoal and concentrated. Upon cooling, the sucrose crystallizes out. The remaining solution is concentrated again and yields more sucrose, brown sugar, and molasses.

9. Description

Colorless crystals, crystalline masses or blocks, or a white, crystalline powder. It is odorless and has a sweet taste.

SEM: KY-57
Excipient: Sucrose
Manufacturer: Great Western Sugar Co.   **Lot no:** 1-2-80

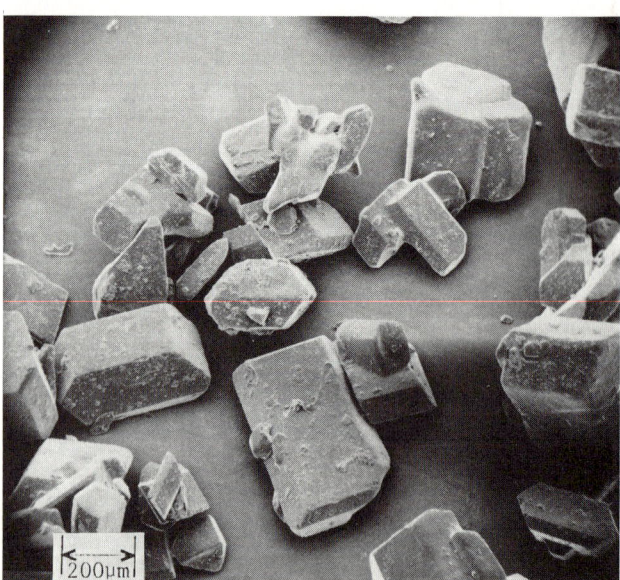

Magnification: 60× **Voltage:** 10 kV

SEM: KY-57
Excipient: Sucrose
Manufacturer: Great Western Sugar Co.   **Lot no:** 1-2-80

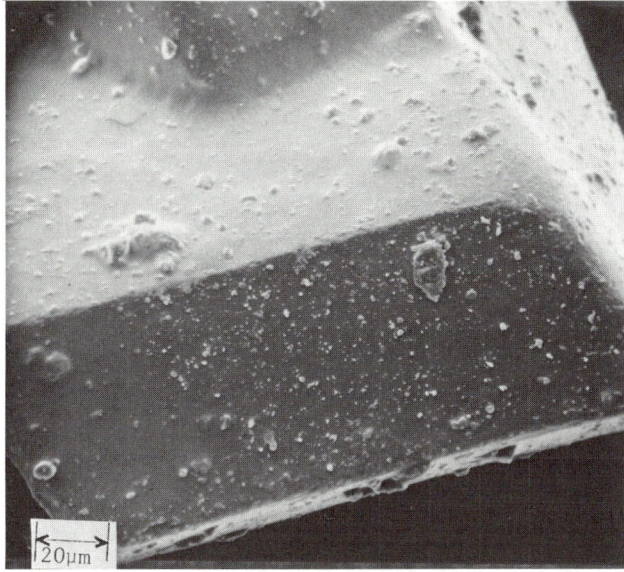

Magnification: 600× **Voltage:** 10 kV

SEM: KY-61
Excipient: Holly extra fine sugar
Manufacturer: Holly Sugar Corp.   **Lot no:** TNG-2-2

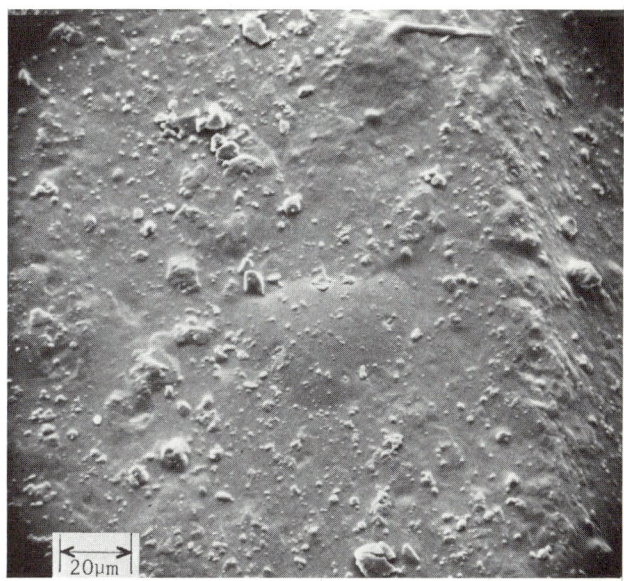

Magnification: 600× **Voltage:** 10 kV

SEM: KY-61
Excipient: Holly extra fine sugar
Manufacturer: Holly Sugar Corp.   **Lot no:** TNG-2-2

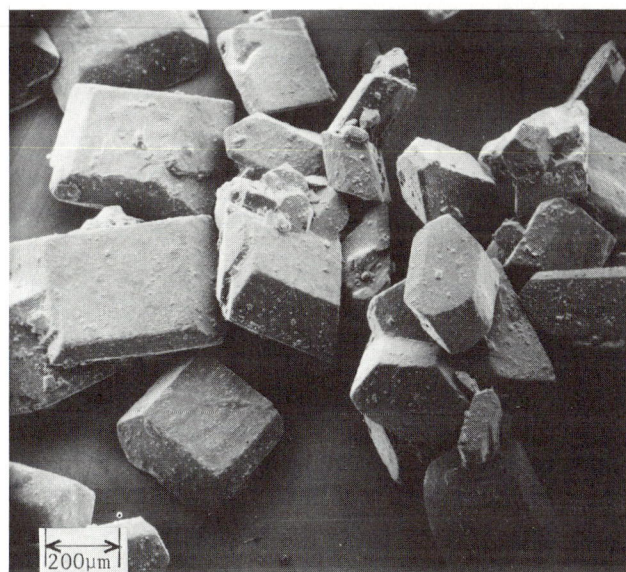

Magnification: 60× **Voltage:** 10 kV

10. Pharmacopeial Specifications

Test	NF	BP/EP
Identification	—	+
Specific optical rotation	—	+66.2 - +66.8°
Specific rotation	≥ +65.9	—
Residue on ignition	≤0.05%	≤0.05%
Heavy metals	≤5 ppm	—
Lead	—	≤0.5 ppm
Chloride	≤0.0035%	—
Sulfate	≤0.006%	—
Sulfated ash	—	≤0.02%
Invert sugar	+	—
Calcium	+	—
Acidity or alkalinity	—	+
Clarity, odor and color of solution	—	+
Barium	—	+
Sulfite	—	+
Dextrins	—	+
Foreign coloring matter	—	+
Glucose and invert sugar	—	+
Foreign sugars	—	+

11. Typical Properties

Compression characteristics: Crystalline sucrose: See Figure 1; compression machine used: Manesty E2; speed of compression: 50 strokes per minute (machine lubricated after each compression.); diameter of compacts: 12.5 mm; weight range of compacts: 675 ± 10 mg; tablet strength instrument: Schleuniger; no lamination was encountered.
Density: Particle, 1.56 g/cm³ (crystalline sucrose); helium pycnometry, 1.56 g/cm³ (powdered sucrose); bulk, 0.93 g/cm³ (crystalline sucrose), 0.60 g/cm³ (powdered sucrose); tapped, 1.03 g/cm³ (crystalline sucrose), 1,250 taps 0.82 g/cm³ (powdered sucrose)

Flowability: Free flowing (crystalline sucrose); cohesive solid (powdered sucrose)

Melting point: 168°C - 186°C (with decomposition)

Moisture content: (a) Karl Fischer: 0.1%; (b) Moisture sorption isotherm (samples dried initially at 60°C over silica gel for 24 hrs.); See Figures 2 and 3

Particle size: Powdered sucrose—white granular powder, angular and irregular; crystalline sucrose—colorless granular solid, crystalline and roughly cubic

Particle size distribution: See Figures 4 and 5

Solubility:

Solvent	S (g in 100 ml solvent) (at 25°C)	(at 60°C)
Water	200	333
Aqueous buffers (Teorell and Stenhagen phosphate-citrate-borate)	200	333
Ethanol (100%)	0.25	
(96%)	0.27	
Propan-2-ol	0.25	

Specific surface area: 0.41 m²/g (crystalline sucrose); 0.77 m²/g (powdered sucrose); (micromeritics model 2205)

Color: Hunter Colorlab Tester

Powdered sucrose: L = 83.4
                    a = +0.4
                    b = +0.9

Crystalline sucrose: L = 73.1
                      a = +2.5
                      b = +0.7

Specific gravity: d_4^{25} 1.587. d_4^{20} of aqueous solutions (g/100g); 2%, 1.0060; 6%, 1.0219; 10%, 1.0381; 20%, 1.0810; 30%, 1.1270; 40%, 1.1764; 50%, 1.2296; 60%, 1.2865; 70%, 1.3471; 76%, 1.3854.

Refractive index: n_D^{20} of 10% solution = 1.34783

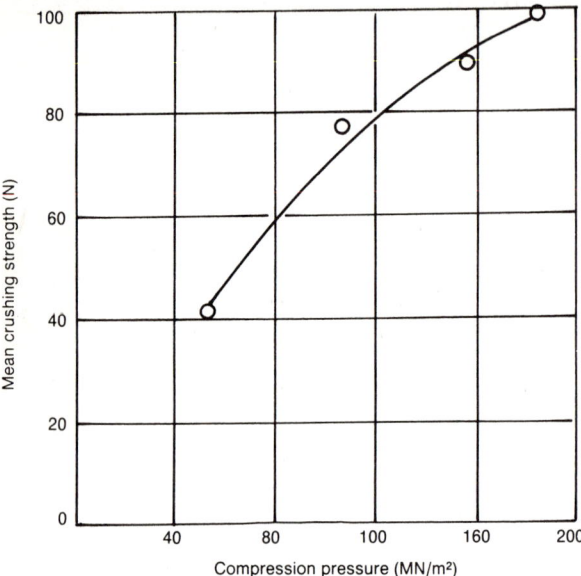

Figure 1: Compression characteristics (crystalline sucrose)

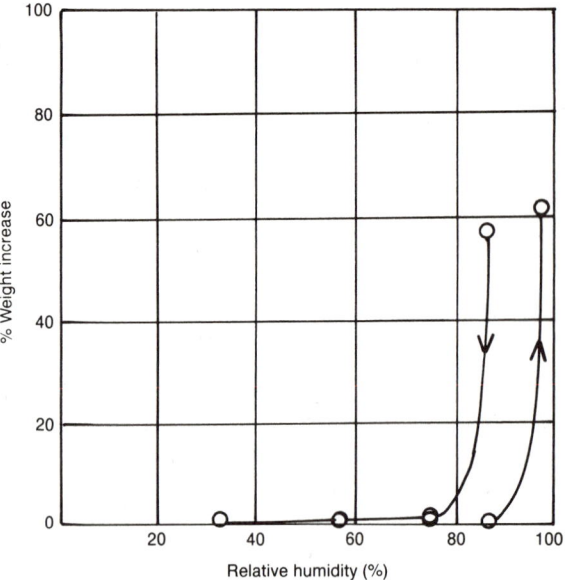

Figure 2: Moisture sorption-desorption isotherms (crystalline sucrose)

NOTE: At 97% relative humidity, sufficient water was absorbed to cause dissolution of the solid.

Figure 3: Moisture sorption-desorption isotherms (powdered sucrose)

NOTE: At 90% relative humidity, sufficient water was absorbed to cause dissolution of the solid.

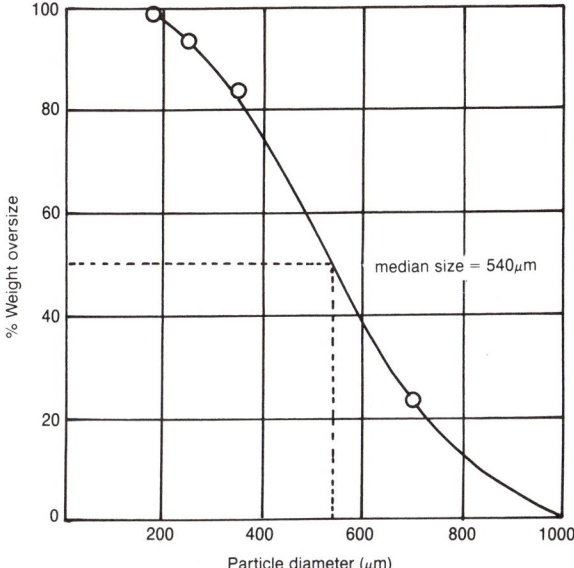

Figure 4: Particle size distribution (crystalline sucrose)

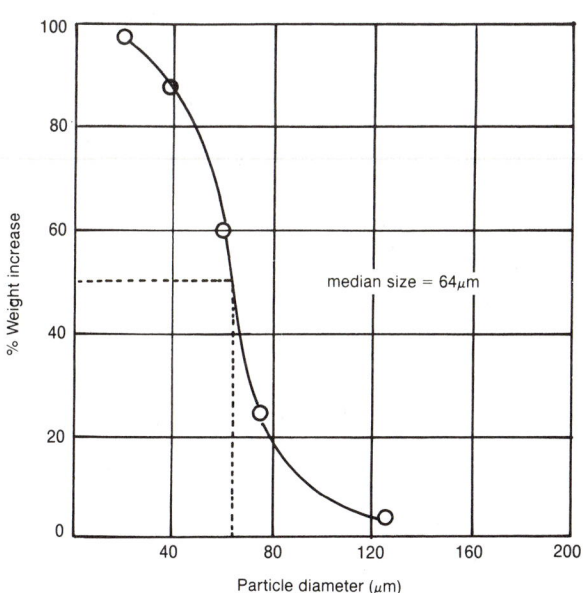

Figure 5: Particle size distribution (powdered sucrose)

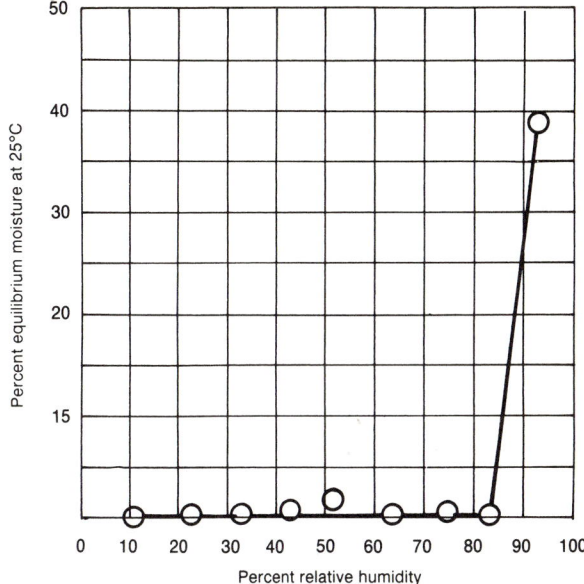

Sucrose USP, (Amstar, Lot No 51995)
Figure: 10-EMC-5   **Method**: EMC-1

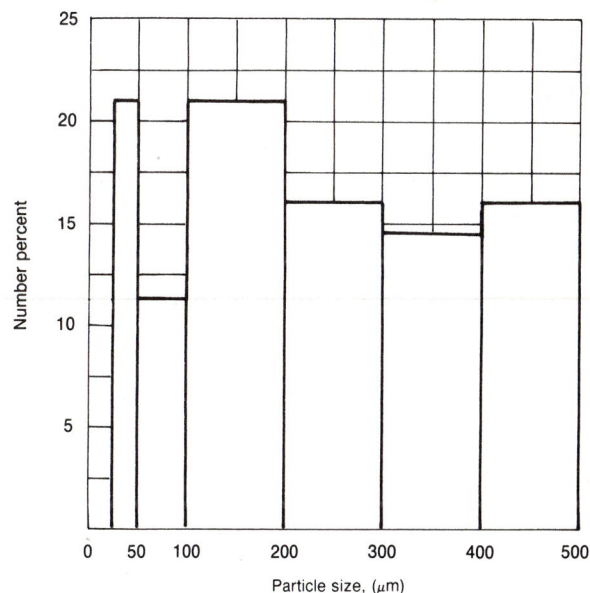

Sucrose
Figure: 3-PSD-3   **Method**: PSD-9

Academy HPE Laboratory Project Data			
	Method	**Lab #**	**Results**
Moisture content	MC-10	10	<0.10%[a]
Moisture content	MC-8	5	0.15%[c]
Density	DE-1	7	1.62 ± 0.02g/cm³[b]
Particle friability	PF-1	36	0.010%[c]
Average flow rate	FLO-2	3	46.9g/sec.[c]
EMC plot	EMC-1	10	Fig:10-EMC-5[a]
PSD plot	PSD-9	3	Fig:3-PSD-3[a]

Suppliers: Amstar[a]; C&H Sugar[b]; Great Western[c]

12. Stability and Storage Conditions

Good stability at room temperature and at moderate relative humidity. Absorbs up to 1% moisture, which is given up upon heating to 90°C. Caramelizes when heated to temperatures above 160°C. Dilute solutions are liable to attack by microorganisms. Store in a well-closed container.

13. Incompatibilities

Powdered sucrose is often contaminated with traces of heavy metals. This can lead to incompatibility with active ingredients (for instance, ascorbic acid). Sucrose may also be contaminated with sulfite (from the refining process). With high sulfite content, color changes can occur in coated tablets. There is a limit for sulfite content in certain coating colors: maximum, 1 ppm (calculated as sulfur). In the presence of dilute or concentrated acids, sucrose is hydrolyzed or inverted to glucose and fructose (invert sugar). Dilute solutions are subject to attack by microorganisms.

14. Safety

Sucrose should be administered with care to patients with diabetes mellitus. Acute oral LD_{50} is 35.4 ± 7 g/kg in males and $29.7 \pm$ g/kg in females. Although these levels may be extrapolated to the equivalent of a pound of candy in a 25-pound child, the acute gastroenteritis observed in animals would surely produce vomiting in humans. The intravenous use of 50% solutions (200 to 300 ml) to produce diuresis or to lower intracranial pressure carries a grave risk of renal damage. Sucrose is considered to be more cariogenic than other carbohydrates because it is more easily converted to dental plaque, and this plaque could hold acid fermentation products in contact with the enamel. Some studies have shown an increase in coronary disease and myocardial infarction in patients consuming more sucrose than control subjects.

15. Handling Precautions

A nontoxic nuisance dust; threshold limit value, 10 mg/m³

16. Regulatory Acceptance

NF XVI; BP/EP 1980

17. Applications in Pharmaceutical Formulation or Technology

Tableting: Sucrose (as syrup 50-67%) is used as a binding agent for wet granulation. In powder form, it serves as a dry binder (2-20%) or as a bulking agent and sweetener in chewable tablets and lozenges. Tablets which contain large amounts of sucrose may harden to give poor disintegration.

Use	Concentration
Tablet binder (wet granulation)	2-20%
Tablet binder (dry granulation)	2-20%
Tablet coating (syrup)	≤85%
Viscosity syrup	≤85%
Sweetening agent	≤85%

Coating: In coating syrups sucrose is included at concentrations between 50 and 80%. Typical boiling point values for such syrups (without inversion of the sugar) are as follows.

Sucrose (%)	Boiling point (°C)
50	101.5
60	103
64	104
72	105.5
75	107
77.5	108.5
80	110.5

With higher concentrations, partial inversion of the sugar occurs. Inverted sugar at concentrations greater than 5% makes sugarcoating difficult.

Liquid dosage forms: Syrups containing sucrose (e.g., syrup BP 66.7% w/w or syrup NF 85% w/v) are used as vehicles to enhance palatability or to increase viscosity.

18. Related Substances

Compressible sugar NF; confectioner's sugar NF.
Sugar beadlets or nonpareil seeds contain 65-85% sucrose with starch and invert sugar.

19. Comments

—

20. Specific References

1. J. Yudkin, Sugar and disease, *Nature*, 239: 197 (1972).
2. A. O. Onyekweli and N. Pilpel, Effect of temperature change on the densification and compression of griseofulvin and sucrose powders, *J. Pharm. Pharmacol.*, 33: 397-381 (1983).
3. R. H. Barry, M. Weiss, J. B. Johnson and E. DeRitter, Stability of phenylpropanolamine hydrochloride in liquid formulations containing sugars, *J. Pharm. Sci.*, 71(1): 116-118 (1982).

USA: W. T. Gloor*; J. Russo**; Z. Chowhan**
UK: N. A. Armstrong

Compressible Sugar

1. Nonproprietary Name
NF: Compressible sugar

2. Functional Category
NF: Sweetening agent tablet and/or capsule diluent.

3. Synonyms
Direct compacting sucrose *Nu-Tab*; *Di-Pac*; *Sugartab*

4. Chemical name and CAS Registry Number
—

5. Empirical Formula
Primarily $C_{12}H_{22}O_{11}$. Contains not less than 95.0% and not more than 98.0% of sucrose.

6. Structural Formula
—

7. Commercial Availability
USA
Amstar Corporation
Desmo Chemical Co.
Edward Mendell
Ingredients Technology Corp.
Sucrest Corporation

UK
Forum Chemicals
Wilfred Smith, Ltd.

8. Method of Manufacture
Not reported by the manufacturers.

9. Description
Nu-Tab: Composed of processed sucrose, about 4% invert sugar, and 0.1% to 0.2% each of corn starch and magnesium sterate.
Di-Pac: Crystallized product consisting of about 98% sucrose and 2% higher saccharides (dextrins).
Sugartab: An agglomerated sugar product containing approximately 90-93% sucrose, the balance being invert sugar.

10. Pharmacopeial Specifications

Test	NF
Identification	+
Microbial limits	Absence of *E. coli* and *Salmonella* species
Loss on drying	0.25-1.0% by wt.
Residue on ignition	≤0.1%
Chloride	≤0.014%

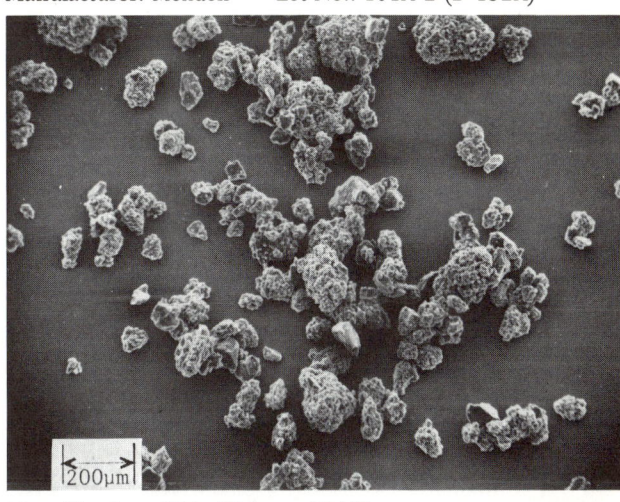

SEM: KY-58
Excipient: Compressible Sugar (Sugartab)
Manufacturer: Mendell   **Lot No.:** 101A-2 (D-132X)

Magnification: 60×   **Voltage:** 20 kV

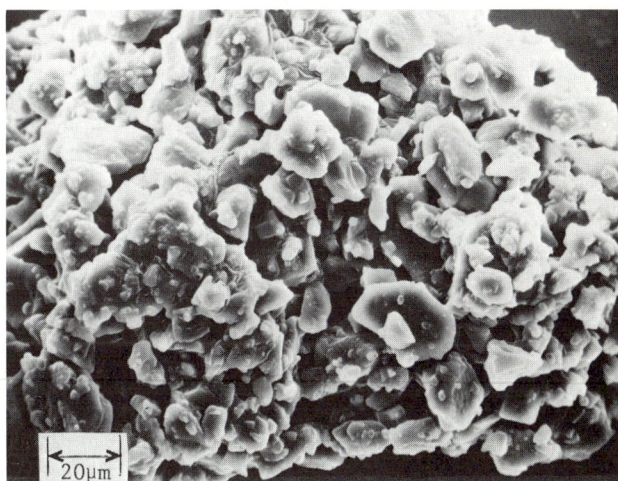

Magnification: 600×   **Voltage:** 20 kV

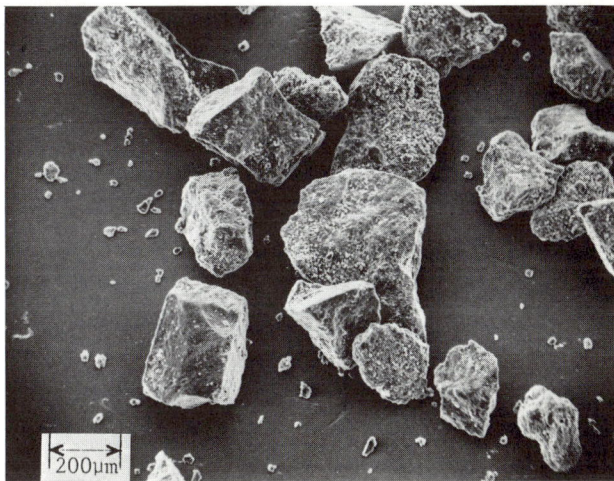

SEM: KY-60
Excipient: Compressible Sugar (Nutab)
Manufacturer: ITE   **Lot No.:** 101A-3 (10-105)

Magnification: 60×   **Voltage:** 20kV

SEM: KY-60
Excipient: Compressible Sugar (Nutab)
Manufacturer: ITE   Lot No.: 101A-3 (10-105)

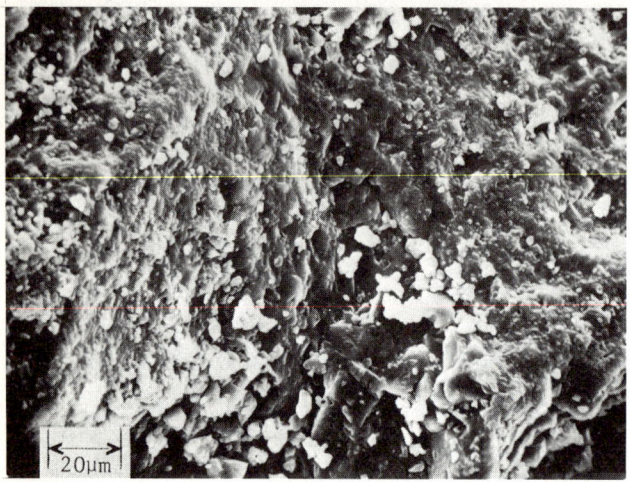

Magnification: 600×   **Voltage:** 20 kV

SEM: KY-60
Excipient: Compressible Sugar (Di-Pac)

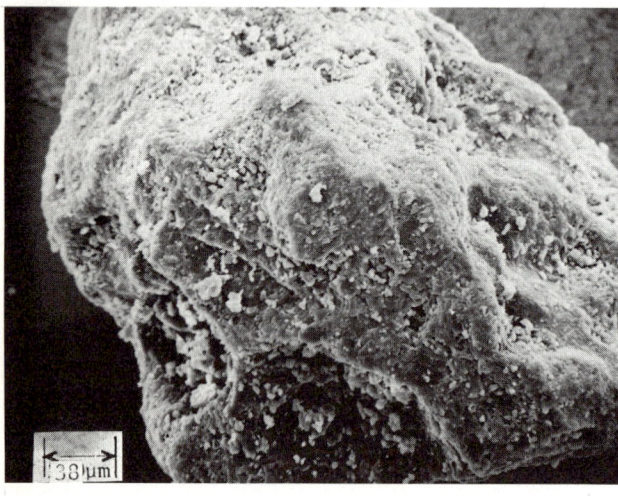

SEM: KY-60
Excipient: Compressible Sugar (Di-Pac)

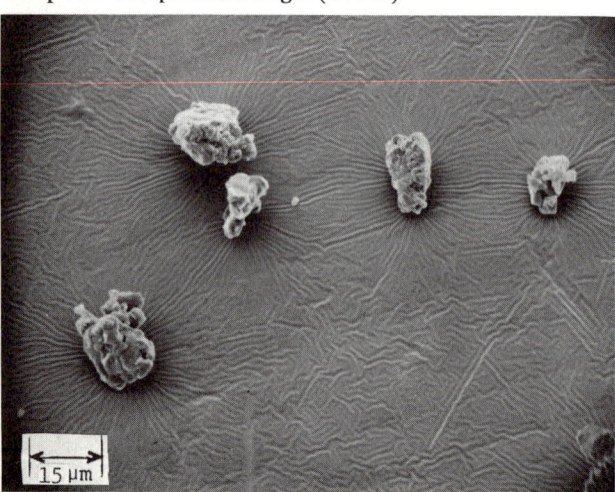

Test	NF
Sulfate	≤0.010%
Calcium	+
Heavy metals	≤5 ppm
Assay	95.0 - 98.0%

11. Typical Properties

Bulk density: Nu-Tab—approximately 1.2 g/ml.
Solubility: The sucrose portion is completely water soluble.
Particle size: Sugartab—30% on #20 mesh screen; 3% passes a #30 mesh screen.
Nu-Tab—50% max. on #60 mesh screen; 20% max. through #120 mesh screen.
Di-Pac—3% max. on #40 mesh screen; 75% min on #100 mesh screen; 5% max. through #200 mesh screen.

Academy HPE Laboratory Project Data

	Method	Lab #	Results
Moisture Content	MC-3	33	0.57%
	MC-4	33	0.20%
Bulk/Tap Density	BTD-1	1	B:0.602g/ml
			T:0.685g/ml
	BTD-7	14	B:0.740g/ml
			T:0.770g/ml
Particle Friability	PF-1	36	0.141%
Average Flow Rate	FLO-2	3	42.7g/sec.
PSD Plot	PSD-9	3	Fig:3-PSD-4

Supplier: Mendell

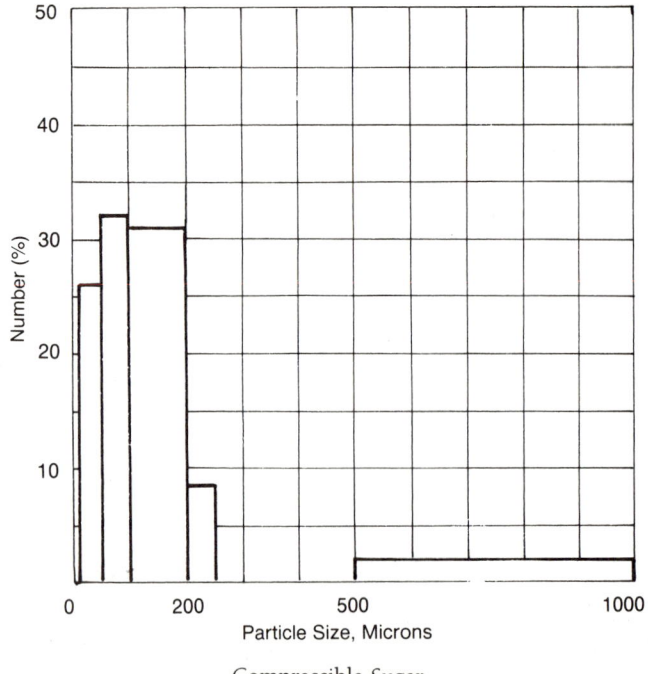

Compressible Sugar

Figure: 3-PSD-4   **Method:** PSD-9

12. Stability and Storage Conditions

Compressible sugar should be preserved in a well-closed container. Compressible sugar is stable in air under normal storage conditions of room temperature and low relative humidity.

13. Incompatibilities

Dilute acids cause the hydrolysis of sucrose to invert sugar. Alkaline earth hydroxides react with sucrose to form sucrates.

14. Safety

Sucrose is contraindicated in diabetic patients. There is some evidence that through a high dietary intake of sugar and the accompanying bacterial fermentation to acids in plaques on teeth, dissolution of dental enamel and dentine can take place.

15. Handling Precautions

None.

16. Regulatory Acceptance

NF XVI

17. Applications in Pharmaceutical Formulation or Technology

Use	Concentration (%)
As a binder in tablet formulations (dry binder)	5-20
As a filler in regular and chewable tablets	20-60
As a sweetener in chewable tablet formulations	10-50

18. Related Substances

Sucrose NF; confectioners sugar NF

19. Comments

Compressible sucrose is used primarily in the preparation of direct-compression chewable tablets. The tableting properties of compressible sugar can be influenced by small changes in moisture level.

20. Specific References

1. Product literature—Edward Mendell Co.
2. Product literature—Mallinckrodt Chemical Works
3. Product literature—Amstar Corporation
4. NU-TAB as a chewable direct compression carrier, *Drug and Cosmetic Industry,* Dec. 1974.
5. A.B. Rizzuto, A.C. Chen and M.F. Vega, *Pharmaceutical Technology,* 8, 32-53 (1984).

USA: D. Savello*; P. Nadkarni**

Confectioner's Sugar

1. Nonproprietary Name
NF: Confectioner's sugar

2. Functional Category
NF: Sweetening agent; tablet and/or capsule diluent
Others: Sugar coating adjunct

3. Synonyms
Icing sugar

4. Chemical Name and CAS Registry Number
—

5. Empirical Formula   Molecular Weight
Primarily sucrose ($C_{12}H_{22}O_{11}$)   —

6. Structural Formula
—

7. Commercial Availability
USA
Amstar Corporation
ICN Nutritional Biochemicals
Rugar Chemical Co., Inc.
Sucrest Corporation

UK
Forum Chemicals, Ltd.
Independent Chemists Marketing, Ltd.

8. Method of Manufacture
Confectioner's sugar is manufactured by pulverizing a mixture of refined granulated sugar and food-grade, re-dried starch (most common anti-caking agent) to fine powder. Other anti-caking agents, such as tricalcium phosphate and various silicates, are used, but are uncommon.

9. Description
A fine, white, odorless powder having a sweet taste.

SEM:KY-59
Excipient Confectioner's sugar

Manufacturer: Frost   **Lot No:** 101A-1

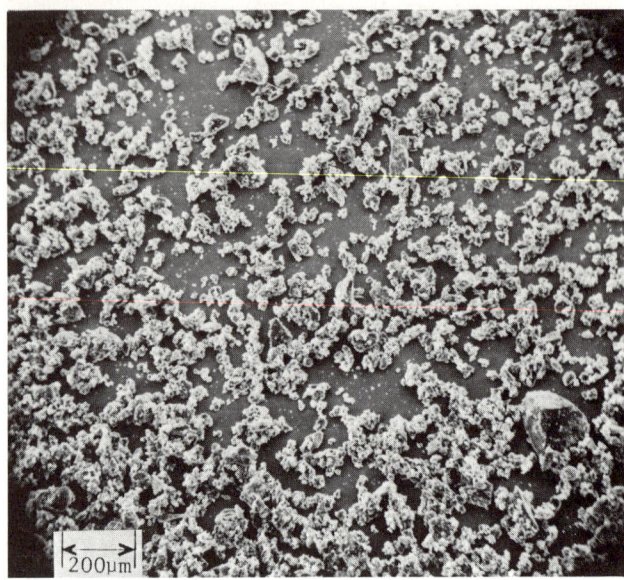

Magnification: 60×   **Voltage:** 20 kV

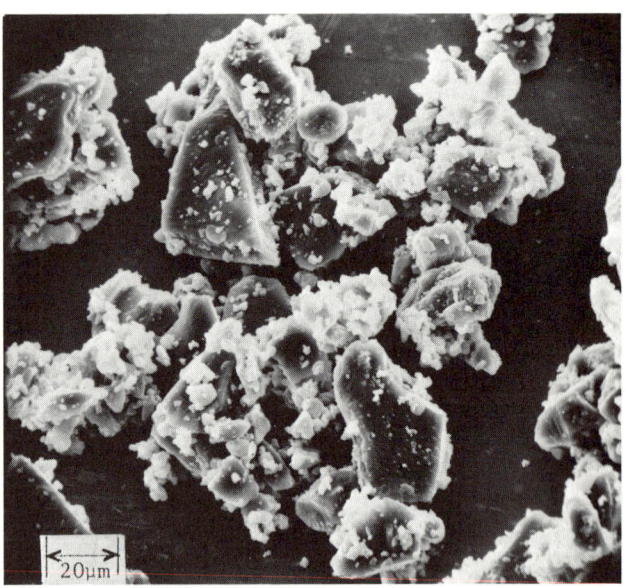

Magnification: 600×   **Voltage:** 20 kV

10. Pharmacopeial Specifications

Test	NF
Identification	+
Specific rotation	$\geq +62.6°$
Chloride	0.014%
Calcium	+
Sulfate	$\leq 0.006\%$
Heavy metals	≤ 5 ppm
Microbial limits	Absence of *E. coli* and *Salmonella* species
Loss on drying	$\leq 1.0\%$
Residue on ignition	$\leq 0.08\%$
Assay	$\geq 95.0\%$ Sucrose

11. Typical Properties

Physical: Particle size: 6X confectioner's sugar—retained on a Tyler sieve #100—1.0% max. Through a Tyler sieve #200—94% min. 10X confectioner's sugar—greater than 98% passes through a Tyler sieve #200. Sometimes it will contain as much as 50% of an anti-caking agent (starch).
Ash: Not usually specified because of variability of starch.
Solubility: The sucrose portion is completely water soluable.
Microbiological: Per 10 grams of dry substance—Yeast: 10 max. Mold: 10 max. Mesophiles: 100 max.

Academy HPE Laboratory Project Data

	Method	Lab #	Results
Moisture content	MC-3	33	0.31%
Moisture content	MC-4	33	0.10%
Bulk/Tap Density	BTD-1	1	B:0.43lg/cm³ T:0.694g/cm³
	BTD-7	14	B:0.560g/cm³ T:0.710g/cm³
Particle Size Dist.	PSD-7	24	14.3µm
Average flow rate	FLO-2	3	NO FLOW
PSD plot	PSD-9	3	Fig: 3-PSD-5
Compression	COM-3	20	POOR FLOW

Supplier: Frost

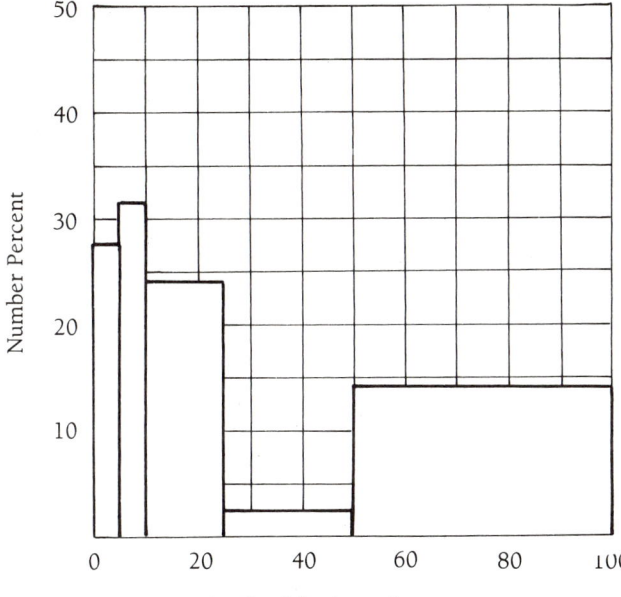

Figure 3: 3-PSD-5   Method: PSD-9

12. Stability and Storage Conditions

Confectioner's sugar should be preserved in a well-closed container. It is stable in air under normal storage conditions.

13. Incompatibilities

Dilute acids cause the hydrolysis of sucrose to invert sugar. Alkaline earth hydroxides react with sucrose to form sucrates.

14. Safety

Sucrose is contra-indicated in diabetic patients. There is some evidence that, through high dietary intake of sugar and the accompanying bacterial fermentation to acids in plaques on teeth, dissolution of enamel and dentine of the teeth can take place.

15. Handling Precautions

None

16. Regulatory Acceptance

NF XVI

17. Applications in Pharmaceutical Formulation or Technology

Use	Concentration (%)
Sugar coating	As desired
Sweetening agent in tablets	10-20
Tablet excipient	10-50

18. Related Substances

Powdered sugar.

19. Comments

Confectioner's sugar is not used widely in pharmaceutical formulations. It is used when sugar with a small particle size is desirable in a formulation. The poor flow properties of this material prevent it from being used in direct compression formulations.

20. Specific References

1. Literature from Sucrest Corporation, 120 Wall Street, New York, New York.

USA: D. Savello*; P. Nadkarni**

Suppository Bases (Semi-Synthetic Glycerides)

1. Nonproprietary Name
BP/EP: Hard fat

2. Functional Category
BP/EP: Pharmaceutical aid
Others: Suppository base

3. Synonyms
Adeps neutralis; Semi-synthetic; glycérides; hydrogenated vegetable glycerides; massa ad suppositoria
Hydrofol glyceride; Massa estarinum; Wecobee; Witepsol; Suppocire; Massupol; Massa Estarinum; IV Novata

4. Chemical Name and CAS Registry Number
—

5. Empirical Formula   Molecular Weight
Hard fat suppository bases consist of mixtures of the triglyceride esters of higher saturated fatty acids (mainly C_{10} to C_{18}) with varying proportions of mono- and diglycerides.
Special grades may contain additives such as beeswax, lecithin, polysorbates, ethoxylated fatty alcohols and ethoxylated partial fatty glycerides.

6. Structural Formula

Where $R_1 = -OH$ or $-O-\overset{O}{\overset{|}{C}}-(CH_2)_N-CH_3$
$R_2 = -OH$ or $-O-\overset{O}{\overset{|}{C}}-(CH_2)_N-CH_3$
$R_3 = -OH$ or $-O-\overset{O}{\overset{|}{C}}-(CH_2)_N-CH_3$
N = 8 to 16
Not all R's can be −OH at the same time.

7. Commercial Availability
USA
A&S Corporation
Ashland Chemicals
Kay-Fries Chemicals, Inc.
PVO International, Inc.

UK
Alfa Chemicals, Ltd.
Chemicals Trading Co., Ltd.
Croklaan VB, The Netherlands
Dynamit Nobel (UK), Ltd.
Ets Gattefossé, France
Henkel Chemicals, Ltd.

8. Method of Manufacture
The most common method involves hydrolysis of natural vegetable oils (e.g., coconut or palm kernel), fractional distillation of the free fatty acids produced, hydrogenation of the C_{12} to C_{18} fractions and, finally, re-esterification under controlled conditions with glycerin to form a mixture of tri-, di- and mono-glycerides of the required characteristics and hydroxyl value (e.g., *IV Novata, Witepsol*). In an alternative procedure, selected grades of vegetable oils are directly hydrogenated and then subjected to heat treatment during which some triglycerides are split into mono- and di-glycerides. The free fatty acids which are released may participate in trans-esterification reactions (e.g., *Suppocire*).

9. Description
White, brittle, solid; almost tasteless and odorless; unctuous to the touch. On warming, melts to a colorless or slightly yellow liquid.

10. Pharmacopeial Specifications

Test	BP/EP
Melting point	33-36°C
Acid value	≤0.5
Hydroxyl value	≤50
Iodine value	≤3
Peroxide value	≤6
Saponification value	225-245
Unsaponifiable matter	≤0.5%
Alkaline impurities	+
Decomposition products	+
Ash	≤0.05%

Additionally, the EP specifies that, when tested for odor, hard fat is free from rancidity.

11. Typical Properties
Acid value (BP method): See Table 1.
Color number:

IV Novata	
Massa Estarinum	≤3 (Iodine color index number)
Witepsol	
Suppocire (excluding "L" grades)	≤3 (Gardner scale)
Suppocire "L" grades	≤5

Density (at 20°C):

IV Novata	0.955-0.975 g/cm³
Massa Estarinum	
Suppocire	0.950 - 0.960 g/cm³
Witepsol	0.950 - 0.980 g/cm³

Heat for melting (22° - 40° C):

IV Novata	approx 125 kJ/kg/K
Massa Estarinum	approx 145 kJ/kg/K
Witepsol	
Suppocire	100 - 130 kJ/kg/K

Hydroxyl value (BP method): See Table 1.
Iodine value (BP method): See Table 1.
Melting point: See Table 1.
Values for *Suppocire* were determined by the method of the French Pharmacopeia (capillary U tube). Other determinations were carried out by the EP method (open-ended capillary tube).

Moisture content (Karl Fischer):

IV Novata	≤0.1%
Massa Estarinum }	≤0.2%
Witepsol	
Suppocire	≤0.5%

Peroxide value (BP method):

IV Novata	
Massa Estarinum }	≤3
Witepsol	
Suppocire	≤1.2

Saponification value (BP method): See Table 1.

Solidification point (Shukkoff flask method): (see also EP, Vol. II, method for freezing point) See Table 1.

Solubility (at approx 22°C): All grades of *IV Novata, Massa Estarinum, Witepsol* and *Suppocire*.

Solvent:

Water	Practically insoluble
Ethanol (96%) }	
Carbon tetrachloride	
Chloroform	Freely soluble
Toluene	
Xylene	
Ether	Varies between grades
Petroleum spirit (40°-60°)	from slightly soluble to very soluble

Specific heat (0° - 20°C):

IV Novata	1.9-2.1 kJ/kg/K
Massa Estarinum }	approx 2.6 kJ/kg/K
Witepsol	
Suppocire	1.7 - 2.5 kJ/kg/K

Unsaponifiable matter (BP method): See Table 1.

Table 1—Typical Properties of Suppository Bases

Product		Acid value	Hydroxyl value	Iodine value	Melting point (°C)	Saponification value	Solidification point (°C)	Unsaponifiable matter (%)
IV Novata	A	≤0.3	35-45	≤3	33.5-35.5	225-240	29-31	≤0.3
	AB	≤0.3	25-40	≤3	29-31	230-245	26.5-28.5	≤0.3
	B	≤0.3	20-30	≤3	33.5-35.5	225-240	31-33	≤0.3
	BBC	≤0.3	20-30	≤3	34-36	225-240	30.5-32.5	≤0.3
	BC	≤0.3	30-40	≤3	33.5-35.5	225-240	30.5-32.5	≤0.3
	BCF	≤1	20-30	≤3	35-37	225-240	30-32	≤0.3
	BD	≤0.3	≤15	≤3	33.5-35.5	230-245	30-32	≤0.3
	C	≤0.3	20-30	≤3	36-38	220-235	33-35	≤0.3
	D	≤0.3	30-40	≤3	40-42	220-235	38-40	≤0.3
	E	≤1	45-60	≤3	34-36	215-230	29-31	≤2
	299	≤0.3	≤5	≤3	33.5-35.5	235-250	31.5-33.5	≤0.3
Massa Estarinum	A	≤0.5	35-45	≤3	33.5-35.5	225-240	29-31	≤0.3
	AB	≤0.3	25-40	≤3	29-31	230-245	26.5-28.5	≤0.3
	B	≤0.3	20-30	≤3	33.5-35.5	225-240	31-33	≤0.3
	BB	≤0.3	18.5-28.5	≤3	33.5-35.5	225-240	31.5-33.5	≤0.3
	BC	≤0.3	30-40	≤3	33.5-35.5	225-240	30.5-32.5	≤0.3
	BCF	≤0.3	25-30	≤3	35-36.5	225-240	30.5-32.5	≤0.3
	BD	≤0.3	≤15	≤3	33.5-35.5	225-240	32-34	≤0.3
	C	≤0.3	20-30	≤3	36-38	225-235	33-35	≤0.3
	D	≤0.3	30-40	≤3	40-42	220-230	38-40	≤0.3
	E	≤1	45-60	≤3	34-36	215-230	29-31	≤2
	299	≤0.3	≤2	≤3	33.5-35.5	240-255	32-34.5	≤0.3
Massupol				≤2	34-36	240-250	31-32.5	
Massupol 15				≤3	35-37	220-230	31-33	
Suppocire	A	≤0.5	20-30	≤2	35-36.5	225-245		≤0.6
	AM	≤0.2	≤6	≤2	35-36.5	225-245		≤0.6
	AML	≤0.5	≤6	≤3	35-36.5	225-245		≤0.6
	AIML	≤0.5	≤6	≤3	33-35	225-245		≤0.6
	AS$_2$	≤0.5	15-25	≤2	35-36.5	225-245		≤0.6
	AS$_2$X	≤0.5	15-25	≤2	35-36.5	225-245		≤0.6
	AT	≤0.5	25-35	≤2	35-36.5	225-245		≤0.6
	AP	≤1.0	30-50	≤1	34-37	200-220		≤0.5
	B	≤0.5	20-30	≤2	36-37.5	225-245		≤0.6
	BM	≤0.2	≤6	≤2	36-37.5	225-245		≤0.6
	BML	≤0.5	≤6	≤3	36-37.5	225-245		≤0.6
	BS$_2$	≤0.5	15-25	≤2	36-37.5	225-245		≤0.6
	BS$_2$X	≤0.5	15-25	≤2	36-37.5	220-240		≤0.6
	BT	≤0.5	25-35	≤2	36-37.5	225-245		≤0.6
	BP	≤1.0	30-50	≤1	36-37.5	200-220		≤0.5
	C	≤0.5	20-30	≤2	38-40	220-240		≤0.6

Table 1—Typical Properties of Suppository Bases (continued)

Product		Acid value	Hydroxyl value	Iodine value	Melting point (°C)	Saponification value	Solidification point (°C)	Unsaponifiable matter (%)
	CM	≤0.2	≤6	≤2	38-40	220-240		≤0.6
	CS$_2$	≤0.5	15-25	≤2	38-40	220-240		≤0.6
	CS$_2$X	≤0.5	15-25	≤2	38-40	220-240		≤0.6
	CT	≤0.5	25-35	≤2	38-40	220-240		≤0.6
	CP	≤1.0	≤50	≤1	38-40.5	200-220		≤0.5
	D	≤0.5	20-30	≤2	42-45	220-240		≤0.6
	DM	≤0.2	≤6	≤2	43-45	220-240		≤0.6
	NA	≤0.5	≤40	≤2	35.5-37.5	225-245		≤0.5
	NB	≤0.5	≤40	≤2	36.5-38.5	225-245		≤0.5
	NC	≤0.5	≤40	≤2	38.5-40.5	220-240		≤0.5
	OSI	≤0.5	20-30	≤2	33-35	225-245		≤0.6
Witepsol	H5	≤0.2	≤5	≤2	34-36	235-245	33-35	≤0.3
	H12	≤0.2	≤15	≤3	32-33.5	240-255	29-33	≤0.3
	H15	≤0.2	≤15	≤3	33.5-35.5	230-240	32.5-34.5	≤0.3
	H19	≤0.2	20-30	≤7	33.5-35.5	230-240	32-35	≤0.3
	H32	≤0.2	≤3	≤3	31-33	240-250	30-32.5	≤0.3
	H35	≤0.2	≤3	≤3	33.5-35.5	235-250	32-35	≤0.3
	H37	≤0.2	≤3	≤3	36-38	225-245	35-37	≤0.3
	H39	≤0.2	≤3	≤3	38-40	220-240	37-39.5	≤0.3
	H42	≤0.2	≤3	≤3	41-43	220-240	40-42.5	≤0.3
	H175	≤0.7	≤15	≤3	34.5-36.5	225-245	32-34	≤1.0
	H185	≤0.3	≤15	≤3	38-39	220-235	34-37	≤0.3
	W25	≤0.3	20-30	≤3	33.5-35.5	225-240	29-33	≤0.3
	W31	≤0.3	25-35	≤3	35-37	225-240	30-33	≤0.5
	W32	≤0.3	40-50	≤3	31-33	240-255	28-31	≤0.3
	W35	≤0.3	40-50	≤3	33.5-35.5	225-235	27-32	≤0.3
	W45	≤0.3	40-50	≤3	33.5-35.5	225-235	29-34	≤0.3
	S51	≤1.0	55-65	≤7	30-32	210-225	26-28	≤2.0
	S55	≤1.0	50-65	≤3	33.5-35.5	215-230	28-33	≤2.0
	S58	≤1.0	60-70	≤7	32-33.5	215-225	27-29	≤2.0
	E75	≤1.3	≤15	≤3	37-39	220-230	32-36	≤3
	E76	≤0.3	30-40	≤3	37-39	220-230	31-35	≤0.5
	E85	≤0.3	≤15	≤3	42-44	220-230	37-42	≤0.5

Typical properties of molded suppository bases are shown in Table 2. Samples for these tests were prepared by melting the bases at 40° - 50°C and pouring into 2 g molds. When set, the suppositories were removed and stored at 20°C for 3 days prior to testing.

Fracture index: Determined by using the Erweka apparatus at room temperature (22°C).

Handling properties: Determined by using an apparatus similar to that described by Setnikar and Fantelli (*J. Pharm. Sci.*, 52: 38-43, 1963). The method used here differed from that described in the literature in that the test was started at 28°C (not 30°C) and used a 500 g weight (not 460 g) and a 50 g rod (not 40 g).

ST is the softening temperature (i.e., 5 mm displacement) and LT is the liquefaction temperature (i.e., 9 mm displacement).

Liquefaction time: Determined by the method described by Krowczynski (*Diss. Pharm.*, 11: 269-273, 1959). The times quoted are for a 15 mm displacement of the glass rod.

Note: These data should only be used as a guide. The tests are highly empirical, and the results can be influenced by factors such as the manufacturing conditions and storage history of the test sample, the physicochemical properties of the base, their location in either the middle or the ends of the defined ranges, and the presence of any drugs or adjuvants.

Table 2—Typical Properties of Molded Suppository Bases

Product		Fracture index (kg)	Handling properties ST (°C)	Handling properties LT (°C)	Liquefaction time (min.)
IV Novata	A	5.4+	33.7	35.3	15.3
	AB	5.4+	31.6	32.6	10.5
	B	5.4+	33.1	35.0	14.6
	BBC	5.4+	33.1	34.6	12.1
	BC	5.4+	33.2	35.0	14.0
	BCF	5.4+	34.4	35.8	20.4
	BD	5.4+	33.7	34.9	14.8
	C	5.4+	35.7	37.4	60.0+
	D	5.4+	40+	—	60.0+
	E	5.4+	32.9	35.5	14.0
	299	5.4+	33.9	35.9	11.7

Table 2—Typical Properties of Molded Suppository Bases (continued)

Product		Fracture index (kg)	ST (°C)	LT (°C)	Liquefaction time (min.)
Massa					
Estarinum	A	5.4+	32.9	34.5	9.8
	AB	5.4+	31.4	32.2	6.2
	B	5.4+	32.8	34.8	12.6
	BB	5.4+	33.3	35.0	12.1
	BC	5.4+	33.0	34.7	13.8
	BCF	5.4+	33.6	35.4	12.6
	BD	5.4+	32.9	34.6	13.7
	C	5.4+	35.5	36.9	60.0+
	D	5.4+	40.0	40.0+	60.0+
	E	5.4+	33.1	35.2	14.4
	299	4.9	32.1	35.4	8.1
Suppocire	A		32.4	34.7	7.8
	AM	5.4+	32.7	35.0	8.7
	AML	5.4+	32.2	34.5	8.6
	AIML	4.3	31.4	33.9	5.3
	AS₂	4.4	32.2	34.6	9.9
	AS₂X	2.4	31.9	34.0	9.9
	AT	5.4	32.3	34.8	11.3
	AP	4.2	32.7	35.0	9.5
	B	5.4+	32.5	35.5	13.1
	BM	5.4+	33.0	35.7	13.1
	BML	5.4+	33.1	35.7	16.4
	BS₂	4.3	32.6	35.4	17.0
	BS₂X	1.4	32.4	35.0	14.0
	BT	3.2	33.4	36.3	29.3
	BP	3.9	32.8	35.4	16.0
	C	4.6	34.4	37.8	60.0+
	CM	5.4+	35.2	37.7	60.0+
	CS₂	5.4+	35.5	37.5	44.4
	CS₂X	5.4+	35.0	37.2	60.0
	CT	5.4+	34.7	37.4	60.0
	CP	5.4+	34.6	37.5	60.0
	D	5.4+	38.0	40.0+	60.0
	DM	5.4+	37.9	40.0+	60.0
	NA	5.4+	33.6	35.3	13.4
	NB	5.4+	34.7	36.7	22.9
	NC	5.4+	37.4	40.0+	60.0+
	OSI	1.0	31.4	33.8	10.1
Witepsol	H5	5.4+	34.2	35.2	13.8
	H12	5.4+	30.0	32.7	3.7
	H15	5.4+	33.2	35.2	11.2
	H19	5.4+	33.1	34.8	14.9
	H32	4.1	31.0	33.0	7.2
	H35	5.4+	33.7	34.7	17.4
	H37	5.4+	34.8	38.5	40.1
	H39	5.4+	35.6	39.0	60.0+
	H42	5.4+	34.7	38.3	50.2
	H175	5.4+	33.7	35.5	12.9
	H185	5.4+	35.5	37.0	48.8
	W25	5.4+	32.4	34.4	14.6
	W31	5.4+	34.9	36.5	31.0
	W32	4.3	31.5	34.3	8.7
	W35	5.4+	32.8	34.5	14.0
	W45	5.4+	32.6	34.3	12.9
	S51	3.2	30.3	32.8	6.8
	S55	5.4+	33.1	35.7	13.0
	S58	5.4+	31.5	33.7	7.7
	E75	5.4+	34.6	36.9	32.5
	E76	5.4+	34.9	38.0	60.0+
	E85	5.4+	39.0	40.0+	60.0+

12. Stability and Storage Conditions

Hard fat bases are fairly stable towards oxidation and hydrolysis. Peroxide values are a measure of their resistance to oxidation and rancidity. Water content is usually low (in *Witepsols*, below 0.05%), and deterioration due to hygroscopicity is infrequent. Melting characteristics, hardness and drug release profiles alter with time, and the melting point may rise by 0.5°C after storage for several months. Due to the complexity of bases, elucidation of the mechanisms which induce these changes on aging is difficult. Evidence has been presented which supports a finite transition from amorphous to crystalline forms in which polymorphism, may or may not contribute, whereas other workers have found melting point changes to be closely associated with the conversion of triglycerides to more stable polymorphic forms. Before melting point determinations are made, bases are "conditioned" to a stable crystalline form. The BP specifies heating at 15° to 22°C for 24 hours, but refrigerated storage for shorter periods has also been recommended. Suppository bases should be stored in air-tight containers, protected from light. Suppositories which are not effectively packaged may develop a "bloom" of powdery crystals at the surface. This is usually due to the presence of low melting point components in the base and can often be overcome by the use of a different base.

13. Incompatibilities

The large range of suppository bases now available has reduced the incidence of incompatibilities, and therefore they have not been extensively documented. A chemical reaction occurring between hard fat bases and drugs is relatively rare. The potential reactivity of a base is usually indicated by the magnitude of its hydroxyl value. For example, the risk of hydrolysis of aspirin may be reduced by the use of a base with a low hydroxyl value and, additionally, by minimization of the water content of both base and aspirin. There is evidence that aminophylline reacts with glycerides in some hard fat bases to form diamides. On aging or exposure to elevated temperatures, degradation is accompanied by hardening, and suppositories tend to exhibit a marked increase in melting point. The ethylene diamine content is also reduced. Certain fat-soluble medications, such as chloral hydrate, may depress the melting point when incorporated into bases. When large amounts of active content, whether solid or liquid, have to be dispersed in a base, the rheological characteristics of the resultant suppository may be changed with concomitant effects on release and absorption. Careful selection of bases or the inclusion of additives may be necessary.

14. Safety

High hydroxyl values are reported to produce irritation.

15. Handling Precautions

Slight fire hazard when exposed to heat or flame.

16. Regulatory Acceptance

BP/EP 1980; Many grades are accepted by the FDA.

17. Applications in Pharmaceutical Formulation and Technology

The primary application of semi-synthetic glycerides is as a vehicle for the rectal administration of a variety of drugs, either to exert local effects or to achieve systemic absorption. Selection of a suppository base cannot usually be made in the absence of knowledge of the physicochemical properties and intrinsic thermodynamic activity of the drug substance. Other drug-related factors that can affect release and absorption and which must therefore be considered are the particle size distribution of insoluble solids, the oil-water partition coefficient and the dissociation constant. The displacement value should also be known as well as the ratio of drug to base. Properties of the suppository base which may or may not be modified by the drug or which can influence drug release are the melting characteristics, chemical reactivity and rheology. The presence of additives in the base can also affect performance.

Melting characteristics: Fatty-based suppositories intended for systemic use should liquefy at just below body temperature. Softening or dispersion may be adequate for suppositories intended for local action or modified release. High melting point bases may be indicated for fat-soluble drugs which tend to depress the melting point of bases or for suppositories used in warm climates. Drugs which dissolve in bases when hot may create problems if they deposit as crystals of different form or increased size on cooling or on storage. Low melting point bases, particularly those which melt to liquids of low viscosity, can be of value when large volumes of insoluble substances are to be incorporated. There is a risk of sedimentation in such instances. An important factor during processing is the time required for setting. This is affected by the temperature difference between the melting point and the solidification point.

Chemical reactivity: Although the use of bases with low hydroxyl values (low partial ester content) is indicated to minimize the risk of interaction with chemically reactive compounds, formulators should be aware that hydroxyl values are also related to hydrophilic properties which, in turn, can modify both release and absorption rates. Bases with low hydroxyl values tend to be less plastic than those with higher values and, if cooled rapidly, may become excessively brittle. Peroxide values give a measure of the resistance of the base to oxidation, and are a guide to the onset of rancidity.

Rheology: The viscosity of the melted base can affect the uniformity of distribution of suspended solids during manufacture. It can also influence the release and absorption of the drug in the rectum. Further reduction of particle size of insoluble solids is the method of choice to minimize the risk of sedimentation. However, the presence of a high content of fine, suspended particles is likely to increase viscosity. It may also make pouring difficult, delay melting and induce brittleness on solidification. Additives are sometimes included to modify rheological properties and to maintain homogeneity, but the extent of their effect on drug release should first be assessed. Release from a base in which viscosity has been enhanced by an added thickener may vary and be related to the aqueous solubility of the drug itself.

Additives: Some grades of commercial bases already contain additives, and these are usually identified by the manufacturers by means of suitable letters or numbers. Additives may also be incorporated by formulators. Properties of suppositories which have been modified and additives or types of additives that have been used are listed below.

1. Melting range	Ethoxylated partial fatty glycerides
	Saturated glyceride mixtures
2. Viscosity	Aluminum monostearate also di- and tri-stearates
	Bentonite
	Glyceryl monostearate
	Magnesium stearate
	Silicon dioxide, colloidal (*Aerosil*)

3. Plasticity (plasticizers and hardeners)

Cetyl alcohol
Glyceryl monostearate
Myristyl alcohol
Polysorbate 80, 85
Propylene glycol
Stearic acid
Stearyl alcohol

4. Hygroscopicity (reduction)

Silicon dioxide, colloidal (*Aerosil*)

5. Dispersants, release and/ or absorber enhancers

Surface active agents

Water is undesirable as an additive because it enhances oxidation and the potential for a chemical reaction between suppository constituents. In low concentration it plays little part in drug release, and it can serve as a medium for microbial growth. General guidance on the characteristics and potential applications of various grades of hard fat suppository bases appears in the following tables.

IV Novata
A: General purpose suppository base suitable for use in both automatic and hand molding processes; rapid cooling can be used. The base has emulsifying properties.
AB: Low melting range base used for formulations containing large quantities of powdery, active ingredients; forced cooling can be used.
B: General purpose base for small- or large-scale production equipment with or without forced cooling.
BBC: Similar to type B, but with a lower solidification point and a higher melting point. Large quantities of powdery ingredients can be incorporated.
BC: Particularly suitable for large-scale production and for the incorporation of crystalline substances with minimal sedimentation.
BCF: Similar to type B, but with a higher melting range. Useful with active ingredients that produce a reduction in melting point or with dense crystalline substances. The base has emulsifying properties.
BD: Material with low hydroxyl value; can be used in large-scale equipment, although forced cooling should be avoided.
C: Higher melting point base; suitable for large-scale equipment but forced cooling should be avoided.
D: High melting range base which can be used to adjust the melting point of suppository formulations.
E: Base with good emulsifying properties, suitable for formulations containing up to 30% water, 20% alcohol or 40-50% glycerol; can be processed with forced cooling.
299: Base with a particularly low hydroxyl value for use with reactive ingredients; can be used in automatic equipment, but forced cooling should be avoided.

Massa Estarinum
A: Base with good emulsifying and dispersing properties, suitable for use on automatic production equipment; rapid cooling can be used.
AB: Similar to type A, but with a lower melting range, and thus suitable for formulations containing a high proportion of solid active ingredient.
B: General purpose base suitable for use with both automatic and non-automatic equipment.
BB: Similar to type B, but more suitable for formulations containing large quantities of solid active ingredient.
BC: Similar to type B, but designed to reduce the sedimentation of crystalline medications.
BCF: Similar to type BC, but with a lower hydroxyl value.

BD: Base with a low hydroxyl value; suitable for automatic equipment, but rapid cooling should not be used.
C: Material with a high melting range.
D: Similar to type C, but with a higher melting range.
E: Material containing a non-ionic, surface active agent which improves dispersing and emulsifying properties.
299: Base with a very low hydroxyl value, for use with particularly reactive substances.

Massupol
Massupol: Very hard base which sets rapidly on cooling.
Massupol$_{15}$: Base designed for cold molding.

Suppocire
A: General purpose base suitable for both automatic and semi-automatic equipment.
AM: Material with a low hydroxyl value; can be used on large-scale automatic equipment, but forced cooling should be avoided.
AML: Similar to type AM, but contains phospholipid. Particularly suitable for formulations containing large quantities of powdery ingredients; can be used on automatic equipment.
AIML: Similar to type AML, but with a lower melting range.
AS$_2$: Similar to type A, but more suitable for use with automatic equipment with (or without) forced cooling.
AS$_2$X: Similar to type AS$_2$, but contains a non-ionic surfactant; can be used for formulations containing up to 10% water.
AT: Material with intermediate hydroxyl value, suitable for large-scale production with forced cooling.
AP: Lower melting range base with increased hydrophilic properties (intended to improve bioavailability).
B: General purpose suppository base similar to type A, but with a higher melting range.
BM: Similar to type AM, but with a higher melting range.
BML: Similar to type AML, but with a higher melting range.
BS$_2$: Similar to type AS$_2$, but with a higher melting range.
BS$_2$X: Similar to type AS$_2$X, but with a higher melting range.
BT: Similar to type AT, but with a higher melting range.
BP: Similar to type AP, but with a higher melting range.
C: General purpose suppository base similar to type B, but with a higher melting range.
CM: Similar to type BM, but with a higher melting range.
CS$_2$: Similar to type BS$_2$, but with a higher melting range.
CS$_2$X: Similar to type BS$_2$X, but with a higher melting range.
CT: Similar to type BT, but with a higher melting range.
D: General purpose base similar to type C, but with a higher melting range.
DM: Similar to type CM, but with a higher melting range.
NA: Material with increased plasticity intended to improve the handling properties of formulations that are brittle or tend to fracture easily.
NB: Similar to type NA, but with a higher melting range.
NC: Similar to type NB, but with a higher melting range.
OSI: Base with a low melting range and medium hydroxyl value. Particularly suited for ingredients which react with hydroxyl groups and/or produce an increase in the melting range. Can be processed on automatic equipment with forced cooling.

Witepsol
H5: Base with a low hydroxyl value; rapid cooling should be avoided.
H12: Material suitable for formulation with large amounts of crystalline or powdery ingredients; rapid cooling should be avoided.
H15: Standard base designed to minimize the sedimentation of active material during processing; rapid cooling should be avoided.

H19: Base containing an additive intended to protect the rectal mucosa and thereby reduce the likelihood of irritation.

H32: Material with a very low hydroxyl value.

H35: Similar to type H15, but with a very low hydroxyl value.

H37: Similar to type H35, but with a higher melting range.

H39: Similar to type H37, but with a higher melting range.

H42: Similar to type H39, but with a higher melting range.

H175: Base with a low hydroxyl value.

H185: Base with a low hydroxyl value and a high melting range.

W25: General purpose base suitable for use on both automatic and non-automatic production equipment; rapid cooling can be used.

W31: Similar to type W25, but with a higher melting range.

W32: General purpose base for use with large quantities of powdery ingredients.

W35: General purpose base with a high hydroxyl value suitable for manufacture on large-scale automatic equipment; rapid cooling can be used.

W45: Similar to type W35, but with a shorter setting time.

S51: Material with added surface-active agent which improves dispersibility of active constituents. The base has a low melting range to allow for the incorporation of large amounts of medication; rapid cooling can be used.

S55: Similar to S51, but with a higher melting range.

S58: Similar to S55, but containing an additive intended to protect the rectal mucosa.

E75: High melting range base; rapid forced cooling should be avoided.

E76: Similar to type E75, but more suitable for use with automatic equipment; forced cooling is recommended.

E85: Very high melting range base used to adjust the melting range of suppository formulations; rapid cooling should be avoided.

18. Related Substances

Theobroma oil: a fat of natural origin comprising a mixture of fatty acid triglycerides with linoleic acid and saturated acids; guerbet alcohols: linked fatty alcohols with 32 to 36 carbon chains, e.g., 2-tetradecyloctadecanol.

19. Comments

Semi-synthetic glyceride suppository bases of various compositions are described in the pharmacopeias of the following countries: Austria, Belgium, West Germany, Hungary, Italy, Nordic countries and Portugal.

20. Specific References:

1. N. Senior. In: "Advances in Pharmaceutical Sciences," Vol. 4, H.S. Bean, A.H. Beckett and J.E. Carless, Eds., Academic Press, London, 1974, pp. 363-435.

2. N. Senior, Review of rectal suppositories, *Pharm. J.*, 203: 703, 706, 732, 736 (1969).

3. J. Anschel and H.A. Lieberman. In: "The Theory and Practice of Industrial Pharmacy," 2nd Ed., L. Lachman, H.A. Lieberman and J.L. Kanig, Eds., Lea and Febiger, Philadelphia, 1976, pp. 245-269.

4. A.J.M. Schoonen, F. Moolenarr and T. Huizinga, Release of drugs from fatty suppository bases: I. The release mechanism, *Inter. J. Pharm.*, 4:141, 152 (1979).

5. L.J. Coben and N.G. Lordi, Physical stability of semi-synthetic suppository bases, *J. Pharm. Sci.*, 69:955, 960 (1980).

6. J.F. Brower, E.C. Juenge, D.P. Page and M.L. Dow, Decomposition of aminophylline in suppository formulations, *J. Pharm. Sci.*, 69:942, 945 (1980).

7. G.G. Liversidge, D.H.W. Grant and J.M. Padfield, Influence of physicochemical interactions on the properties of suppositories I. Interactions between the constituents of fatty suppository bases, *Inter. J. Pharm.*, 7:211, 223 (1981).

8. J.B. Taylor and D.E. Simpkins, Aminophylline suppositories: *In vitro* dissolution and bioavailability in man, *Pharm. J.*, 227:601 (1981).

USA: Z. Chowhan**

UK: M. C. Meyer*; M. Lynch*

Talc

1. Nonproprietary Names
USP: Talc
BP/EP: Purified talc

2. Functional Category
USP: Tablet and/or capsule lubricant; glidant and/or anti-caking agent
BP: Talc dusting powder
Others: Antiadhesive

3. Synonyms
French chalk; purified talc; talcum; soapstone; steatite

4. Chemical Name and CAS Registry Number
Native, hydrous magnesium silicate may contain a small amount of aluminum silicate [14807-96-6]

5. Empirical Formula   Molecular Weight
$Mg_6(Si_2O_5)_4(OH)_4$ —

6. Structural Formula
—

7. Commercial Availability
USA
J. T. Baker Chemical Co.
Beacon CMP Corp.
Charles B. Chrystal Co.
McKesson Chemical Co.
M. F. Moreland Neal & Co.
Ruger Chemical Co.
L. A. Salomon & Bro., Inc.
Thompson-Hayward Chemical Co.
Whittaker, Clark & Daniels, Inc.

UK
Frederick Allen & Sons (Chemicals), Ltd.
D. F. Anstead, Ltd.
Richard Harrison Baker, Ltd.
Bromhead & Denison, Ltd.
L. J. Rickards & Co., Ltd.

8. Method of Manufacture
The naturally occurring hydropolysilicate is pulverized and subjected to flotation processes to remove various mineral substances. Talc is then finely powdered and treated with dilute hydrochloric acid, washed with water and dried.

9. Description
A very fine, white to grayish white, impalpable, odorless, crystalline powder; unctuous; adheres readily to skin; soft to touch and free from grittiness.

SEM:KY-62
Excipient: Talc USP
Manufacturer: Whittaker   **Lot No.:** 102A-4 (1745)

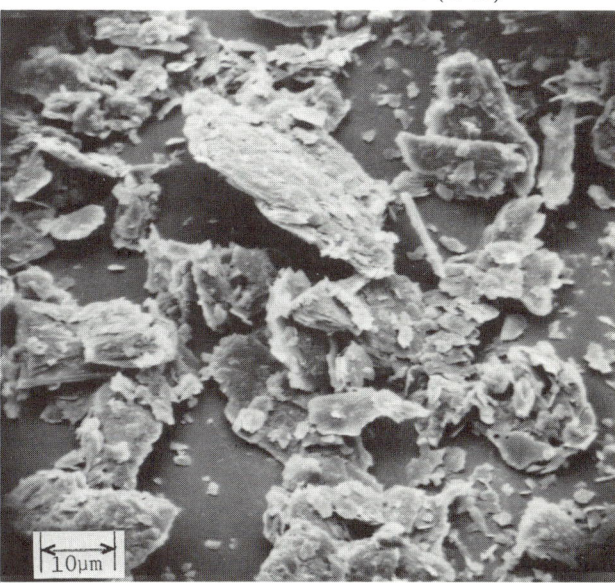

Magnification: 1200× **Voltage:** 10 kV

SEM:KY-63
Excipient: Talc (USP Supreme)
Manufacturer: Cyprus   **Lot No.:** 102A-5(375G)

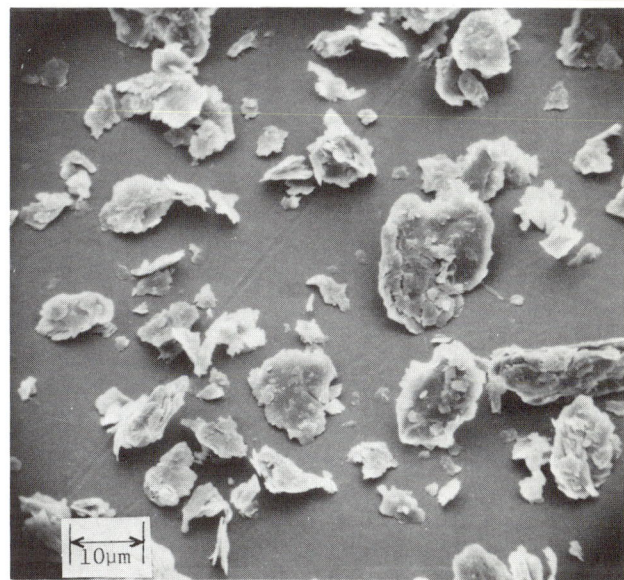

Magnification: 1200× **Voltage:** 10 kV

SEM:KY-64
Excipient: Talc (Purtalc USP MC)
Manufacturer: Chrystal   **Lot No.**: 102A-1

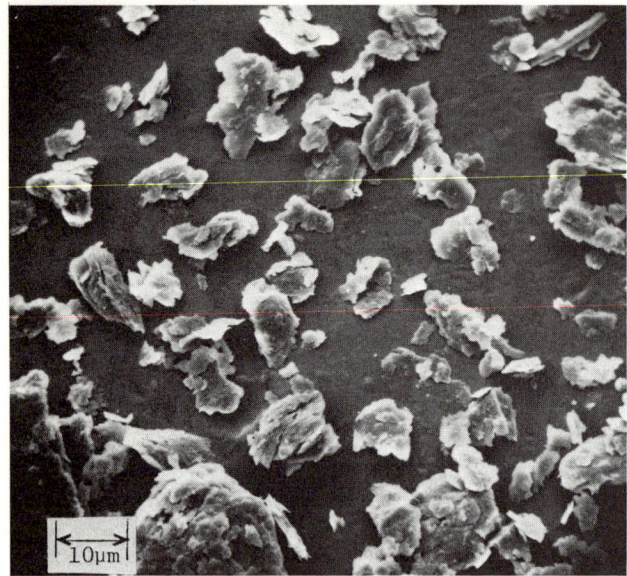

Magnification: 1200× **Voltage**: 10 kV

SEM:KY-66
Excipient: Talc (Purtalc #325)
Manufacturer: Chrystal   **Lot No.**: 102A-2

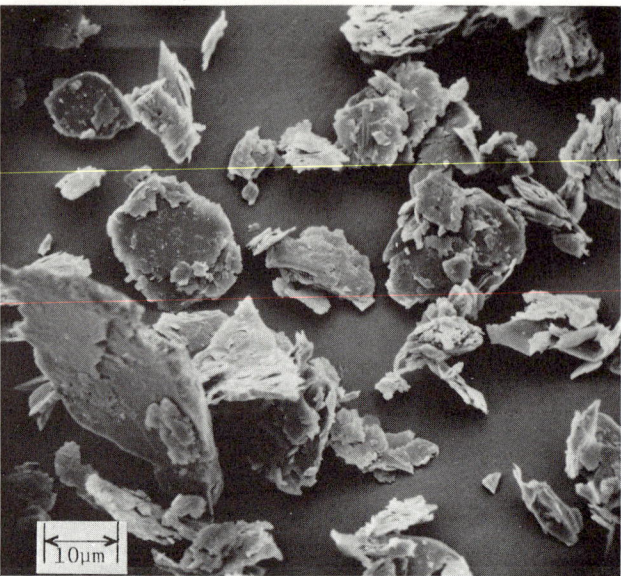

Magnification: 1200× **Voltage**: 10 kV

SEM:KY-65
Excipient: Talc (USP)
Manufacturer: Mallinckrodt   **Lot No.**: 102A-3(KJBN)

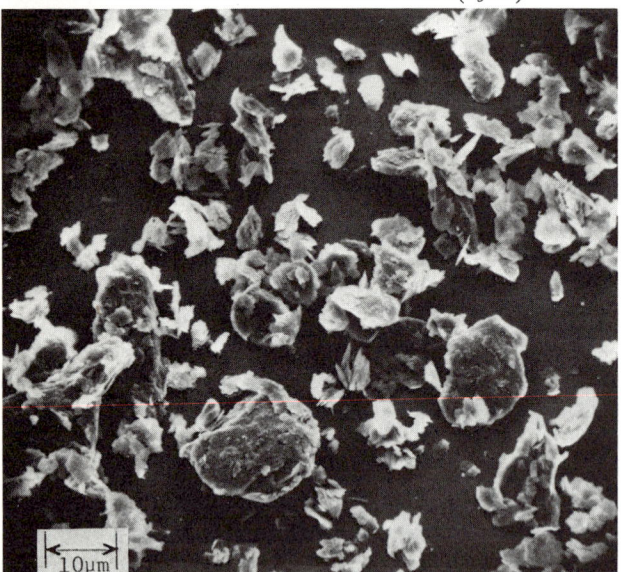

Magnification: 1200× **Voltage**: 10 kV ˈ

10. Pharmacopeial Specifications

Test	USP	BP
Identification	+	+
Loss on ignition	≤6.5%	—
Acid-soluble substances	≤10 mg (2.0%)	≤10 mg
Reaction and soluble substances	≤0.1%	—
Water-soluble iron	+	≤200 ppm
Microbial limit	≤500/g	—
Carbonate	—	+
Chloride	—	≤100 ppm
Readily carbonizable substances	—	+
Loss on drying	—	≤1%
Arsenic	≤3ppm	—
Heavy metals	≤0.004%	—
Lead	≤0.001%	—
Iron	—	≤200 ppm

11. Typical Properties

Adsorbed moisture: <1% (approximately)
Density (loose, CTFA-C8-1): 19-24 lb/ft³
Density (tapped, CTFA-C7-1): 48-62.5 lb/ft³
Microbiological: May contain bacteria. Can be sterilized by dry heat at 160°C for not less than 1 hour or by exposure to ethylene oxide.
pH (1:5 dilution): 6.5-10
Solubility: Insoluble in water, organic solvents, cold acids and dilute alkalis
Specific gravity: 2.7-2.8
Brightness, % (relative to MgO): 86-92%
Particle size distribution: Varies with the source and grade
Less than 2.0μm: 73-90%
Chemical analysis: See Table 1.

Table 1—Typical Chemical Analyses of Representative Samples of Talc from Various Sources

	USA (Alabama) USP/BP	French (Lusenac)		Italian (Val Chisone)		Indian 'Finex'
		OOSP	No. 1	MT 120	Extra 'A'	
Loss on ignition (H_2O + CO_2)	—	4.53	6.48	5.51	5.69	4.90
Silica (SiO_2)	61.22	8.49	60.52	7.52	0.47	62.20
Aluminum oxide (Al_2O_3)	0.42	2.96	3.08	1.27	1.55	0.30
Ferric oxide (Fe_2O_3)	0.58	0.87	0.83	1.03	1.32	0.30
Calcium oxide (CaO)	0.05	0.71	0.53	0.53	0.65	0.10
Magnesium oxide (MgO)	32.36	32.87	31.60	31.75	30.75	32.20
Lead (Pb)	20 ppm	2 ppm	2 ppm max	2 ppm	—	—
Arsenic (As)	2 ppm	0.2 ppm	0.3 ppm	0.51 ppm	—	—

Optical properties: Talc exhibits three indices of refraction. For pure talc, the indices are $2c$ = 1.539; y = 1.589; and z = 1.589. It has a small and variable optic axial angle.

Surface properties: Depending on the source from which it is mined, talc shows different surface characteristics. The Montana talcs are hydrophobic in nature, whereas the California talcs are predominantly hydrophilic.

Surface area: In general, talc exhibits a large surface area in relation to its mass because of its platelike structure. The values, to a large extent, depend on the fineness of the product (typical value: 12 m^2/g).

Basic physical and chemical properties: Typical properties of commercially important cosmetic talcs appear below:

Origin	Chemical purity (hydrous magnesium silicate)	Principal impurities	Color	Slip	Softness
Italy	95	Calcium Magnesium silicate	E	E	F
India	98	Aluminum iron oxides	G	E	F
France	97	Aluminum oxide	G	G	G
Manchuria	98	Aluminum oxide	G	G	E
California	96	Calcium carbonate	G	G	E
Montana	98	Iron oxide	F	G	E
North Carolina	93	Aluminum iron oxides	G	E	G
Alabama	97	Aluminum oxide	F	G	G

E = excellent; G = good; F = fair.

Italian cosmetic talc has been the western world's standard for centuries. No matter what the origin, however, high-quality cosmetic talcs share three common characteristics: high chemical purity, a clean white color and good "slip."

Academy HPE Laboratory Project Data	Method	Lab #	Results
Moisture content[b]	MC-13	18	0.163%
Moisture content[b] (pure talc)	MC-13	18	0.239%
Moisture content[a]	MC-23	21	0.06%
Bulk/tap density	BTD-1	1	B: 0.538 g/cm^3 [b] T: 0.862 g/cm^3 [b]
	BTD-7	14	B: 0.570 g/cm^3 [b] T: 0.710 g/cm^3 [b]
	BTD-1	1	B: 0.510 g/cm^3 [b] T: 0.833 g/cm^3 [b]
	BTD-7	14	B: 0.530 g/cm^3 [b] T: 0.610 g/cm^3 [b]
	BTD-1	1	B: 0.417 g/cm^3 [e] T: 0.667 g/cm^3 [e]
	BTD-1	1	B: 0.439 g/cm^3 [d] T: 0.694 g/cm^3 [d]
Particle size distribution	PSD-5A	21	LT 44μm: 87%[a] 44-74μm: 13%[a]
Solubility (Water)	SOL-1	1	0.028%[b]
(Alcohol)	SOL-1	1	0.010%[b]
(n-Hexane)	SOL-1	1	0.000%[b]
(Water)	SOL-1	1	0.031%[b]
(Alcohol)	SOL-1	1	0.001%[b]
(n-Hexane)	SOL-1	1	0.000%[b]
(Water)	SOL-1	1	0.006%[c]
(Alcohol)	SOL-1	1	0.000%[c]
(n-Hexane)	SOL-1	1	0.000%[c]
(Water)	SOL-1	1	0.000%[e]
(Alcohol)	SOL-1	1	0.000%[e]
(n-Hexane)	SOL-1	1	0.000%[e]
(Water)	SOL-1	1	0.000%[d]
(Alcohol)	SOL-1	1	0.000%[d]
(n-Hexane)	SOL-1	1	0.000%[d]
Compression (at 15.5-180 MN/m^2)	COM-1	21	No compacts formed[a]
Compression	COM-7	12	no compacts[f]
PSD plot	PSD-5A	21	Fig. 21-PSD-4[a]

Suppliers: [a]Bate Chemical Co.; [b]Chrystal Co.; [c]Mallinckrodt; [d]Morelan; [e]Whittaker, Clark & Daniels, Inc.; [f]Pfizer

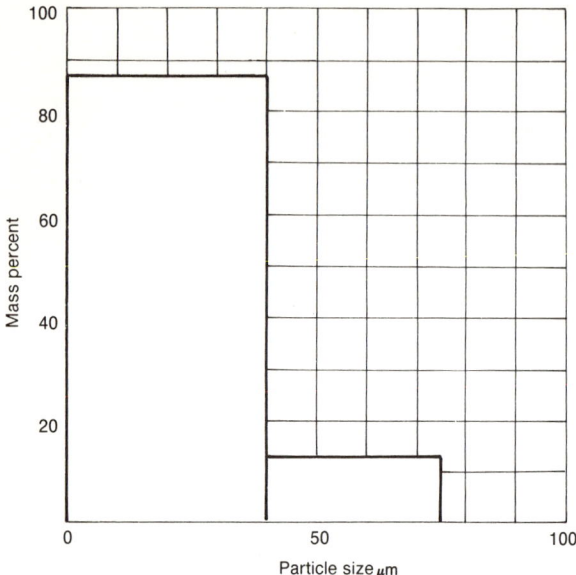

Talc (Bate, Canada, Lot #A2349)
Figure: 21-PSD-4   **Method:** PSD-5A

12. Stability and Storage Conditions

Stable. Preserve in a well-closed container.

13. Incompatibilities

Quaternary ammonium compounds

14. Safety

The available data indicate that talc dust exposure in the modern mining process does not appear to be injurious to health. Contamination of tissues with talc is liable to cause granulomas. Talc should not be applied to open wounds or used on surgical gloves. Prolonged and intense exposure to talc may produce p*neumoconiosis*. The talc should not be inhaled. Being unreactive, talc may be considered practically nontoxic on ingestion. The limit of asbestos impurities, apparently suggested by the FDA and as quoted by a *Wall Street Journal* report (Feb. 26, 1973), is 1%. This figure represents the lowest level detectable by current techniques.

15. Handling Precautions

Avoid inhalation. Use a safety face mask.

16. Regulatory Acceptance

USP XXI; BP 1980

17. Applications in Pharmaceutical Formulation or Technology

Use	Concentration (%)
Lubricant or glidant in tablet and capsule manufacture	1-4
Filler for tablets and capsules	5-30
Dusting powder	90-99

18 Related Substances

—

19. Comments

Talc should not be used as a dusting powder on surgical gloves because it is very irritating to the peritoneal cavity. Talc USP varies in chemical composition according to its source and method of preparation. Different talcs varied significantly in their effects on the stability of aspirin. Aspirin stability was improved by acid washing. In searching for sources of fibers ubiquitous to our everyday environment and of respirable size, 22 talcum products commonly available on retail shelves were examined, and fiber contents ranging from 8-33% by count, with an average of 19%, were found. Fibrous particulates were generally under 1 μm in diameter, with lengths ranging from 1.5 to 6.0 mm.

20. Specific References

1. A. Gold and J. A. Campbell, Effects of selected USP talcs on acetylsalicylic acid stability in tablets, *J. Pharm Sci.*, 53:52 (1964).
2. R. W. Grexa, and C. J. Pamentier, Cosmetic talc properties and specifications, *Cosmetics and Toiletries*, 94:29 (1979).
3. G. Hildick-Smith, Talc: Recent epidemiological studies. In: "Inhaled Particles," 6:919, 1977, p. 123.
4. H. P. Blejer and R. Arlon, Talc: a possible occupational and environmental carcinogen, *J. Occupational Medicine*, 15:92 (1973).
5. L. J. Craley, M. M. Key, D. H. Groth, W. S. Lainhart, and R. M. Ligo, Fibrous and mineral content of cosmetic talcum products, *American Industrial Hygiene Association Journal*, 29:350 (1980).

USA: E. A. Holstius*; Z. Chowhan*; D. Sanvordeker**
UK: P. C. Record*

Thimerosal

1. Nonproprietary Names

USP: Thimerosal
BP: Thiomersal

2. Functional Category

USP: Antimicrobial preservative
BP: Antiseptic; antimicrobial preservative

3. Synonyms

Mercurothiolate; thiomersalate; sodium ethylmercurothiosalicylate

4. Chemical Names and CAS Registry Number

Mercury, ethyl(2-mercaptobenzoato-*S*)−, sodium salt
Ethyl(sodium *o*-mercaptobenzoato)mercury
Sodium (2-carboxyphenylthio)ethylmercury
Sodium (*o*-ethylmercurithio)benzoate
[(*o*-Carboxyphenyl)thio]ethylmercury sodium salt
[54-64-8]

5. Empirical Formula   Molecular Weight

$C_9H_9HgNaO_2S$ 404.81

6. Structural Formula

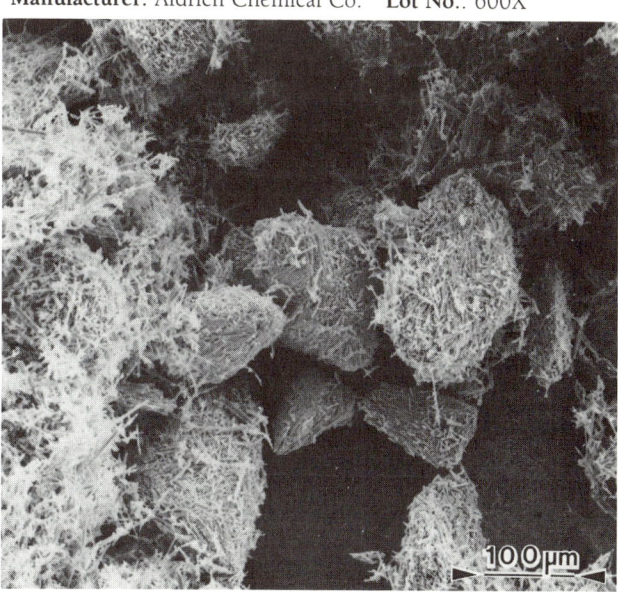

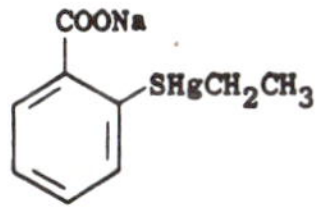

$COONa$ / $SHgCH_2CH_3$

7. Commercial Availability

USA

American Roland Corp.
Atomergic Chemetals Corp.
Austin Chemical Co.
Eli Lilly & Co.
ICN K & K Labs, Inc.
Pfaltz & Bauer, Inc.
Ruger Chemical Co.
Uhe Co., George
United States Biochemicals Corp.

UK

Aldrich Chemical Co. Ltd.
BDH Chemicals Ltd.

8. Method of Manufacture

Thimerosal is prepared by the interaction of ethylmercuric chloride (or hydroxide), thiosalicylic acid and sodium hydroxide in alcohol. It may be prepared by treating 2-mercaptobenzoic acid with ethylmercuric chloride and converting the product to the sodium salt.

9. Description

Light cream-colored crystalline powder; orthorhombic crystals. Slight, characteristic odor.

SEM-MF-27
Excipient: Thimerosal
Manufacturer: Aldrich Chemical Co.   **Lot No.:** 600X

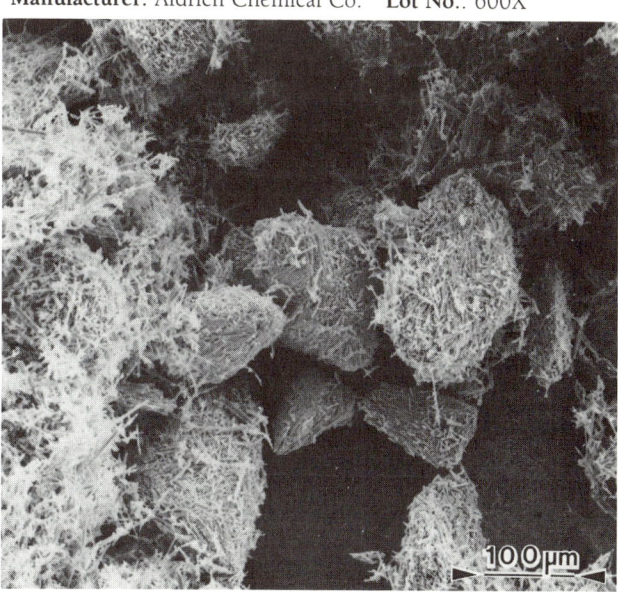

Magnification: 120X

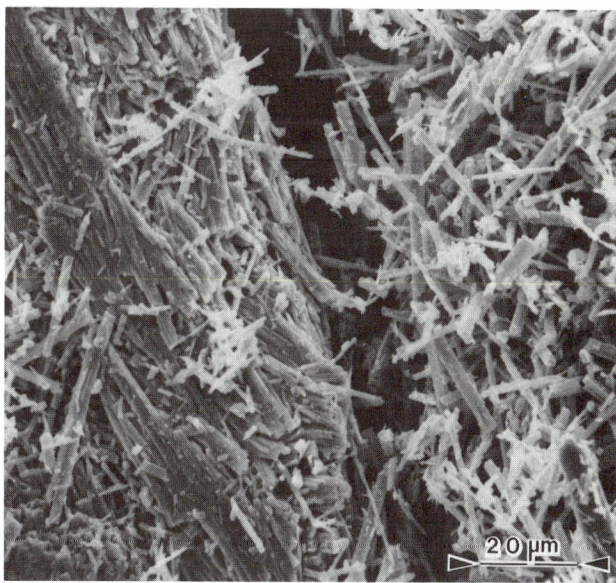

Magnification: 600X

10. Pharmacopeial Specifications

Test	USP	BP
Identification	+	+
pH (1% w/v solution)	—	6.0–8.0
Loss on drying	≤0.5%	≤0.5%
Ether soluble substances	≤0.8%	≤0.6%
Mercury ions/mercuric salt	≤0.7%	+
Readily carbonizable substances	+	—
Assay range	97–101%	≥98%

11. Typical Properties

Bulk density: <0.33 g/cm³
Decomposes between 205-230°C
Magnetically attracted particles: ≤5/100 g
Microbiological: (1) Bactericidal in acidic medium; (2) bacteriostatic and fungistatic in alkaline or neutral medium; (3) not effective against spore-forming organisms.
Solubility: Freely soluble in water; soluble in ethanol; almost insoluble in ether, benzene.
pKa (at 25°C): 3.05

Academy HPE Laboratory Project Data

	Method	Lab #	Results
Solubility	SOL-6	23	*g/ml*
(Water 25°C)			1.007
(Water 37°C)			1.758
(Alcohol 25°C)			0.098-0.104
(Alcohol 37°C)			0.104-0.115
(Propylene glycol 25°C)			0.425-0.675
(Propylene glycol 37°C)			0.425-0.675
(Hexane 25°C)			0.005
(Hexane 37°C)			0.006

Supplier: Eli Lilly & Co.

12. Stability and Storage Conditions

Compatible with alcohols, soaps and physiological salt solutions. Light sensitive in aqueous solutions. Rate of oxidation is greatly increased in the presence of trace copper or other metals. Slightly acidic solutions might be precipitated as the corresponding acid, which would undergo slow decomposition with the formation of insoluble products. Store in fiber drums with polyethylene liners. Protect from light. Protect from ultraviolet light and reducing agents. Ethyl mercury ion forms mercaptides with available sulfhydryl groups. This may be a problem with plastics.

13. Incompatibilities and Inactivation

Incompatibility: Aluminum; phenylmercuric compounds; quaternary ammonium compounds (≥0.01%)
Inactivation: Rubber caps pretreated with thimerosal were as capable as untreated caps of removing thimerosal from solutions in contact with them. The inactivation of thimerosal in 1, 5 and 10 ml rubber-sealed vials was dependent on the following factors: type of rubber, temperature, and ratio of volume of liquid to surface area of rubber exposed to the solution. The residual thimerosal present in 5 and 10 ml after 18 months was sufficient to provide adequate bacteriostasis, but was insufficient in 1 ml vials.
Stability of solutions: Dilute aqueous solutions of thimerosal were fairly stable to heat but labile to light; less stable when alkaline than when acid; most stable to light at pH 5 to 7; and unstable to heat but not to light in the presence of Cu, Fe, or Zn ions, but not Ca or Mg ions. Thimerosal was adsorbed by rubber caps even at 0°C. It was concluded that eye drops containing thimerosal should be stored in light-resistant containers with no direct contact with rubber caps and that they should be buffered at pH 6 to 7. It is strongly adsorbed by plastics, especially polyethylene and by rubber stoppers.

14. Safety

Toxic effects and treatment: As for mercury. Hypersensitivity reactions, usually with erythema and papular or vesicular eruptions, occasionally occur. A patient suffered a burn 5 cm in diameter at the site of contact with an aluminum foil diathermy electrode after preoperative preparation with thimerosal 0.1% in 50% alcohol. Subsequent investigation showed that considerable heat was generated when such a solution came into contact with aluminum. Reports of six cases of poisoning, five of them fatal, have occurred, resulting from the presence of 1,000 times the normal quantity of thimerosal in a preparation of chloramphenicol for intramuscular injection. Thimerosal has been reported to be ototoxic.
Hypersensitivity: Of 100 patients with allergic contact dermatitis, 2 gave positive reactions to patch testing with thimerosal. Delayed hypersensitivity reactions to intradermal injections of thimerosal 1 in 10,000 were noted in 9 of 44 patients. The reactions to old tuberculin have been attributed to the presence of thimerosal. In 63 subjects with positive thimerosal reactions, nearly all had positive reactions to old tuberculin, but 23 had negative reactions to purified protein derivative, which contained no thimerosal. 50 ml of a 1% solution has been injected intravenously in man with no chills or later injurious effects.

15. Handling Precautions

Avoid ingestion, inhalation and contact with skin, nose and mouth.

16. Regulatory Acceptance

USP XXI; BP 1980

17. Applications in Pharmaceutical Formulation or Technology

Use	Concentration (%)
Preservative for biologicals	0.01-0.02
Preservative for eye drops	0.01

18. Related Substances

Other mercurial preservatives

19. Comments

A discrepancy appears to exist between references 6, 7, and 8, which state that thimerosal is strongly absorbed by polyethylene stoppers. Eli Lilly and Company recommends that the product be stored in polyethylene-lined drums.

20. Specific References

1. R. Benesch and R. E. Benesch, *J. Amer. Chem. Soc.*, 73: 3391 (1951).
2. R. Thompson and T. Hoffman, *J. Pharm. Sci.*, 64: 1863 (1975).
3. S. Wiener, *J. Pharm. Pharmac.*, 7: 118 (1955).
4. J. Birner and J. R. Garnet, *J. Pharm. Sci.*, 53: 1426 (1964).
5. K. Tsuji *et al.*, *Arch. Pract. Pharm.*, 24:110 (1964), per *Int. Pharm. Abstr.*, 2: 1166 (1965).
6. H. Hess, *Informationsdienst A.P.V.*, 14: 129 (1968).
7. F. S. Skinner, *Informationsdienst A.P.V.*, 18: 256 (1972).
8. E. Bann, *Informationsdienst A.P.V.*, 18: 246 (1972).
9. H. T. Jones, *Br. Med. J.*, 2: 504 (1972).
10. J. H. M. Axton, *Postgrad. Med. J.*, 48: 417 (1972).
11. J. L. Honigman, *I.C.I. Pharmaceuticals* (letter), *Pharm. J.*, 2: 523 (1975).
12. A. A. Fisher *et al.*, *Archs Derm.*, 104: 286 (1971).
13. H. Mizutari (letter), *New Engl. J. Med.*, 289: 1424 (1973).
14. H. Hansson and H. Möller, *Scand. J. Infect. Dis.*, 3: 169 (1971), per *Abstr. Hyg.*, 47: 29
15. H. Hanson and H. Möller, *Acta Allerg.*, 26: 150 (1971), per *Abstr. Wld. Med.*, 45: 883 (1971).

16. W. A. Jamieson and H. M. Powell, Merthiolate as a preservative for biological products, *Am. J. Hyg.*, 14(1): 218-224, (1931).

17. E. O. Davisson, personal communication: Physical Chemistry Research Department, Eli Lilly and Company.

18. T. Smazynski and L. Krowcynski, *Dissnes Pharm. Warsz.*, 19: 591 (1967), per *Int. Pharm. Abstr.*, 5: 124 (1968).

19. L. Pine *et al.*, *Mycopath. Mycol. Appl.*, 37: 1 (1969), per *Abstr. Hyg.*, 44: 736 (1969).

20. R. M. E. Richards and J. M. E. Reary, *J. Pharm. Pharmac.*, 24 Suppl. 84 (1972).

21. J. D. Abrams *et al.*, *Br. J. Ophthal.*, 49: 146 (1965).

USA: Anthony Palmieri III*; D. Sanvordeker**; Z. Chowhan**
UK: B. J. Meakin*

Titanium Dioxide

1. Nonproprietary Names
USP: Titanium dioxide
BP: Titanium dioxide

2. Functional Category
USP: Coating agent
BP: Protective and pharmaceutical aid
Others: Pigment, U.V. absorber

3. Synonyms
Titanic anhydride; titanium oxide; anatase titanium dioxide; rutile titanium dioxide; octahedrite titanium dioxide; ilmenite titanium dioxide; brookite titanium dioxide; CI 77891

4. Chemical Name and CAS Registry Number
Titanium oxide (TiO₂) [13463-67-7]

5. Empirical Formula   Molecular Weight
TiO₂   79.88

6. Structural Formula
None

7. Commercial Availability
USA
Aceto Chemical Co.
Degussa Corp.
du Pont de Nemours & Co., E.I.
Gulf & Western Natural Resources Group
Kohnstamm & Co., H.
Pfaltz and Bauer, Inc.
Rhone-Poulenc, Inc.
Ruger Chemical Co.
S.S.T. Corp.
Sun Chemical Corp.
Whittaker, Clark & Daniels, Inc.

UK
D.F. Anstead
N.L. Chemicals (UK) Ltd.
Rhodia (UK) Ltd.
Tioxide (UK) Ltd.

8. Method of Manufacture
Titanium dioxide may be prepared by direct combination of titanium and oxygen; by treatment of titanium salts in aqueous solution; by the reaction of volatile inorganic titanium compounds with oxygen; and by oxidation or hydrolysis of organic compounds of titanium.

9. Description
White, amorphous, odorless, tasteless powder.

SEM-KY-67
Excipient: Titanium Dioxide—Atlas white
Supplier: H. Kohnstamm

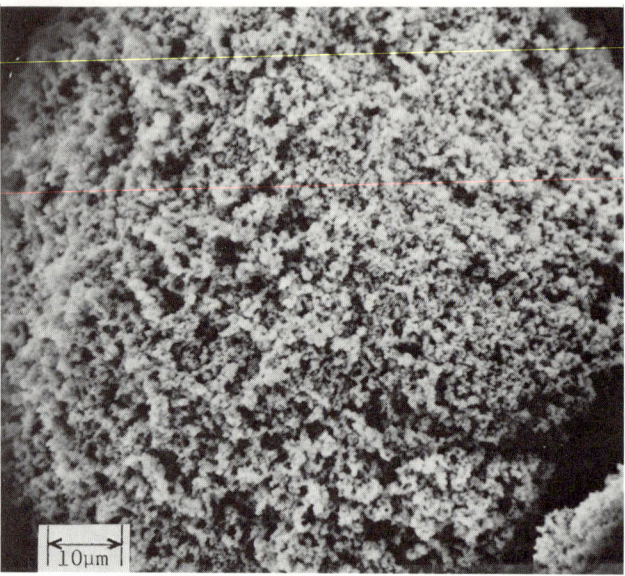

Magnification: 1200× **Voltage:** 10 kV

SEM-KY-68
Excipient: Titanium Dioxide—Kowet

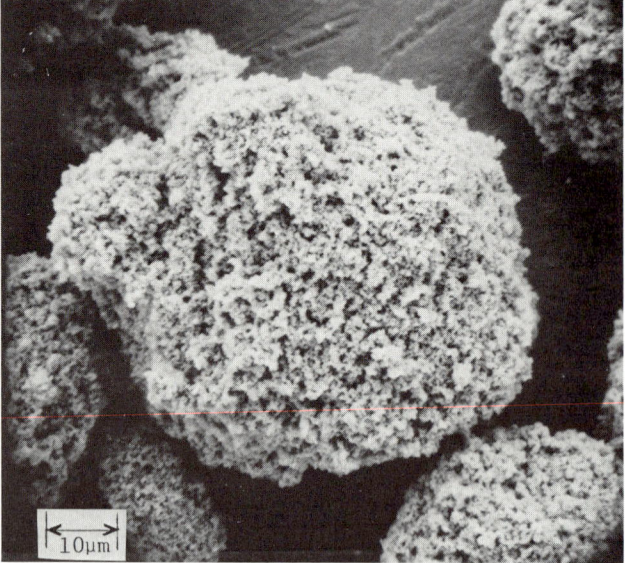

Magnification: 1200× **Voltage:** 10 kV

SEM-KY-69
Excipient: 3328 Titanium Dioxide USP

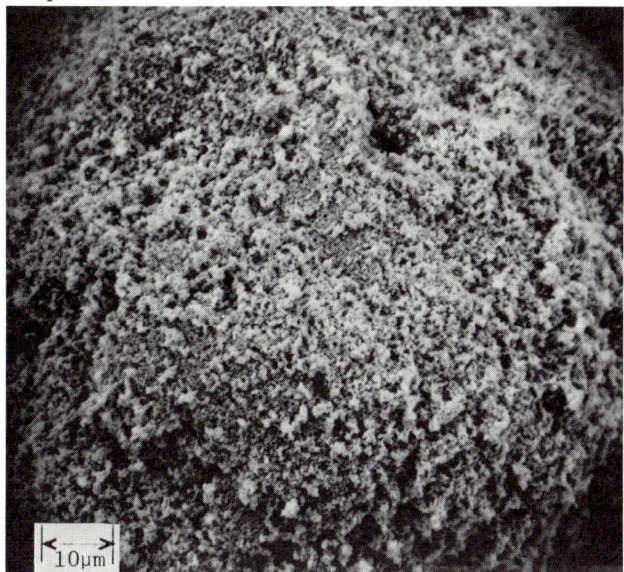

Magnification: 1200× **Voltage:** 10 kV

10. Pharmacopeial Specifications

Test	USP	BP/EP
Identification	+	+
Acidity or alkalinity	–	+
Loss on drying	≤0.5%	–
Loss on ignition	≤0.5%	–
Water-soluble substances	≤0.25%	≤0.25%
Heavy metals	–	≤20 ppm
Acid-soluble substances	≤0.5%	–
Arsenic	≤8 ppm	≤5 ppm
Iron	–	≤200 ppm
Lead	≤0.002%	–
Antimony	–	≤100 ppm
Barium	–	+
Assay range	99.0–100.5%	98.0–100.5%
Clarity & color of solution	–	+

11. Typical Properties

	Mineral Source	
Property	Anatase	Rutile
Appearance	Brilliant white powder	Brilliant white powder
Density (g/cm³)	3.8-4.1	3.9-4.2
Particle size avg. (μm)	0.3	0.2-0.3
Refractive index	2.55	2.76
Tinting strength (Reynolds)	1200-1300	1650-1900
Compressibility coeff. (10⁶cm²/kg)	–	0.53-0.58
Dielectric constant	48	114
Hardness (moh)	5-6	6-7
Melting point (°C)		
In air	–	1830±15
At higher % of O₂	–	1879±15
Specific heat (cal °C/g)	0.17	0.17

Solubility: Insoluble in water, HCl, HNO₃ and dilute H₂SO₄. Soluble in hot, concentrated H₂SO₄ and HF. The reactivity depends on a previous heat treatment; prolonged heating produces a less-soluble material.

Academy HPE Laboratory Project Data

	Method	Lab #	Results
Moisture content	MC-3	33	0.44%[a]
Moisture content	MC-4	33	0.00%[a]
Bulk/Tap density	BTD-1	1	B: 0.431 g/cm³[a]
		1	T: 0.625 g/cm³[a]
	BTD-7	14	B: 0.620 g/cm³[a]
		14	T: 0.830 g/cm³[a]
(Food grade)	BTD-6	8	Volume: 20.5%[a]
			Weight: 21.0%[a]
(Food grade)	BTD-6	8	Volume: 21.5%[a]
			Weight: 22.0%[a]
(CR-A33)	BTD-6	8	Volume: 22.0%[b]
			Weight: 23.0%[b]
Particle size dist.	PSD-4	17	[a]

Sieve Size US Standard	Particle Size (S. μm)	Weight % ± SD
	S 1000	13.53 ± 1.97
18	590 S 1000	11.85 ± 0.83
30	297 S 590	21.05 ± 0.23
50	210 S 297	12.95 ± 0.57
70	149 S 210	10.20 ± 0.51
100	74 S 149	19.94 ± 0.58
200	S 74	10.48 ± 0.71

	Method	Lab #	Results
Solubility (Water 25°C)	SOL-4	10	0.000%[a]
(Water 37°C)	SOL-4	10	0.000%[a]
(Alcohol 25°C)	SOL-4	10	0.0004%[a]
(Alcohol 37°C)	SOL-4	10	0.0004%[a]
(Prop. glycol 25°C)	SOL-4	10	0.0004%[a]
(Prop. glycol 37°C)	SOL-4	10	NA[a]
(n-hexane 25°C)	SOL-4	10	0.000%[a]
(n-hexane 37°C)	SOL-4	10	0.000%[a]
Density	DE-2	36	3.461 g/cm³[a]
PSD Plot	PSD-8	33	Fig:33-PSD-4[a]

Suppliers: Kerr-McGee[a] Whittaker, Clark & Daniels, Inc.[b]

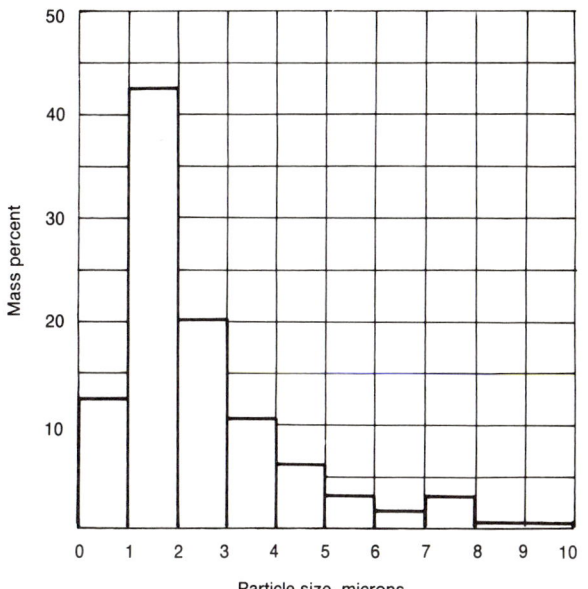

Titanium dioxide (Whittaker, Clark & Daniels, Lot #402302)

Figure: 33-PSD-4 **Method:** PSD-8

12. Stability and Storage Conditions

Titanium dioxide is extremely stable at high temperatures (mp 1800°C) and slow to react. The exceptional stability is due to the strong bond between the tetravalent titanium ion and the bivalent oxygen ions. Titanium dioxide can lose small, unweighable amounts of oxygen by interaction with radiant energy. This oxygen can easily recombine again as a part of a reversible photochemical reaction, particularly if there is no oxidizable material available. These small oxygen losses are important because they can cause significant changes in the optical and electrical properties of the pigment. Preserve in a well-closed container.

13. Incompatibilities

Possible effect on certain active substances, which may be due to a catalytic effect.

14. Safety

High concentrations of the dust may cause irritation to the respiratory tract.

15. Handling Precautions

None

16. Regulatory Acceptance

USP XXI; BP/EP 1980

17. Applications in Pharmaceutical Formulation or Technology

White pigment for film and sugar-coated tablets and for gelatin capsules. Addition to dermatological preparations for topical protection. Scatters UV light at 290-700 nm.

18. Related Substances

None described.

19. Comments

Titanium dioxide, an opacifier used in aqueous film coating solutions, can exist in several polymorphic modifications, each with a different hardness. Rutile has a hardness on the Moh's scale of 5.5-6, whereas anatase has a hardness of 6-6.5. Coating solution containing more rutile was found to cause abrasion or wear of the coating pan surface, causing black specks on the white tablets.

20. Specific References

1. J. Barksdale, "Titanium," 2nd Ed., Ronald, New York, 1966, 1949.
2. *Kronos Guide*, European Titanium Pigment Division, National Lead Company, 1968.
3. P. B. Mitton, L. W. Vejnoska, *et al.*, Hiding power of white pigments—theory and measurement, Part I, *Offic. Dig. Fed. Soc. Paint Technology*, 33:(441), 1264-1287 (1961).
4. F. B. Stieg, Jr., The geometry of white hiding power, *Offic. Dig. Fed. Soc. Paint Technol.*, 34:(453), 1065-1079 (1962).
5. *The Handbook*, Titanium Pigment Division, National Lead Co., New York, New York, 1964.
6. W. A. Kampfer, Titanium dioxide. In: "Pigment Handbook—Properties and Economics," T. C. Patton (Ed.), Vol. 1, John Wiley & Sons, New York, 1973.
7. N. A. Lange and G. M. Forker, "Lange's Handbook of Chemistry," Handbook Publishers, Inc., Sandusky, Ohio, 1946.
8. M. Rosoff and P. Sheen, Pan abrasion and polymorphism of titanium dioxide in coating suspensions, *J. Pharm. Sci.*, 72:(12), 1485 (1983).

USA: R. Gibson*; G. Cuff*; Z. Chowhan**
UK: J. E. Hogan*

Tragacanth

1. Nonproprietary Name
NF: Tragacanth
BP/EP: Tragacanth

2. Functional Category
USP: Suspending and/or viscosity-increasing agent

3. Synonyms
Gum tragacanth; tragacantha; trag; gum dragon; goat's thorn; tragant; persian tragacanth

4. Chemical Name and CAS Registry Number
—

5. Empirical Formula   Molecular Weight
—   About 840,000

6. Structural Formula
—

7. Commercial Availability
USA
Botanicals International, Inc.
Celanese Plastics and Specialties Co.
Chart Corp.
V. L. Clark Chemical Co.
Colony Import and Export Corp.
Eastern Mohair and Trading Co., Inc.
Foralac Co.
Gumix International, Inc.
Kraft Chemical Co.
Dr. Madis' Laboratories, Inc.
Meer Corp.
Ruger Chemical Co.
Strauch Chemical Distributors, Inc.
Tic Gums, Inc.
George Uhe Co., Inc.
Water Soluble Polymers Div.

UK
A.F. Sutter & Co.
Kimpton Brothers Ltd.

8. Method of Manufacture
Tragacanth is the dried, gummy exudation obtained by incision from *Astragalus gummifer* (Labillardere) and other Asiatic species of *Astragalus*.

9. Description
Flattened, lamellated, frequently curved fragments or straight or spirally twisted linear pieces from 0.5 mm to 2.5 mm in thickness. A white to weak yellow, translucent, odorless substance with an insipid mucilaginous taste. In its powdered form it appears white to yellowish.

SEM-MF-26
Excipient: Tragacanth Grade III Powder
Supplier: Sigma Chemical Co. **Lot No.** N.A.

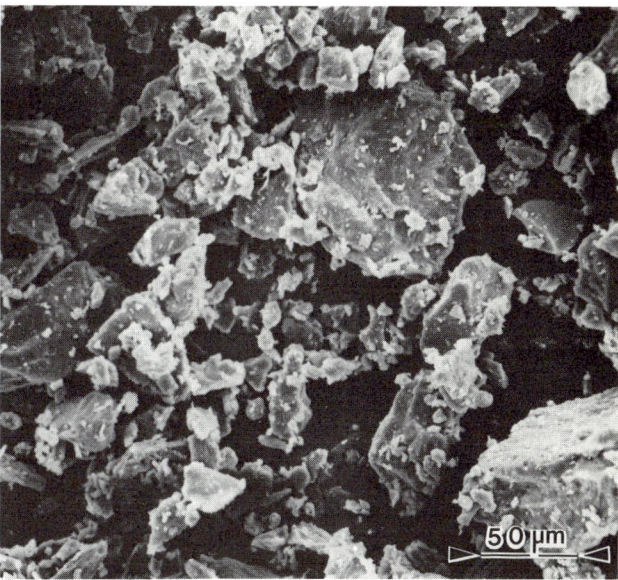

Magnification: 240×

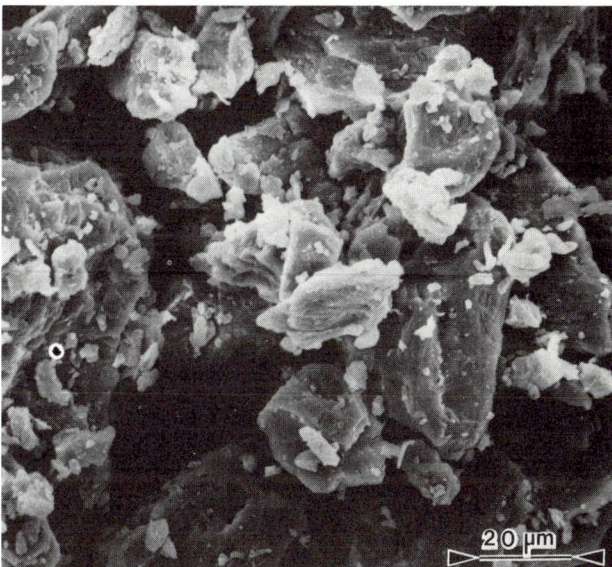

Magnification: 600×

10. Pharmacopeial Specifications

Test	NF XV (Tears or Powder)	BP/EP (Tears)	BP/EP (Powder)
Identification	+	+	+
Microbial limit	Absence of Salmonella and E. coli	—	1.0 g free from E. coli
Arsenic	≤3ppm	—	—
Lead	≤0.001%	—	—
Heavy metals	≤0.004%	—	—
Karaya gum	Absent	—	—
Dextrin	—	Absent	Absent
Agar	—	Absent	Absent

Test	NF (Tears or Powder)	BP/EP (Tears)	BP/EP (Powder)
Acacia and other soluble gums	—	Absent	Absent
Sterculia	—	Absent	Absent
Foreign matter	—	≤1.0%	≤1.0%
Sulfated ash	—	≤4.0%	≤5.0%
Apparent viscosity	—	—	+

11. Typical Properties

Physical: Powder, finer than 80 mesh with approximately 50% finer than 200 mesh. When 1 g is added to 50 ml of water, it swells to form a smooth, nearly uniform, opalescent mucilage. A 0.5% solution shows viscosity ranging from 120 to 600 cps, depending on the type of tragacanth obtained from supplier. It is insoluble in alcohol.

Chemical: When mixed with water it turns into a soluble portion, which is a complex mixture of polysaccharides containing D-galacturonic acid, other sugars and traces of starch and cellulose; and an insoluble portion which swells to a gel and consists of 60 to 70% bassorin.

12. Stability and Storage Conditions

Both tears and powdered tragacanth are stable if stored in airtight containers. Tragacanth gels may be sterilized by autoclaving. It is liable to microbial contamination with enterobacterial species, and stock solutions should contain suitable preservatives.

13. Incompatibilities

Not known.

14. Safety

Sensitization to tragacanth has occurred rarely. An acceptable daily intake could not be evaluated on the toxicological data available.

15. Handling Precautions

Use masks.

16. Regulatory Acceptance

NF XVI; BP/EP 1980

17. Applications in Pharmaceutical Formulation or Technology

Emulsifier and suspending agent in emulsions and suspensions. Concentration varies according to viscosity and type of product.

18. Related Substances

Hog gum, from species of *prunus* (Fam. Rosaceae), and sterculia gum are used in industry as substitutes for tragacanth.

19. Comments

In the preparation of aqueous dispersions, powdered tragacanth should first be triturated with alcohol before adding the water.

20. Specific References:

1. P. C. Eisman, J. Cooper and D. Jaconia, Influence of gum tragacanth on the bacterial activity of preservatives, *J. Am. Pharm. Assoc.*, Sci. Ed., 46: (2), 144-147 (1957).
2. J. W. Fairbairn, The presence of peroxidases in tragacanth, *J. Pharm. Pharmacol*, 19: (3), 191 (1967).
3. A. Taub, Conditions for the preservation of gum tragacanth jellies, *J. Am. Pharm. Assoc.*, Sci. Ed., 47: (4), 235-239 (1958).

USA: D. Hsia*; W. Rix**
UK: H. Burlinson**

Trichloromonofluoro-methane

1. Nonproprietary Names

NF: Trichloromonofluoromethane
BP: Trichlorofluoromethane

2. Functional Category

NF: Aerosol propellant
BP: Aerosol propellant

3. Synonyms

Propellant 11; refrigerant 11; *Freon; Genetron; Ucon*

4. Chemical Names and CAS Registry Number

Methane, trichlorofluoro
Trichlorofluoromethane [75-69-4]

5. Empirical Formula   Molecular Weight

C-Cl$_3$-F   137.37

6. Structural Formula

—

7. Commercial Availability

USA

Allied Chemical Corp.
E. I. DuPont De Nemours & Co.
Union Carbide Corp.

UK

I.C.I. Plc
ISC Chemicals Ltd.

8. Method of Manufacture

See monograph on dichlorodifluoromethane.

9. Description

See monograph on dichlorodifluoromethane.

10. Pharmacopeial Specifications

Test	NF	BP
Identification	+	+
Boiling temperature	24°C, approx.	Approx. 23.7°C
Water	≤0.001%	≤0.001%
High boiling residues (matter)	≤0.01%	≤0.01%
Inorganic chlorides (chloride)	+	+
Acidity	—	≤2ppm
Solubility	—	Immiscible with water
Distillation range	—	0.3°C

11. Typical Properties

Boiling point (1 atm.): 74.7°F; 23.7°C
Freezing point: −168°F; −111°C
Vapor pressure (psia)*: 13.4 at 70°F
          39.0 at 130°F
Liquid density (g/ml): 1.485 at 70°F
          1.403 at 130°F
Liquid viscosity (Centipoise): 0.439 at 70°F
          0.336 at 130°F
Surface tension (dynes/cm.): 19 at 77°F
Solubility in water (weight %): 0.11 at 77°F
Limits of inflammability: Noninflammable
* psia = 14.7 + psig

12. Stability and Storage Conditions

See monograph on dichlorodifluoromethane. Trichloromonofluoromethane is subject to hydrolysis in the presence of water and will form traces of hydrochloric acid, which may be irritating to the skin or may cause corrosion when used in a metallic container. It will also react with aluminum in the presence of ethyl alcohol to cause corrosion within the container, with the formation of hydrogen gas.

13. Incompatibilities

See monograph on dichlorodifluoromethane.

14. Safety

See monograph on dichlorodifluoromethane.

15. Handling Precautions

See monograph on dichlorodifluoromethane.

16. Regulatory Acceptance

NF XVI; BP 1980

17. Applications in Pharmaceutical Formulation or Technology

See monograph on dichlorodifluoromethane.

18. Related Substances

Dichlorodifluoromethane; dichlorotetrafluoroethane

19. Comments

This fluorocarbon possesses a distinct carbon tetrachloride-like odor, which may limit its use. Blends of propellant 11/12 produce vapor pressures of 15-70 psig at 21°C, which adequately cover the range of pressure required for satisfactory aerosol products.

20. Specific References:

1. J. J. Sciarra, Pharmaceutical and cosmetic aerosols, *J. Pharm. Sci.*, 63: 1815-1836 (1974).
2. Y. M. Amiin, E. B. Thompson, W. L. Chiou, Fluorocarbon aerosol propellants XII: Correlation of blood levels of trichloromonofluoromethane to cardiovascular and respiratory responses in anesthetized dogs, *J. Pharm. Sci.*, 68: 160-163 (1979).

USA: J. J. Sciarra*; Z. Chowhan*
UK: P.J. Davies*

Triethanolamine

1. Nonproprietary Names
NF: Trolamine
BP: Triethanolamine

2. Functional Category
NF: Alkalizing agent, emulsifying and/or solubilizing agent

3. Synonyms
Trihydroxytriethylamine; tris(hydroxyethyl)amine; triethylolamine; TEA

4. Chemical Names and CAS Registry Number
Ethanol,2,2',2''-nitrilotris
2,2',2''-Nitrilotriethanol [102-71-6]

5. Empirical Formula   Molecular Weight
$C_6H_{15}NO_3$ 149.19

6. Structural Formula
$(HO-CH_2-CH_2)_3 \equiv N$

7. Commercial Availability
USA
Ashland Chemical Co.
ICN K & K Labs, Inc.
McKesson Chemical Co.
Olin Chemicals
Pfaltz & Bauer, Inc.
Protameen Chemicals, Inc.
Ruger Chemicals Co.
Stoney-Mueller, Inc.
Thompson-Hayward Chemical Co.
Union Carbide Corp., Chemicals & Plastics
United States Biochemicals Corp.

UK
Shell Chemicals (UK), LTD
UNALCO, LTD

8. Method of Manufacture
Production of the ethanolamines is accomplished by reacting ethylene oxide with ammonia to yield a mixture of the three compounds. By a series of separation procedures, monoethanolamine, diethanolamine and triethanolamine are obtained.

9. Description
A clear, colorless to pale yellow viscous liquid having a slight ammoniacal odor.

10. Pharmacopeial Specifications

Test	NF	BP
Identification	+	+
Specific gravity	1.120-1.128	1.120-1.130
Refractive index (20°C)	1.481-1.486	1.482-1.485
Water	≤0.5%	—
Residue on ignition	≤0.05%	—
Sulphated ash	—	≤0.1%
Content of alkanolamines	99.0-107.4%	99%-110%
Content of triethanolamine (assay)	—	≥80%
Related substances		
(a) Monoethanolamine	—	≤3%
(b) Diethanolamine	—	≤12%
(c) Others	—	≤5%
(d) Equivalent of total bases		≤110.0%

11. Typical Properties
Academy HPE Laboratory Project Data

	Method	Lab #	Results
Moisture content	MC-3	25	0.09%

Supplier: Olin Chemicals

Melting point, °C: 21.2
Flash point (open cup), °C: 185
Vapor pressure, 20°C, mm Hg: 0.01
Viscosity (absolute), 20°C, cps: 1013
Surface tension, 20°C, dynes/cm: 47.5
pKa, 25°C: 9.5
pH (0.1N solution): 10.5
Solubility: Miscible with water, methanol, acetone. Solubility at 25°C: in benzene: 4.2%; in ether: 1.6%; in carbon tetrachloride: 0.4%; in n-heptane: <0.1%.
Hygroscopicity: Very hygroscopic.
Chemical properties: The ethanolamines are characterized by the presence of a basic nitrogen atom and hydroxyl group(s). Thus, they are capable of undergoing reactions typical for both amines and alcohols. The amine group usually exhibits the greater activity, whenever it is possible for a reaction to take place at either the amine or hydroxyl group. Triethanolamine is a tertiary amine and displays the usual properties of this class of nitrogen bases.

12. Stability and Storage Conditions
The ethanolamines present no unusual problems in handling under ordinary conditions. In general, it is advisable to store them in tight containers protected from light, and the storage temperature should not exceed 50°C. Storage in mild steel is satisfactory for a limited time. However, stainless steel should be used if prolonged storage is anticipated. This will prevent color development. The color may develop due to absorption of atmospheric oxygen. Thus, storage tanks should also be gas padded, if color is important. Ethanolamines are hygroscopic. If water content is to be minimized, a dry, inert gas pad under pressure should also be used when stored in tanks. Pure ethanolamines may solidify at room temperature or slightly below. The 85% grade of triethanolamine tends to stratify below 15°C. Homogeneity can be restored by warming.

13. Incompatibilities

Triethanolamine will react with acids to form salts and esters. Triethanolamine reacts with copper to form complex salts. Discoloration and precipitation will take place in the presence of heavy metal salts. Triethanolamine can react with reagents such as thionyl chloride to replace the hydroxyl groups by halogens. The products of the reactions are very toxic, resembling other nitrogen mustards.

14. Safety

All of the ethanolamines are capable of producing severe eye injuries. They may be health hazards primarily because of their instant action on the skin and in eyes. The mono- and diethanolamines are also considered to be slightly hazardous from the standpoint of oral administration. The hazard from triethanolamine in this respect would be negligible.

Insofar as absorption through the skin is concerned, only pure monoethanolamine has a definite toxicity. In this respect di- and triethanolamine are much less toxic. The table below summarizes the acute toxicity of triethanolamine.

Acute oral LD_{50}, g/kg	8
Acute dermal toxicity LD_{50}, g/kg	>2

15. Handling Precautions

Personal protective equipment should be used by personnel handling concentrated solutions of ethanolamines.

16. Regulatory Acceptance

NF XVI; BP 1980

17. Applications in Pharmaceutical Formulation or Technology

Triethanolamine forms soaps with free fatty acids. These soaps have valuable properties as detergents and emulsifiers. They are neutral (pH approximately 8.0), and thus should be free from irritating effects upon the skin. The soaps form very stable emulsions of almost any oil, fat or wax for external use.

Concentrations usually used for emulsification are 2-4% of triethanolamine and 2-5 times as much fatty acid. For mineral oils the amount of the aminoalcohol is increased to 5% with an appropriate increase in the amount of fatty acids.

Preparations made with triethanolamine soaps tend to darken on storage. Avoiding light and contact with metal can reduce the discoloration. Triethanolamine is also used in salt formation for injectable solutions. Other general uses are as buffers, polymer plasticizers and humectants.

18. Related Substances

Diethanolamine, NF; monoethanolamine, NF

19. Comments

There are various grades of triethanolamine. The standard grade contains 15% of diethanolamine and 0.5% of monoethanolamine. The superior grade contains 98-99% triethanolamine.

One volume part of triethanolamine with 5-7 parts of a mixture of CaO_2 and ZnO_2 was used as a filling material which enhanced the restorative process in periodontal tissues. (I. I. Volnov, O. I. Kruglyakev and A. I. Marchenko, *C. A.*, 77: 52373h, 1972.) Triethanolamine was also claimed to have been used with other ingredients as a lubricant on rubber gloves for use in operations. (K. Asano and M. Sawatari *C.A.*, 86: 127325r, 1977).

20. Specific References

1. "Ethanolamines," technical brochure, Jefferson Chemical Company, Inc., 1972.
2. "Ethanolamines," product data, Olin Chemicals "Triethanolamine," material safety data, Olin Chemicals, 1977.
3. "Triethanolamines S.," technical leaflet, BASF AG, 1976.
   "Alkanolamines," BASF AG, 1972.

USA: E. Shek*, G. S. Brenner**

Pharmaceutical Waters
(Water for Pharmaceutical Purposes)

1. Nonproprietary Names

USP/BP: Purified water (distilled, de-ionized or demineralized water)
USP/BP: Water for injection
USP: Bacteriostatic water for injection
USP: Sterile water for injection
USP: Sterile water for inhalation
USP: Sterile water for irrigation

2. Functional Category

USP: Sterile vehicle—water for injection, bacteriostatic solvent—purified water
Others: Vehicle and solvent for drug substances and excipients

3. Synonyms

Aqua; aqua pura; aqua distillata; aqua purificata; aqua pro injectionibus

4. Chemical Names and CAS Registry Number

Water [7732-18-5]
Hydrogen oxide

5. Empirical Formula   Molecular Weight

H_2O 18.02

6. Structural Formula

H_2O

7. Commercial Availability

The potable water supply for pharmaceutical manufacturing used in the preparation of official pharmaceutical waters is covered by the U.S. Public Health Service Drinking Water Standards set forth in sub-part J of 42 CFR Part 72 and sub-part C of the current Good Manufacturing Practice for Finished Pharmaceuticals 21 CFR Part 211, April 1, 1979.

8. Method of Manufacture

Drinking water undergoes very important purification processes in civilized communities prior to the preparation of water for pharmaceutical purposes. The steps are listed as follows:

1. Removal of insoluble matter through coagulation, settling and filtering processes.

2. Destruction of pathogenic micro-organisms by aeration, chlorination and other means. Water may also be rendered free of micro-organisms by active boiling for 15 to 20 minutes.
3. Improved palatability through aeration and charcoal filtration.

Distillation: A wide variety of stills are available to produce purified or distilled water. Such a distillation unit consists of an evaporator, vapor separator and compressor. The distilland (raw feed water) is heated in the evaporator to boiling. The vapor produced is separated from entrained distilland in the separator. The vapor then enters a compressor where the temperature of the vapors is raised to 107°C. Superheated vapors are then condensed on the outer surface of the tubes of the evaporator containing cool distilland circulating within. The heat of condensation is used efficiently to bring feed water in the tubes to boiling. High purity can be obtained with properly constructed stills. Vapor compression stills are available in sizes ranging from 50 to 2,800 gallons/hour. High-quality distillate, such as water for injection, can be obtained if water is first demineralized. The best stills are constructed of types 304 or 316 stainless steel and coated with pure tin, or made with chemical-resistant glass.

Demineralization: Resins are used to purify water. They remove dissolved ions from mineral, mineral acid and alkali sources by ion exchange. Dissolved gases are also removed while chlorine, in concentrations generally found in potable water, is destroyed by the resin itself. Some organics and colloidal particles are removed by adsorption and filtration. Resin beds may foster microbial life and produce pyrogenic effluent unless adequate precautions are taken to prevent contamination. Mixed bed units produce purer water (decreased conductivity) than stills. However, the organic matter content is usually higher. Ion exchange units are normally used today to treat raw feed water prior to distillation or to reverse osmosis processing.

Reverse Osmosis: Water is forced through a semi-permeable membrane in the opposite direction to normal osmotic diffusion. A very small proportion of inorganic salts passes through but undissolved materials (bacteria and large molecules, such as viruses, pyrogens and high molecular weight organics) are removed.

9. Description

Water is a clear, colorless, odorless liquid.

10. Pharmacopeial Specifications

See Table I. Specifications and testing methods presently used to establish the quality and purity of compendial waters should be revised in order to take advantage of more modern analytical procedures and instrumentation.

Table I — Classification of Water for Pharmaceutical Purposes

Test	Water (USP XVIII)	Purified Water USP	Purified Water Add. 1982 BP/EP	Water for Injection USP/BP	Water for Injection Add. 1982 BP/EP	Bacteriostatic Water for Injection USP	Sterile Water for Injection USP	Sterile Water for Inhalation USP	Sterile Water for Irrigation USP
Identification	—	—	—	—	—	—	—	—	—
pH	—	5.0-7.0	+	5.0-7.0	—	4.5-7.0	5.0-7.0	4.5-7.5	5.0-7.5
Chloride	—	+	+	1-0.5 ppm[2]	—	+	0.5 ppm	0.5 ppm	0.5 ppm
Sulfate	—	+	+	+	—	+	+	+	+
Ammonia (Ammonium)	—	0.3 ppm	+	0.3 ppm	—	—	≤0.3 ppm[7] ≤0.6 ppm[8]	+	≤0.3 ppm[7] ≤0.6 ppm[8]
Calcium	—	+	+	+	—	+	+	+	+
Magnesium	—	—	+	—	—	—	—	—	—
Carbon dioxide	—	+	—	+	—	+	+	+	+
Zinc	+	—	—	—	—	—	—	—	—
Heavy metals	+	+	≤0.1 ppm	+	—	+	+	+	+
Oxidizable substances	no odor	+	+	+	—	—	+	+	+
Non-volatile matter	—	—	≤0.001	—	≤0.004%[2] ≤0.003%[3]	—	—	—	—
Nitrates	—	—	≤0.2 ppm	—	≤0.2 ppm	—	—	—	—
Total solids	0.1%	0.001%	—	0.001%	—	0.001%	≤0.004%[4] ≤0.003%[5] ≤0.002%[6]	—	≤0.004%[4] ≤0.003%[5] ≤0.002%[6]
Bacteriological purity	Complies with US EPA regulations[1]	Complies with 40 CFR 141.14 and 141.21	—	Not required	—	Not required	Not required	Not required	Not required
Pyrogens	—	—	—	+	—	+	+	—	+
Sterility	—	—	—	—	—	+	+	+	+
Antimicrobial preservative effectiveness	—	—	—	—	—	+	—	—	—
Bacterial endotoxins	+	—	—	—	—	+	+	+	+
Particulate matter	—	—	—	—	—	+	+	—	+

[1]Not more than 50 bacteria/100 ml on three successive days, and no coliform bacteria
[2]Containers of 10 ml or less
[3]Containers of 10 ml or more
[4]Containers of 30 ml or less
[5]Containers of 30-100 ml
[6]Containers of 100 ml or more
[7]Containers of 50 ml or less
[8]Containers of 51 ml or more

11. Typical Properties

Boiling point: 100°C
Melting point: 0°C
Critical temperature: 374.2°C
Critical pressure: 218.3 atmospheres
Critical volume: 56.3 cc/g-mole
Critical compressibility: 0.232
Vapor pressure: 23.76 mm of mercury at 25°C
Heat of vaporization: 590 calories/g, or 1100 BTU/lb
Heat capacity (vapor): 0.45 calories/g (°C) or 0.45 BTU/°F
(liquid): 1.02 calories/g (°C) or 1.02 BTU/°F
Specific gravity: 0.9971 at 25°C
Surface tension: 71.97 dynes/cm at 25°C
Viscosity: 0.8904 centipoise at 25°C
Thermal conductivity: 14.6×10^{-4} cal/sec/cm at 25°C
Heat of formation: −55 Kcalories/mole at 25°C
Refractive index: 1.3325 at 25°C
Dielectric constant: 78.54 at 25°C
Dipole moment: 1.84 debye
Ionization constant: 1.008×10^{-14} at 25°C
Solvent properties: Miscible and soluble with most polar solvents and electrolytes

12. Stability and Storage Conditions

Considered chemically stable in all physical states (ice, liquid water and steam).

Table II — Storage Requirements

Type	Storage Requirements*
Water	Preserve in tightly sealed containers.
Purified water	Preserve in tightly sealed containers.
Water for injection	Preserve in tightly sealed containers.
Bacteriostatic water for injection	Preserve in single-dose and multiple-dose containers, preferably of Type I or Type II glass, of not larger than 30 ml size.
Sterile water for injection	Preserve in single-dose containers, preferably of Type I or Type II glass, not more than 1000 ml size.
Sterile water for inhalation	Preserve in single-dose containers, preferably of Type I or Type II glass.

*To prevent evaporation and to maintain quality.

13. Incompatibilities

Pharmaceutical waters react with drugs and ingredients that are susceptible to hydrolysis (decomposition in the presence of water or moisture) at ambient room (15-30°C; 59-86°F) and elevated temperatures. They react violently with alkali metals and rapidly with alkaline metals and their oxides (calcium, magnesium, etc.). They react with anhydrous salts and materials to form hydrates of various compositions and with certain organic materials and calcium carbide.

14. Safety

Water is the basis for many biological life forms, and its safety is unquestioned as long as it meets standards of quality for potability and microbial content. Plain water is considered slightly more toxic upon injection to laboratory animals than physiological salt solutions (normal saline, Ringer's, etc.).

15. Handling Precautions

No restrictions specified except for the use of suitable packaging materials to prevent moisture vapor phase transmission through packaging films and plastic containers.

16. Regulatory Acceptance

USP XX; BP 1980

17. Applications in Pharmaceutical Formulation or Technology

Type	Use (up to 100% concentration)
Water	Solvent and vehicle for the manufacture of drug substances and excipients
Purified water	Vehicle and solvent in the manufacture of drug products and pharmaceutical preparations
Bacteriostatic water for injection	Diluent for ophthalmic and multiple-dose injections
Sterile water for injection	Diluent for injectables
Sterile water for inhalation	Diluent for inhalation therapy products
Sterile water for irrigation	Diluent for internal irrigation therapy products

18. Related Substances

Soft water: Equivalent to not more than 60 mg/liter of calcium carbonate.
Hard water: Equivalent to not less than 120 mg/liter and not more than 180 mg/liter of calcium carbonate.
De-aerated water: Purified water that has been boiled vigorously for 5 minutes and cooled to reduce the air (oxygen) content.
Carbon dioxide-free water: Purified water that has been boiled vigorously for 5 minutes and allowed to cool while protecting it from absorption of atmospheric carbon dioxide.

19. Comments

The term "water" now refers to purified or distilled water in most pharmacopeias. Without further purification, "water" may be unsuitable for certain pharmaceutical uses. For example, the presence of calcium in water affects the viscosity and gel strength of algins and pectin dispersions. The use of drinking water affects the clarity and quality of cough mixtures and the stability of antibiotic liquid preparations. Water commonly contains salts of calcium, iron, zinc, aluminum, magnesium, potassium and sodium. Toxic substances such as arsenic, mercury, barium, cadmium, chromium, cyanide, lead and selenium may constitute a danger to health if present in excess. Ingestion of water containing high amounts of nitrate and calcium are also contra-indicated. The World Health Organization (WHO) has issued revised limits for toxic substances which should not be exceeded in piped water supplies.

Table III — Standards for Drinking Waters

Inorganics	WHO	EPA
	(mg/liter)	(mg/liter)
Sodium	—	No limit
Potassium	—	No limit
Calcium	75	—
Magnesium	30	—
Barium*	1,000	1,000
Copper	50	1,000
Zinc	5	5,000
Iron	100	300
Manganese	—	300
Chromium*	50	50
Silver*	—	50
Lead*	100	50
Arsenic*	50	50
Selenium*	10	10
Cadmium*	10	10
Mercury*	1	2
Chloride	200	250,000
Sulfate	—	250,000
Nitrogen	—	10,000
Cyanide*	50	—

Limits have also been placed on detergents, phenolics, chlorinated phenolics and other toxic organic substances.
*Considered to be more toxic.

20. Specific References

1. W. H. Thomas and H. Harvey, Achieving purity in pharmaceutical Water, *Mfg. Chem. & Aerosol News*, Oct. (1976).
2. B. Holtz, Assuring water quality, *Food Product Development*, December (1976).
3. World Health Organization, *International Standards for Drinking Water*, 3rd Edition (1971).
4. United States Environmental Protection Agency (EPA) Safe Drinking Water Act, *Code of Federal Regulations*, Title 40, Sections 141.14 and 141.21 (1974).
5. R. Rossler, Water and air in the manufacture of sterile pharmaceuticals, *Arzneimittel-Forschung*, 130 (1976).

USA: R. Nash*; I. Nagy**
UK: K. Ridgway*

Carnauba Wax

1. Nonproprietary Names
NF: Carnauba wax
BP: Carnauba wax

2. Functional Category
USP: Tablet coating agent.
BP: Pharmaceutical aid.
Others: Cosmetic formulations, such as creams and depilatory sticks. Sustained-release tablet formulations, tablet polishing agent.

3. Synonyms
Caranda wax; Brazil wax

4. Chemical Name and CAS Registry Number
—

5. Empirical Formula   Molecular Weight
—   —

6. Structural Formula
—

7. Commercial Availability
USA
Durachem
International Wax Refining Co.
Koster Keunen, Inc.
M. Argueso and Co., Inc.
Mutchler Chemical Co.
Strahl & Pitsch, Inc.

UK
G. Eggar & Co., Ltd.
Kimpton Bros., Ltd.
Poth Hillea Co., Ltd.

8. Method of Manufacture
Carnauba wax is obtained by treating the leaf buds and leaves of *Copernicia cerifera* Mart. (Farm Palmae) with hot water. The leaves are dried and beaten to shreds. The wax is then removed with the addition of hot water.

9. Description
Light-brown to pale yellow, moderately coarse flakes or powder, possessing a characteristic bland odor and free from rancidity. There are various types and grades.

10. Pharmacopeial Specifications

Test	NF	BP
Melting range	81-86°C	78°-85°C
Residue on ignition	≤5 mg (0.25%)	—
Heavy metals	≤0.004%	—
Acid value	2-7	≤12.0
Saponification value	78-95	75-95
Iodine value	—	7-14

11. Typical Properties
Ester number: 75-85
Flash point: 570°F min.

Refractive index: U$_D^{90}$ 1.450
Solubilities: Alcohol (boiling): slightly soluble; benzene (warm): freely soluble; chloroform (warm): soluble; ether: soluble; toluene (warm): soluble; water: insoluble
Specific gravity: 0.996-0.998 (25°C)
Unsaponified matter: 50-55%

12. Stability and Storage Conditions
Store in a well-closed container.

13. Incompatibilities
No citations in the literature.

14. Safety
Purified bleached carnauba wax is dermatologically innocuous. It is neither a primary irritant nor a sensitizer.

15. Handling Precautions
No restrictions specified.

16. Regulatory Acceptance
NF XVI; BP 1982 Add.

17. Applications in Pharmaceutical Formulation or Technology
Carnauba wax has been used in sustained-release formulations with stearyl alcohol, and either alone or in combination with various drug entities (10 to 50% w/w). It is used as a polishing agent for sugarcoated tablets. Aqueous emulsions may be prepared (10%) by mixing with an ethanolamine compound and oleic acid. These emulsions will dry with a good luster without rubbing.

18. Related Substances
No citations in the literature.

19. Comments
The specifications from the American Wax Importers and Refiners Assn. for genuine pure carnauba wax, October 1976 (supersedes specifications of October 1960) are as follows:
Scope: These specifications cover the following types and grades:

Brazilian designation	American designation
Type 1 - Flor	= Flor
Primeira	= Prime or No. 1 Yellow
Type 2 - Mediana	= Medium or No. 2 Yellow
Type 3 - Cauipe	= Cauhype
Gorda Clara	= Gorda Clara
	Light Fatty
	No. 2 North Country
Type 4 - Gordarosa	= Fatty Grey or No.3
	North Country

Color: The color of types 1, 2, and 3 shall be no darker than that of the official color card of the American Wax Importers and Refiners Assn., or unless otherwise agreed upon by the seller and the purchaser.
Composition and properties: The wax shall be of an original virgin product made directly from the powder obtained from the leaves of the carnauba palm (*Copernicia cerifera*). It shall be free of extenders or admixtures of other substances, shall conform to the following requirements and shall be so guaranteed by the seller.

| | Crude | | Centrifuged | Filter press refined | |
	Yellow types 1 & 2	Fatty types 3 & 4	Fatty type 4	Yellow types 1 & 2	Fatty types 3 & 4
Melting point - minimum	83°C	82.5°C	82.5°C	83°C	82.5°C
	181.4°F	180.5°F	180.5°F	181.4°F	180.5°F
Flash point - minimum	310°C	299°C	299°C	310°C	299°C
	590°F	570°F	570°F	590°F	570°F
Volatile matter (moisture included) - max. percent	2.0	1.5	1.0		
Insoluble impurities (moisture included) - max. percent	1.0	2.0	0.5	Negligible	Negligible
Acid number - minimum	2.0	4.0	4.0	2.0	4.0
Acid number - maximum	6.0	10.0	10.0	6.0	10.0
Saponification number - minimum	78.0	78.0	78.0	78.0	78.0
Saponification number - maximum	88.0	88.0	88.0	88.0	88.0
Paraffinic hydrocarbons - maximum percent	2.0	2.0	2.0	2.0	2.0
Acetone soluble resinous matter - maximum percent at 15°C	5.0	3.5	3.5	5.0	3.5
Benzene solubility - maximum percent at 25°C	8.0	8.0	8.0	8.0	8.0

20. Specific References

1. E.G. Wiseman, and N.J. Federici, Development of a sustained release aspirin tablet, *J. Pharm. Sci.*, 51: 1535 (1968).
2. C.M. Prasad, and G.P. Srivastava, Study of some sustained release granulations of aspirin, *Indian J. Hosp. Pharm.*, 8: 21 (1971).
3. S.C. Dave, *et al.*, Sustained release tablet formulations of diphenhydramine hyrochloride, part 2, *Indian J. Pharm.*, 36: 94 (1974).
4. K. Kumar, *et al.*, Sustained release tablet formulations of diethycarbamazine citrate, *Indian J. Pharm.*, 37: 57 (1975).

USA: N.H. Kobayashi*, W. McKeehan, L.C. Lappas**
UK: P.C. Record**

Emulsifying Wax

1. Nonproprietary Name
NF: Emulsifying wax [nonionic]
BP: Emulsifying wax [anionic]

2. Functional Categories
USP: Emulsifying and/or solubilizing agent; stiffening agent.

3. Synonyms
Crodex A; *Lanette wax SX BP*; *Cyclonette Wax*; *Collone SEC*; *Polawax*

4. Chemical Name and CAS Registry Number
—

5. Empirical Formula   Molecular Weight
—   —

6. Structural Formula
—

7. Commercial Availability
USA

Croda, Inc.

UK

ABM Chemicals, Ltd.
Albright & Wilson, Ltd.
Croda Chemical, Ltd.
Ronsheim and Moore, Ltd.
Witco Chemicals, Ltd.

8. Method of Manufacture
Emulsifying wax BP contains cetostearyl alcohol and sodium lauryl sulfate or sodium salts of similar sulfated higher primary aliphatic alcohols. A suitable preparation may be obtained by the following process:

Cetostearyl alcohol   90 g
Sodium lauryl sulfate   10 g
Purified water   4 ml

Melt the cetostearyl alcohol and heat to about 95°C. Add the sodium lauryl sulfate mix, add the purified water, heat to 115°C and maintain at this temperature, stirring vigorously until frothing ceases and the product is translucent. Cool quickly.

Proprietary brands of emulsifying wax, may contain different sodium alkyl sulfates; e.g., in *Collone SEC*, sodium cetyl sulfate is used.

Emulsifying wax NF contains cetostearyl alcohol and a polyoxyethylene derivative of a fatty acid ester of sorbitan.

9. Description
An almost white, or pale yellow, waxy solid which when warmed becomes plastic before melting. Odor—faintly waxy; taste—bland.

10. Pharmacopeial Specifications

Test	NF	BP
Melting range	48–52°C	—
pH (3 in 100 dispersion)	5.5–7	—
Hydroxyl value	178–192	—
Iodine value	≤ 3.5	≤ 3.0
Saponification value	≤ 14.0	≤ 2.0
Identification	—	+
Acidity	—	+
Alkalinity	—	+
Sodium alkyl sulfate	—	≥ 8.7
Unsaponifiable matter	—	≥ 86.0
Water	—	≤ 4.0
Alcohols	—	+

11. Typical Properties
Density: 0.97 g/cm³
Melting range: 47-61°C
Solubility: Water: insoluble; ethanol (96%): partially soluble; ether: partially soluble; chloroform: partially soluble; fixed oils: soluble on warming; liquid paraffin: soluble on warming

12. Stability and Storage Conditions
Chemically stable in the solid state, but iron vessels should not be used when heating emulsifying wax. Stainless steel containers are satisfactory. There are no special storage requirements.

13. Incompatibilities
Incompatibilities of emulsifying wax BP are essentially those of sodium alkyl sulfates; i.e., cationic compounds (quaternary ammonium compounds, acriflavine, ephedrine hydrochloride, antihistamines and other nitrogenous compounds); salts of polyvalent metals (aluminum, zinc, tin and lead); and thioglycollates. Compatible with most acids (unless the pH is below 2.5); also with alkalis and hard water. Emulsifying wax, NF, is compatible with non-ionic, anionic and cationic medications, due to its non-ionic nature.

14. Safety
Cetyl alcohol is non-irritating; both cetyl and stearyl alcohols are classified as practically non-toxic. Sodium lauryl sulfate is known to irritate the skin at high concentrations; sodium cetyl sulfate is claimed to be less irritating. Nonionic emulsifying wax NF is claimed to be non-irritating.

15. Handling Precautions
—

16. Regulatory Acceptance
NF XVI; BP 1980.

17. Applications in Pharmaceutical Formulation and Technology
Emulsifying agent: A general purpose (oil-in-water) self-emulsifying agent for external use. In concentrations of about 2%, emulsions are pourable; stiffer emulsions contain up to 10% of emulsifying wax (e.g., aqueous cream, BP). Creams should be adequately preserved. They can usually be sterilized by autoclaving.

Ointment base: Anhydrous ointment bases may be prepared which contain 3-30% emulsifying wax with soft and liquid paraffins (e.g., emulsifying ointment, BP). A preparation of 80% emulsifying wax in white soft paraffin has been used as a soap substitute in the treatment of eczema.

Suppository base: Emulsifying wax (10%) has been added to theobroma oil to give a suppository base with a melting point of 34°C.

Aerosol foam: Emulsifying wax NF is a suitable surface-active agent for the preparation of quick-breaking aerosol foams.

18. Related Substances

A number of proprietary emulsifying waxes are available which contain different sodium alkyl sulfates and may not meet the official specifications; for example, *Collone SEC* contains sodium cetyl sulfate.

19. Comments

BP emulsifying wax is anionic, while NF emulsifying wax is non-ionic in nature. They are therefore not interchangeable in a given composition. Emulsifying wax is also included in the pharmacopeias of India, Yugoslavia, Nordic countries and Switzerland. A similar preparation which contains cetostearyl alcohol (90%) and sodium cetostearyl sulfate (10%) is official in the pharmacopeias of Belgium and West Germany.

20. Specific References

1. *Pharmaceutical Emulsions and Emulsifying Agents*, 4th Edition, R. F. White, Ed. *Chemist and Druggist*, London, 1964.

USA: J. Mullins**
UK: A. J. Winfield*

Microcrystalline Wax

1. Nonproprietary Name

NF: Microcrystalline wax

2. Functional Category

NF: Coating agent
Others: Stiffening agent in semisolid products such as creams and ointments

3. Synonyms

Petroleum wax (microcrystalline); amorphous wax; petroleum ceresin; *Microwax*; *Multiwax*

4. Chemical Name and CAS Registry Number

A mixture of straight-chain, branched-chain and cyclic hydrocarbons.

5. Empirical Formula

Empirical Formula	Molecular Weight
—	580 to 900

6. Structural Formula

—

7. Commercial Availability

USA

Boler Petroleum Co.
Durachem Division of Dura Commodities Corp.
Industrial Raw Materials Corp.
International Wax Refining Co., Inc.
Ishihara Corp.
Kaster Keunen, Inc.
Lux Chemical Co.
Micro Powders, Inc.
Moore and Munger Marketing, Inc.
Multi-Chem, Inc.
National Wax Co.
Petrolite Corp.
Ruger Chemical Co., Inc.
Shamrock Chemical Corp.
Strahl and Pitsch, Inc.
Sun Petroleum Products Co.
Witco Chemical Corp.

UK

A. F. Sutter & Co. Ltd.

8. Method of Manufacture

Microcrystalline wax is prepared by solvent fractionation of the still bottom fraction of petroleum by suitable dewaxing or de-oiling.

9. Description

Solid, microcrystalline waxy material, colorless to light yellow and without odor or taste.

10. Pharmacopeial Specifications

Test	NF
Color	+
Melting range	54 to 102°C
Consistency	3 to 100
Acidity	+
Alkalinity	+
Residue on ignition	≤0.1%
Organic acids	+
Fixed oils, fats, and rosin	Absent

11. Typical Properties

Freezing range: 60 to 75°C
Viscosity: 10 to 30 cps (100°C)
Solubility: Insoluble in water; slightly soluble in anhydrous ethanol; soluble in ether, benzene, and chloroform. When melted, miscible with volatile oils and most warm fixed oils.

Academy HPE Laboratory Project Data

	Method	Lab #	Results
Solubility	SOL-4	10	
Water, 25°C			0.0000%
Water, 37°C			0.0000%
Alcohol, 25°C			0.0003%
Alcohol, 37°C			0.0003%
Propylene glycol, 25°C			0.0001%
Hexane, 25°C			0.0053%
Hexane, 37°C			0.0088%

Supplier: International Wax Refining Co.

12. Stability and Storage Conditions

Stable in the presence of acids, alkalis, light and air. NF specifies storage in tight containers.

13. Incompatibilities

—

14. Safety

Nontoxic and nonirritating

15. Handling Precautions

—

16. Regulatory Acceptance

NF XVI; complies with FDA requirements of CFR 121.1156 as a direct food additive or component.

17. Applications in Pharmaceutical Formulation or Technology

Microcrystalline waxes modify the crystal structure of other waxes present in a mixture (particularly paraffin) so that change in crystal structure, usually exhibited over a period of time, does not occur. Also, they minimize the sweating or bleeding of oils from blends of oils and waxes. They also generally have higher melting points and higher viscosities when molten, thereby increasing the consistency of creams and ointments when incorporated. They are also used in chewing gums and food.

18. Related Substances

Paraffin (NF)

19. Comments

—

20. Specific References

1. Technical Data Sheets of Witco Chemical, Sonneborn Division, New York.

USA: D. Pasquale*; M. J. Akers**

White Wax

1. Nonproprietary Names
NF: White wax
BP/EP: White beeswax

2. Functional Categories
NF: Stiffening agent (in ointment and suppositories)
Others: Emulsion stabilizer (w/o), water-absorbing ointment constituent, melting-point modifier in suppositories.

3. Synonym
Bleached wax

4. Chemical Name and CAS Registry Number
—

5. Empirical Formula   Molecular Weight
—   —

6. Structural Formula
—

7. Commercial Availability
USA
International Wax Refining Company, Inc.
Frank B. Ross Co.
Koster Keunen, Inc.

UK
British Wax Refining Co.
Poth Hille & Co., Ltd.
Kimpton Bros. Ltd.

8. Method of Manufacture
The source of beeswax is the honeycomb of the bee [*Apis mellifera* Linné (Fam. Apidae)], from which it is separated by melting and filtration. Subsequent treatment with oxidizing agents provides the bleaching effect, which yields the desired color.

9. Description
White or slightly yellow sheets with some translucence, or fine granules. The odor is faintly honey-like.
Beeswax consists of 70-75% of a mixture of various esters from C_{26}-C_{32} alcohols, particularly palmitic, hydroxypalmitic, d-β-dehydropalmitic and cerotic acids. Also present are free acids (about 14%) and, carbohydrates (about 12%) as well as approximately 1% free wax alcohols and stearic esters of fatty acids.

10. Pharmacopoeial Specifications

Test	NF	BP/EP
Melting range	62-65°C	61-65°C
Saponification cloud test	+	—
Fats, or fatty acids, Japan wax, rosin and soap	+	—
Ceresin, paraffin and certain other waxes	—	+
Acid value	17-24	17-24
Ester value	72-79	70-80
Ratio number	—	3.3-4.3
Saponification value	—	87-104
Glycerol and other polyhydric alcohols (as glycerol)	—	≤0.5%

11. Typical Properties
Solubility: Soluble in chloroform, ether and both fixed and volatile oils. Partly soluble in cold benzene or carbon disulfide, but soluble at temperatures above 30°C.
Specific gravity: Approximately 0.95
Peroxide value: ≤8
Iodine value: 8-11
Unsaponified matter: 52-55%

Academy HPE Laboratory Project Data			
	Method	Lab #	Results
Density	DE-1	7	0.958 ± 0.006 g/cm³

12. Stability and Storage Conditions
Store in a well-closed container.

13. Incompatibilities
Oxidizing substances

14. Safety
Hypersensitivity reactions have been reported.

15. Handling Precautions
—

16. Regulatory Acceptance
NF XVI; BP/EP 1980

17. Applications in Pharmaceutical Formulation or Technology
Increases the consistency of creams and ointments and stabilizes water-in-oil emulsions. Also used for the polishing of sugarcoated tablets and for adjusting the melting point of suppositories.

18. Related Substance
Yellow wax

19. Comments
—

20. Specific References
See yellow wax

USA: L. Bighley*; M. Bornstein**; Z. Chowhan**
UK: P. C. Record**

Yellow Wax

1. Nonproprietary Names
NF: Yellow wax
BP: Yellow beeswax

2. Functional Category
USP: Stiffening agent
Other: Ingredient of ointments and oil emulsions

3. Synonym
Yellow wax

4. Chemical Names and CAS Registry Number
—

5. Empirical Formula   Molecular Weight
—   —

6. Structural Formula
—

7. Commercial Availability
USA

Frank B. Ross, Inc.
International Wax Refining Company, Inc.
Koster-Keunen, Inc.

U.K.

British Wax Refining Co. Ltd.
Kimpton Bros. Ltd.
Poth Hille & Co., Ltd.

8. Method of Manufacture
Yellow wax is a natural secretion of bees (*Apis mellifera* and other species). On a large scale, the honey is abstracted from the combs by shaving off the ends of the cells, then draining and placing them in centrifuges. The honey is rapidly whirled out, water is added and the wax is thoroughly and quickly cleaned. After melting and straining, it is run into flat dishes or molds to cool and harden.

9. Description
Yellow or light brown pieces or plates with a fine-grained matt; noncrystalline fracture; becomes soft and pliable when warmed. The odor is faint and characteristic.
Beeswax consists of 70-75% of a mixture of various esters from C_{26}-C_{32} alcohols, particularly palmitic, hydroxypalmitic, *d*-β-dehydropalmitic and cerotic acids. Also present are free acids (about 14%) and carbohydrates (about 12%) as well as approximately 1% free wax alcohols and stearic esters of fatty acids.

10. Pharmacopeial Specifications

Test	NF	BP/EP
Melting range	62-65°C	61-65°C
Saponification cloud test	+	—
Fats, or fatty acids, Japan wax, resin and soap	+	—
Acid value	17-24	17-22
Ester value	72-79	70-80
Ratio number	—	3.3-4.3
Saponification value	—	87-102
Glycerin and other polyhydric alcohols (as glycerin)	—	≤0.5%
Ceresin, paraffin and certain other waxes	—	+

11. Typical Properties
Solubility: Soluble in chloroform, ether and both fixed and volatile oils. Partly soluble in cold benzene or carbon disulfide, but soluble at temperatures above 30°C.
Density: 0.950-0.960 g/cm^3
Fracture index: n_D^{25} 1.440-1.445
Iodine number: 8-11
Peroxide value: ≤8
Unsaponified matter: 52-55

12. Stability and Storage Conditions
Protect from light; store in a well-closed container.

13. Incompatibilities
Oxidizing substances

14. Safety
Hypersensitivity reactions have been reported.

15. Handling Precautions
None specified

16. Regulatory Acceptance
NF XVI; BP/EP 1980, Addendum 1983

17. Applications in Pharmaceutical Formulation or Technology
Stiffening agent in ointments and creams: 5-20%
Polishing agent for sugar-coated tablets; emulsion stabilizer; forms a soap with borax

18. Related Substance
White wax

19. Comments
None

20. Specific References
1. Product Bulletin, International Refining Company, Inc.
2. E. Cronin, *J. Soc. Cosmet. Chem.*, 18: 681 (1967).
3. H. W. Rothenborg, *Archs. Derm.*, 95: 381 (1967).

USA: L. Bighley*; M. Bornstein**; Z. Chowhan**
UK: P.C. Record*

Xylitol

1. Nonproprietary Name
Xylitol

2. Functional Category
Sweetener

3. Synonyms
Pentapentol; *Xylit*; *Xilitol*; *Xylitolo*; *Klinit*

4. Chemical Names and CAS Registry Number
1,2,3,4,5-Pentanpentol
Xylitol [87-99-0]

5. Empirical Formula   Molecular Weight
$C_5H_{12}O_5$ 152.15

6. Structural Formula

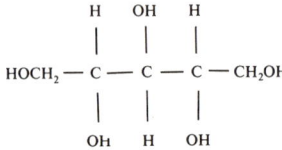

7. Commercial Availability

USA

Hoffmann-La Roche
Edward Mendell Co.
Sigma Chemical Co.

UK

Eisai, Co., Ltd.
Hoffmann-LaRoche Inc., Roche Chemical Div.
Xyrofin, Ltd.

8. Method of Manufacture
Xylitol is derived from various types of cellulose products, such as wood, straw, cane pulp, seed hulls and shells. These usually contain 20-35% xylan, which is readily converted to xylose by hydrolysis and then to xylitol through hydrogenation. The final step is purification and crystallization. It can be made biologically through yeast fermentation. It can also be made by oxalic acid treatment of the cellulose products.

9. Description
White, granular solid comprising crystalline, equi-dimensional particles having a mean diameter of 0.5-0.7 mm; odorless, with a sweet taste that imparts a cooling sensation. It is also available in powder form.

SEM: Xylitol

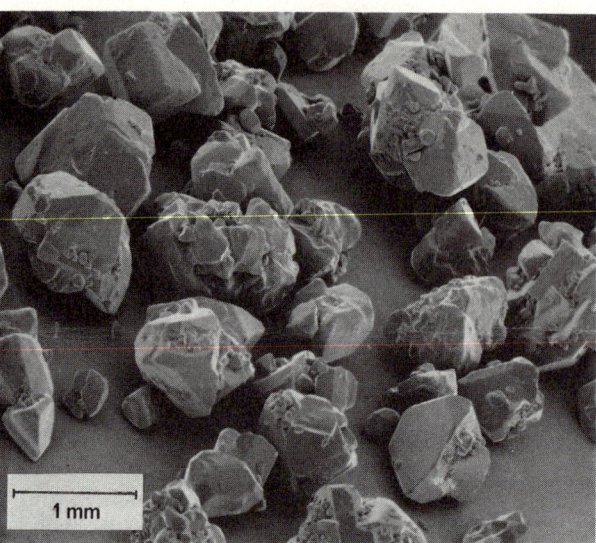

Magnification: 20X

10. Pharmacopeial Specifications
Not official

11. Typical Properties
Boiling point (stable form): 215 - 217°C
Density (at 20°C): 1.52 g/cm³ (particle)
Melting point: (stable) 92-95°C; (metastable) 61-61.5°C
Moisture content: Equilibrium moisture content:* 0.1% (at 20°C and 52% RH); loss on drying: ≤0.5% (4 hours at 80°C in vacuum over P_2O_5); moisture sorption isotherm determined at 20°C (see Figure 1).
Optical activity: none.
Solubility (at 20°C):

Solvent	g/100 ml	Solvent	g/100 g
Water	64.2	Propylene Glycol	6.7
Ethanol	1.2	Glycerol	<0.1
Methanol	6.0	Propan-2-ol	0.2
Pyridine	soluble	Arachis oil	<0.1

Stability of crystals: Crystallization from alcohol yields metastable rhombic crystals or monoclinic crystals which are stable.
pH: 5 - 7 (5% aqueous solution)
Purity (typical values): arsenic ≤3 ppm; heavy metals ≤5 ppm; reducing sugars ≤0.2%; assay ≥98.5% (on dry basis).
Viscosity: 20.63 mN s/m² (60% solution at 20°C).

*May vary with purity, source and particle size.

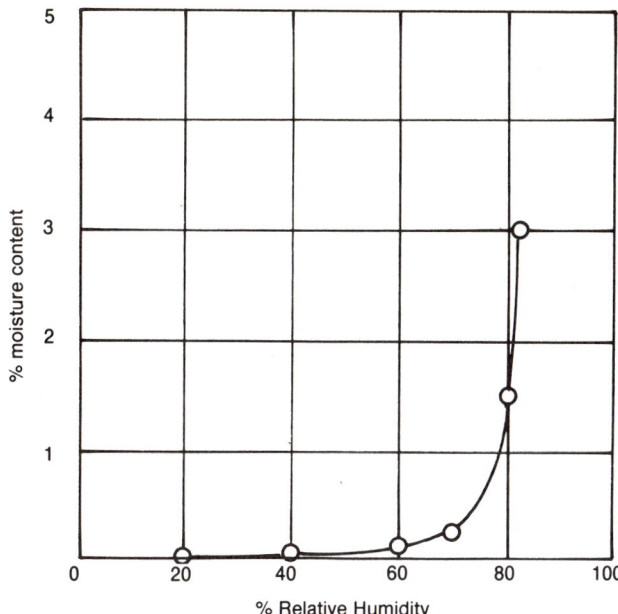

Fig. 1: Moisture sorption isotherm

12. Stability and Storage Conditions

Metastable forms exist. Aqueous solution has been reported as being stable even on prolonged heating and storage. Since it is not utilized by most micro-organisms, products made with xylitol are usually safe from microbial attack. Nonfermentable. Store below 75% RH.

13. Incompatibilities

No incompatibilities or inactivation reported. Possible impurities are mannitol, sorbitol, galactol or orabitol.

14. Safety

Tolerance of 200 g oral doses daily. Laxative in large doses. (See also #16).

15. Handling Precautions

None specified

16. Regulatory Acceptance

Not official in USP/NF and BP. The safety aspects of Xylitol have been reviewed from time to time. The material has been approved for use in foods in the United Kingdom (Food Additives and Contaminants Committee, Report on the Review of Sweeteners in Food FAC/REP/34 HMSO 1982). Xylitol is permitted for use in certain foods in the following countries: Argentina, Belgium, Canada, Colombia, Denmark, Finland, German Dem. Rep., German Fed. Rep., Israel, Italy, Mexico, the Netherlands, New Zealand, Norway, Peru, Spain, Sweden, Switzerland, Taiwan, South Africa, USA, USSR, Venezuela and Yugoslavia.

17. Applications in Pharmaceutical Formulation or Technology

Used as a sweetener in tablets, syrups, coatings. Certain coating procedures are covered by: German Patent Application 2,913,555, Jan. 4, 1979.

18. Related Substances

—

19. Comments

Sweetening power approximately equal to sucrose, although it has been shown to be pH-, concentration- and temperature-dependent. It is 2.5 times as sweet as mannitol. Xylitol does not promote dental caries.

20. Specific References:

1. A. Emodi, "Xylitol: Its Properties and Food Applications," *Food Technology*, 28 (1978).
2. F. Voirol, Xylitol—A new substitute for sugar in foods. In: "Proc. IV International Congress Food Sci. and Technol., 1, 9 (1974).
3. U. Manz, E. Vanninen and F. Voirol, Food Research Association Symposium on "Sugar and Sugar Replacements," London, 1973, p. 22.
4. N. J. Counsell, "Xylitol," Applied Science Publishers, Ltd., London, 1978.
5. K. K. Makinen, "Xylitol and Oral Health," 25, 137, 158 (1979).
6. R. Ylckahri, Metabolic and nutritional aspects, *Adv. Food Res.*, 25, 159, 180 (1979).
7. A. Scheinin, Xylitol in relation to oral and general health, *Dent. J.*, 29 (3), 237, 243 (1979).
8. H. Iwaco, A review of the synthesis, and physical and chemical properties (Nat'l. Inst. Nutr., Tokyo, Japan), *Kagaku To Jikken*, 31 (12), 20, 24 (1980).

USA: A. Palmieri III*; J. Mullins**; Z. Chowhan**

UK: H.C. Worthington*

Zein

1. Nonproprietary Name
Merck Index: Zein

2. Functional Category
Wet granulation binder; coating agent; extended release agent

3. Synonyms
Zein

4. Chemical Name and CAS Registry Number
A prolamine of corn gluten —

5. Empirical Formula   Molecular Weight
Not known   Approximately 38,000

6. Structural Formula
Not known

7. Commercial Availability
USA

Colorcon, Inc.
Freeman Industries, Inc.

UK

BDH Chemicals, Ltd.
Colorcon, Ltd.

8. Method of Manufacture
Zein is extracted from corn gluten meal with dilute isopropanol.

9. Description
Granular, straw to pale yellow-colored, amorphous powder or fine flakes; bland in taste; characteristic odor.

10. Pharmacopeial Specifications
None

11. Typical Properties
Assay (% N X 6.25 dry basis): 88%
Moisture (105°C - 1 hr.): 6.5% max.
Oil: 7.0% max.
Melting point: 180-200°C
Color Cv (mostly xanthophyl 11): 250 mg/lb.
Particle size (through 20 mesh): 100%
Ash: <2.0%
Heavy metals: 5 ppm max.
Arsenic: 2 ppm max.
Solubility: Water: insoluble; *isopropanol, hydrous:* soluble; *acetone:* insoluble; *acetone/water 60-80%:* soluble.

Solubility test: A 15% w/w solution in 85% isopropanol does not gel after standing for one week at room temperature.

Microbiological (max.):

Aerobic plate count	10,000/g
Yeast or mold	100/g
Coliform	50/g
Salmonella	Negative
Staphylococcus aureus	Negative
E. coli	Negative
Pseudomonas aeruginosa	Negative
Shigella	Negative
Streptococcus	Negative

Amino acid content (approximate):

Alanine	8.3%	Lysine	0.0%
Arginine	1.8%	Methionine	2.0%
Asparagine	4.5%	Phenylalanine	6.8%
Cystine	0.8%	Proline	9.0%
Glutamic Acid	1.5%	Serine	5.7%
Glutamine	21.4%	Threonine	2.7%
Glycine	0.7%	Tryptophane	0.0%
Histidine	1.1%	Tyrosine	5.1%
Isoleucine	6.2%	Valine	3.1%
Leucine	19.3%		

12. Stability and Storage Conditions
Information not available.

13. Incompatibilities
No citations in the literature.

14. Safety
Safe for use in food and in pharmaceuticals.

15. Handling Precautions
No restrictions specified.

16. Regulatory Acceptance
GRAS list

17. Applications in Pharmaceutical Formulation or Technology

Use	Concentration (%) w/w
Wet granulation binder	30
Tablet sealer	20
Tablet coater	15

18. Related Substances
—

19. Comments
—

20. Specific References
1. Carter, Reck, German Patent 2,002,337 (Nutrilite Prod., 1971).
2. Mosse, Review article, *Ann. Physiol. Vegetale* Vol. 3:105 (1961).

USA: W. Feinstein*; R. O. Zimmerer, Jr.**

Zinc Stearate

1. Nonproprietary Names

USP: Zinc stearate
BPC: Zinc stearate

2. Functional Category

USP: Tablet and/or capsule lubricant
Others: Dusting powder; thickener

3. Synonyms

None

4. Chemical Names and CAS Registry Number

Octadecanoic acid, zinc salt, but containing zinc salts of related fatty acids
Zinc stearate [557-05-1]

5. Empirical Formula

$C_{36}H_{70}O_4Zn$

Molecular Weight

632.33

6. Structural Formula

$Zn[CH_3(CH_2)_{16}COO]_2$

7. Commercial Availability

USA

Diamond Shamrock Corp., Process Chemical Div.
Mallinckrodt, Inc.
Mathe Div., The Norac Co., Inc.
Petrochemicals Company, Inc.
Synthetic Products Company, Division of Port Industries
Tenneco Chemicals Specialty and Commodity Chemicals
Witco Chemical Corporation

UK

Durham Chemicals, Ltd.
Stancourt Sons & Muir, Ltd.

8. Method of Manufacture

An aqueous solution of zinc sulfate is added to a sodium stearate solution, and the precipitate is washed with water and then dried. Prepared from stearic acid and zinc chloride.

9. Description

Fine, white, bulky hydrophobic powder, free from grittiness. Has a faint, characteristic odor. It is neutral to moistened litmus paper.

SEM-MF-30
Excipient: Zinc Stearate

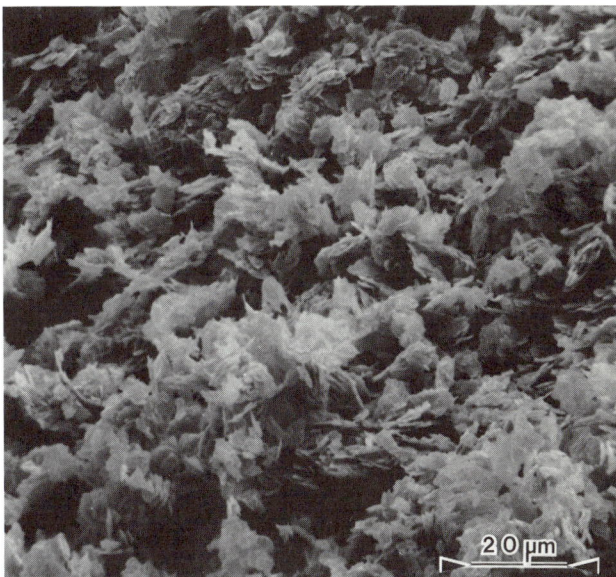

20 µm

Magnification: 600×

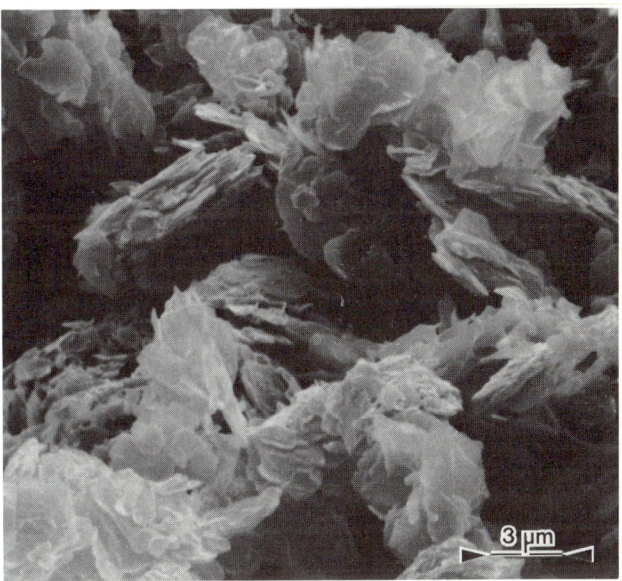

3 µm

Magnification: 2,400×

10. Pharmacopeial Specifications

Test	USP	BP
Identification	+	+
Acidity or alkalinity	—	≤0.01 meq/g
Alkalis and alkaline earths	≤1.0%	≤2.0%
Arsenic	≤1.5 ppm	—
Ether-soluble matter	—	≤1.0%
Lead	≤0.001%	—
Sulfate	—	≤0.6%
Assay range	12.5-14.0% ZnO	10.45-12.45% Zn

11. Typical Properties

Melting range: 120-122°C
Particle size: 100% thru #325 mesh
Solubility: Insoluble in water, alcohol or ether, but is soluble in benzene; decomposed by dilute acids
Specific gravity: 1.095
Flash point: 530°F
Auto-ignition temperature: 790°C

12. Stability and Storage Conditions

Stable. Store in a well-closed container.

13. Incompatibilities

No citations in the literature.

14. Safety

On the GRAS list. Inhalation reported as causing pulmonary fibrosis. Poisoning has been reported in infants when the powder has been inhaled. Food grade product must be made from chickedema-free fatty acid. Combustible material: slight fire hazard when exposed to heat or flame.

15. Handling Precautions

Zinc stearate should not be inhaled or applied to infants.

16. Regulatory Acceptance

USP XXI; BPC 1973

17. Applications in Pharmaceutical Formulation or Technology

Use	Concentration (%)
Compound calamine cream	2.5
Water repellent ointments	2.5
Tablet lubricant	0.5–1.5

18. Related Substances

None

19. Comments

None

20. Specific References

1. Mallinckrodt, Inc., data sheet.

USA: S. M. Tuthill*; J. Mullins **

APPENDIX I

Suppliers

A

ABM Chemicals Ltd., Poleacre Lane; Woodley, Stockport, Cheshire SK6 1PQ, England

AKZO Chemie, Armak Co., Agent, 300 S. Wacker, Chicago, IL 60606 (312-786-0400)

AKZO Chemie (U.K. Ltd.) 12 St. Ann's Crescent; London SW18 2LS, England (01-874 7761)

A&S Corp., P.O. Box 339, 819 Edwards Road, Parsippany, NJ 07054 (201-575-6330)

Abbott Laboratories Ltd., Queensborough, Kent ME11 5EL, (0795-663371)

Accurate Chemical & Scientific Grp., 300 Shames Dr., Westbury, NY 11590 (516-433-4900)

Aceto Chemical Co., Inc., 126-02 Northern Blvd.; Flushing, NY 11368 (212-898-2300)

Aeropres Corp., 1108 Petroleum Tower, Shreveport, LA 71106.

Air Products & Chemicals Inc., Box 538, Allentown, PA 18105 (215-481-4911)

Air Products, Ltd., Hersham Place, Molesey Road, Walton-on-Thames, Surrey KT12 4RZ, England (0932-49200)

Alba Chemical, Inc., 285 County Road, Tenafly, NY 07670

Albright & Wilson Ltd., P.O. Box 3, Hagley Road West, Oldbury, Warley, West Midlands B68 0NN, England (021-429 4942)

Alcohols Ltd., Imperial Buildings, 56 Kingsway, London, WC2B 6DX, England (01-242 0596)

Alcolac, Inc., 3440 Fairfield Rd.; Baltimore, MD 21226 (301-355-2600)

Aldrich Chemical Co., Ltd., The Old Brickyard, New Road Gillingham, Dorset SP8 4JL, England (074-762211)

Alembic Products Ltd., Oaklands House, Oaklands Drive, Sale, Manchester M33 1WS, England (061-962 4423)

Alfa Chemicals Ltd., Broadway House, Shute End, Wokingham, Berks. RG11 1BH, England (0734-792566)

Alginate Industries Ltd., 22 Henrietta St., London WC2E 8NB, England (01-240 5161)

Allied Chemical Corp., P.O. Box 2064R, Morristown, NJ 07960 (201-455-4400)

Allied Colloids Ltd., P.O. Box 38, Low Moor, Bradford, West Yorkshire BD12 0JZ, England (0274-671267)

Alltech Associates, Inc., 202 Campus Drive, Arlington Heights, IL 60004

Alwitt Ltd., Zelide House, 2 Mount Ephraim, Tunbridge Wells, Kent TN4 8AS, England (0892-36111)

Amerchol Corporation, P.O. Box 351 Talmadge Rd., Amerchol Park, Edison, NJ 08818 (201-287-1600)

American Cyanamid Co., One Cyanamid Plaza, Wayne, NJ 07470 (201-831-1234)

American Hoechst Corporation, Chemical Div., P.O. Box 73875, Baton Rouge, LA 70807 (504-775-0150)

American International Chemical, Inc., 209 West Central St.; Nattick, MA 01760 (617-655-5805)

American Lecithin, 32-35 61st Street, Woodside, Long Island, NY 11377

American Maize-Products Co., 1100 Indianapolis Blvd., Hammond, IN 46320 (219-659-2000)

American Research Products Co., P.O. Box 21009, South Euclid, OH 44121 (216-587-5100)

American Roland Corp., 157 Chambers Street, New York, NY 10007

American Scientific & Chemical, 3259 20th Ave., West Seattle, WA 98199 (206-282-2133)

Amstar Corporation, 1251 Avenue of the Americas, New York, NY 10020

Anachemia Chemicals Inc., P.O. Box 87, Champlain, NY 12919 (518-298-4444)

Angelo Rhodes Ltd., Corolin Road, Lower Tuffley, Glos GL2 6DQ, England (0452-35021)

Anheuser Busch, Inc., Industrial Products Division, 10877 Watson Road, St. Louis, MO 63127

D.F. Anstead Ltd., Victoria House, Radford Way, Billericay Essex CM12, ODE, England (027-7453131)

Apache Chemicals, Inc., P.O. Box 126, Seward, IL 61077

Arco Chemical Co., Div., Atlantic Richfield Co., 1500 Market Street; Philadelphia, PA 19101 (215-557-3240)

Armak Co. Industrial Chemical Div., Poleacre Lane; Woodley, Stockport, Cheshire SK6 1PQ, England (061-430 4391); 300 S. Wacker, Chicago, IL 60606 (312-786-0400)

Aroma Resources Div. of Biddle Sawyer Corp., 2 Pen Plaza, Suite 2355, New York, NY 10121

Ashland Chemical Co., Box 2219; Columbus, OH 43216 (614-889-3333)

Astor Chemical Ltd., Tavistock Road, West Drayton, Middlesex UB7 7RA, England (08954-45511)

Atlantic Gelatin, General Foods Corp., Woburn, MA 01801 (617-933-2800)

Atlas Chemical Division, DuPont Building, Wilmington, DE 19899

Atlas Chemical Industries (UK) Ltd., Cleeve Road, Leatherhead, Surrey KT22 7SW, England (03723-76122)

Atomergic Chemetals Corp., 100 Fairchild Ave.; Plainview, NY 11803 (516-349-8800)

Austin Chemical Co., 205 West Touhy Ave., Norwalk, CT 06854

Avebe America Inc., P.O. Box 427, 1767 Morris Ave., Union, NJ 07083

B

BASF AG, Carl-Bosch-Strasse 38, 6700 Ludwigshafen, W. Germany (0621-1601)

BASF (UK) Ltd., Earl Road, Cheadle Hulme, Cheadle, Cheshire SK8 6QG, England (061-485 6222)

BASF Wyandotte Corp., 100 Cherry Hill Road, Parsippany, NJ 07054 (201-263-3400)

BBL Microbiology Systems, P.O. Box 243, Cockeysville, MD 20130

BDH Chemicals Ltd., Broom Road, Poole, Dorset BH12 4NN, England (0202-745520)

BF Goodrich Chemical Company, 6100 Oak Tree Blvd., Cleveland, OH 44131 (216-447-6000)

BP Chemicals Ltd., Sun Alliance House, Wellington Road North, Stockport, Cheshire SK4 1AT, England (061-477 0011)

BTP Cocker Chemicals Ltd., Hayes Road, Cadishead, Manchester M30 5BX, England (061-775-3945)

Bage, Inc., 3117 N. Clybourn, Chicago, IL 60618

Baker Chemical Co., J.T., Pershing Square Building, 100 East 42nd Street, New York, NY 10017 (212-867-0200)

Batewell Ltd., Meadow Cottage, Speldhurst, Tunbridge Wells, Kent TN3 0NS, England (089-286 2443)

Bayer, UK Ltd., Bayer House, Richmond, Surrey TW9 1SJ, England (01-940 6077)

Beacon CMP Corp., 1485 Morris Ave., Union, NJ 07083

Becpharm Ltd., Patman House, George Lane, South Woodford, London E18 2LS, England (01-989 8461)

Becton Dickinson Immuno Diagnostics, Mountain View Ave., Orangeburg, NY 10962 (914-359-2700)

Bentex Chemicals, Inc., One Main Street, P.O. Box 639, Chatham, NJ 07928

Berje Chemical Products, Inc., 43-10 23rd St., Long Island City, NY 11101 (212-937-1280)

Berk Spencer Acids Ltd., Canning Road, Stratford, London E15 3NX, England (01-534 5162)

Beta Chemical Corp., P.O. Box 40, Haddon Heights, NJ 08035

J. Bibby & Sons Ltd., Edible Oils Division, 57 Great Howard Street, Liverpool, England 051-236 6671)

Biddle Sawyer Corp., (Shin-Etsu Chemical Co.) 2 Penn Plaza, New York, NY 10121

Biochemical Laboratories, Inc., 14422 S. San Pedro St., Gardenia, CA 90248 (213-515-1919)

Bio-rad Laboratories, 2200 Wright Ave., Richmond, CA 94804 (415-234-4130)

Blagden Cambell Chemicals Ltd., AMP House, Dingwall Road, Croydon, Surrey CR9 3QU, England (01-681 1341)

Blythe, William & Co. Ltd., Holland Bank Works, Church, Accrington, Lancs BB5 4PD, England (0254 37211)

Bofors (Great Britain) Co., Ltd., Ramsden Heath, Billericay, Essex, England (0268-710731)

Boots Co., Ltd., 1 Thane Road, W., Nottingham NG2 3AA, England (0602 5611)

Borden Chemical, 180 East Broad St., Columbus, OH 43215 (614-225-4000)

Brampton Co., J.W., 71 Allen Blvd., Farmingdale, NY 11735

Branwell, Arthur & Co. Ltd., Ibex House, Minories, London EC3N 1HP, England (01-488 4141)

Brenntag (UK) Ltd., Brenntag House, High Street, Hampton Wick, Kingston-Upon-Thames, Surrey, England (01-943 0711)

British Ceca Co. Ltd., 17-27 Garratt Lane, Wandsworth, London SW18 4AE (01-874 7272)

British Celanese Ltd., P.O. Box 5, Spondon, Derby DE2 7BP, England (0332-661422)

British Gypsum Ltd., Ruddington Hall, Loughborough Road, Ruddington, Nottingham NG11 6LX, England (0602-844 844)

British Saccharin Sales Co., Thane Road, Nottingham NG2 3AA, England (0602-51165)

British Salt Ltd., Cledford Lane, Middlewich, Cheshire CW10 0JP, England (06084-2881)

British Sugar Corporation Ltd., 39 Sackville Street, London W1X 1DB, England (01-439 9741)

British Traders & Shippers Ltd., 6 Merrie Lands Crescent, Dagenham, Essex RM9 65L, England (01-595 4211)

British Wax Refining Co., Ltd., 29 St. John's Road, Redhill, Surrey RH1 6DT, England (0737-61242)

Bromhead & Denison Ltd., 7 Stonebank, Welwyn Garden City, Herts AL8 6NQ, England (07073-31031)

Brown Company, Berlin Gorham Div., 555 Fifth Ave., New York, NY 10017

Browning Chemical Corp., 330 Madison Ave., New York, NY 10017

Buckeye Scientific Co., Inc., P.O. Box 30837, Columbus, OH 43230

Burlington Bio-Medical Corp., 100 Fairchild Ave., Plainview, NY 11803

Burmah-Castrol Industrial Ltd., Burmah House, Pipers Way, Swindon, Wilts SN3 1RE, England (0793-30151)

Burrough, James Ltd., Beafeater House, 60 Montford Place, Kennington Lane, London SE11, England (01-735 8131)

Burtonite Co., Inc., P.O. Box 749, Frankline Ave., Nutley, NJ 07110

Bush, Boake, Allen Ltd., Blackhorse Lane, London E17 5QP, England (01-531 4211)

Byron Chemical Co., 40-11 23rd Street, Long Island, NY 11101 (212-786-8441)

C

Cabot Corporation, 125 High Street, Boston, MA 02110

Calbiochem-Behring Corp., P.O. Box 12087, San Diego, CA 92112 (714-453-7331).

Calcium Carbonate Co., 3150 Garner Expressway, Quincy, IL 62301

California & Hawaii Sugar Co., San Francisco, CA 94106

Calor Group Ltd., Key West Windsor Road, Slough, Berks SL1 2EQ, England (0723 23824)

Cambridge Stereoscan Mark IIA, Cambridge Ltd., Cambridge, England

Camilli, Albert & Laloue, 230 Brighton Road, Clifton, NJ 07012

Canada Packers Inc., Chemical Div., 5100 Timberlea Blvd., Mississauga, Ontario, Canada L4W 255

Capital City Products Co., Div. of Stockely-Van Camp, Inc., 525 West First Ave., Columbus, OH 43216

Carless Chemicals Ltd., All Saints Refinery, Cargo Fleet Road, Middlesbrough, Cleveland TS3 6AF, England (0642-248559)

Carson Chemical, Inc., 2779 East El Presidio, Long Beach, CA 90810

Central Soya Co., Inc., 1300 Fort Wayne National Bank Building, Fort Wayne, IN 46802 (219-425-5100)

Chalk Products Ltd. 14a Langley Park Road, Sutton, Surrey SM1 4TB, England (01-642 2310)

Chance & Hunt, P.O. Box 4, Rutland House, Runcorn, Cheshire WA7 2MI, England

Chemcentral Corp., 7050 W. 71st Street, Chicago, IL 60638.

Chemical Dynamics Corp., P.O. Box 395, Hadley Road., South Plainfield, NJ 07080 (201-753-5000)

Chemical Exchange (UK) Ltd., Chemexel House, 11 Sunderland Road, London SE23 2PS, England (01-699 0466).

Chemical Service Inc., 660 Tower LA, P.O. Box 194, West Chester, PA 19380 (215-692-3026)

Chemicals Trading Co. Ltd., 25 Berkeley Square, London WIX 6DH, England (01-499-1246)

Chemisphere Corp., P.O. Box 96, Boonton, NJ 07005 (201-335-6972)

Chrystal Co., Chales B., Inc., 53 Park Place, New York, NY 10007

Ciba-Geigy Corp. Dyestuffs & Chemicals Div., 410 Swing Road, Greenboro, NC 27409 (919-292-7100)

Ciba-Geigy (UK) Ltd., Industrial Chemical Division, Tenax Road, Trafford Park, Manchester M17 IWT England (061-872 2323)

Clinton Corn Processing Co., Div. Nabisco Brand, Inc., 600 Three First National Plaza, Chicago, IL 60602 (312-269-5300)

Coalite Group Ltd., P.O. Box 21, Chesterfield, Derbys S44 6AB, England (0246-822281)

Colgate-Palmolive Co., 300 Park Ave. New York, NY 10022 (212-310-2000)

Colloids, Inc., 394-8 Frelinghuysen Ave., Newark, NJ 07114 (201-926-6100)

Colloides Naturels, P.O. Box 561, Route 202 & Dumont Rd., Far Hills, NJ 07931

Colony Import & Export Corp., New York, NY 10017

Colorcon Inc., Moyer Blvd., West Point, PA 19486

Colorcon Ltd., Murray Road, St. Pauls Cray, Orpington, Kent BR5 3QY England. (0689 38301)

Comerican International, Inc., 260 Madison Ave., New York, NY 10016

Connock, A. & E. (Perfumery & Cosmetics) Ltd., Alderholt Mill House, Fordingbridge, Hants SP6 1PU, England (0425 53367)

Conoco Chemicals Co., P.O. Box 19029, 15990 N. Barkers Landing Road, Houston, TX 77224 (713-531-3200)

Continental Chemical Co., 270 Clifton Blvd., Clifton, NJ 07015 (201-472-5000)

Continental Water Systems Corp., P.O. Box 20018, El Paso, TX 79998

Cooper, Peter, Corp., Gowanda, NY 14070

Corn Products Company, A Div. of CPC North America International Plaza, Englewood Cliffs, NJ 07632 (201-894-4000)

Costec, Inc., 800 East Northwest Highway, Suite 314, Palatine, IL 60067

Courtin & Warner Ltd., 19 Phoenix Place, Lewes, East Sussex BN7 1JX England (07916 3202)

CPC (UK) Ltd., Industrial Division Trafford Park, Manchester M17 1PA, England (061-872 5959)

Croda Chemicals, Inc., 183 Madison Ave., New York, NY 10016

Croda Chemicals Ltd. & Croda Universal Ltd., Cowick Hall, Snaith, Goole, North Humberside DN14 9AA, England (0405-860551)

Croda Synthetic Chemicals Ltd., Four Ashes Works, Four Ashes, Wolverhampton, Staffordshire, England (0902-791479)

Crosfield & Sons, Joseph, Ltd., P.O. Box 26, Warrington, Cheshire WA5 1AB England (0925 31211)

Croxton and Garry Ltd., Curtis Road, Dorking, Surrey RH4 1XA, England (0306-886688)

Cyanamid of Great Britain Ltd., Farehem Road, Gosport, Hants PO13 OAS, England (0329-236131)

Cyclo Chemicals Corp., 7500 N.W. 66th Street, Miami, FL 33166 (305-592-6700)

D

Dairy Crest Foods, Thames Ditton, Surrey England (01 398 4155)

Degussa, Inc., Rt. 46 at Hollister Road, PO Box 2004, Teterboro, NJ 06708 (201-288-6500)

Degussa Ltd., Paul Ungerer House, Earl Road, Stanley Green, Handforth, Wilmslow, Cheshire SK9 3RL, England (061-486 6211)

Degussa Pigments Division, P.O. Box 2644, 6000 Frankfurt 1, W. Germany (0611-2181)

Delamar, Inc., 2653 Greenleaf Avenue, Elk Grove Village, IL 60007 (312-437-9560)

Desno Chemical Corp., 8 Westchester Plaza, Elmford, NY 10523

Dey Duncan & Co., Ltd., Haddon House, Hindhead Road, Haslemere, Surrey GU27 1LH, England (0428 51331)

Diamond Shamrock Corp., 7171 N. Harwood Street, Dallas, TX 75201 (214-745-2000)

Diamond Shamrock Europe Ltd., Emerson House, Albert Street, Eccles, Manchester M30 OLJ, England (061-707 3244).

Dihoval Ltd., 54 Dundonald Road, London SW19 3PH, England (01-543 3755)

Distillers Co. Ltd., 12 Torphichen Street, Edinburgh EH3 8YT, Scotland (031-229-2468)

Distillers Co., The (Carbon Dioxide) Ltd., 39 London Road, Reigate, Surrey RH2 9QE England (07372-41133)

Diversified Chemical & Propellant Co., 350 E. Ogden Ave., PO Box 447, Westmont, IL 60559-0447

Dormar Chemicals Inc., Box 1859, Paterson, NJ 07509 (201-345-6780)

Dow Chemical Company, 2020 Dow Center, Barstow Building, Midland, MI 48640 (517-636-1000)

Dow Chemical Co. Ltd. Meadow Bank, Bathroad, Hounslow, Middlesex TW5 9QY, England (01-759 2600)

Dumas Chemicals (Tunbridge Wells) Ltd. Pantiles House, Neville Street, Tunbridge Wells, Kent, England (0892-38981)

Dunn Bros. (Manchester) Ltd., Heywood Old Road, Middleton, Manchester M24 4SA, England (061-653 3677)

DuPont De Nemours & Co., E.I., Brandywine Building, Wilmington, DE 19898 (302-774-2421)

DuPont (UK) Ltd. Wedgwood Way, Stevenage, Herts SGI 4QN, England. (0438-734000)

Durham Raw Materials Ltd., 1 Great Tower Street, London EC3R 5AA, England (01-626 4333)

Durkee Industrial Foods/SCM Corp., 900 Union Commerce Building, Cleveland, OH 44115

Dynamit Nobel (UK) Ltd. Dist: Chemicals Trading Co. Ltd. Gateway House, 302 High Street, Slough, Berks SL1 1HF, England (07533 71851)

E

Eastern Chemical, PO Box 2500, Smithtown, NY 11787 (516-273-0900)

Eastern Chemical, Div. of Guardian Chemical Corp., 230 Marcus Blvd., Hauppage, NY 11787

Eastman Chemical International AG, PO Box 66, Kodak House, Station Road, Hemel Hempstead, Herts HP1 1JU, England (0442 41171)

Eastman Chemicals Product, Inc., PO Box 431, Kingsport, TN 37662 (800-251-0351)

Eastman Organic Chemicals, Eastman Kodak Co., Rochester, NY 14650

ECC International Ltd., John Keay House, St. Austell, Cornwall PL25 40J, England (0726 4482)

Eggar & Co. (Chemicals) Ltd., Goring Heath, Reading, Berks RG8 7SX, England (0491 680402)

Eisai Co. Ltd., 6-10 Koishikawa 4 Chome, Bunkyo-Ku, Tokyo 112, Japan (03-813-1151)

E.M. Laboratories Inc., E. Merck Germany Associate, 560 Executive Blvd., Elmsford, NY 10523 (914-592-4660)

Emco International Corporation, Route 52, Carmel, New York 10512

Emery Industries, Chemical Specialties Group, 15 Logan Avenue, Lock Haven, PA 17745 (717-748-9502)

Emery Industries, Personal Care Product Group, 8733 S. Dice Rd., Santa Fe Springs, CA 90670 (213-685-5664)

Engelhard Minerals & Chemical Corp. Menlo Park CN 28, Edison, NJ 08818 (201-321-5000)

Esso Chemicals Ltd., Arundel Towers, Portland Terrace, Southhampton S09 2GW, England (0703 34191)

ETS Gattefossé France, Dists: Alfa Chemicals Ltd., Jacobson Van den Berg & Co. (UK) Ltd.

Exxon Company, U.S.A., PO Box 2180, Houston, TX 77001

F

Fallek Chemical Co., 460 Park Ave., New York, NY 10022 (212-752-0250)

Fanning Corp., The, 3117 N. Clybourn Ave., Chicago, IL 60618

Fina Chemicals Ltd., Petrofina House, York Road, London SE1 7NT, England. (01-928 8000)

Finetex Inc., P.O. Box 216, 418 Falmouth Ave., Elmwood Park, NJ 07407 (201-797-4686)

Fisher Scientific Co., 711 Forbes Ave., Pittsburgh, PA 15219 (412-562-8300)

Fisons Ltd., 12 Derby Road, Loughborough, Leics LE11 OBB, UK (0509 263113)

Florasynth Inc., 410 East 62nd Street, New York, NY 10021 (212-371-7700)

Floressence Perfumes Oils, Inc., 21 South Mall, Plainview, NY 11803

Fluorochem Ltd., Dinting Vale Trading Estate, Dinting Lane, Glossop, Derbys SK13 9NU, England (04574 62518)

FMC Corporation, 2000 Market Street, Philadelphia, PA 19103 (215-299-8000)

Food Industries Ltd., Bromborough Port, Wirral, Merseyside L62 4SU, England (051-645 2060)

Foremost McKesson Foods Group, Crocker Plaza, One Post Street, San Francisco, CA 94104

Forum Chemicals Ltd., Lonsdale House, 7 High Street, Reigate, Surrey RH2 9RR, England (07372 22256)

France Coleur, SA, 198-212 rue de Muaux, 93410 Vaujours, France

Frederick Allen and Sons (Chemicals) Ltd., Hatherley Wharf, Bow Common Lane, London E3 4 AX, England. (01-987 1260).

G

GAF (Great Britain) Ltd., Chemical Division, Tilson Road, Roundthorn, Wynthenshawe, Manchester M23 9PH, England. (061-998 1122)

GAF Corp., 140 West 51st St. New York, NY 10020 (212-621-5000)

Gallard-Schlesinger Chemical Mfg. Corp. 584 Mineola Avenue, Carle Place, NY 11514 (516-333-5600)

Gattefossé, Ets, 36 Chemin de Genas, 69800 St. Priest, France (7890-6311)

Gelatin Mfg. Ins. of Amer., 516 Fifth Ave., RM 507, New York, NY 10036

General Mills Chemical, Inc., Minneapolis, Minn. 55435

Genrichem Corp., 85 Main St., PO Box J, Little Falls, NJ 07424 (201-256-9266)

Georgia Kaolin Co., 433 North Broad Street, Elizabeth, NJ 07207 (201-352-9800)

Gerhardt Pharmaceuticals, Ltd., Thornton House, Hook Road, Surbiton, Surrey KT6 5AR, England (01-397 9478)

Gibco Laboratories, 3175 Staley Road, Grand Island, NY 14076 (716-773-0700)

Givaudan Corp., 100 Delawanna Ave., Clifton, NJ 07014 (201-365-8000)

Givaudan & Co. Ltd., Godstone Road, Whyteleafe, Surrey CR3 OYE, England (08832 2241)

Glyco Inc., PO Box 700, Greenwich Office Park No. 1, Greenwich, CT 06836 (203-622-1500)

Goodrich, B.F. Chemical Co., 6100 Oak Tree Blvd., Cleveland, OH 44131 (216-447-6000)

Goldschmidt Chemical Corp., 920 Randolph Rd., PO Box 1299, Hopewell VA 23860

Grace, W.R. Ltd., Cryovac Division, Northdale House, North Circular Road, London NW10 7UH, England (01-965 0611)

Grayslake Gelatin Co., PO Box 248, Grayslake, IL 60030 (312-223-8141)

Great Western Sugar Co., Denver, CO 80202

Greeff, K & K Chemical Group Ltd., Suffolk House, George Street, Croydon CR9 3QL UK (01-686-0544)

Greeff & Co., R.W., 1445 E. Putnam Ave., Old Greenwich, CT 06870

Grinsted Products AS, Edwin Rahrs Vej 38, 8220 Braband, Denmark (06-253366)

Gross, A. and Co., A Millmaster Onyx Group, Kewanee Industries, Inc., 4001 Raleigh St., Charlotte, NC 28206 (704-333-0737)

H

Hamburger, M. and Sons Ltd., Tannery Lane, Send, Nr Woking, Surrey GU23 7HB, England (0483 223501)

Hammil Gillespie, Inc., PO Box 104, Livingston, NJ 07039

Hampden Color & Chemical Co., 126 Memorial Drive, Springfield, MA 01104

Hardy, M.W. & Co. Ltd., Hardy House, Northbridge Road, Berkhamsted Herts HP4 1EF, England (04427-3366)

Harshaw Chemicals Ltd., London Road, Daventry, Northants, England (03272-2161)

Henkel Chemicals Ltd. Merit House, Edgeware Road, London NW9 5AB, England (01-205 6004)

Henkel Corporation, 4620 W. 77th. Minneapolis, MN 55435 (612-830-7831)

Hercules Inc., Hercules Plaza, Wilmington, DE 19894, (302) 594-6500

Hercules Ltd., 20 Red Lion Street, London WC1R 4PB, England. (01-404 4000)

Hexcel Corp. Specialty Chemicals Div., 205 Main St., Lodi, NJ 07644

Hicks Bros (Produce) Ltd., 19 Earl Street, London EC2A 2AH, England. (01-377-9700)

Highgate and Job Ltd., 60 Murray Street, Paisley, Strathclyde PA3 1QH, Scotland (041-889 3207)

Hilton Davis Chemical Group, 2235 Langdon Farm Road, Cincinnati, OH 45237.

Hodag Chemical Corp., 7247 N. Central Park Ave., Skokie, IL 60076.

Hoechst UK Ltd., Hoechst House, Salisbury Road, Hounslow, Middlesex TW4 6JH, England (01-570 7712)

Hoffmann-LaRoche, Inc., 340 Kingsland Street, Nutley, NJ 07110 (201-235-5000)

Hollandsche, B.V. Melksuikerfabriek, Uitgeest, Netherlands

Holly Sugar Co., Colorado Springs, CO 80902

Honeywill & Stein Ltd., Greenfield House, 69 Manor Road, Wallington, Surrey SM6 OBP, England (01-669-4433)

Hooker Chemical Company, P.O. Box 19601, Irvine CA 92713 (714-957-7806)

Hopkin & Williams, PO Box 1, Romford, Essex RM1 1HA, England (01-590 7700)

Hughes & Hughes Ltd., Elms Industrial Estate, Church Road, Harold Wood, Romford, Essex RM3 OHR, England (04023 49017)

Hubinger, 1 Progress Street, Keokuk, IA 52632

Humko Products (Div. of Kraft Foods) Ltd., Regina House, 259 Old Marylebone Road, London NW1, England (01-723 2084)

Humko Sheffield Chemical, P.O. Box 630, Norwich, NY 13815

I

ICC Industries, Inc., 720 Fifth Ave., New York, NY 10019.

ICD Group, Inc., 641 Lexington Ave., New York, NY 10022

ICI Americas, Inc., 608 Ferry Blvd., Stratford, CT 06497 (203-378-7303)

I.C.I. Plc, Pharmaceutical Div., Alderley House, Alderley Park, Macclesfield, Cheshire SK10 4TF England (0625-582828)

ICN Pharmaceuticals, Inc. 222 North Vincent Ave., Covina, CA 91722 (213-967-0771)

Ideal Chemical & Supply Co., P.O. Box 18439, Memphis, TN 38118

Impag (Great Britain) Ltd., Lyon Industrial Estate, Lyon Road, Kearsley, Bolton, Lancs BL4 8TG, England (0204 78224)

Imperial Sugar Co., Sugarland, TX 11478

Indiana Botanic Gardens Inc., 626 177th Street, PO Box 5 Hammond, IN 46325.

Industrial Hydrocarbons Inc., 175 W. Bonita Ave., San Dimas, CA 91773

Ingredients Technology Corp. Fragrance & Flavor Div., 10 Pelham Pkwy, Pelham Manor, NY 10803

Ingredients International, Inc., 2265 27th Street, Santa Monica, CA 90405

Inolex Chemical Co., Jackson & Swanson Sts., Philadelphia, PA 19148 (215-271-6400)

International Wax Refining Co., 181 E. Jamaica Ave., PO Box 221, Valley Stream, NY 11582

ISC Chemicals Ltd., St. Andrew's Road, Avonmouth, Bristol BS11 9HP, England (0272 823631)

Isolab Inc., Drawer 4350, Akron, OH 44321

J

Jacobson Van Den Berg & Co. (UK) Ltd., 231 The Vale, London W3 7RN, England (01-743-9121)

Janca's Jojoba Oil & Seed Co., 20 Southern Ave., Mesa, AZ 85202

Johnson Matthey Chemicals Ltd., Orchard Road Royston, Herts SG8 5HE, England (0763-44161)

Jonas Chemical Corp., Five Beekman Street, New York, 10038 (212-732-1818)

Jordan Chemical Co., 1830 Columbia Ave., Folcroft, PA 19032

J&W Starches, Ltd., Unit N1/7, Heywood Industrial Estate, Heywood, Lancs, England (0706-621341)

K

Kalama Chemical, Inc., Suite 1110, Bank of California Center, Seattle, WA, 98164 (206-682-7890)

Kay-Fries, Inc., 10 Link Drive, Rockleigh, NJ 07647 (800-526-0339)

Kelly's, John (London) Ltd., Prescot House, Prescot Street, London E1 8BB, England (01-481 2110)

Kelco Co., Div. Merck & Co., 8355 Aero Dr., San Diego, CA 92123 (714-292-4900)

Kelco/AIL International, 22 Henrietta Street, London WC2E 8NB, England (01-240 5161)

Kerax Ltd., Cowling Road, Chorley, Lancs PR6 9DR, England (02572 78321)

Keystone Gelatin Col. 2350 Kerper Blvd., Dubuque, IA 52001

Kimpton Bros. Ltd., Berkshire House, 168 High Holborn, London WCIV 7AF, England (01-379 6422)

Kind & Knox Gelatin Co., 900 Kings Highway, Cherry Hill, NJ 08034

Kingsley & Keith Ltd., Suffolk House, George St., Croydon, Surrey CR9 3QL, England

K & K Greeff Chemicals Ltd., Suffolk House, George St., Croydon CR9 3QL, England (01-686 0544)

Knoll Fine Chemicals Div., Knoll Pharmaceutical Co., 120 East 56th St., New York, NY 10022 (212-752-9520)

Koch-Light Laboratories Ltd., 2 Willow Road, Colnbrook, Slough, Berks SL3 0BZ, England (02812 2262)

Kodak Ltd., Chemical Div., Acornfield Road, Kirkby, Liverpool L33 7UF England (051-546 2101)

Kohnstamm & Co., H., Inc., Kearney, NJ 07032

Koppers Company, Inc., 1250 Koppers Building, Pittsburgh, PA 15219 (412-227-2296)

Koster Keunen, Inc., PO Box 383, Sayville, NY 11782

Kraft Chemical Co., 1975 North Hawthorne, Melrose Park, IL 60160

L

Lachat Chemicals, Inc., 10500 N. Port Washington Rd., Mequon, WI 53092 (414-241-3872)

Laing-National Ltd., Ashburton Road East, Trafford Park, Manchester M17 1BJ, England (061-872 6161)

Lambson Ltd., Aire and Calder Works, Cinder Lane, Castleford, Yorkshire, England

Lanatex Products Inc., 151-157 Third Ave., Elizabeth, NJ 07206

Lankro Chemicals Group Ltd., P.O. Box 1, Emerson House, Albert Street, Eccles, Manchester M30 0BH (061-789 7300)

La Pine Scientific Co., 6001 South Knox Ave., Chicago, IL 60629

LaPorte Industries Ltd., 11, Camford Way, Sundon Park, Luton, Beds LU3 3AN, England (0582 584884)

Leek Chemicals Ltd., Bridge End Works, Leek, Staffs ST13 8LG, England (0538-382124)

Leiner Gelatin Ltd., Treforest Mid-Glamorgan, Wales (044-385-2464)

Leiner P. and Sons America, Inc., 20101 Nine Mile Road, St. Clair Shore, MI 48080

Lever Brothers Company, 390 Park Ave., New York, NY 10022 (212-688-6000)

Lilly, Eli, & Co., P.O. Box 618, Indianapolis, IN 46206 (317-261-2000)

Lippo Chemicals Inc., 207 19th Avenue, Paterson, NJ 07504 (201-345-8600)

Liquid Carbonic Company, Subsidiary of Houston Natural Gas, Chicago, IL

Lonza, Inc., 22-10 RT. 208, Fairlawn, NJ 07401 (201-794-2400)

Lovelock Ltd., Oaklands House, Manchester N33 1WS (061-962 4423)

Lowenstein Dyes & Cosmetics, Inc., 420 Morgan Ave., Brooklyn, NY 11222

Luscombe, W. R. Ltd., Luscombe House, 481 Green Lanes, London N13 4BU, England (01-886 1456)

Lusochimica S.P.A., Via Carnia 26, 20132 Milan, Italy (02-2894-841)

M

Mabrook, Inc., Box 11, Oradell, NJ 07649

Dr. Madis Laboratories, Inc., 375 Huyler Street, South Hackensack, NJ 07606 (201-440-5000)

Madron Products Ltd., Whitehaven, UK

Mallinckrodt Ltd., Laynes House, 526 Watford Way, London NW7 4RS (01-906 0911)

Mallinckrodt, Inc., Second and Mallinckrodt Street, St. Louis, MO 63147 (314-895-2000)

Malmstrom Chemical—Emery Industries, PO Box 587, Linden, New Jersey

Manchem Ltd., Ashton New Road, Manchester M11 4AT, England (061-223 7100)

Mantrose-Haeuser Co., Millmaster Onyx Group, 99 Park Ave., New York, NY 10016

Marathon Morco Co., PO Drawer C, Dickinson, TX 77539 (713-337-1534)

Maruzen Fine Chemicals Inc., 353 Cider Ave., Mooristown, NJ 08057

Matheson Gas Products, P.O. Box 85, East Rutherford, NJ 07073 (201-933-2400)

Matthey, Johnson Chemicals Ltd., Orchard Road, Royston, Herts SG8 5HE (0763-44161)

May and Baker Ltd., Rainham Road South, Dagenham, Essex RM10 7XS, England (01-592 3060)

Mazer Chemicals Inc., 3938 Porett Drive, Gurnee, IL 60031 (312-244-3410)

MC & B Manufacturing Chemists, 2909 Highland Ave., Norwood, OH 45212

McKesson Chemical Co., Crocker Plaza, 1 Post Street, San Francisco, CA 94104

McKesson & Robbins, 8 Wilton Road, Haine Industrial Estate, Ramsgate ET12 5HF, UK (0843-22399)

Meer Corporation, 9500 Railroad Ave., North Bergen, NJ 07047 (201-861-9500)

Megret Ltd., Customs House, NE Toxteth Dock, Liverpool L3 4AS England (051-708 7034)

Die Melkindustrie Veghel, P.O. Box 13, 5460 BA Veghel, Netherlands

Mendell Co., Edward, Route 52, Carmel, NY 10512

Methylating Co. Ltd., Devonshire House, Mayfair Place, London WIX 6AY, England (01-629 8867)

Michel, M. & Co., 90 Broad St., New York, NY 10004

Miles Laboratories, Inc., P.O. Box 932, Elkhart, IN 46515 (219-262-7453)

Mitsui & Co. Europe s.p.a., Piazza Del Liberty 2, 20121 Milan, Italy

Mitsubishi International Corp., 277 Park Ave., New York, NY 10017

Mobay Chemical Corp., PO Box 419, Hawthorne, NJ 07507 (201-942-3232)

Modre and Munger Marketing, Inc., Fairfield Office Center, 140 Sherman St., Fairfield, CT 06430 (203-359-7861)

Monroe Chemical Co., Saville Ave. at 4th Street, Eddystone, PA 19013

Monsanto Industrial Chemicals Co., 800 N. Lindbergh Blvd., St. Louis, MO 63167 (314-694-1000)

Morton Salt, Div. Morton ThioKol Inc., 110 N. Wacker Dr., Chicago, IL 60606-1555

Mutchler Chemical Co., Inc., 259 Broadway, New York, NY 10007

N

Naarden International USA, Inc., Third Ave., New York, NY 10022

Napp Chemicals, 199 Main Street, Lodi, NJ 07644 (201-773-3900)

National Starch & Chemical Corp., 10 Finderne Ave., Bridgewater, NJ 08807 (201-685-5000)

Neal & Co., M.F., P.O. Box 24, Richmond, VA 23201

New Cheshire Salt Works Ltd., Wincham, Northwich, Cheshire CW9 6DD, England (0606-2361)

Nipa Laboratories Ltd., Nipa Industrial Estate, Llantwit Fardre, Nr Pontypridd, Mid-Glamorgan CF38 2SN, Wales (0443-205311)

NL Chemicals/NL Industires, Inc., P.O. Box 700, Hightstown, NJ 08520 (609-443-2000)

Norda, Inc., 140 Route 10, East Hanover, NJ 07936

O

Olin Chemicals Corporation, 120 Long Ridge Road, Stamford, CT 06904 (203-356-2000)

Onyx Cheical Co., 190 Warren Street, Jersey City, NJ 07302 (201-434-1700)

Orbis Products Corp., 140 Route 10, East Hanover, NJ 07936 (201-887-5600)

Organon, Inc., West Orange, NJ 07052

Oury, Millar & Co. Ltd., 16A Poyle, Guildford, Surrey GUI 35J, England (0483 32231)

P

Page, Charles & Co. Ltd., Acorn House, Victoria Road, London W3 6XU, England (01-992 5500)

Pardee Co., The, 485 Fifth Ave., New York, NY 10017

Paulaur Corp., PO Box 673, Princeton/Windsor Inc. Park, Princeton Jct., NJ 08550

Pechiney Ugine Kuhlmann Ltd., 259 Euston Road, London NW1, England

Pechiney Ugine Kuhlmann Ltd., Tour Manhattan, La Defense 2, 6 Place de L'Iris, 92400 Courbevoie, Paris, France (01-773-3456)

Penick & Ford Ltd., 920 First Street SW, Cedar Rapids, IA 52406

Penick, S.B. & Co., 1050 Wall Street, Lyndhurst, NJ 07047

Penreco, Division of Pennzoil Company, PO Box 671, Butler, PA 16001 (412-283-5600)

Perny, Inc., PO Box 721, Ridgewood, NJ 07451

Petrochemicals Company, Inc., PO Box 2199, Fort Worth, TX 76113 (817-625-2111)

Petrolite Corp., 369 Marshall Ave., St. Louis, MO 63119 (314-961-3500)

Pfaltz & Bauer, Inc., 375 Fairfield Ave., Stamford, CT 06902 (203-357-8700)

Pfanstiehl Laboratories Inc., 1219 Glen Rock Ave., Waukegan, IL 60085 (312-623-0370)

Pfizer, Inc., Chemical Div., 235 East 42nd St., New York, NY 10017 (212-573-2323)

Pfizer Ltd., Ramsgate Road, Sandwich, Kent CT13 9NJ, England (0304 616161)

Phillips Chemical Co., Drawer "O", Borger, TX 79007 (800-858-4327

P-L Biochemicals Inc., 1037 West McKinley Ave., Milwaukee, WI 53205 (414-347-7442)

Polarome Mfg. Co., 22 Ericsson Pl., New York, NY 10013

Polyesther Corp., PO Drawer BBBB, Southampton, NY 11968 (516-283-4400)

Poth Hille Co. Ltd., 37 High Street, London E15 2QD, England (01-534 7091)

PPG Industries Inc., Chemical Divs.; One Gateway Center, Pittsburgh, PA 15222

Proctor & Gamble Distributing Co., PO Box 599, Cincinnati, OH 45201 (513-562-2641)

Proctor and Gamble Ltd., Industrial Chemical Div., PO Box 9, Hayes Gate House, Hayes, Middlesex, England (01-848 9671)

Protameen Chemicals, Inc., 409 Minnisink Road, Totowa, NJ 07511 (201-256-4374)

Publicker Industries, Inc., 777 West Putnam Ave., Greenwich, CT 06830 (203-531-4500)

PVO International, Inc., 14 Ridgedale Ave., Suite 26, Cedar Knolls, NJ 07927 (201-285-0900)

Q

Quad Chemical—Lonza Specialty Chemicals, Lonza, Inc., 22-10 RT 208, Fairlawn, NJ 07410 (201-794-2400)

R

Ransom, William & Son Ltd., Hitchin Herts SG5 1LY, England (0462 4575)

Reisman Corp., H., 377 Crane St., Orange, NJ 07051

Rhodia (UK) Ltd., Hulton House, Fleet Street, London EC4, England (01-353 5033)

Rhone-Poulenc, Inc., Black Horse Lane, Monmouth Junction, NJ 08852 (201-297-0100)

Richardson Co., Organic Chemical Div., 2400 East Devon Ave., Des Plaines, IL 60018

Richard Harrison Baker Ltd., 253 Cranbrook Road, Ilford, Essex IG1 4TQ, England (01-554 0102)

Riches-Nelson, Inc., 254 Mill Street, Greenwich, CT 06830 (203-869-3088)

Rickards, L. J. & Co. Ltd., Mackenzie House, 221-241 Beckenham Road, Beckenham, Kent BR3 4UF (01-659 2345)

Riker Laboratories, Morley Street, Loughborough, Leics LE11 1EP, England (0509-268181)

Robeco Chemicals, Inc., 99 Park Ave., New York, NY 10016 (212-986-6410)

Robinson Wagner Co., Inc., 628 Waverly Ave., Mamaroneck, NY 10543

Roche Products Ltd. (Fine Chemicals Div.), 318 High Street North, Dunstable, Beds. LU6 1BG, England (0582 605961)

Rohm & Haas Co., Independence Mall West, Philadelphia, PA 19105 (215-592-3000)

Rohm & Haas (UK) Ltd., Lennig House, 2 Mason's Avenue, Croydon CR9 3NB, England (01-686 8844)

Rohm Tech, Inc., 195 Canal Street, Malden, MA 02148 (716/322-0358)

Ronsheim & Moore Ltd., Ings Lane, Castleford, West Yorkshire WF10 2JT, England (0977-556565)

Roquette (UK) Ltd., Pantiles House, 2 Nevill Street, Tunbridge Wells, Kent TN2 5TT, England (0892 40188)

Ross Co., Frank B., PO Box 4085, 6-10 Ash Street, Jersey City, NJ 07304 (201-433-4512)

Roussel Corp., 155 East 44th St., New York, NY 10017 (212-697-5820)

Roussel Laboratories Ltd., Chemical Sales Div., Roussel House, Wembley Park, Middlesex HA9 0NF, England (01-903 1454)

Rousselot Ltd., Colthorp Lane, Thatchan, Newbury, Belks RG13 4XH, England (0635-65660)

R.I.T.A. Corp., 332 Virginia St., PO Box 556C, Crystal Lake, IL 60014

Ruger Chemical Co., Inc., PO Box 806, Hillside, NJ 07205 (201-926-0331)

S

Salomon Bros., Inc., L.A., PO Box 828, Port Washington, NY 11050

Salsbury Laboratories, Inc., Chemical Dept., 2000 Rockford Road, Charles City, IA 50616 (800-247-1833)

Sandoz Colors & Chemicals, Route 10, East Hanover, NJ 07936

Santell Chemical Co., 1600 South Canal Street, Chicago, IL 60613

Scherer North America, R.P., 2725 Scherer Dr., St. Petersburg, FL 33702

Sheffield Products, PO Box 630, Norwich, NY 13815

Shell Chemical, Co., One Shell Plaza, Houston, TX 77002 (713-241-6161)

Shell Chemicals (UK) Ltd., Northumberland House, Trafalgar Sq., London WC2N 5LF, England (01-839 1277)

Sherex Chemical Co., Box 646, Dublin, OH 43017 (614-764-6500)

Sherwin-Williams Chemicals, PO Box 6520, Cleveland, OH 44101 (216-566-2344)

Siegle, G & Co. GmbH, Sieglestrasse 25, 7 Stuttgart 30, W. Germany

Sigma (London) Chemical Co. Ltd., Fancy Road, Poole, Dorset BH17 7NH, England (0202 733114)

Sipon Products Ltd., Tretol House, Edgware Road, Colindale, London NW9, England

Sitco (Shah International Trading Corp.), 318 Cleveland Ave., Highland Park, NJ 08904 (201-846-6000)

Smith, Warner G., Inc., 1730 Train Ave., Cleveland, OH 44173 (216-861-3676)

Smith, Wilfred, Ltd., Gemini House, High Street, Edgware, Middlesex HA8 7ET, England (01-952 6655)

Sonoco Products Co., Hartsville, SC 29550 (803-383-7000)

Specialty Chemical Div., Benzol Product Department, Meadow Road, Edison, NJ 08817

Spencer-Kellogg, 120 Delaware Ave., PO Box 807, Buffalo, NY 14240 (716-852-5850)

Speywood Labs Ltd., Ash Road, Wrexham Industrial Estate, Wrexham, Clwyd, England (0978 61181)

S.S.T. Corp., Clifton, NJ 07015

Staley Mfg. Co., A.E., Box 151, Decatur, IL 62525

Stancourt, Sons and Muir Ltd., County House, 76 St. John's Road, Tunbridge Wells, Kent TN4 9PH, England (0892 39277)

Starchem Corporation, 60 East 42nd Street, New York, NY 10017

Starches, J&W, Ltd., Unit N1/7 Heywood Industrial Estate, Heywood, Lanc, England (0706 621341)

Stauffer Chemical Co., Westport, CT 06881

Stavely Chemicals Ltd., Stavely Works, Chesterfield, Derbys S43 2PB, England (0246-77251)

Steetley Chemicals Ltd., Berk House, PO Box 56, Basing View, Basingstoke, Hants RG21 2EG, England (0256 29292)

Stein-Hall & Co., Inc., New York, NY 10016

Stepan Chemical Co., Northfield, IL 60093 (312-446-7500)

Sterling Organics, Div. Sterling Drug Inc., 90 Park Avenue, NY, NY 10016 (212-972-2632)

Stevenson Brothers & Co., Inc., 1039 West Venanco Street, Philadelphia, PA 19140 (215-223-2600)

Stoney-Mueller, Inc., Page & Newark Avenues, Lyndhurst, NJ 07071

Strahl & Pitsch, Inc., 230 Great East Neck Road, West Babylon, NY 11704

Stuart Pharmaceuticals (Div. of ICI US Inc.), Wilmington, DE 19897

Sturge Ltd., John & E., Denison Road, Selby, N. Yorks. Y08 8EF, England (021-440 3271)

Suburban Chemical Co., PO Box 485, River Street Station, Paterson, NJ 07524

Sun Chemical Corp., 200 Park Ave., New York, NY 10166 (212-986-5500)

Sun Petroleum Products Co., 1801 Market Street, Philadelphia, PA 19103 (215-977-3746)

Suncrest Corp., 120 Wall St., New York, NY 10005

Supelco, Inc., Supelco Park, Bellefonte, PA 16823 (814-359-2732)

Surfactants, Inc., 48 Liberty St., Metuchen, NJ 08840

Surgikos Ltd., Kirkton Campus, Livingston, West Lothian EH54 7AT, Scotland (0506 37441)

Suter, A. F. & Co. Ltd., Swan Wharf, 60 Dace Road, London E3 2NQ, England (01-986 8218)

Swift Edible Oil Co., Food Ingredients Products, 115 W. Jackson Blvd., Chicago, IL 60604

Synthetic Products Co., Div. of Port Industries, Inc., 1636 Wayside Rd., Cleveland, OH 44112

T

Takeda-Fallek Sales, Inc., 400 Park Ave., New York, NY 10022

Tamms Industries Co., Drawer C, 1222 Ardmore Ave., Itasca, IL 60143

Tate & Lyle Refineries Ltd., Leon House, High Street, Croydon CR9 3NH, England (01-686 5656)

Technical Petrolatum Co., 6233 N. Pulaski Road, Chicago, IL 60646

Ted Pella, Inc., Box 510, Tustin, CA 92680

Tennants (Lancashire) Ltd., Hazelbottom Road, Cheetham, Manchester M8 7GR, England (061-205 4454)

Tenneco Chemicals, Inc., PO Box 365, Turner Place, Piscataway, NJ 08854 (201-981-5000)

Tenneco Organics Ltd., Rockingham Works, Avonmouth, Bristol BS11 0YT, England (0272 3611)

Tensia Ltd., North Road Industrial Estate, Bridgend, Mid-Glamorgan, Wales (0656 58921)

Thew, Arnott & Co., Ltd., Flodden Works, 270 London Road, Wallington, Surrey SM6 7DJ, England (01-669 3131)

Thompson-Hayward Chemical Co., PO Box 2383, 5200 Speaker Road, Kansas City, KS 66106 (913-321-3131)

Thomson & Joseph Ltd., 119 Plumstead Road, Norwich, Norfolk, England (0603 39511)

TIC Gums, Inc., 144 E. 44th Street, New York, NY 10017

Tonra Ltd., Flodden Works, 270 London Road, Wallington, Surrey SM6 7DJ, England (01-669 3131)

Toyomenka (America) Inc., Suite 4011, One World Trade Center, New York, NY 10048 (212-466-4680)

Tragacanth Importing Corporation, New York, NY 10017

Trask, Arthur C., Corp., 7207 W. 65th Street, Chicago, IL 60638

Tridom Chemical, Inc., 255 Oser Ave., Hauppague, NY 11787

Tri-K Industries, Inc., 99 Kinderkamack Rd., Westwood, NJ 07675

Tunnel Avebe Starches Ltd., Avebe House, Otterham Quay, Rainham, Kent ME8 7UU, England (0634 373551)

Tunnel Refineries Ltd., Thames Bank House, Tunnel Ave., London SE10 0PA, England (01-858 3033)

U

Ubichem Ltd., 281 Hithermoor Road, Stanwell Moor, Staines, Middlesex TW19 6AZ, England (02812 511719)

Uhe Co., George, Inc., 76 Ninth Ave., New York, NY 10011 (212-929-0870)

Unalco Ltd., 215 Tunnel Avenue, East Greenwich, London SE10 0PU, England (01-858-8631)

Ungerer & Co., 4 Bridgewater Lane, Lincoln Park, NJ 07035 (201-628-0600)

Unichema Chemicals Ltd., Bebington, Wirral, Merseyside L62 4UF, England (051-645-2020)

Union Carbide Corp., PO Box 60369, Jacksonville, FL 32205 (904-783-2180)

Union Carbide Ltd., 95 High Street, Rickmansworth, Herts WD3 1RB, England (0923-720366)

United States Biochemicals Corp., PO Box 22400, Cleveland, OH 44122

Universal Oil Products Co., State Highway 17, East Rutherford, NJ 07073

Unwin, R.W. & Co., Ltd., 10 Prospect Place, Welwyn, Herts AL6 9EW, England (043-871 6441)

Uromilk, 32 St. Mary-at-Hill, London EC3 3AJ, England (01-623 9333)

U.S. Gypsum Co., Chemical Div., 101 South Wacker Dr., Chicago, IL 60606

U.S.I. Chemicals National Distillers & Chemical Corporation, Boston, MA 01460 (212-949-5700)

U.S. Industrial Chemicals Co., 99 Park Ave., New York, NY 10016 (212-949-5700)

V

Vanderbilt, R. T., Co., Inc., 30 Winfield Street, Norwalk, CT 06855 (203-853-1400)

Van Dyk & Co., Inc., Main and Williams Streets, Belleville, NJ 07109 (201-759-3225)

Velisicol Chemical Corp., 341 East Ohio St., Chicago, IL 60611 (312-670-4500)

VGF Chemical Corp., 420 Lexington Ave., New York, NY 10017

Virginia Chemicals Co., 3340 West Norfolk Road, Portsmouth, VA 23703 (804-483-7000)

Vitamins, Inc., 200 East Randolph Dr., Chicago, IL 60601 (312-861-0700)

Vyse Gelatin Co., 5010 N. Rose St., Schiller Park, IL 60176

W

Wagner Company, Inc., Charles, A., 4457 North 6th Street, Philadelphia, PA 19140

Ward Blenkinsop Trading Ltd., Townsend House, 160 Northolt Road, South Harrow, Middlesex HA2 0HJ, England (01-422 1244)

Watts, R.A., Ltd., 36 Woodcote Road, Wallington, Surrey SM6 0NN, England (01-647 1073)

Welch, Holme & Clark Co., Inc., 1000 South 4th Street, Harrison, NJ 07029

Westbrook Lanolin Co., Argonaut Works, Laisterdyke, Bradford, West Yorkshire BD4 8AU, England (0274 663331)

Whey Products Ltd., P.O. Box 150, By The Sea Road, Trowbridge, Wiltshire BA14 8HS, England (02214 3611)

Whiting, Peter (Chemicals) Ltd., 5 Lord Napier Place, Upper Mall, London W6 9UB, England (01-741 3107)

Whittaker Clark and Daniels, Inc., 100 Coolridge St., South Plainfield, NJ 07080

Wickhen Products, Inc., Big Pond Road, Huguenot, NY 12746

Williams (Hounslow Ltd.), Greville House, Hibernia Road, Hounslow, Middlesex TW3 3RX, England (01-570 7766)

Witco Chemical Corp., 520 Madison Ave., New York, NY 10022 (212-605-3800)

Witco Chemical Co. Ltd., Union Lane, Droitwich, Worcs WR9 9BB, England (0905-772454)

Woodward & Dickerson Inc., 2 Girard Plaza, Philadelphia, PA 19102

Wynmouth Lehr & Fatoils Ltd., 158 City Road, London ECIV 2PA, England (01-253 5871)

X

Xyrofin Ltd., 6340 Baar, Switzerland

Z

Zimmerli, Aaburg, Switzerland

Zimmermann Hobbs Ltd., Dawson Road, Bletchley, Milton Keynes MK1 1JR, England (0908 71821)

APPENDIX II

HPE Laboratory Methods

Compression Characteristics

COM-1: Lab #21

Instrumentation and Calibration of a Manesty B3B Rotary Tablet Press

Compressional force was monitored from a remote site using pairs of metal foil strain gauges[1] (in Wheatstone bridge configuration) bonded to turned-down sections on opposite sides of the pressure rod. The unbalance in the bridge circuit caused by elongation of the pressure rod during tablet compression was monitored using a carrier amplifier,[2] that also served to activate the bridge. Compression events were recorded on a storage-type oscilloscope.[3] Responses were read directly as units of scope deflections that were later converted into units of force.

The instrumented site was previously calibrated against an upper punch that has been instrumented by bonding strain gauges[1] (in Wheatstone bridge configuration) to turned down sections on opposite sides of the punch. Bridge excitation voltage was provided by a DC power supply.[4] Bridge unbalance voltage was amplified by one of the differential amplifiers of the oscilloscope. The punch was calibrated in a Carver press[5] by observing scope deflection *vs* applied compressional force. The punch was then inserted into the tablet press and scope deflection from the punch and pressure rod were recorded simultaneously and compared while manually turning the press under varying compressional loads. The signal deflection produced by the pressure rod was found to be directly proportional to the punch compressional force.

COM-2: Lab #21

Use of the Carver Press in the Preparation of Compacts
Apparatus:
Carver Press Model
Stainless steel baseplate
Flat faced plug for bolt hole in press head
½″ round die (from tests using rotary press)
½″ round lower punch (from tests using rotary press)

Method:
1. The die, baseplate and punch face are lubricated with a 10% solution of stearic acid in chloroform, applied using a cotton-tipped applicator.
2. The die and baseplate are centered on the platen and a measured amount of powder is introduced into the die cavity.
3. The plug is inserted into the bolt hole and the punch inserted into the die cavity.
4. Desired pressure is applied and released immediately.
5. While holding the die with the punch inverted, the head of the punch is tapped on the base of the press to force the tablet from the die.
6. The die, baseplate, and punch face are re-lubricated prior to formation of the next compact.
A diagram of the assembly is seen in Figure 1.

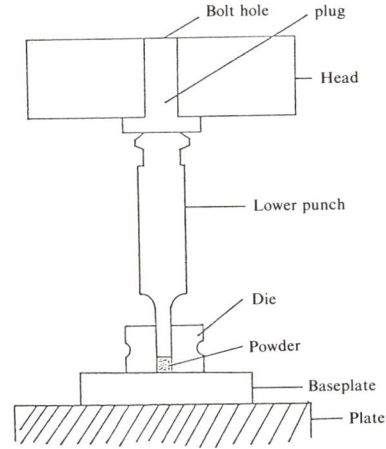

Figure 1: Set up of the Carver Press for Compact Formation

COM-3: Lab #20

Procedure for Compression-Hardness Testing
1. Approximately 1 Kg of each material was blended with 0.25% magnesium stearate (Mallinckrodt lot #2Z55) for 5 minutes in an Erweka cube blender.
2. Compression was accomplished on a 16-station Stokes B-2 rotary press using 4 stations set up with 7/16-inch standard concave tooling.
3. Compression and ejection forces were monitored through strain gauges on a Tektronix dual-beam storage oscilloscope.
4. Edge thicknesses were measured with a vernier caliper.
5. Hardnesses were measured with a Schleuniger model 2E hardness tester.
6. Each reported data point is the mean of 20 determinations.
7. Profiles were drawn as a 2nd degree regression curve with a Tektronix programmable calculator and X-Y plotter, except in the cases of microcrystalline cellulose PH 101 an 102, which were drawn by 3rd degree regression.

COM-4: Lab #29

Procedure for Stokes, Model F, Single Punch Press
Equipment: Stokes Model F-single punch press equipped with ½ inch, round, flat-faced tooling and instrumented with piezo electric transducers leading to an instrument panel with an oscilloscope and to a computer.
Procedure
1. Adjust fill volume (lower punch) to obtain compacts of 600 mg.
2. Preliminary Test—Operate under machine power to determine that tablet weight is reasonably uniform. (Collect in groups of 10 tablets)
3. Test—Collect 10 tablets compressed under machine power.
4. Record applied compressional force reading from computer output.
5. Repeat steps 3 and 4 at other pressure settings. (Adjust to approximate pressure setting *via* oscilloscope.)
NOTE: Press operating at 60 tablets per minute.

COM-5: Lab #29: Unlubricated Carver Press, Manual Oper.

Equipment and procedure are the same as COM-6.

COM-6: Lab #29: Lubricated Carver Press, Manual Oper.

Equipment: Hydraulic press ½ inch, round, flat-faced upper and lower punches and the appropriate die supports for the die with lower punch at a constant height to allow for the die fill.
A pressure gauge, graduated to 10,000 pounds with 100 pound increments.

Procedure

1. Apply a 5% w/w solution of stearic acid in denatured alcohol to the punch face and sides and to the die bore.
2. Place the die on the supports with lower punch in place.
3. Transfer a pre-weighed 600 mg increment material to the die cavity.
4. Position top punch in the die cavity.
5. Apply pressure manually to specified setting; hold at maximum for 5 seconds and release.
6. Remove the upper punch and invert the assembly on the supports.
7. Pushing against the lower punch, use the press to eject the compact downward without causing undue stress on the structural strength of the compact.
8. Repeat the process four times at each level of applied force.

COM-6: Lab #29-1: Physical Property Measurements

Tablet Weight
1. Weigh tablets individually on Mettler H₂O T semi-micro analytical balance.
2. Record tablet weight in mg.

Tablet Thickness
1. Measure tablets individually with Ames Dial Comparator calibrated in 0.01 mm.
2. Record tablet thickness in mm.

Tablet Breaking Strength
Method A—For Tablets less than 16 kg
1. Measure tablets individually in Heberlein electric hardness tester.
2. Record breaking strength in Kg.

Method B—For tablets greater than 16 kg
1. Measure tablets individually using the Stokes Gun equipped with heavy duty spring.
2. Record initial and final readings.
3. Calculate breaking strength in Kg by the following formula (Reading$_{final}$–Reading$_{initial}$) × 3 = Breaking Strength.

COM-7: Lab #12: Compression Characteristics

Procedure

Evaluations of compression characteristics were carried out with a Model B Carver Laboratory Press[5]. A set of 16/32″ F.F.B.E. punches and appropriate die was fitted into the standard Carver Press retention chuck. Five hundred mg of test material or, depending on the material evaluated, sufficient powder to fill the die to 70-80% of capacity was weighed into the die. Pressure at the required compression force was applied and immediately released when the desired value was obtained.

At least five tablets were prepared at a minimum of four different compression forces if acceptable tablets could be compressed. Dies were lubricated with a 10% stearic acid in chloroform solution. Tablet hardness values were obtained using the Schleuniger Model 2E hardness tester.

---

[1] FAET 25-B-35-56-E half bridge T-rosettes, Type SR-4, BLH Electronics, Waltham, MA.
[2] Sanborn Model 311A, Hewlett Packard Col, Palo Alto, CA.
[3] Model 5113 with 4B12N time base and two 5A26 dual differential amplifiers, Tektronic Inc. Mf. Co., Beaverton, OR.
[4] Model 21-200 Calex Mfg. Co., Pleasant Hill, CA.
[5] Fred S. Carver, Inc., Summit, NJ.

Consistency (Penetrometer)

PEN-1: Lab #4

The consistency values were determined by the method given in the USP XX (p. 603).

Density

DE-1: Lab #7 & Lab. #31

Helium Air Pycnometry (Micromeritic Instrument Corp.)

DE-2: Lab #36

Pycnometer method for solids insoluble and heavier than water (*Remington's Pharmaceutical Sciences*, 15th Ed., Page 94): Titanium dioxide.

DE-3: Lab #36

Sinker method for solids insoluble and lighter than water (*Remington's Pharmaceutical Sciences*, 15th Ed., Page 95). Each sample was first melted and resolidified prior to determination, and stearic acid saturated water was used as the displaced liquid: Stearic acid.

DE-4: Lab #36

Pycnometer method for solids soluble in water using heptane as the displaced liquid (*Remington's Pharmaceutical Sciences*, 15th Ed., Page 95): Lactose, anhydrous.

DE-5: Lab #30

30 ml, capillary bore stopper, pycnometer; exact volume determined by weighing water at 24° in accord with standard data tables that correlate density with temperature.

Bulk and Tap Density or Volume

BTD-1: Lab #1 & Lab #14

Samples were passed through a #20 mesh screen prior to density determination. Bulk density was performed by pouring 25 g material into a 100 ml graduated cylinder and measuring the volume to the nearest ml. Tapped density was performed by placing the graduated cylinder in the Tap-Pak Volumeter* and operating the unit through a series of taps until the powder contained in the graduated cylinder attained a constant tapped volume. Results presented represent an average of two determinations per sample.

BTD-2: Lab #1

25 g were placed in a 250 ml graduated cylinder.

BTD-3: Lab #1

The samples were not passed through a #20 mesh screen prior to density determination.

BTD-4: Lab #1

Six g were placed in a 250 ml graduated cylinder.

BTD-5: Lab #6

Weighed samples of not more than 130 g to not less than 40 g were placed in a 250 ml graduated cylinder using a glassine type weighing paper to facilitate ease of flow. Transfer of the weighed powder to the cylinder was done as rapidly as flow would permit with the cylinder being held at approximately 45° angle. The cylinder containing the sample was brought to the vertical and given a sharp shake to level the volume for reading.

After reading the loose bulk volume, each sample was placed on the Tap-Pak device* and run in 100 tap increments from 100 through 500 taps and then 1000 taps. At 1000 taps, the sample was run in 1000 tap increments up to a total of 4000 taps. The volume of each tap increment was recorded in ml.

The data indicated that a relative constant volume was achieved between 3000 to 4000 taps using this apparatus.

After each one hundred taps the volume was recorded until the three consecutive readings were the same which was defined as the tap volume of this sample.

BTD-8: Lab #36

1. A weighed portion of each sample was gently poured through a glass funnel into a 250 ml graduated cylinder supported at an angle of 45° on a ring stand.
2. The graduated cylinder was then rotated to an upright position, the powder surface gently leveled and the bulk volume of the sample was recorded.
3. The graduated cylinder loaded with the powder sample was then subjected to the action of an apparatus (Tap-Pak Volumeter, Model 2, Shandon Scientific Co., Inc., Sewickley, PA) which was adjusted to operate for 100 taps.

---

*Model No. JEL ST2 manufactured by J. Engelsmann A.F. of Ludwigshafen a. Rh. West Germany. Available through Shandon Scientific Company, Sewickley, Pennsylvania.

Flowability

FLOW-3: Lab #24

The powder flowmeter used in this evaluation consisted of an aluminum pan attached to a beam equipped with four strain gauges capable of measuring weight differences in microseconds, a strain gauge activation and measuring unit which converts the strain gauge signal to an electrical impulse measurable by a 10 in. strip chart recorder with variable speed. The sample to be evaluated is placed in a cone (70°C) suitably held above the pan and equipped with an electrically triggered trap door. The strip chart recorder is adjusted so that 250 g would be represented by 100% of scale. The sample is allowed to flow onto the pan and the time required for the sample to empty from the funnel is recorded. The rate of flow is determined from the strip chart recorder and expressed as a flow rate in g/sec.

All samples are passed through a 30 mesh screen to remove any lumps. All measurements are repeated three times.

Moisture Content

MC-1: USP XX, Water Determination, Chapter 921, Page 987, Gravimetric, Method III, 5 hours at 60°.

MC-2: USP XX, Water Determination, Chapter 921, Page 987, Gravimetric, Method III, 16 hours at 60°.

MC-3: USP XX, Water Determination, Chapter 921, Page 988, Method I, Titrimetric.

MC-4: USP XX, Loss on Drying, Chapter 731, Page 960, Thermogravimetric.

MC-5: USP XX, Loss on Drying, Chapter 731, Page 960, 2 hours at 60°.

MC-6: USP XX, Loss on Drying, Chapter 731, Page 960, 3 hours at 60°.

MC-7: USP XX, Loss on Drying, Chapter 731, Page 960, 3 hours at 105°.

MC-8: USP XX, Loss on Drying, Chapter 731, Page 960, 4 hours at 105°.

MC-9: USP XX, Loss on Drying, Chapter 731, Page 960, 5 hours at 105°.

MC-10: USP XX, Loss on Drying, Chapter 731, Page 960, 16 hours at 105°.

MC-11: USP XX, Loss on Drying, Chapter 731, Page 960, 17 hours at 105°.

MC-12: USP XX, Loss on Drying, Chapter 731, Page 960, heat to constant weight at 105°.

MC-13: USP XX, Loss on Drying, Chapter 731, Page 960, heat to constant weight at 110°.

MC-14: USP XX, Loss on Drying, Chapter 731, Page 960, 2 hours at 105°.

MC-15: USP XX, Loss on Drying, Chapter 731, Page 960, 4 hours at 120°.

MC-16: USP XX, Loss on Drying, Chapter 731, Page 960, 1 hour at 105°, then 3 hours at 120°.

MC-17: USP XX, Loss on Drying, Chapter 731, Page 960, 2 hours at 105°, then 16 hours at 120°.

MC-18: USP XX, Loss on Drying Under Vacuum, Chapter 731, Page 960.

MC-19: USP XX, Loss on Drying Under Vacuum, Chapter 731, Page 960, 8 hours at 45°.

MC-20: USP XX, Loss on Drying Under Vacuum, Chapter 731, Page 960, 16 hours at 60°.

MC-21: USP XX, Loss on Drying Under Vacuum, Chapter 731, Page 960, 17 hours at 60°.

MC-22: USP XX, Loss on Drying Under Vacuum, Chapter 731, Page 960, 20 hours at 60°.

MC-23: USP XX, Loss on Drying Under Vacuum, Chapter 731, Page 960, 3 hours at 105° and 10mm Hg.

MC-24: USP XX, Loss on Drying Under Vacuum, Chapter 731, Page 960, 3 hours at 200° and 76mm Hg.

MC-25: USP XX, Loss on Ignition, Chapter 733, Page 960.

MC-26: American Association of Official Analytical Chemists, AOAC, 12th Ed., Page 221.

MC-27: Food Chemicals Codex, 2nd Edition, Loss on Drying, Page 163.

MC-28: USP XX, Residue on Ignition, Chapter 281, Page 911.

MC-29: Accurately weigh approximately 1 g of the sample on a watch glass; dry for 24 hours at 110° and weigh; dry for an additional 24 hours and weigh again. Convert loss on drying to percent moisture content.

MC-30: No direct method for water content in dibasic calcium phosphate dihydrate is available. In compendial tests, the loss on ignition is used. This loss includes loss of free water, water of hydration and the elimination of one mole of water for every two moles of $CaHPO_4$ as it converts to the prophosphate ($Ca_2P_2O_7$). The following calculation was used to arrive at the stated values:

$$\%H_2O = \frac{\text{gram sample} - (\text{Residue on ignition} \times \frac{272.12}{254.12}) \times 100}{\text{g sample}}$$

where $272.12 = 2(CaHPO_4)$
$254.12 = Ca_2P_2O_7$
H_2O = Water of crystallization and absorbed water

Theory for $CaHPO_4.2H_2O$ is 20.9% H_2O

MC-31: USP XX, Water Determination, Chapter 94, Page 987, Gravimetric, Method III, 16 hours at 105°.

Equilibrium Moisture Content

EMC-1: Lab #2, 10, 15, 18 and 22

Materials

Nine plastic desiccators, Nalge/Sybron Corporation, approximately 9 inches in diameter, were obtained from a local laboratory supply house. Glass desiccators of equivalent size may be substituted for the plastic containers.

A supply of glass analytical weighing bottles with standard taper covers (25 mm O.D. × 40 mm ht. with 12 ml capacity) were used to contain samples for testing. Samples were weighed on an analytical balance to the nearest 0.1 mg. A series of saturated salt solutions were prepared as described in Table I.

Table I. Saturated Salt Solutions for Maintaining Constant Relative Humidity Conditions in Desiccators

Saturated Salt* Solution*	Percent Relative Humidity at Temperatures (9-11)			
	20°C	25°C	30°C	37°C
Lithium chloride	12	11	11	11
Potassium acetate	24	23	23	23
Magnesium chloride	33	33	32	31
Potassium carbonate	44	43	42	41
Magnesium nitrate	53	52	52	51
Sodium nitrite	66	64	63	62
Sodium chloride	76	75	75	75
Potassium bromide	84	83	82	81
Potassium nitrate	94	93	92	91

*Prepared from reagent grade salts dissolved in purified water.

Procedure

EMC determinations were made by placing accurately weighed samples of each material (100-200 mg) in 2 or 3 open, tared, and numbered weighing bottles and then into a labeled desiccator containing one of the saturated salt solutions described in Table I. A liberal amount of the saturated salt solution (with excess crystals) was placed in the well of the desiccator.

Samples were stored in each of the nine securely closed individual desiccators, each containing a different moisture atmosphere. At equilibrium (7 days storage at controlled room temperature 25° ± 2°C) the samples were removed from the desiccators and the moisture increase or decrease determined for each sample by obtaining the final equilibrium weight with the aid of an analytical balance. These data were recorded on moisture analysis data sheets.

EMC values were calculated from P (% moisture dry basis). Initial moisture content (A) of each excipient was accurately determined by a suitable method, such as loss on drying to constant weight and used to calculate P. EMC values, at each relative humidity tested, were tabulated and plotted, using co-ordinate graph paper, to obtain EMC vs relative humidity curves.

Particle Friability

PF-1: Lab #36

Procedure

A 50 g portion of each sample was sieved through a series of selected standard sieves with the aid of a Ro-Tap Testing Sieve Shaker (The W.S. Tyler Company, Cleveland, Ohio) for 5 minutes. The powder retained on each sieve was weighed to obtain a weight-size distribution of the sample. The arithmetic mean particle size was calculated. (Reference: E. Parrott and W. Saski, "Experimental Pharmaceutical Technology," 3rd Ed., Burgess Publishing Company, Minneapolis, MN 1971, p. 286).

A second 50 g portion of each sample was attritioned by placing 100 g of 5 mm glass beads and the sample in the sieve collector and subjecting both to the action of the Ro-Tap Testing Sieve Shaker for 5 minutes.

The weight size distribution of the attritioned sample was determined by the method outlined above, and the arithmetic mean particle size was calculated.

The difference between the arithmetic mean particle sizes obtained before and after attrition was divided by the size before attrition to obtain a number which was defined as Friability Index.

Particle Size Distribution Methods

PSD-1: Lab #1

Sieve analysis using a Syntrol Sieve Shaker, Model TSS-31-C. Amplitude was set at 0.080″ and sieving time was 15 minutes. All sieves were U.S. Standard Sieve Series (ASTM Designation E11). Samples identified as PSD-1S were passed through a #20 mesh screen to break up lumps before analysis.

PSD-2: Lab #5

Sieve analysis using USP XX Method for Powder Fineness, Page 971 with U.S. Standard Sieves (Fisher Scientific Co.) made of stainless steel. Sample size was approximately 10 g and each sample was screened for 35 minutes on a mechanical sieve shaker (Fritsch Co.). The arithmetic mean diameter, d_{av}, was determined by Eq1 (see "The Theory & Practice of Industrial Pharmacy," 2nd Ed., Lea and Febiger, Philadelphia 1976, Page 466). Weight size is the product of the arithmetic mean size of the openings and the percentage retained on the smaller sieve.

$$d_{av} = \frac{\Sigma(nd)}{\Sigma n} \text{ (Eq1)}$$

PSD-3: Lab #12

Place a 100 g sample in the top screen of a series on a Cenco Meinzer Sieve Shaker (Central Scientific Co., Cat. #18480). Shake at Intensity #7 for 5 minutes. The results are reported as percentage retained on each screen size.

PSD-4: Lab #17

Determine the tare weight of each sieve and the pan used in the ATM Sonic Sifter (ATM Corporation). Weigh 4 g of the excipient and transfer to the top sieve of the sieve assembly. Run the sifter for 2 minutes using the Sift/Pulse Mode, with the amplitude of sift = 8 on a scale of 10. After the sifting, weigh each sieve and the pan. Calculate the net weight and the weight percent of excipient retained on each sieve. Run the analysis in triplicate and report the weight percent and standard deviation retained on sieves of different opening sizes.

PSD-5A: Lab #21

The Alpine Air Jet Sieve, Model 200, is operated at "8" reading on the manometer using water. The 10 g sample is run for 10 minutes per screen size and the results are reported as percentage retained on each sieve.

PSD-5B: Lab #21

The 10 g sample is placed on a nest of sieves which has previously been wetted. A stream of cold distilled water is passed over the sample until no more passes through the sieve. The retained material on each sieve is dried and weighed.

PSD-6: Lab #23

Accurately weigh a 100 g sample and place it on the top sieve of a sieve series (Tyler Sieves) with meshes 35, 48, 60, 80, 100, 150, 200 and the Pan. Obtain the tare weight of each sieve and the pan. Place the nest of sieves on the Tyler Portable Sieve Shaker, Model RX21. Operate for 5 hours and accurately weigh each sieve and the pan. Operate the nest of sieves for an additional 2 hours. If there is no change in the weights, convert the weight of the excipient retained on each sieve to percent of total weight.

PSD-7: Lab #24

The Fisher Sub-Sieve Particle Size Analyzer operates on the air-permeability principle for measuring the average particle size of powders. Particles in the path of a regulated air flow will affect that air flow in relationship to their size. This principle finds its basis in the fact that a current of air flows more readily through a bed of coarse powder than through an otherwise equal bed of fine powder that is equal in shape of bed, apparent volume, and percentage of voids; but by reason of difference in general coarseness of material and (differing in average pore diameter and in total interstitial surface), measurements of average particle sizes are obtained. The particle size data reported represent an average of 3 determinations and lie within ± 0.3 micron.

PSD-8: Lab #33

The Micromerograph (Sharples Type XC) was used to determine the particle size distribution of the samples with the data represented in terms of equivalent spherical diameters in microns. The principle involved is sedimentation in an air column. Samples of hydrogenated castor oil and Dehydag Wax O (Witepsol) were unsuitable for particle size distribution measurement because of their physical properties.

PSD-9: Lab #3

The method used, microscopy, is considered to be adequate for narrowly distributed samples, whereas highly dispersed samples will be prone to errors due to sampling. The parameter obtained in this case is simply a supporting parameter. A small sample of the excipient, 20 mg at the most, was dispersed in 3 to 4 drops of mineral oil, and a sample of this dispersion further diluted with mineral oil and transferred to a hemocytometer slide, so that the concentration was sufficiently large to allow counting but not too large to prevent counting. A cover slip was placed on the sample and care taken not to entrap air. The slide was then mounted on the microscope and photographed using a Polaroid Land Camera. Particle size distributions were then determined from the photograph.

Scanning Electron Microscopy

The purpose of this study is to obtain a topographical characterization of pharmaceutical excipients through the use of scanning electron microscopy. Photomicrographs are included in the Handbook.

Methodology

The aluminum stubs used for SEM were first polished with a metal polish (Wenol[1]) and ultrasonified for 5 minutes in a bath of acetone. The stubs were rinsed with ethyl alcohol and coated with a thin layer of adhesive (Mikrostik[1]). Prior to the evaporation of the adhesive, the excipient sample was placed uniformly on the stub. By this procedure, the excipient sample was fastened to the surface of the stub. A thin layer of gold was then coated on the surface in a vacuum evaporator and the SEM micrographs were taken with a Cambridge Scanning Electron Microscope[2] at the required magnifications.

---

[1] Tedd Pella Inc.
[2] Cambridge Stereoscan Mark IIA.

Solubility Methods

SOL-1: Lab #1

An excess of each excipient was added to approximately 30 ml of purified water, alcohol or n-hexane. The excipient-solvent mixtures were agitated on a wrist-action shaker for 1 hour. The mixtures were then filtered through 0.45 micron Millipore-MF filters in the case of alcohol and n-Hexane. Ten (10) ml of the filtrates were pipetted into tared culture dishes and the solvents permitted to evaporate at ambient conditions. The dishes were reweighed and examined for residue until all of the solvent evaporated.

SOL-2: Lab #1

Weighed increments of each excipients were added to 1.0 ml of purified water, alcohol and n-Hexane. The mixtures were agitated on a Vortex Genie until the material dissolved. Since the mixtures were warmed by the Vortex Genie, each mixture was allowed to cool to room temperature. The mixtures were examined to determine if the excipient dissolved and remained in solution. If a precipitate was present or if the solution became cloudy, the previous increment was considered to be the limit of solubility. In the case of Povidone, reported solubilities in purified water and alcohol are not maximum solubilities, but are values limited by high viscosities which made mixing impossible.

SOL-3: Lab #10

A saturated solution of the excipient was either filtered or decanted; 10 ml of the clear solution was evaporated to dryness and the residue weighed. Most determinations were performed in quadruplicate and weighings made on a single-pan analytical balance (accuracy 0.1 mg). In the absence of any measurable residue, the material was considered as insoluble.

SOL-4: Lab #10

For solubility in propylene glycol, an excess of weighed material was dissolved and suspended in a measured volume of solvent. When no more of the excipient would dissolve, the suspension was filtered through a medium pore, tared, sintered glass funnel. The filtrate was then used to rinse all suspended material into the funnel. When all of the material was in the funnel, the funnel and its contents were briefly rinsed with cold water (none of these materials was appreciably soluble in water), the funnel was dried and the recovered material was dried to determine the solubility.

The above procedure was not feasible at 37°. Considering the negligible solubility of these excipients in propylene glycol at room temperature, and the difficulties of using this procedure at 37°, this aspect of the work was not performed.

The measurement of the solubility of stearyl alcohol in hexane presented problems due to its high solubility, its tendency to supersaturate, and its considerable tendency to crystallize upon a very slight temperature change such as inevitably would occur during an attempt to filter a saturated solution. Therefore, this solubility point was estimated by preparing a series of concentrated solutions and noting the highest concentration attainable after making sure that the solution was not supersaturated.

SOL-5: Lab #11

The general method involved the equilibration of a large excess of solid solute in the solvent. Samples were drawn with warmed glass pipettes possessing glasswool wrapped tips. Solutions were maintained at specified temperatures by placing the containers in jacketed beakers and circulating water at the indicated temperatures within the jacket. Control of temperature was within 0.1°. Vigorous magnetic stirring of the slurries continued until sampling time. With this method, equilibrium was obtained in less than one hour.

Experimental data on the aqueous solubility of benzoic acid was determined in water acidified with HCl to a pH of 2.14. The analytical method employed in all cases was spectrophotometry with appropriate standards, i.e., Beer's Law Plots in each solvent.

Experimental data on the aqueous solubility of sodium benzoate was determined at the natural pH taken by the excipient. Determination of the solubility of sodium benzoate in propylene glycol proved to be difficult as a cloudy, colloidal (in appearance) supernatant was obtained. Filtering through glasswool was tested and found to be satisfactory. The data reported represent the combined values of two trials. Only the solubility of saccharin in alcohol is reported by this laboratory.

SOL-6: Lab #23

For purified water, alcohol and hexane, a known volume of saturated solvent was placed in a weighing pan and the solvent evaporated. For propylene glycol, a solute was added to the solvent in accurately weighed increments until dissolution failed to take place within 48 hours. All determinations were performed in duplicate and reported as the combined values of the two trials.

SOL-7: Lab #32

The solubility determinations at 25° and 37° were carried out using the four analytical techniques of gas chromatography (GC), UV spectroscopy (UV), gravimetric analysis (GA) and visual estimation (VE), as follows:
1. *Butylated hydroxyanisole:* water (GC); ethanol (UV); hexane (GC), propylene glycol (UV)
2. *Butylated hydroxytoluene:* Same as #1
3. *Cetyl alcohol:* water (insoluble); ethanol (GC); hexane (GC); propylene glycol (VE)
4. *Hydroxypropyl cellulose:* water (VE); ethanol (GA); hexane (GA); propylene glycol (VE)
5. *Pluronic F68:* Same as #4
6. *Sodium lauryl sulfate:* Same as #4
7. *Polyoxyl-40 stearate:* Same as #4 (Lipal 39S)
8. *Polyoxyl-40 stearate:* (Myrj 52S) same as #4

SOL-8: Lab #30

Solubility was determined by preparing saturated solutions at 24°, evaporating the solvent and weighing the residues.

Sorption-Desorption Plots

SDI-1: Lab #14

Moisture Equilibration:

A known weight of each material (200-300 mg) contained in a labeled 10 ml beaker was stored in a desiccator which contained a saturated salt solution to control the relative humidity in a 25° oven. The beaker was reweighed periodically and the weight gain was calculated as the percent total water uptake at that relative humidity. This procedure was repeated after storage in each higher RH chamber and then back again through each lower RH chamber to identify any hysteresis effects. Determinations were made on two separate samples by two separate analysts in order to assess slight variations in handling technique. Table 2 shows the saturated salt solutions used and the resultant chamber RH.

Table 1: Salt used to prepare saturated solution for control of Relative Humidity at 25°[1]

Salt Used	Relative Humidity
LiCl	10.2
$MgCl_2$	33.0
$Na_2Cr_2O_7$	54.0
NaCl	75.3
KNO_3	92.5

[1]*Lange's Handbook of Chemistry*, 12th Ed., McGraw-Hill Book Company, New York (1979), p. 10-84.

Results: Latent moisture content was significant for all batches of excipients except those labelled "anhydrous." Moisture uptake was significant in most cases and percent water absorbed increased in all cases with increase in relative humidity.

SDI-2: Lab #26

Samples of all excipients except PEG 4000 and PEG 6000 were weighed into open tared Petri dishes and dried to constant weight at 70°. PEG 4000 and PEG 6000 were dried at 40° so as not to cause any physical changes by melting or softening them. The dried samples were placed in dessicators at room temperature containing salt solutions producing the relative humidities given below. These particular salt solutions produce nearly constant relative humidities over a range of temperatures (5-40°).

Table 2: Resultant chamber RH and the salt solutions used

RH	SALT	RH	SALT
11%	Lithium chloride	57%	Sodium bromide
23%	Potassium acetate	67%	Cupric chloride
33%	Magnesium chloride	75%	Sodium chloride
43%	Potassium chloride	83%	Potassium bromide
52%	Magnesium nitrate		

When the samples reached constant weight, the quantity of water absorbed by each was calculated as a percent of the dry weight. Similarly, other samples of the dried excipients were equilibrated at 83% RH in desiccators. These samples were then placed at lower humidity conditions. Upon attainment of constant weight, the amount of water desorbed was calculated as a percent of dry weight.

Note: Only the PEG samples did not exhibit adsorption/desorption hysteresis.

Sorption Isotherm

SI-1: Lab #13

Samples of the excipients were dried to constant weight at temperature between 60-105°C. Eight 1.000 g samples of each excipient were weighed into each of 8 petri dishes of approximately 4.5 cm diameter. The samples were placed in a desiccator containing the saturated salt solution of known relative humidity. The desiccators were immersed and maintained in a constant temperature bath at 25 ± 1.0°C. After 5-7 day intervals, the petri dishes were quickly removed from the desiccators and rapidly weighed and the weight change recorded. Weighings were continued until there was no further change in weight. The weight gain, therefore, represented the amount of water absorbed and the percent moisture gain was plotted versus percent relative humidity.

Viscosity Methods

VIS-1: Lab #27

Viscosity was measured using the Brookfield Model LVT Syncho-Lectric viscometer equipped with the U.L. adapter and mounted on a Brookfield laboratory stand. All fluids except glycerin were tested with the U.L. adapter.

The U.L. adapter using the closed tube is attached by a sequence of steps where the spindle coupling nut is screwed onto the viscometer coupling screw followed by insertion of the adapter body over the pivot housing of the viscometer. The spindle link is attached and the spindle hung from the loop. The closed tube is placed over the spindle and pushed up, matching the vertical slot on the side of the tube with the screw on the side of the adapter, until the horizontal groove in the tube coincides with the screw. The tube is rotated slightly to lock in place. The viscometer can then be operated in its normal fashion.

Viscosity measurements were preceded by proper leveling of the viscometer using adjustments provided with the Brookfield laboratory stand and the bubble level on the viscometer. All fluids were handled so as to prevent the entrapment of air bubbles. The temperature of measurement was ambient temperature. For the U.L. adapter the fluid volume was 18 ml. The measurements were obtained according to the normal procedure where the clutch is depressed and the viscometer turned on, then the clutch is released to allow the dial to rotate to a stable point. The viscosity in centipoise is determined from the product of the dial reading and the multiplication factor supplied by Brookfield. The accuracy of the readings is within 1% of the full scale. The reported viscosities are the average of two trials plus or minus the absolute error computed from the multiplication factor.

For the glycerin viscosities the viscometer was calibrated using Castor Oil USP as a standard fluid and using Spindle 3. To have sufficient depth of fluid, a 50 ml graduated cylinder was used instead of the regular 600 ml beaker. By using the formula to find the multiplying factor for the 50 ml graduate the following values were obtained:*

	Multiplication Factor for Castor Oil USP	
rpm	600 ml beaker	50 ml graduate
12	10.2	96.3
30	40.8	38.95
60	20.4	19.24

The viscosities of the glycerin were obtained according to the normal procedure for use of the Brookfield viscometer with attachment of the spindle to the lower shaft of the viscometer and immersion of the spindle into the fluid to the immersion groove.

The PEG samples were prepared as 2% w/w aqueous solutions. The weight of each solution was 100 g. Sufficient distilled deionized water was placed in a 250 ml beaker and with stirring the PEG sample added slowly in divided portions and stirred until solution was complete.

$$*\text{Factor}_{50\,ml} = \eta_{600\,ml} \frac{}{\text{Dial reading}_{50\,ml}}$$

VIS-2: Lab #30

Viscosity was determined with the use of cleaned Ostwald tube viscometers, stopwatch and glycerin viscosity as a standard. Correlation between temperature (24°C) and viscosity was based upon the standard data tables.

VIS-3: Lab #28

Using the Brookfield Model LVT viscometer, attach the selected spindle to the lower shaft. Insert the spindle in the test material until the fluid level comes up to the immersion groove cut in the spindle shaft. Level the viscometer with the aid of the bubble level. Depress the clutch and turn on the viscometer motor. Release the clutch and allow the dial to rotate until the pointer on the dial stabilizes at a fixed position on the dial. Determine the viscosity of the preparation in centipoise from the dial reading using the slide rule type factor finder supplied with the viscometer.

Note: Selection of spindle size and speed of spindle rotation are dependent on the viscosity properties of the test sample. The viscometer's operation may be calibrated by measuring the viscosity of known standard viscosity solutions supplied by Brookfield.

VIS-4: Lab #6

Major parameters in this study included the following:
1. Instrumentation for viscosity determinations were the Brookfield Synchro-Lectric Viscometers, Models RVF and HBT.
2. All dispersions for testing were prepared as % w/v, using 200 ml of water.
3. The Natrosol and Algum S 15/600 materials were prepared using water at room temperature. Klucel materials were prepared using the hot water (50-60°C) method as described by the product brochure (800-4A 11-76 6M 73672H), Method 1.
4. All materials[1] were dried at 105°C for 3 hours and used without correcting for moisture content.
5. All dispersions were equilibrated at 25° ± 0.5°C in a water batch, re-mixed for 60 seconds by mechanical stirring and then read after a 3 minute rotation cycle of the viscometer combination of speed and spindle.

Data were recorded for each material concentration prepared using both the RVF and HBT model Brookfield Synchro-Lectric viscometers. All on-scale readings were recorded over the entire range of speeds and spindles used. This monograph contains those data related to the development of viscosity profiles which were most consistant over each viscometer series.[2].

Methods
Sample Materials
1. All sample materials were dried at 105°C for 3 hours. Materials used for dispersion preparation were then weighed without moisture correction.

Dispersion Preparation
1. Each dispersion was prepared as percent weight/volume (% w/v) in 200 ml capacity beakers.

2. Dispersion was prepared mechanically using electronic controlled mixer and propeller type stirrer device.

3. Both the sodium alginate and the hydroxyethyl cellulose materials were prepared using water at room temperature (23-24°).

4. The hydroxypropyl cellulose materials were prepared by the hot water dispersion method as described under Method 1 in the Klucel brochure[3].

5. Each dispersion was mixed for NLT 30 minutes at a speed to adequately disperse the material without causing aeration.

6. Dispersions were covered and placed in a constant temperature bath (25 ± 0.5°C) for NLT 30 minutes prior to reading the viscosity.

7. All dispersions were re-mixed using a mechanical stirrer for 60 seconds after being removed from the water bath prior to making viscosity readings.

8. Samples were run on both RVF and HBT model Brookfield Synchro-Lectric viscometers using a three-minute rotation cycle before reading.

9. Viscosities were determined from the data supplied by the Brookfield Factor-Finder Chart.

Equipment

1. Viscometers, Brookfield[4] Synchro-Lectric
   a. Model RVF: 4 speeds, 7 spindles, 28 ranges
      Viscosity Range: Minimum: 0-500 cps
      Maximum: 0-2,000,000 cps
   b. Model HBT: 8 speeds, 7 spindles, 56 ranges
      Viscosity Range: Minimum: 0-800 cps
      Maximum: 0-64,000,000 cps

2. Vessels: 250 ml capacity Pyrex glass beaker, Griffin (Corning 1000)

3. Mechanical stirrer: G.H. Heller, electronic controlled laboratory stirrer, Model GT 21

4. Stirring Device: standard 3-prong propeller

---

[1] Study samples supplied by Merck, Sharp and Dohme Research Laboratories West Point, Pennsylvania.

[2] Series used here to define a set of spindles and speed combinations used on a specific viscometer model to produce on-scale readings.

Larger dispersion volumes must be used in those cases where the No. 1 and No. 2 spindle sizes are required to provide reasonable readings without incurring possible vessel sidewall effects. When attempting to profile very low viscosities, the LV type Brookfield viscometer should be used. Vendor supplier's procedures and suggestions should be reviewed and followed as closely as possible.

[3] Klucel Chemical and Physical Properties, product brochure of 1976, edition 800-4A 11-76 73672H.

[4] Brookfield Engineering Laboratories, Inc., Stoughton, Massachusetts.

Index

Trade names are in italics